THE VITAMINS

Chemistry, Physiology, Pathology, Methods

SECOND EDITION

VOLUME V

VOLUME I—VOLUME V

Edited by

W. H. SEBRELL, JR. and ROBERT S. HARRIS

VOLUME VI and VOLUME VII

Edited by

PAUL GYÖRGY and W. N. PEARSON

THE VITAMINS

Chemistry, Physiology, Pathology, Methods

SECOND EDITION
VOLUME V

Edited by

W. H. SEBRELL, JR.
Institute of Nutrition Sciences
Columbia University
New York, New York

ROBERT S. HARRIS
William F. Lasby Professor in the
Health Sciences
University of Minnesota
Minneapolis, Minnesota

ACADEMIC PRESS   New York and London

1972

ACADEMIC PRESS, INC.
111 Fifth Avenue, New York, New York 10003

United Kingdom Edition published by
ACADEMIC PRESS, INC. (LONDON) LTD.
24/28 Oval Road, London NW1

LIBRARY OF CONGRESS CATALOG CARD NUMBER: 66-26845

PRINTED IN THE UNITED STATES OF AMERICA

Contents

CHAPTER 14. *Riboflavin*

CHAPTER 15. *Thiamine*

CHAPTER 16.   *Tocopherols*

CHAPTER 17. *New and Unidentified Growth Factors*

Contributors to Volume V

Numbers in parentheses indicate the pages on which the authors' contributions begin.

STANLEY R. AMES (218, 225, 233, 312), Biochemical Research Laboratories, Distillation Products Industries, Division of Eastman Kodak Company, Rochester, New York

ANNETTE BAICH (320, 322, 398), Department of Biochemistry, Southern Illinois University, Edwardsville, Illinois.

GENE M. BROWN (122), Division of Biochemistry, Department of Biology, Massachusetts Institute of Technology, Cambridge, Massachusetts

G. BRUBACHER (248, 255), Department of Vitamin and Nutritional Research, F. Hoffman- La Roche and Colk Ltd., Basel, Switzerland

VERNON H. CHELDELIN (320, 322, 392, 393, 394, 398), Oregon State University, Corvallis, Oregon

G. S. FRAENKEL (329), Department of Entomology, University of Illinois, Urbana, Illinois

STANLEY FRIEDMAN (329), Department of Entomology, University of Illinois, Urbana Illinois

J. GREEN (252, 259), Beecham Research Laboratories, Vitamins Research Station, Walton Oaks, Dorking Road, Tadworth, Surrey, England

ROBERT HARRIS (3, 98, 166), William F. Lasby Professor of Health Sciences, University of Minnesota, Minneapolis, Minnesota

M. K. HORWITT (46, 49, 50, 52, 53, 85, 88, 272, 293, 309, 316), Department of Biochemistry, St. Louis University, School of Medicine, St. Louis, Missouri

O. ISLER (168), F. Hoffmann-La Roche and Co., Ltd., Grenzacherstrasse, Bassel, Switzerland

B. C. P. JANSEN (99, 145, 148, 156), Institut vor Volksvoeding, J. D. Meÿerplein 3, Amsterdam, Holland.

MERTON P. LAMDEN (110, 114, 120, 134), Department of Biochemistry, College of Medicine, University of Vermont, Burlington, Vermont

KARL E. MASON (272, 293, 309), Nutrition Program Director, National Institute of Arthritic and Metabolic Disorders EP, Westwood Building, National Institute of Health, Bethesda, Maryland

H. Mayer (168), F. Hoffmann-La Roche and Co., Ltd., Grenzacherstrasse, Basel, Switzerland

R. A. Morton (355), Emeritus Professor of Biochemistry, Zoology Department, The University of Liverpool, Liverpool, England

Edward F. Rogers (130), Merck Sharp and Dohme Research Laboratories, Division of Merck and Co., Inc., Rahway, New Jersey

P. Schudel* (168), F. Hoffmann-La Roche and Co., Ltd., Basel, Switzerland

W. H. Sebrell, Jr., (162), Institute of Nutrition Sciences, Columbia University, New York, New York

E. E. Snell (71), Department of Biochemistry, University of California, Berkeley, California

Klaus R. Unna (150), Department of Pharmacology, University of Illinois, College of Medicine, Chicago, Illinois

Theodor Wagner-Jauregg (3, 43), Bottenwilerstrasse, Zofingen, Switzerland

O. Wiss (248, 255), F. Hoffmann-La Roche and Co., Ltd. Basel, Switzerland

L. A. Witting (53), Address unknown.

H. M. Wuest (104), Sloan-Kettering Institute for Cancer Research, New York, New York

*Present address: Givaudan-Esrolko Ltd., Research Company, CH- 8600 Dubendorf-Zurich.

Preface

We are pleased to present this second edition of "The Vitamins." The many years that have passed since publication of the first edition have been filled with diligent search by many scientists for an understanding of how each vitamin functions in animals and plants. The content of "The Vitamins" has broadened and deepened, and the vast amount of new information has created a need for a nearly complete rewriting of the first edition. Since most of the recent advances have been concerned with chemistry, biochemistry, and physiology, it is understandable that these biodisciplines have received special emphasis in this second edition.

We have followed the same general principles as guided us in the first edition. The writing of each section of each chapter has been assigned to a scientist who is especially expert on the subject. Current knowledge concerning the chemistry, industrial production, biogenesis, biochemistry, deficiency effects, requirements, pharmacology, and pathology of each of the vitamins has been emphasized, and considerable space has been devoted to bibliographic material since this is essentially a reference work. Extensive discussion of clinical manifestations of vitamin deficiency or treatment has been omitted since this is well covered in clinical publications.

Little space was given in the first edition to methods of measurement and assay of the various vitamins. This important aspect of vitamin science has been consolidated and is presented in Volumes VI and VII of this treatise.

We hope that this critical summary of current vitamin knowledge will assist teachers, students, investigators, and practitioners toward a better understanding of the role of the vitamins in biology.

We take this opportunity to express our appreciation to the many authors who have contributed to these volumes and to Academic Press for patient collaboration and cooperation in the production of these volumes.

W. H. Sebrell, Jr.
Robert S. Harris

Contents of Other Volumes

Page 360 last sentence should read:

Comparisons with the spectra of other substituted toluquinones confirmed the positions of the alkoxy groups:

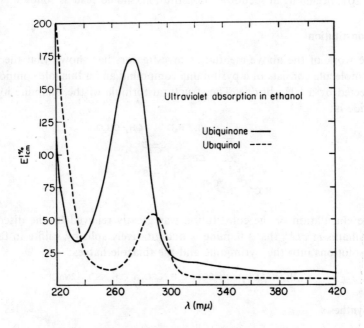

Ultraviolet absorption of ubiquinone (50) and ubiquinol (50).

THE VITAMINS
Chemistry, Physiology, Pathology, Methods
SECOND EDITION, VOLUME V

Edited by

W. H. SEBRELL, JR.   ROBERT S. HARRIS

Page 101, beginning at section C. Constitution, should read as follows:

C. Constitution

The work of the above-mentioned investigators has shown that the thiamine molecule consists of a pyrimidine compound and a thiazole compound, connected by a CH_2 bridge. The structural formula of the thiamine hydrochloride is:

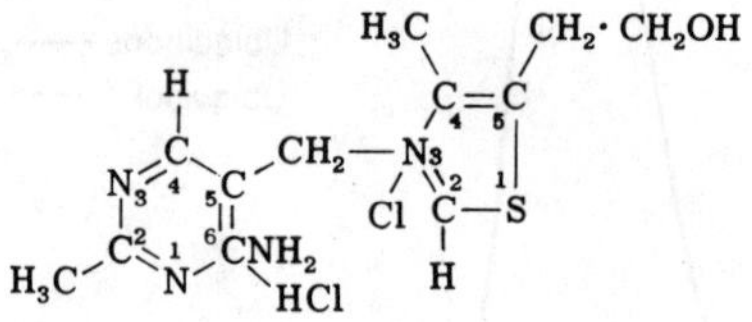

The elucidation of the constitution was greatly relieved by the discovery of Williams et al.[11] that thiamine is quantitatively split by sulfite in faintly acid solutions into the pyrimidine and the thiazole halves:

$$C_{12}H_{18}ON_4SCL_2 + Na_2SO_3 = C_6H_9N_3SO_3 + C_6H_9NSO + 2NaCl$$

D. Synthesis

The synthesis of thiamine has been performed in different ways. It is possible to synthesize the pyrimidine nucleus and the thiazole nucleus separately and afterwards to connect both parts. It is also possible to synthesize one of the nuclei with an extra side branch and afterwards to build up the other ring from this side branch.

For synthesizing the pyrimidine part, ethyl formate and ethyl-β-ethoxy propionate may be condensed with Na.

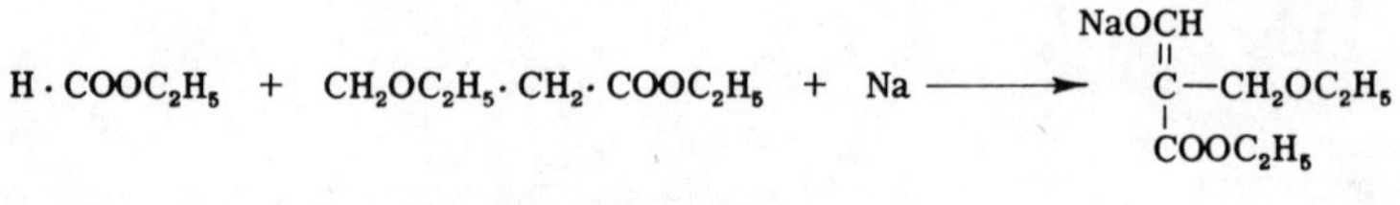

This product is condensed with acetamidine.

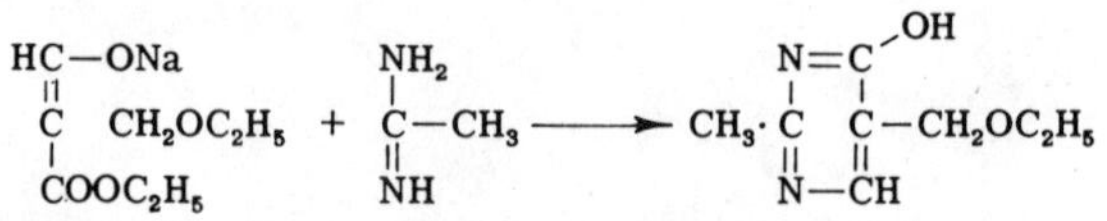

The hydroxyl group is converted into an NH_2 group by treating first with

[11] R. R. Williams, E. R. Buchman, and A. E. Ruehle, J. Amer. Chem. Soc. 57, 536 (1935).

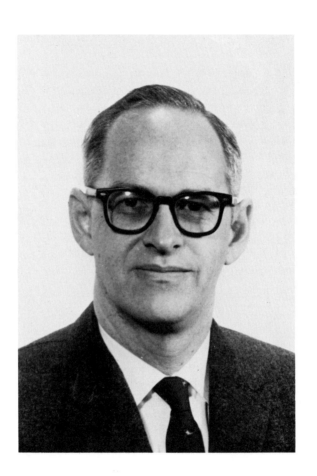

WILLIAM N. PEARSON

January 5, 1924–November 28, 1968

This volume of the second edition of "The Vitamins" is dedicated to William N. Pearson, coeditor of Volumes VI and VII, whose sudden and tragic death occurred on Thanksgiving Day, November 28, 1968. At the time of his death he was Professor of Biochemistry and Associate Director of the Division of Nutrition, Vanderbilt University School of Medicine, and Editor-Elect of the *Journal of Nutrition*. He had just completed a term as Secretary of the American Institute of Nutrition and was serving as a member of the National Institutes of Health Study Section on Nutrition. He was on the Committee on Recommended Dietary Allowances of the Food and Nutrition Board, as well as on a Committee of the Council on Foods and Nutrition of the American Medical Association. He was a special consultant to the Nutrition Program, U.S. Public Health Service, and was Organizing Chairman of the Second Western Hemisphere Nutrition Congress (August, 1968) held in San Juan, Puerto Rico.

Bill Pearson's capability as a scientist was matched only by the kindly warmth and delightful humor that ever pervaded his relationships with colleagues at all levels. His scientific contributions illustrated his versatility and included major contributions to the selection, standardization, and testing of biochemical methods and interpretation of nutrition survey data accumulated throughout the world; to understanding of bound niacin and the influence of fat and other dietary factors on niacin requirements; to the assessment of nutritional quality of protein foodstuffs and investigation of amino acid imbalance, and the relationship of the latter to tryptophan metabolism in pellagra; to the studies on the site and mechanism of absorption of iron and of zinc; to a series of investigations on the metabolism of selenium; and to a major program of research on the metabolism of thiamine. For these studies he received the 1967 Mead Johnson Award of the American Institute of Nutrition.

His near-encyclopedic knowledge of the nutrition literature coupled with a critically keen analytic sense made Bill Pearson a particularly effective writer of informative and clarifying reviews. His interest in the preparation of educational material in the field of nutrition reflected his exceptional devotion to teaching—an activity that he clearly enjoyed and conscientiously undertook. He motivated students at all levels—medical students, graduate students, students in the allied medical fields—to have a serious interest in the subject.

He indelibly influenced the career of many with whom he came into contact. His effectiveness as a teacher stemmed in large part from the unselfish contribution of the teacher himself. Of students he expected the same qualities of diligence, integrity, thoughtfulness, knowledge of the literature, originality, and persistence that he exemplified. Gently, but firmly, always with good humor, he brought forth these qualities in his younger associates.

His death has left a void in the life of all of his colleagues, in the science of nutrition, and among the editors and contributors to this treatise.

CHAPTER 14

RIBOFLAVIN

1

I. Nomenclature

Robert S. Harris

Accepted names: riboflavin (U.S. Pharmacopeia); riboflavine (British Pharmacopoeia and IUPAC).

Obsolete names: Vitamin B_2, vitamin G, lactoflavin, ovoflavin, lyochrome, uroflavin, hepatoflavin.

Empirical formula: $C_{17}H_{20}N_4O_6$

Chemical name: 6,7-Dimethyl-9-(D-1'-ribityl)isoalloxazine

Structural formula:

Riboflavin (old numbering system)

Riboflavin (new numbering system)

II. Chemistry[1]

Theodor Wagner-Jauregg

A. Name and Discovery

Lactoflavin was the original name of riboflavin, and this term is sometimes still used in Europe. Ovoflavin, hepatoflavin, uroflavin, etc., also are historical names, indicating the origin of the preparation. Riboflavin, the American designation, indicates that the naturally occurring flavin is a derivative of D-ribose. This name was adopted in 1952 by the International Commission for the Reform of Biochemical Nomenclature.

Riboflavin is identical with vitamin B_2. Formerly in the United States, the term vitamin G was also used for this nutritional factor.

After vitamin B_1 had been obtained in pure form, the isolation of crystallized riboflavin became one of the most fascinating chapters in the chemistry of the water-soluble vitamins. For the sake of its historical interest, the story of the discovery of riboflavin will be told here briefly.

In 1927, Paul György, at that time at the pediatric clinic of the University of Heidelberg, began investigations on the curative factor for egg white injury, which he called vitamin H[2]. In 1931, he and Edgar Lederer, who worked with Richard Kuhn at the Kaiser Wilhelm Institute for Medical Research, Heidelberg, attempted to isolate this vitamin. Vitamin H deficiency in rats is characterized by a dermatitis. Since pellagra is another avitaminosis connected with skin symptoms, it seemed useful and interesting to make a comparative study of the nutrition factor connected with this disease. A lack of vitamin B_2, the heat-

---

[1] During the last 9 years, the following comprehensive articles on riboflavin appeared: J. P. Lambooy, in Compr. Biochem, 11, 23 (1963); T. W. Goodwin, "The Biosynthesis of Vitamins and Related Compounds," pp. 24–68. Academic Press, New York, 1963; F. Wagner and K. Folkers, "Vitamins and Coenzymes," pp. 46–71, Wiley (Interscience) New York, 1964; I. Fragner, "Vitamine, Chemie und Biochemie," G. Fischer, Jena, 1964; G. W. E. Plaut, in "The Encyclopedia of Biochemistry" (R. J. Williams and E. M. Lansford, Jr., eds.), pp. 728–730. Van Nostrand-Reinhold, Princeton, New Jersey, 1967; H. Beinert and P. Hemmerich, in "The Encyclopedia of Biochemistry" (R. J. Williams and E. M. Lansford, Jr., eds.), pp. 331–336. Van Nostrand-Reinhold, Princeton, New Jersey, 1967; "Flavins and Flavoproteins" (E. C. Slater, ed.), 549 pp., Elsevier, Amsterdam, 1966; "Flavins and Flavoproteins" (K. Yagi, ed.), University of Tokyo Press, Tokyo, and University Park Press, Baltimore, 1968; "Flavins and Flavoproteins" (H. Kamin, ed.), 286 pp., University Park Press, Baltimore, 1970; A. H. Neims and L. Hellermann, in Annual Review of Biochemistry, Vol. 39, pp. 867–888. American Review, Inc., Palo Alto, California, 1970; Th. Wagner-Jauregg, in "Ammon-Dirscherl: Fermente–Hormone–Vitamine," 3 Auflage Band III, Teil 1 (in press).

[2] In 1940 P. György, V. du Vigneaud, and D. Melville identified this vitamin with the yeast growth-promoting factor biotin, which had been isolated some years before by F. Kögl and B. Tönnis.

stable companion of the heat-labile vitamin B_1, at that time was considered to be the cause of pellagra. Therefore, at the beginning of 1932, Th. Wagner-Jauregg started the isolation of so-called vitamin B_2 at R. Kuhn's institute. György performed the biological tests on rats, according to the method of Sherman and Bourquin; later on, when our preparations became purer, the diet of the animals had to be modified somewhat, since it was lacking not only in vitamin B_2 but also in another member of the B-vitamin complex.

The literature contained very little and vague data on the concentration of vitamin B_2 from yeast and liver, which turned out to be of little value for the procedure of isolation. For the adsorption of the vitamin, fuller's earth in acid solution had been recommended. Another valuable adsorbent soon was found, which adsorbed vitamin B_2 already from neutral solution; this was " Frankonit KL " (a bleaching earth produced by the Pfirschinger Mineralwerke, Kitzingen/Main, Franconia), which since that time has been used frequently in biochemical work. Before the vitamin B_2 investigation a sample of this adsorbent lay forgotten in one of the laboratory closets, after I had tried it with little success for the polymerization of isoprene.

None of the known methods was suitable for elution of the vitamin from the adsorbent in yields worth mentioning.

Finally a wrong hypothesis about the chemical nature of vitamin B_2 helped me to find the right trail. In one paper it had been assumed that vitamin B_2 might contain iron. With regard to the biological properties of hemin derivatives, one would be inclined to guess that iron porphyrin complexes were involved. Since pyridine is a solvent for compounds of this type, this substance, diluted with water and alcohol, was tried out for the elution of vitamin B_2 adsorbates. This attempt was a full success. The later progress of our investigation made it clear that iron has nothing to do with vitamin B_2, but the wrong hypothesis had proved useful.

The successful elution drove the isolation procedure one essential step forward. It soon became evident that all eluates that were active in the animal experiments were greenish yellow and showed a yellowish green fluorescence in the light of a quartz lamp. Therefore, I speculated that vitamin B_2 itself might be colored, and the investigation was continued with attention to this assumption.

It still was difficult to obtain purified preparations of the vitamin from extracts of yeast, liver, heart, or kidney because of the presence of large amounts of accompanying substances. An 80% methanol extract of egg white turned out to be a much better starting material. The concentrated, greenish yellow eluates on precipitation with $AgNO_3$ gave a brownish red crude silver salt of the vitamin. In later experiments, a precipitation with Tl_2SO_4 was inserted for further purification. This salt had been chosen with regard to the chemical relationship of certain thallous and silver salts. The first few milligrams of crystallized " ovoflavin " became available for analysis shortly before Christmas, 1932. The animal tests proved without any doubt the growth-promoting nature of the substance.

At this stage of the investigation, we learned that the pharmacologist Ph. Ellinger in Düsseldorf, working on the fluorescence of animal organs, had prepared from skimmed milk a colored concentrate, which obviously was similar to ovoflavin. Our methods of purification proved to be particularly applicable to whey. We therefore changed over to this starting material. It was, however, not possible to handle the large amounts of liquid in the laboratory. Therefore, the first step of the concentration, the adsorption, was carried out in a large cheese dairy in Bavaria. With this procedure we soon were able to obtain 1 gm of crystallized " lactoflavin " from 5400 liters of whey, thus opening a way for the elucidation of the chemical structure of vitamin B_2.

Other investigators had obtained impure preparations of flavin. As early as 1879, A. W. Blyth isolated from whey a resinous preparation of a red-orange color which he called "lactochrom." In 1925, B. Bleyer and O. Kallmann attempted the purification of the yellow pigment of whey. In 1932, I. Banga and A. Szent-Györgyi obtained a golden yellow pigment from heart muscle, the colored component of which they called "cytoflav." In 1933, Ellinger and Koschara described impure, crystalline preparations of flavin ("llyochrome") at the same time as the isolation of pure, crystallized lactoflavin was reported by György, Kuhn, and Wagner-Jauregg.[2a] The vitamin nature of the pigment was unknown before the investigations of the latter authors. Soon Karrer at Zurich followed with the isolation of riboflavin from various natural sources. Also in 1933, L. E. Booher in the United States described a concentrate from whey powder with the chemical and biological properties of riboflavin.

For the understanding of the biochemical function of riboflavin, the discovery of the "yellow enzyme" by Warburg and Christian in 1932 was of extraordinary importance. The same authors described lumiflavin, a photochemical degradation product of riboflavin, which proved to be of great value for the elucidation of the chemical structure of riboflavin (Kuhn, Wagner-Jauregg, and co-workers, 1933–34). The synthesis of riboflavin by Kuhn and Weygand and by Karrer and his co-workers in 1934 finally confirmed the structural formula.

B. Occurrence and Isolation

For the occurrence and concentration of riboflavin in various natural materials see Sections IV and V.

A high concentration of riboflavin is contained in the eyes of many fish,[3] in certain crabs,[4] *Hemopis sanguisuga*,[5] *Tineola bisselliella*,[6] the Malpighian tube of fireflies (*Luciola cruciata*)[7] (117.8 µg/gm of dry substance) and of cockroaches[8] (the concentration being 40 times higher than in beef liver), and in the seminal vesicles of some bulls.[9] Crystals of riboflavin are formed in cells of the fungus of *Eremothecium ashbyii*[10] and the brilliant golden colored tapetum of a lemur (*Galago crassicaudatus agisymbanus*) which is made of crystalline riboflavin.[11] The tapetum is the basis of eyeshine in animals; it may be be made up of crystals or of regularly arranged fibers. Many fish, for example, have tapeta made of crystals of guanidine; carnivores have tapeta crystals of a complex of zinc-cysteine,[12] and herbivores, such as the sheep or the cow, have fibrous tapeta. Man and the higher apes have no tapetum.

[2a] P. György, Th. Wagner-Jauregg, and R. Kuhn, *Mitt. Kaiser Wilhelm Ges.* **2**, 1/4 (1933); R. Kuhn and Th. Wagner-Jauregg, *Ber. Deut. Chem. Ges.* **66**, 1577 (1933); Th. Wagner-Jauregg, *Verhandl. Schweiz. Naturforsch. Ges., Altdorf.* 1933, s. 349.

[3] H. von Euler and E. Adler, *Hoppe-Seyler's Z. Physiol. Chem.* **228**, 1 (1934).

[4] R. G. Busnel, *C. R. Acad. Sci.* **214**, 189 (1942); **216**, 85, 162 (1943).

[5] G. Ferrari, *Boll. Soc. Ital. Biol. Sper.* **26**, 144 (1950).

[6] R. G. Busnel and A. Drilhon, *C. R. Acad. Sci.* **216** 213 (1943).

[7] H. Nakamura, *Science (Japan)* **14**, 254 (1944) [*Chem. Abstr.* **44**, 10937 (1950)].

[8] R. L. Metcalf and R. L. Patton, *J. Cell. Comp. Physiol.* **19**, 373 (1942).

[9] I. G. White and G. J. Lincoln, *Nature (London)* **182**, 667 (1958).

[10] A. Guilliermond, "The Cytoplasm of the Plant Cell." Chron. Bot., New York, 1941.

[11] A. Pirie, *Nature (London)* **183**, 985 (1959).

[12] G. Weitzel, E. Buddecke, *et al.*, *Hoppe-Seyler's Z. Physiol. Chem.* **299**, 193 (1955); S. Heller, *Hoppe-Seyler's Z. Physiol. Chem.* **348**, 1211 (1967). The reflecting material of seatrouts (Sciænidse) is a lipid, H. J. Arnott, et al. *Nature* **233**, 130 (1971).

Riboflavin occurs, in its free dialyzable form only, in the retina of the eye, in whey, and in urine. In organs, tissues, and other living cells, riboflavin is present as riboflavin monophosphoric acid (FMN) and as riboflavin adenine dinucleotide (FAD). The riboflavin in human milk is present as FAD.[13] The two phosphates account for practically all the riboflavin present in rat kidneys, and 70–90% of the total riboflavin in all tissues is present in the form of the dinucleotide.[14] However the ratio of FAD:FMN in the native state is still a matter under discussion.[15] Spleen contains an enzyme that rapidly degrades the phosphate-bound forms of riboflavin to the free vitamin.[16]

It has been shown that riboflavin phosphoric acid is able to form loose, non-dialyzable complexes—for instance, with a solution of pseudoglobulin or albumin from horse serum. The separation of the flavin component and the protein in this case can be achieved by precipitation of the protein with ammonium sulfate.[17] In serum, riboflavin and its phosphate are mainly bound to albumin.[17a]

In order to liberate riboflavin from its natural protein-bound forms, it is necessary to treat the mashed tissues with suitable solvents at room temperature or at the boiling point of the solvent. Methanol, ethanol, acetone undiluted or diluted with water, and aqueous acid solutions have been used for extraction of the vitamin. For instance, riboflavin from fresh or dried plants has been extracted in good yields by boiling the material with 70% methanol for 45 minutes.[18]

For the isolation of riboflavin from the extracts, it is sometimes useful first to remove lipids by extraction with ether, in which the vitamin is insoluble. Salts and glycogen in some cases can be eliminated from riboflavin concentrates by fractionate precipitation with alcohol or acetone. Impurities from fermentation liquors may be precipitated by means of acetone, and crude riboflavin can be recovered from the concentrated filtrate by the addition of more acetone.[19] The vitamin can be extracted with butanol and then precipitated from the extract by the addition of petroleum ether.[20] In the isolation

[13] V. Modi and E. C. Owen, *Nature (London)* **178**, 1120 (1956); K. Gupte et al., *Experientia* **19**, 400 (1963).

[14] O. A. Bessey, O. H. Lowry, and R. H. Love, *J. Biol. Chem.* **180**, 775 (1949).

[15] Z. Kaninga and C. Verger, *Biochim. Biophys. Acta* **77**, 339 (1963).

[16] J. L. Crammer, *Nature (London)* **161**, 349 (1948); R. S. Comline and F. R. Whatley, *Nature (London)* **161**, 350 (1948).

[17] Th. Wagner-Jauregg and H. Arnold, *Biochem. Z.* **299**, 280 (1938), appendix.

[17a] H. Baker et al., *Nature* **215**, 84 (1967); W. J. Jusco and G. Levy, *J. Pharm Sci.* **58**, 58 (1969) and *Am. J. Physiol.* **218**, 1046 (1970); S. Christensen, *Acta Pharmacol. Toxicol.* **29**, 428 (1971).

[18] H. Roth, *Biochem. Z.* **320**, 355 (1950).

[19] Merck and Co., Brit. Patent No. 621,401 (Aug. 15, 1946) [*Chem. Abstr.* **43**, 7189 (1949)].

[20] Merck and Co., U.S. Patent No. 2,355,220 (Aug. 8, 1944) [*Chem. Abstr.* **38**, 6488 (1944)].

of riboflavin from whey, the accompanying creatinine has been removed by picric acid precipitation.

Precipitation of riboflavin occurs with lead acetate and with silver nitrate in neutral solution, or with phosphotungstic acid in 1 N H_2SO_4; from the latter precipitate the phosphotungstic acid can be extracted with amyl alcohol. Silver nitrate or mercuric sulfate in acid solution leaves the vitamin in solution but precipitates some accompanying substances.

Good adsorbents for riboflavin are fuller's earth in acid solution, Florisil, Floridin XXF, and Frankonit in neutral solution. One of the best eluants is pyridine diluted with aqueous methanol or ethanol[21]; ammonia, triethanolamine, 0.1 N NaOH in 60% ethanol, boiling 60% ethanol, 80% acetone, and polyhydric alcohols[22] have also been used for elution. Vitamin B_2 is adsorbed very strongly by charcoal; however, elution is difficult from this adsorbate. Adsorption occurs also with lead sulfide when this is precipitated in a riboflavin solution; the vitamin can be extracted with hot water from the precipitate. Riboflavin is not adsorbed by kieselguhr, kaolin, talc, aluminum oxide, or calcium carbonate.

A combination of precipitation and adsorption methods usually will be necessary to isolate pure riboflavin. As examples might be mentioned the isolation of riboflavin from egg white,[23] egg yolk,[25] liver, [24, 25] whey,[26] and urine.[27] A general method for the preparation of pure D-riboflavin from natural sources has been described which is based on adsorption on fuller's earth, fractionation with immiscible solvents and acetone, and crystallization from an aqueous acetone–petroleum ether mixture; aqueous alcohol solutions have been used for elution of the adsorbates.[28]

The reduced forms of riboflavin are rather insoluble in water and can be used for isolation purposes.[29]

[21] P. György, R. Kuhn, and T. Wagner-Jauregg (to I. G. Farbenindustrie A.G.), Ger. Patent No. 607,512 (Nov. 22, 1932).

[22] S. H. Rubin and E. DeRitter, *J. Biol. Chem.* **158**, 639 (1945); Commercial Solvents Corp., U.S. Patent No. 2,343, 254 (March 7, 1944) [*Chem. Abstr.* **38**, 3093 (1944)].

[23] R. Kuhn, P. György, and T. Wagner-Jauregg, *Ber. Deut. Chem. Ges.* **66**, 576 (1933).

[24] R. Kuhn and T. Wagner-Jauregg, *Ber. Deut. Chem. Ges.* **67**, 1770 (1934).

[25] P. Karrer, H. Salomon, and K. Schopp, *Helv. Chim. Acta* **17**, 735 (1934).

[26] R. Kuhn, P. György, and T. Wagner-Jauregg, *Ber. Deut. Chem. Ges.* **66**, 1034 (1933); R. Kuhn, H. Rudy, and T. Wagner-Jauregg, *Ber. Deut. Chem. Ges.* **66**, 1950 (1933).

[27] W. Koschara, *Ber. Deut. Chem. Ges.* **67**, 761 (1934).

[28] R. D. Greene and A. Black, *J. Amer. Chem. Soc.* **59**, 1820 (1937).

[29] G. E. Hines, Jr., U.S. Patent No. 2,367,644 (Jan. 1945); R. J. Hickey, *Arch. Biochem.* **11**, 259 (1946). S. Umemoto, Jap. Patent No. 180,228 (Sept. 3, 1949) [*Chem. Abstr.* **46**, 1222 (1952)] and loc. cit. 14a, page 45.

C. Chemical and Physical Properties[29a]

$C_{17}H_{20}N_4O_6$: molecular weight 376.4; C 54.25%, H 5.36%, N 14.89%.
Riboflavin crystallizes from 2 N acetic acid, alcohol, water, or pyridine in
fine orange-yellow needles. The decomposition point is 278°–282° (darkening
at about 240°). Values for the decomposition point between 271° and 293° can
be found in the literature. The vitamin is odorless and has a bitter taste.

Riboflavin is soluble in water only to the extent of 10–13 mg in 100 ml at
25°–27.5°, 19 mg in 100 ml at 40°, and 230 mg in 100 ml at 100°.[30] The
vitamin dissolves in ethanol to 4.5 mg/100 ml and is slightly soluble in amyl
alcohol, cyclohexanol, benzyl alcohol, and phenol or amyl acetate. The
impure material has a much higher solubility than the pure substance.
Alkali dissolves the vitamin well, but these solutions are unstable. There is no
solubility in ether, acetone, chloroform, or benzene. Formic acid dissolves
more than 1% of riboflavin.[30]

In order to obtain more concentrated solutions, riboflavin has been dissolved together with other compounds that increase its solubility[31].

For intravenous administration, sterile, supersaturated solutions of riboflavin in normal saline have been employed. By heating to the boiling point, a
temporary concentration of 1 mg/ml is said to be attained. The supersaturated solution of riboflavin is fairly stable; it takes a day to crystallize.

Today, aqueous solutions of the sodium salt of riboflavin-5′-phosphoric
acid are generally used for injections. Other water-soluble derivatives of
riboflavin include esters with sulfuric, gallic, aminoacetic, phthalic, succinic,
citric, malic, tartaric, and levulinic acids, and methylol and acetal derivatives.[32] In the synthesis of methylol derivative, preparations with as high as
55% microbiological activity can be obtained in a short reaction time, when
only 1 mole of formaldehyde is combined with 1 mole of riboflavin. Upon
addition of 2 or more moles of formaldehyde, the activity falls off rapidly. As
in the case of tri- and tetrasuccinates, the sulfate is microbiologically active
only after previous hydrolysis. Riboflavin mono- and disuccinates have
vitamin B_2 activities for the rat which are 100% and 65%, respectively, of the
activity of riboflavin. Both the mono- and diacetone derivatives of riboflavin
are active in the nutrition of rats. Riboflavin 5′-phosphate is fully as active in
the rat as riboflavin (oral and parenteral administration), as well as in the
microbiological test. The same is true for flavin adenine dinucleotide.

[29a] G. R. Penza, G. K. Radda, J. A. Taylor, and M. B. Taylor, in "Vitamins and Hormones" (R. S. Harris, ed.), Academic Press, New York, 1970.
[30] C. C. Tzong, Hakko Kogaku Zasshi 24, 56, 187 (1946) [Chem. Abstr. 44, 5975 (1950)].
[31] For literature references, cf. the first edition of this volume and the book of Vogel and
H. Knobloch, "Chemie u. Technik d. Vitamine Vol. 2, (II), 1955. pp. 196–197, I. F.
Enke Verlag, Stuttgart, where a table of the solubility increases is given.
[32] M. F. Furter, G. J. Haas, and S. H. Rubin, J. Biol. Chem. 160, 293 (1945); Merck and
Co., U.S. Patent No. 2,358, 356 (Sept. 19, 1944) [Chem. Abstr. 39, 1514 (1945)].

Neutral solutions of riboflavin are a greenish yellow. The absorption spectrum shows characteristic absorption maxima at 475, 446, 359–375, 268, and 223 nm. The absorption in the visible part of the spectrum has been used for quantitative determination of riboflavin.

Neutral aqueous solutions of riboflavin display intense yellowish green fluorescence, with a maximum at 565 nm which can be used for quantitative determination of the vitamin. The fluorescence vanishes on the addition of acid or alkali; optimal fluorescence occurs at pH 3–8.[33] The relatively weak fluorescence of FAD may be caused by internal quenching by interaction of the alloxazine and adenine portions of the molecule.[34, 73a]

Riboflavin has an amphoteric character. Its dissociation constants are $K_\alpha = 6.3 \times 10^{-12}$ and $K_\beta = 0.5 \times 10^{-5}$; the isoelectric point corresponds to a pH of 6.0. The pH of the saturated aqueous solution is approximately 6.[33] Below pH 2, a proton is added at N(1); the cation so formed shows only one maximum, at 239 nm. Dissociation of NH(3) at pH 10 affects the spectrum only slightly. By alkylation on NH (3) the molecule becomes extremely alkali labile.

The optical activity of riboflavin in neutral and acid solutions is exceedingly small. In an alkaline medium, the optical rotation is strongly dependent upon the concentration: $[\alpha]_D^{21°} = -70° (c = 0.06\%; 0.1\ N\ NaOH)$; $[\alpha]_D^{21°} = -117°$ $(c = 0.5\%; 0.1\ N\ NaOH)$.[35]

Borate buffer complexes with the ribityl side chain of riboflavin in a reversible 1-to-1 association; the negatively charged complex is more resistant to hydroxylic attack on the isoalloxazine ring.[36] Borate-containing solutions are strongly dextrorotatory: $[\alpha]_D^{20°} = +340°$ (pH 12); in this case the rotation depends only slightly upon the riboflavin concentration.[37]

Neutral aqueous solutions of riboflavin are relatively heat stable if protected from light and can be sterilized by autoclaving for a short time: only slight destruction occurs by heating to 120° for 6 hours. At room temperature (27°) decomposition of buffered solutions (pH 5 and 6) takes place at rates of 3 and 1.2% per month. No appreciable destruction of the vitamin can be observed during the cooking of food,[38] but when milk in bottles is exposed to

---

[33] R. Kuhn and G. Moruzzi, Ber. Deut. Chem. Ges. 67, 888 (1934); F. Kavanagh, Arch. Biochem. 20, 315 (1949); S. G. Schulman, J. Pharm. Sci. 60, 628 (1971). Quenching Studies: A. W. Varnes, R. B Dodson, and E. L. Wehry, Amer. Chem. Soc. 94, 946 (1972).

[34] G. Weber, Biochem. J. 47, 114 (1950); D. Voet, and A. Rich, C.A. 76, 31409p (1972).

[35] R. Kuhn, H. Rudy, and F. Weygand, Ber. Deut. Chem. Ges. 68, 625 (1935). For the rule which governs the rotation of different 9-polyhydroxyalkyl flavins, see F. Weygand, Ber. Deut. Chem. Ges. 73, 1278 (1940).

[36] D. A. Wadke and D. E. Suttmann, J. Pharm. Sci. 53, 1073 (1964).

[37] R. Kuhn and H. Rudy, Ber. Deut. Chem. Ges. 68, 169 (1935).

[38] R. R. Williams and V. H. Cheldelin, Science 96, 22 (1942).

sunlight, more than half of the riboflavin is destroyed within 2 hours.[40, 41] The rate of destruction by light becomes higher with increasing temperature and pH Alkali decomposes riboflavin rapidly.

Riboflavin is stable against acids, air, and the common oxidizing agents (except chromic acid, $KMnO_4$, and potassium persulfate), bromine, and nitrous acid. A very successful method for the purification of crude natural or synthetic flavins is based on this fact: in acid solution impurities are oxidized at a temperature below 100° with use of Cl_2, H_2O_2, HNO_3, or $HClO_3$.[42] But the vitamin is destroyed by hydrogen peroxide in the presence of ferrous ions to form a blue-violet fluorescent substance.[42a,b]

Reducing agents such as sodium dithionite ($Na_2S_2O_4$), zinc in acid solution, catalytically activated hydrogen, and titanous chloride transform riboflavin in alkaline, neutral, or acetic acid solutions directly into an almost colorless, pale yellow dihydroflavin, which is reoxidized on shaking with air. The potential of an equimolecular mixture of riboflavin and its leuco compound at pH 7.0 is -0.185 V (-0.146 V at pH 5.9), pretty much on the negative side. Combination with the enzyme protein has been shown to raise the redox potential from -0.19 V for D-riboflavin 5′-phosphate to -0.06 V for the "old yellow enzyme."[43]

By the action of zinc, tin, or sodium amalgam in strong HCl (pH < 1), a red reduction intermediate, a semiquinone radical, forms.[44, 45] This behavior of riboflavin might be useful for its detection.

With concentrated H_2SO_4, riboflavin gives a red-violet color which changes to yellow on dilution. When heated with 50% NaOH solution, riboflavin produces a green color, changing to red on dilution.[46]

Bacteriostatic effects of riboflavins have been observed only in the light. These may be explained possibly by the formation of toxic products and in part by destruction of needed nutrients. It has been demonstrated that in the presence of riboflavin irradiation causes destruction of tryptophan, pyridoxine,[47] and probably histidine.[48]

[40] W. J. Peterson, F. M. Haig, and A. O. Shaw, *J. Amer. Chem. Soc.* **66**, 662 (1944).

[41] J. A. Ziegler, *J. Amer. Chem. Soc.* **66**, 1039 (1944).

[42] R. Posternack and E. V. Brown (to Charles Pfizer and Co.), U.S. Patent No. 2,324,800 (July 20, 1944) [*Chem. Abstr.* **38**, 221 (1944)].

[42a] A. Leviton, *J. Amer. Chem. Soc.* **68**, 835 (1946).

[42b] S. Sawaki, *Chem. Abstr.* **46**, 1027 (1952).

[43] R. Kuhn and P. Boulanger, *Ber. Deut. Chem. Ges.* **69**, 1557 (1936).

[44] R. Kuhn and T. Wagner-Jauregg, *Ber. Deut. Chem. Ges.* **67**, 361 (1934). See also K. G. Stern, *Biochem. J.* **28**, 949 (1934).

[45] L. Michaelis, M. P. Schubert, and C. V. Smythe, *J. Biol. Chem.* **116**, 587 (1936).

[46] M. Z. Barakat and N. Badran, *J. Pharm. Pharmacol.* **3**, 501 (1951).

[47] M. N. Meisel and E. M. Dikanskaya, *Dokl. Akad. Nauk SSSR* **85**, 1377 (1952) [*Chem. Abstr.* **47**, 2258 (1953)].

[48] J. J. O'Neill, T. Wagner-Jauregg *et al.*, *Fed. Proc. Fed. Amer. Soc. Exp. Biol.* **14**, No. 1 (1955).

injection amounts to 340 mg/kg.[49] The LD_{50} value for rats, with the same form of application, is 560 mg/kg.[50] The administration of 10 gm/kg orally to rats or 2 gm/kg orally to dogs showed no toxic effects.[51]

D. Structure and Reactions

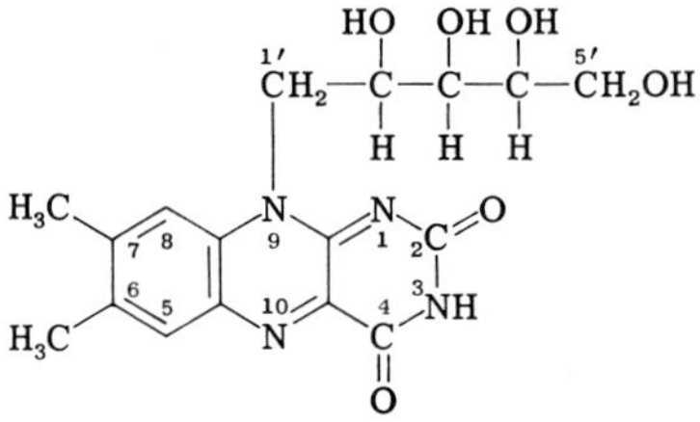

Riboflavin

I

Riboflavin is practically nontoxic. The toxicity to mice by intraperitoneal
The side chain of riboflavin is characterized by the following reactions: Acetylation with acetic anhydride in pyridine gives a chloroform-soluble tetraacetate, melting at 242°–243°. It is easily saponified by diluted alkali at room temperature. The formation of a tetraacetate indicates the presence of four hydroxyl groups.

Formation of a diacetone compound indicates that two hydroxyl groups in pairs are adjacent. Oxidation of riboflavin with lead tetraacetate yields 0.8 mole of formaldehyde. That proves the presence of a primary hydroxyl group in the α position to a secondary hydroxyl group.

The oxygen-containing part of the side chain of riboflavin can be removed by irradiation in alkaline solution. The resulting lumiflavin (m.p. 330°), in contrast to riboflavin, is chloroform soluble.[52] Irradiation of riboflavin in neutral or acid solution removes the entire side chain, yielding lumichrome.[53]

When riboflavin is illuminated anaerobically the yellow color fades and the isoalloxazine ring becomes reduced; on reoxidation the flavin color returns, and on treatment with alkali in the dark the chloroform-soluble lumiflavin is obtained.[53a] The assumption has been made that a "deuteroflavin" is involved in this photoreaction. Recently it was shown that, on anaerobic photobleaching of riboflavin followed by reoxidation with air, a mixture of flavins is

[49] R. H. Kuhn and P. Boulanger, *Hoppe-Seyler's Z. Physiol. Chem.* **241**, 233 (1936).
[50] K. Unna and J. G. Greslin, *J. Pharmacol. Exp. Ther.* **76**, 75 (1942).
[51] V. Demole, *Z. Vitaminforsch.* **7**, 138 (1938).
[52] O. Warburg and W. Christian, *Naturwissenschaften* **20**, 980 (1932); *Biochem. Z.* **266**, 377 (1933).
[53] P. Karrer, H. Salomon, K. Schöpp, E. Schlittler, and H. Fritsche, *Helv. Chim. Acta* **17**, 1010 (1934).
[53a] R. Kuhn and Th. Wagner-Jauregg, *Ber. Deut. Chem. Ges.* **66**, 1950 (1933).

produced, including riboflavin (I), lumiflavin (III), lumichrome (II) and about 10% of 6,7-dimethyl-9-formylmethylisoalloxazine (IV), the latter meeting the description of "deuteroflavin."[54] The anaerobic photochemical fading of riboflavin results from an intramolecular oxidoreduction of the flavin molecule, with cleavage of the ribityl side chain,[54a] probably with the formation of glyceraldehyde and glycolaldehyde.[55]

The photochemical behavior of vitamin B_2 is demonstrated in the following scheme[55a]:

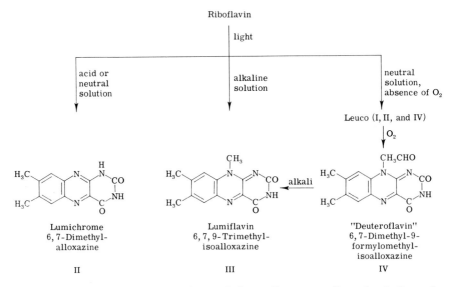

In the photolysis of *9-(2′-hydroxyethyl) isoalloxazine*, alloxazine is formed and the side chain produces acetaldehyde, formaldehyde, and an acid, probably formic acid.[56]

Riboflavin phosphate (FMN) has been shown to participate in photosynthetic phosphorylation in isolated chloroplast systems[56a] and to enhance bioluminescence.[56b]

The photoreduction of flavins by ethylenediaminetetraacetic acid and the

[54] E. C. Smith and D. E. Metzler, *J. Amer. Chem. Soc.* **85**, 3285 (1963); K. Yagi and D. B. McCormick, *J. Amer. Chem. Soc.* **87**, 5763 (1965).

[54a] B. Holmström and G. Oster, *J. Amer. Chem. Soc.* **83**, 1867 (1961); B. Holmström, *Bull. Soc. Chim. Belg.* **71**, 869 (1962).

[55] A. Kocent, *Chem. Listy* **47**, 195 (1953).

[55a] For the photobleaching of riboflavin phosphate and the mechanism of the photoreduction of riboflavin, see B. Holmström, *Ark. Kemi* **22**, 281 (1964). FAD is more stable to light.

[56] M. Halwer, *J. Amer. Chem. Soc.* **73**, 4870 (1951).

[56a] F. R. Whatley et al., *Biochim. Biophys. Acta* **32**, 32 (1959).

[56b] W. D. McElroy and H. H. Seliger, *Advan. Enzymol. Relat. Subj. Biochem.* **25**, (1963).

bleaching of flavin mononucleotide (FMN) under anaerobic conditions is inhibited by 3-(p-chlorophenyl)-1,1-dimethylurea (CMU), which is known to be a highly specific inhibitor of photosynthesis.[57] In the anaerobic photoreduction of FMN, as in riboflavin, the electrons for the reduction are derived from the side chain of the molecule in an intramolecular rearrangement.[57a]

Lumichrome (II) is the 6,7-dimethyl derivative of alloxazine (V), whereas riboflavin and lumiflavin are substitution products of the hypothetical isoalloxazine (VI).

Alloxazine   Isoalloxazine

V   VI

Lumichrome is formed also by stoichiometric oxidation of riboflavin by *Pseudomonas riboflavina*[58] or by mycobacteria;[59] under anaerobic conditions 6,7-dimethyl-9-(2'-hydroxyethyl)isoalloxazine[60] is formed. Tsai *et al.*[61] have demonstrated the aerobic decomposition of riboflavin by cell suspensions of *Pseudomonas riboflavina* as summarized in Fig. 1. The first intermediate is 1-ribityl-2,3-diketo-1,2,3,4-tetrahydro-6,7-dimethylquinoxaline (VII), formed by cleavage of ring C of the isoalloxazine nucleus with formation of urea. Further oxidation leads to ribose and 6,7-dimethylquinoxaline-2,3-dion (VIII). The final production of the oxidation are 3,4-dimethyl-6-carboxy-α-pyrone (IX) and oxamide.

The alkaline hydrolysis of riboflavin gives urea and 1,2-dihydro-6,7-dimethyl-2-keto-1-D-ribityl-3-quinoxalinecarboxylic acid (X). (This acid has been shown to have a depressant action on cardiac and visceral muscles when injected intravenously in the dog.[62]) In the case of lumiflavin, 1,2-dihydro-2-keto-1,6,7-trimethyl-3-quinoxalinecarboxylic acid (XI) is obtained along with urea.[62, 63]

[57] P. Hofmann and H. Gaffron, *Science* **141**, 905 (1963).

[57a] W. M. Moore *et al.*, *J. Amer. Chem. Soc.* **85**, 3367 (1963); G. K. Radda and M. Calvin, *Biochemistry* **3**, 384 (1964).

[58] J. W. Foster, *J. Bacteriol.* **47**, 27 (1944); **48**, 97 (1944) [*Chem. Abstr.* **38**, 1761, 5526 5526 (1944)].

[59] H. C. Hou, *Proc. Soc. Exp. Biol. Med.* **70**, 581 (1949).

[60] H. T. Miles and E. R. Stadtmann, *J. Amer. Chem. Soc.* **77**, 5746 (1955).

[61] L. Tsai, P. Z. Smyrniotis, D. Harkness, and E. R. Stadtmann, *Biochem. Z.* **338**, 561 (1963).

[62] A. R. Surrey and F. C. Nachod, *J. Amer. Chem. Soc.* **73**, 2336 (1951).

[63] R. Kuhn and T. Wagner-Jauregg, *Ber. Deut. Chem. Ges.* **66**, 1577 (1933); R. Kuhn and H. Rudy, *Ber. Deut. Chem. Ges.* **67**, 892, (1934); R. Kuhn, K. Reinemund, and F. Weygand, *Ber. Deut. Chem. Ges.* **67**, 1460 (1943).

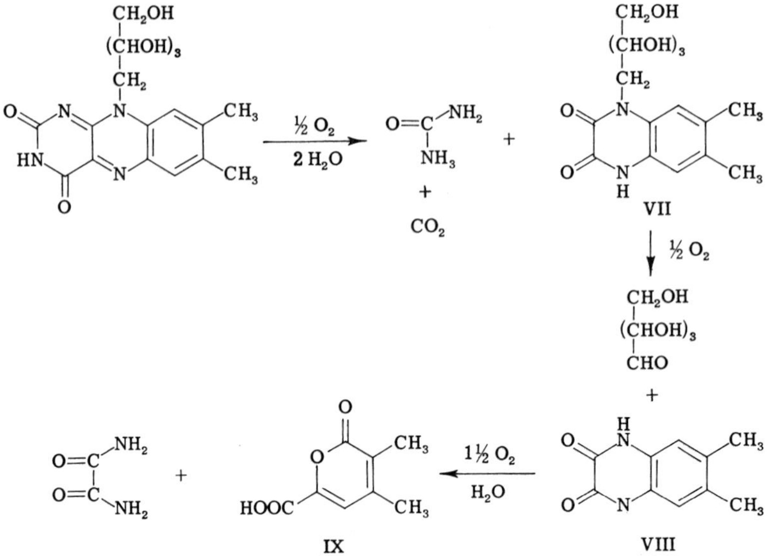

FIG. 1. Degradation of riboflavin by *Pseudomonas riboflavina*.

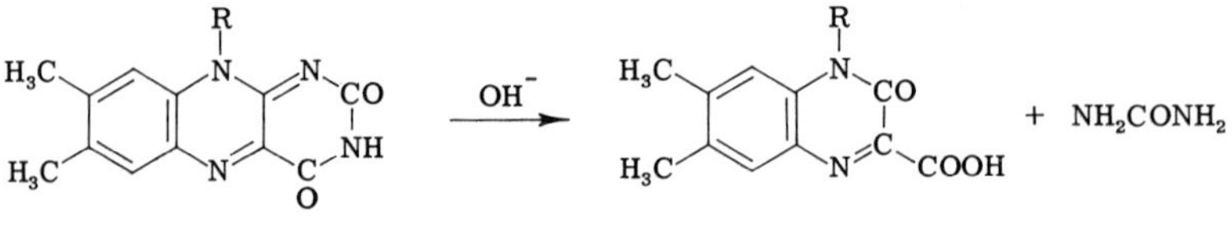

X: R = D-Ribityl
XI: R = CH₃

The oxocarbonic acid (XI) can be decarboxylated by sublimation with formation of the lactam (XII). This, when heated with NaOH, gives 1,2-dimethyl-4-amino-5-methylaminobenzene (XIII).

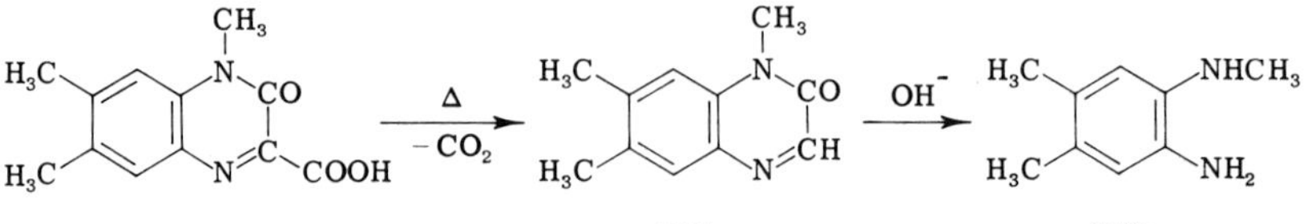

XI   XII   XIII

On reduction, riboflavin readily rakes up two hydrogen atoms with formation of a leuco compound. The pale yellow dihydroriboflavin can be stabilized by acetylation on NH(10); the acetyl group can be hydrolyzed under very mild conditions.

Stronger catalytic hydrogenation of flavins yields octahydroflavins, which are easily oxidized in alkaline solutions by air to the corresponding hexa-hydroflavins.[64]

Flavin   Dihydroflavin

Hexahydroflavin   Octahydroflavin

In acid solution (pH 1) flavins are reduced to dihydroflavins through inter-mediate forms which are *semiquinone radicals*.[64a, 65] This reduction can be formulated as shown in Fig. 2.[66]

The overall process involves the addition of two protons and one electron; the semiquinone radical is an ion radical. This is consistent with the results of spectroscopy and potentiometric titration. Structures XIV and XV differ only in the position of one proton. However, structure XV seems to be prefer-able for several reasons; for instance it is consistent with the electron para-magnetic resonance (EPR) results whereas structure XIV is not.

Three intermediate compounds have been obtained in the crystalline state by stepwise reduction of riboflavin to leucoriboflavin. They consist of para-magnetic molecular compounds of reduced and unreduced and semiquinone radical intermediates.[67] In *verdoflavin*, 1 mole of riboflavin and 1 mole of monohydroriboflavin (with a free valence) are associated; *chloroflavin* is probably partly free monohydroriboflavin and partly a quinhydrone, formed of riboflavin and leucoriboflavin; *rhodoflavin* contains the hydrochlorides of leucoriboflavin and monohydroriboflavin (1:1).

By analysis of the titration curves, Michaelis and Schwarzenbach[68] showed that in solution, at low concentration including the physiological concentration range, there is an intermediate form of reduction entirely represented by a free radical. The maximum ratio of this to the total dye is

[64] P. Karrer and R. Ostwald, *Rec. Trav. Chim. Pays-Bas* **57**, 500 (1938).

[64a] R. Kuhn and T. Wagner-Jauregg, *Ber. Deut. Chem. Ges.* **67**, 361 (1934).

[65] L. Michaelis, M. P. Schubert, and C. V. Smythe, *J. Biol. Chem.* **116**, 587 (1936).

[66] A. V. Guzzo and G. Tollin, *Arch. Biochem. Biophys.* **103**, 231 (1963).

[67] R. Kuhn and R. Ströbele, *Ber. Deut. Chem. Ges.* **70**, 747, 753 (1937).

[68] L. Michaelis and G. Schwarzenbach, *J. Biol. Chem.* **123**, 527 (1938).

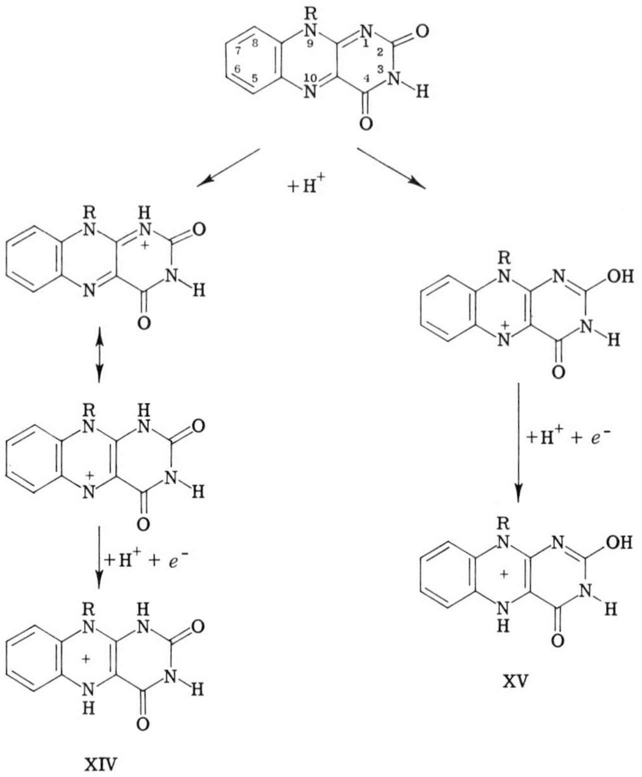

FIG. 2. Alternative pathways for the reduction of the isoalloxazines in dilute HCl.

0.10 at pH 4.62, and 0.14 at pH 6.92 at 30°. In higher concentrations, a partial dimerization of the radical to a bimolecular compound takes place. No other molecular species on an oxidation level between flavin and dihydroflavin could be detected in solution.

Flavoproteins reacting with substrates unfortunately do not form semiquinone species detectable by EPR[69] (with the exception of microsomal NADPH reductase[70]): therefore only direct spectrophotometric and kinetic evidence is available for semiquinone formation. However, semiquinones are readily detected by EPR in metalloflavoproteins and appear to be kinetically significant intermediates in the reactions of these enzymes.[71] Direct interaction between metal and flavin semiquinone in metalloflavoproteins has been demonstrated by spin relaxation studies.[71a]

[69] H. Beinert, *Proc. 6th Int. Congr. Biochem., New York* Sect. IV, p. 285 (1964). For the role of semiquinones in flavoprotein catalysis, see also V. Massey and Q. H. Gibson, *Fed. Proc. Fed. Amer. Soc. Exp. Biol.* **23**, Part I, 18 (1964).

[70] T. Nakamura and Y. Ogura, *J. Biochem. (Tokyo)* **52**, 214 (1962).

[71] H. Beinert and G. Palmer, *Advan. Enzymol.* **27**, 105 (1965).

[71a] H. Beinert and P. Hemmerich, *Biochem. Biophys. Res. Commun.* **18**, 212 (1965).

The structure of the particles connected with the flavin redox system has been discussed.[71b]

Molecular complexes of flavins with adenine,[71c] caffeine and other purines,[72] indole, tryptophan,[71d] serotonin, etc. and with chlortetracycline, phenols,[73] but no other benzene derivatives, have been described. The intramolecular association of riboflavin and adenine portions within FAD has been indicated by numerous investigations, most clearly by observing the optimum for fluorescence of this coenzyme with pH change.[34, 73a]

It was found that the phenolic hydroxyl group combines with FAD in competition with the apoprotein of enzymes containing dissociable flavin coenzymes as a prosthetic group, e.g., D-amino acid oxidase. This suggests that the tyrosyl group of the oxidase protein is the binding site with FAD. The absorption band of the riboflavin–tryptophan complex at 500 nm has been considered to correspond to the absorption band of rhodoflavin at 503 nm.

Probably only in the formation of the phenol—but not the purine or indole complexes—charge-transfer forces are involved.[74] The crystal structure of the charge-transfer complex between riboflavin and hydroquinone has been determined.[74a]

One mole of FMN and 1 mole of $FMNH_2$ form a charge-transfer complex.[75] Charge-transfer complexes were described between enzyme-reduced flavin adenine dinucleotide and oxidized pyridine nucleotide; the complexes had long wavelength bands, associated with a blue-green color.[75a]

A purple compound was isolated under anaerobic conditions in crystalline form; it contained the flavoprotein D-amino acid oxidase and D-alanine.[75b]

[71b] P. Hemmerich, M. C. Veeger and H. C. S. Wood, *Angew. Chem.* Intern. Ed. Engl. **4**, 671 (1965); D. E. Fleischmann and G. Tollin, *Biochim. Biophys. Acta* **94**, 248 (1965); D. E. Fleischmann and G. Tollin, *Proc. Nat. Acad. Sci. U.S.* **53**, 237 (1965).

[71c] K. Uehara, T. Micoguchi, S. Hosomi, T. Fujiwara, and K. Tomita, *J. Biochem.* (*Tokyo*) **64**, 589 (1968).

[71d] H. Mitsuda, H. Tsuge, and F. Kassai, *J. Vitaminol.* **16**, 119 (1970).

[72] I. Isenberg and A. Szent-György, *Proc. Nat. Acad. Sci. U.S.* **44**, 857 (1958); **45**, 1229 (1959); **47**, 245 (1961); H. A. Harbury et al., *Proc. Nat. Acad. Sci. U.S.* **44**, 662 (1958); **45**, 1708 (1959).

[73] K. Yagi, I. Ishibashi, and Y. Matsuoka, *Bitamin* **7**, 874, 935 (1954); K. Yagi, T. Ozawa, and K. Okada, *Biochim. Biophys. Acta* **35**, 102 (1959).

[73a] C. M. Tsibris, D. B. McCormick, and L. B. Wright, *Biochemistry* **4**, 504, 2612 (1965); D. B. McCormick and I. A. Roth, *Proc. Int. Congr. Biochem.*, Tokyo, **1967**

[74] G. Tollin et al., *Biochim. Biophys. Acta* **94**, 248, 258 (1965); A. Wilson, *Biochemistry* **5**, 1351 (1966); J. F. Pereira and G. Tollin, *Biochim. Biophys. Acta* **143**, 79 (1967).

[74a] C. A. Bear, J. M. Waters, and T. N. Waters, *Chem. Communicat.* 702 (1970).

[75] H. Beinert, *J. Amer. Chem. Soc.* **78**, 5323 (1956); Q. H. Gibson, V. Massey, and N. M. Atherton, *Biochem. J.* **85**, 369 (1962).

[75a] V. Massey and G. Palmer, *J. Biol. Chem.* **237**, 2347 (1962); T. Sakurai and H. Hosoya, *Biochim. Biophys. Acta* **112**, 459 (1966).

[75b] K. Yagi and T. Ozawa, *Biochim. Biophys. Acta* **67**, 685 (1963); **81**, 29 (1964); **85**, 300 (1965); **167**, 77 (1967).

Later studies indicated that this purple intermediate is a diamagnetic charge-transfer complex between the enzyme and substrate.[75c]

For other molecular complexes of flavins see the paragraph on analogs of riboflavin with a nitrogen-containing side chain, p. 40–42.

Metal complexes of riboflavin. It has long been known that riboflavin gives a deep-red silver salt.[23] The strong bathochromic shift of the flavin spectra occurring by interaction with Ag^+ can also be obtained with Cu^+ and Hg^{2+} but not with any other metal ions.[76] The red silver and copper flavin complexes have a long wavelength absorption band (pH 1, 492 nm; pH 5.7, 500 nm) quite similar to that of the red protonated flavin free radical "rhodo-flavin" (503 nm).[77] These very strong complexes contain the flavin and the metal ligand anion in a molecular ratio of 1:1. They were first formulated as 4,5-chelates of the 8-hydroxyquinoline type.[78] However, their color very likely is due to a *charge transfer* between the metal and the flavin, this mesomeric state (XVI) being responsible for the specific chelating qualities.[79]

reduced   oxidized

Of the chelates that belong to this group, with Fe(II/III), Mo(V/VI), Cu(I/II), and Ag (I/II), only the last two are stable in the presence of water.

There exists another group of metal complexes, *radical chelates*, with Mn(II), Fe(II), Co(II), Ni(II), Zn(II), and Cd(II); the radical character of the ligands is still conserved in these complexes.[80]

A number of brownish colored, solid "chelates" containing two atoms of metal has been described,[81] but these preparations probably do not correspond to pure substances.[82]

[75c] K. Yagi et al., J. Biochem. **59**, 521 (1966); **65**, 151, 663 (1969).

[76] P. Hemmerich, Experientia **16**, 534 (1960).

[77] H. Beinert, J. Amer. Chem. Soc. **78**, 5323 (1956).

[78] A. Albert, Biochem. J. **47**, XXVII (1950); **54**, 646 (1953). The chelate stability constants published by this author, demonstrating for instance a heightened affinity of riboflavin for Fe^{2+}, have been criticized by P. Hemmerich and S. Fallab, Helv. Chim. Acta **41**, 498 (1958) and by T. H. Harkins and H. Freiser, J. Phys. Chem. **63**, 309 (1959).

[79] I. F. Baarda and D. F. Metzler, Biochim. Biophys. Acta **50**, 463 (1961); P. Bamberg and P. Hemmerich, Helv. Chim. Acta **44**, 1001 (1961); K. H. Dudley, A. Ehrenberg, P. Hemmerich, and F. Müller, Helv. Chim. Acta **47**, 1354 (1964).

[80] A. Ehrenberg and P. Hemmerich, in "Biological Oxidations" (T. P. Singer, ed.), 722 pp. Wiley Interscience, New York, 1968.

[81] W. O. Foye and W. E. Lange, J. Amer. Chem. Soc. **76**, 2199 (1954).

[82] P. Hemmerich and S. Fallab, Helv. Chim. Acta **41**, 498 (1958).

Metal constituents are present in a number of flavoproteins.[83] The structure and function of iron–flavoproteins has been discussed.[84, 85] Molybdenum is contained in addition to iron in xanthine dehydrogenase from calf and chicken liver and *Clostridium cylindrosparterus*. Bovine intestinal xanthine oxidase is a metalloflavoprotein containing iron, copper, and FAD.[85a] A purified preparation of D-lactatecytochromic reductase of aerobic yeast contains Zn^{2+} and FAD in a molar ratio of $3:1$.[86] In the zinc–flavoprotein the metal functions in substrate binding. In all the other cases evidence is available from EPR spectroscopy, that the metal components participate in oxidation reduction. For flavin nucleotide-linked enzymes see ref.[86a]

For a *Survey of Flavoprotein Function, Model Studies on Flavin-Dependent Oxidoreduction* and the *Chemical Properties of Flavins in Relation to Flavoprotein Catalysis,* see ref.[86b] It is not yet known whether metal chelates play a role in the catalysis of metalloflavoproteins.[86c]

E. Synthesis of Flavins[87]

1. CHEMICAL METHODS

In 1891, O. Kühling synthesized alloxazines by condensation of *o*-phenyl-enediamine hydrochloride with alloxan.

[83] H. R. Mahler, *Advan. Enzymol.* **17**, 233 (1956). See also the extensive list of P. Hemmerich, G. Nagelschneider and C. Veeger in *FEBS Letters* **8**, 69 (1970); J. E. Colemann in "Progress in Bioorganic Chemistry," Vol. 1, edited by E. T. Kaiser and F. J. Kézdy, page 229–233 and 317–321 (1971), Wiley–Interscience; K. V. Rajagopalan, F. O. Brady and M. Kanda in *Vitamins and Hormones* **28**, 303–314 (1970), Academic Press, New York.

[84] P. Handler, K. V. Rajagopalan, and V. Aleman, *Fed. Proc. Fed. Amer. Soc. Exp. Biol.* **23**, Part I, 30 (1964).

[85] K. V. Rajagopalan and P. Handler, *J. Biol. Chem.* **239**, 1509 (1964); K. V. Rajagopalan, P. Handler, G. Palmer, and H. Beinert, *J. Biol. Chem.* **243**, 3784, 3797 (1968).

[85a] G. G. Roussos and B. H. Morrow, *Arch. Biochem. Biophys.* **114**, 600 (1966).

[86] C. Gregolin and T. P. Singer, *Biochim. Biophys. Acta* **57**, 410 (1962); T. Cremona and T. P. Singer, *J. Biol. Chem.* **239**, 1466 (1964).

[86a] P. Boyer, H. A. Lardy, and K. Myrback, eds., "The Enzymes," 2nd Ed., Vol. 7. Academic Press, New York, 1963. Also see this volume, p.

[86b] P. Hemmerich in *Vitamins and Hormones* **28**, 467–488 (1970); G. R. Penzer, G. K. Radda, J. A. Tailor and M. B. Taylor, *ibid.* page 441–466.

[86c] A. Ehrenberg, *loc. cit.* 86b, page 489–504.

[87] See also the excellent article of J. P. Lambooy, ref. 1.

Using the same principle, R. Kuhn and P. Karrer worked out methods for the synthesis of flavins, based on o-xylenes, D-ribose, and alloxan as starting

materials. Riboflavin (III) could be obtained by condensation of 1,2-di-methyl-4-amino-5-(D-1'-ribitylamino)benzene (I) with alloxan, which reacts in its lactim form (II). The reaction is carried out in acid solution. Boric acid as a catalyst increases the yield considerably.[88, 89] Other catalysts are H_2S, $SnCl_2$, or alloxantin in the presence of 1 mole of HCl.[90]

Four representative examples of riboflavin synthesis which differ in the preparation of the intermediate I are given below:

1. This intermediate can be prepared by condensation of o-nitroxylidine (IV) with D-ribose[91] and catalytic reduction of the formed riboside (V) to the diamine (I).[92] The yield was 16% riboflavin, calculated on the amount of ribose used.

[88] R. Kuhn, *Angew. Chem.* **49**, 6 (1963).

[89] R. Kuhn and F. Weygand, *Ber. Deut. Chem. Ges.* **68**, 1282 (1935).

[90] Hoffmann-La Roche and Co., Brit. Patent No. 628,410 (Aug. 29, 1949) [*Chem. Abstr.* **44**, 4935 (1950)].

[91] By condensation of aromatic amines with D-ribose, two isomers are obtained which have been considered to be the corresponding N-arylribofuranosylamines (A) and N-arylribopyranosylamines (B); A is converted to B in the presence of water [L. Berger and J. Lee, *J. Org. Chem.* **11**, 75, 84, 91 (1946); G. P. Ellis and J. Honeyman, *Nature (London)* **167**, 239 (1951); G. P. Ellis and J. Honeyman, *J. Chem. Soc.* p. 1490, 2053 (1952)]. The Na_2SO_4 complexes of arylamine-N-D-ribopyranosides can be hydrogenated to the corresponding ribitylamines in excellent yield [Hoffmann-La Roche, Inc., U.S. Patent Nos. 2,384,102 and 2,384,105 (Sept. 4, 1945) [*Chem. Abstr.* **40**, 600, 2854 (1946)].

[92] R. Kuhn and R. Ströbele, *Ber. Deut. Chem. Ges.* **70**, 773 (1937).

Among other flavins 6-ethyl-[93] and 6,7-diethyl-9-(D-1'-ribityl)isoalloxa-zine[94] have been prepared by this method. D-Ribose was found not to combine with 2-nitro-4-chloro-5-methylaniline[95] and 2-nitro-4-methyl-5-chloraniline.

2. o-Nitrochlorobenzenes have been reacted with amino sugars or amino alcohols, and the condensation product was hydrogenated to the diamine.[96] Poor yields are obtained with sugars containing four and five hydroxyl groups, but sugars with shorter chains ($n < 4$) give satisfactory yields.

The required glycamines can be prepared by hydrogenation of the corresponding sugars in liquid ammonia containing 3% of water, over a Raney nickel catalyst at 85° and 200 psi.[97]

9-(β-Hydroxyethyl)isoalloxazine,[96] 6-nitro-9-(β-hydroxyethyl)isoalloxa-zine, 9-(β-diethylaminoethyl)isoalloxazine, 6-nitro-9-(β-diethylaminoethyl) isoalloxazine, and other basically substituted isoalloxazines[98] have been prepared by this method. 9-(Dialkylaminoalkyl)isoalloxazines, the free bases, differ chemically from riboflavin by their solubility in organic solvents, for instance $CHCl_3$.

3. Another method for the synthesis of substituted 2-nitroanilines which are needed for the synthesis of riboflavin is the condensation of substituted o-dinitrobenzene with sugar amines. For instance, o-dinitroxylene and riba-mine are condensed in aqueous alcoholic solution and catalytically reduced to the corresponding diamine. The overall yield of riboflavin amounted to 4.5% of the ribose used.[99]

[93] H. V. Aposhian and J. P. Lambooy, *J. Amer. Chem. Soc.* **76**, 1307 (1954).

[94] J. P. Lambooy, *J. Amer. Chem. Soc.* **72**, 5225 (1950).

[95] E. E. Haley and J. P. Lambooy, *J. Amer. Chem. Soc.* **76**, 5093 (1954).

[96] P. Karrer, H. Salomon, K. Schöpp, and E. Schlittler, *Helv. Chim. Acta* **17**, 1165 (1934); P. Karrer, E. Schlittler, K. Pfaehler, and F. Benz, *Helv. Chim. Acta* **17**, 1516 (1934).

[97] R. B. Flint and P. L. Salzberg, U.S. Patent No. 2,016,962 (1932); F. W. Holly, E. W. Peel, K. Folkers *et al.*, *J. Amer. Chem. Soc.* **72**, 5416 (1950); **73**, 332 (1951); **74**, 4047 (1952).

[98] F. Kipnis, N. Weiner, and P. E. Spoerri, *J. Amer. Chem. Soc.* **69**, 799 (1947).

[99] R. Kuhn and F. Weygand, *Ber. Deut. Chem. Ges.* **68**, 1001 (1935).

$$H_3C \diagdown NO_2 \quad +H_2NR \rightarrow \quad H_3C \diagdown NHR \quad +H \rightarrow \quad H_3C \diagdown NH \cdot R$$
$$H_3C \diagdown NO_2 \qquad\qquad H_3C \diagdown NO_2 \qquad\qquad H_3C \diagdown NH_2$$

3-Methylriboflavin[100] and 6,7-dichloro-9-(1'-D-sorbityl)isoaloxazine and its analogs have been synthesized by this method; a variant uses substituted o-iodonitrobenzenes as starting materials.[101]

4. A fourth method of riboflavin synthesis starts with the condensation of 3,4-xylidine with D-ribose by boiling the amine and the sugar in alcoholic solution.[102–104] The 3,4-xylidine-N-D-riboside formed is catalytically reduced without isolation of the reduction product prior to hydrogenation.[105] Karrer and Meerwein[106] have shown that coupling with phenyldiazonium salt gives the corresponding azo dye, with a yield of 92% of the theoretical amount. The reduction to (2-amino-4,5-dimethylphenyl)-D-1'-ribamine can be performed with 85% of the theoretical yield.[107]

$$H_3C \diagdown NH_2 \quad \xrightarrow[\substack{H_2 \text{ (Ni or} \\ \text{Pd) } 71\%}]{+ \text{D-ribose}} \quad H_3C \diagdown NHCH_2(CHOH)_3CH_2OH$$
$$H_3C \qquad\qquad\qquad\qquad H_3C$$

$$+ p\text{-}RC_6H_4N_2Cl$$

$$H_3C \diagdown NHCH_2(CHOH)_3CH_2OH \quad \xleftarrow{+ Na_2S_2O_4} \quad H_3C \diagdown NHCH_2(CHOH)_3CH_2OH$$
$$H_3C \diagdown NH_2 \qquad\qquad\qquad\qquad H_3C \diagdown N{=}N{-}C_6H_4R\text{-}p$$

This method can be used for the industrial preparation of riboflavin. The yield obtained is very high, 38% calculated for ribose. The method is fit also for the synthesis of analogs of riboflavin,[93, 104, 108] but it is limited to 6,7-substituted flavins, because only m,p-disubstituted aniline derivatives couple with diazonium salts in the ortho position.

[100] R. Kuhn, K. Reinemund, F. Weygand, and R. Ströbele, Ber. Deut. Chem. Ges. 68, 1765 (1935).

[101] F. W. Holly, E. W. Peel, R. Mozingo, J. J. Cahill, F. R. Koniuszy, C. H. Shunk, and K. Folkers, J. Amer. Chem. Soc. 72, 5416 (1950); 74, 4047, 4251 (1952).

[102] P. Karrer et al., Helv. Chim. Acta 18, 1435 (1935); W. A. Wisansky and S. Ansbacher, J. Amer. Chem. Soc. 63, 2532 (1941).

[103] R. Kuhn and L. Birkhofer, Ber. Deut. Chem. Ges. 71, 621 (1938).

[104] E. E. Haley and J. P. Lambooy, J. Amer. Chem. Soc. 80, 110 (1958).

[105] Hoffmann-La Roche, Inc., U.S. Patent No. 2,477,560 (Aug. 2, 1949) [Chem. Abstr. 44, 169 (1950)].

[106] P. Karrer and H. Meerwein, Helv. Chim. Acta. 18, 1130 (1935); 19, 264 (1936).

[107] P. Karrer, Helv. Chim. Acta 30, 2101 (1947).

[108] J. P. Lambooy, J. Amer. Chem. Soc. 80, 110 (1958).

Depending on the R group in the arylazo radical, varying small amounts of material with the azo group in the 6-position will be formed besides the 2-isomer. Separation of the 2- and the 6-azo compounds is difficult and the subsequent steps of synthesis will lead to mixtures of the 6,7-disubstituted and the 5,6-disubstituted isoalloxazines. However, the isomeric impurity, in certain cases, can be removed by repeated recrystallization from water.[109]

D-*Ribose*, needed for the riboflavin synthesis described, can be obtained either from natural sources or by synthetic methods. It has been prepared by hydrolysis of yeast nucleic acid.[110] From 2 kg of yeast, only 1–2 gm of pure D-ribose have been obtained via yeast nucleic acid and guanosine.

The synthetic method starts with glucose, which, via calcium gluconate, is converted to D-ribose through the following steps: D-arabinose, diacetyl-arabinal, D-arabinal. The latter, by oxidation with perbenzoic acid, gives a mixture of D-arabinose and D-ribose, with a yield of 10–17%.[100, 111] The sirupy ribose prepared by this method can be obtained crystallized by conversion to aniline-*N*-D-ribofuranoside and subsequent hydrolysis (Berger and Lee[91]).

Processes have been developed whereby ribose can be prepared directly by electrolytic reduction of ribonolactone. The corresponding acid can be obtained by rearrangement of arabonic acid, which usually is produced by the oxidation of corn sugar in alkaline solution with oxygen or air. By a method of the Northern Regional Research Laboratory, calcium arabonate is obtained with 85% yield by electrolytic oxidation of 2-ketogluconate.[112]

Since the preparation of D-ribose forms a bottleneck in the synthesis of riboflavin, methods have been developed which avoid the use of ribose.

F. Weygand[113] in 1940 showed that it is possible to use D-arabinose for the synthesis of riboflavin. The *N*-D-Arabinoside of xylidine (VI) is transformed by a so-called Amadori isomerization into the isoarabinose derivative VII, which under alkaline conditions (possibly favoring the keto form) can be hydrogenated to the intermediate VIII of the riboflavin synthesis. The yield is about 13% of the pentose used.

[109] J. P. Lambooy, *J. Nutr.* **75**, 116 (1961).
[110] H. Bredereck, *Ber. Deut. Chem. Ges.* **71**, 408 (1938); H. Bredereck, M. Köthnig, and E. Berger, *Ber. Deut. Chem. Ges.* **73**, 956 (1940).
[111] M. Gehrke and F. X. Aichner, *Ber. Deut. Chem. Ges.* **60**, 918 (1927); W. C. Austin and F. L. Humoller, *J. Amer. Chem. Soc.* **56**, 1152 (1934); T. Reichstein and M. Steiger, *Helv. Chim. Acta* **19**, 189, 193 (1936).
[112] C. L. Mehltretter, *Yearb. Agr.* (*U.S. Dep. Agr.*) p. 782 (1950–1951).
[113] F. Weygand, *Ber. Deut. Chem. Ges.* **73**, 1259, 1264 (1940). Based on a similar principle is the modified synthesis of riboflavin described by V. M. Berezovskiĭ, V. A. Kurdyukova, and N. A. Preobrazhanskiĭ, *J. Appl. Chem. USSR* **22**, 527, 533 (1949) [*Chem. Abstr.* **44**, 2530 (1950)]. A variant of Weygand's method forms the object of a patent of the Miles Laboratories, Inc., Brit. Patent No. 594,949 (Nov. 24, 1947) [*Chem. Abstr.* **42**, 2630 (1948)].

VI   VII   VIII

Later, processes of technical importance were developed which avoid the primary use of pentoses altogether and operate with D-ribonic acid or its lactone. This sugar acid can be obtained by pyridine epimerization of D-arabonic acid, which in its turn is prepared from D-glucose.

In the procedure of Pfizer and Co.,[114] D-ribonamide is acetylated and the reaction product is converted into tetraacetylribonic acid by treatment with nitrous acid, which then is reacted with PCl_5 to form the acid chloride. This is reduced to give tetraacetyl-D-ribose, palladium supported on $BaSO_4$ being used as a catalyst. Hydrogenation of tetraacetyl-D-ribose in the presence of o-4-xylidine, with Raney nickel or platinum as catalyst, yields tetraacetyl-1-D-ribityl-o-4-xylidine, which finally is coupled with a phenyldiazonium salt. A similar method uses tetrabutyryl D-ribonamide as a starting material.[115]

A somewhat different method starts with D-ribonolactone, prepared from D-arabonic acid via D-ribonic acid.[116] The lactone is reacted with

[114] Pfizer and Co., Inc., Brit. Patent Nos. 545,360 (May 21, 1942), 551,401 (Feb. 25, 1943) [*Chem. Abstr.* **38**, 5845, 2344 (1944)], and 585,212 (Feb. 3, 1947) [*Chem. Abstr.* **41**, 3815 (1947)].

[115] Merck and Co., U.S. Patent No. 2,424,341 (Sept. 22, 1947) [*Chem. Abstr.* **42**, 211 (1948)].

[116] M. Tishler, N. L. Wendler, K. Ladenburg, and J. W. Wellman, *J. Amer. Chem. Soc.* **66**, 1328 (1944); Merck and Co., U.S. Patent No. 2,420,210 (May 6, 1947) [*Chem. Abstr.* **41**, 5548 (1947)]; Hoffmann-La Roche, Inc., U.S. Patent Nos. 2,438,881 and 2,438,883 (March 3, 1948) [Chem. Abstr. **42**, 5048 (1948)].

xylidine, and the ribonic xylidide, after acetylation, is chlorinated to the imidochloride, which can be reduced smoothly to the amine and then deacetylated.

In another procedure, 3,4-dimethylaniline and tetraacetyl-D-ribononitrile[117] are subjected to catalytic reductive coupling and the resulting acetylated amine is deacetylated.

Alloxan, which was needed for the earlier synthesis of riboflavin, can be obtained by oxidation of uric acid or barbituric acid.

The newer methods use barbituric acid, 5-chloro- or 5,5-dichlorobarbituric acid directly. The condensation with N-(1′-D-ribityl)-2-arylazo-4,5-dimethyl-aniline (the 6-arylazo isomer does not react) can be carried through in the presence of a weak organic acid, such as acetic acid.[117, 118] Large amounts of pure riboflavin and other flavins (e.g., L-lyxoflavin[119]) could be synthesized by this method, as follows.

3,4-Dimethylaniline (IX) is reductively condensed in the presence of a palladium catalyst with tetraacetyl-D-ribononitrile (X) with loss of NH_3. Ribonitrile can be prepared from ribonic acid via the amide. The formed N-tetraacetyl-D-ribitylamino-3,4-dimethylaniline (XI) is coupled with p-nitro-phenyldiazonium chloride, and the product (XII) is reduced in the presence of a platinum catalyst to 1-N-tetraacetylribitylamino-2-amino-4,5-dimethylben-zene (XIII). This compound is then condensed with 5,5-dichlorobarbituric acid (XIV) to form tetraacetylriboflavin (XV), which is then hydrolyzed to riboflavin.

6,7-Dimethyl-9-benzylisoalloxazine can be formed by heating 5,5-dichloro-barbituric acid in pyridine with 1-benzylamino-2-amino-4,5-dimethylbenzene. Similarly, 5-amino-N-ribityl-o-4-xylidine and 5,5-dichlorobarbituric acid give riboflavin in excellent yield. Among other flavins synthesized by this method are $2 - {}^{14}$C-labeled riboflavin[104] and 3,6,7-trimethyl-9(1′-D-ribityl) isoalloxazine[120] (using 2-methylbarbituric acid).

Previously, Bergel et al.[121] converted N-D-ribityl-o-4-xylidine into ribo-flavin by coupling with diazotized aniline and shaking the resulting azo

[117] M. Tishler and J. W. Wellman (to Merck and Co.), U.S. Patent No. 2,261,608 (Nov. 4, 1941) [Chem. Abstr. 36, 1050 (1942)]; K. Ladenburg, M. Tishler, J. W. Wellman, and R. D. Babson, J. Amer. Chem. Soc. 66, 1217 (1944); M. Tishler, J. W. Wellman, and K. Ladenburg, J. Amer. Chem. Soc. 67, 2165 (1945).

[118] M. Tishler and G. H. Carlson, U.S. Patent No. 2,350,376 (1944) [Chem. Abstr. 38, 4963 (1944)]; M. Tishler, K. Pfister, III, R. D. Babson, K. Ladenburg, and A. J. Fleming, J. Amer. Chem. Soc. 69, 1487 (1947).

[119] D. Heyl, E. C. Chase, F. R. Koniuszy, and K. Folkers, J. Amer. Chem. Soc. 73, 3826 (1951).

[120] J. P. Lambooy, E. E. Haley and R. A. Scala, J. Nutr. 74, 466 (1961).

[121] F. Bergel, A. Cohen, and J. W. Haworth, J. Chem. Soc. London p. 165 (1945); Hoffmann La Roche Inc., Brit. Patent Nos. 550,169 (Dec. 28, 1942) [Chem. Abstr. 38, 1247 (1944)] and 550,836 (Jan. 27, 1943) [Chem. Abstr. 38, 1752 (1944)].

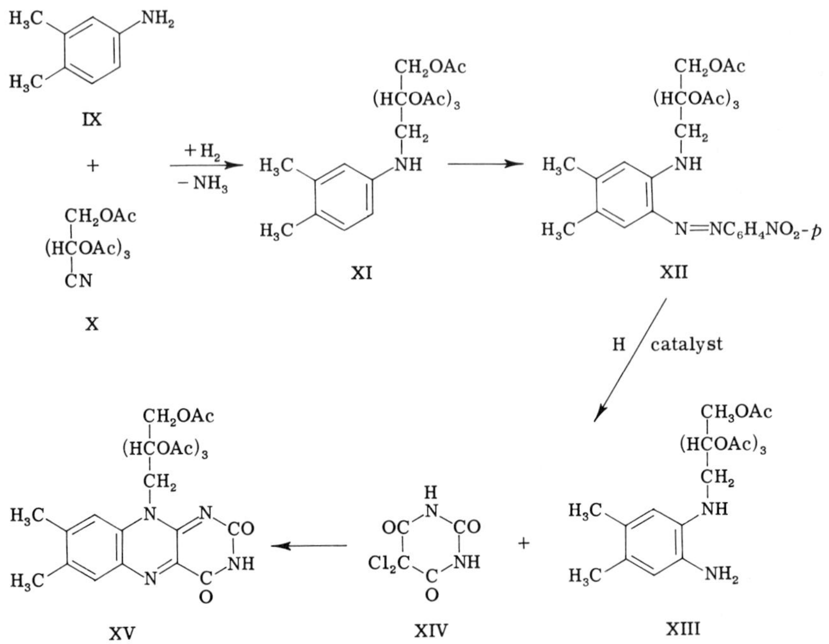

H₃C, NH₂ ... IX

+

CH₂OAc (HCOAc)₃ CN   X

$\xrightarrow[- NH_3]{+ H_2}$

H₃C, NH ... (with CH₂OAc (HCOAc)₃ CH₂)   XI

→

H₃C, NH N=NC₆H₄NO₂-p ... (with CH₂OAc (HCOAc)₃ CH₂)   XII

H / catalyst

XV ← XIV (OC, Cl₂C, NH, CO, H, N, O) + XIII (H₃C, NH, NH₂ with CH₃OAc (HCOAc)₃ CH₂)

XV structure (H₃C, H₃C, N, N, CO, NH, C, O with CH₂OAc (HCOAc)₃ CH₂)

compound with excess alloxantin or dialuric acid in an atmosphere of nitrogen, finally oxidizing any leucoriboflavin by shaking with air.

A reversed mode of synthesis for riboflavin is the condensation of dimeric o-benzoquinone (XVI) with 5-amino-4-D-ribitylaminouracil (XVII), which gives a yield of 29% of the vitamin.[122]

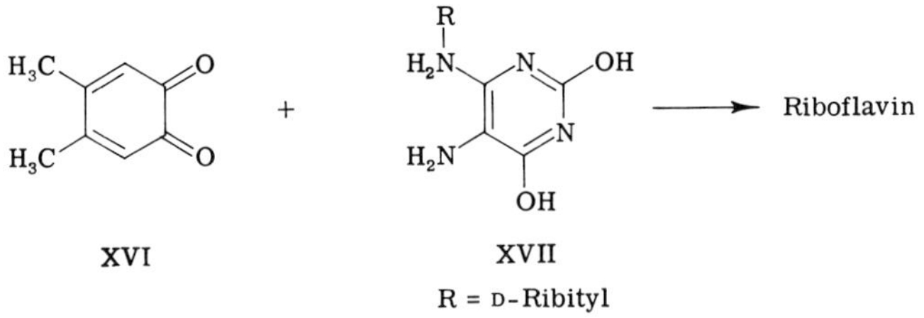

XVI (H₃C, H₃C, O, O) + XVII (R, H₂N, N, OH, H₂N, N, OH) ⟶ Riboflavin

XVI   XVII

R = D-Ribityl

Riboflavin has been made from 6,7-dimethyl-8-ribityllumazine with 55% yield by Rowan and Wood. (loc. cit. 145) (page 30).

10-Deazariboflavin was synthesized from N-ribityl-4,5-dimethylanthranylic aldehyde and barbituric acid.[122a]

[122] R. M. Cresswell, T. Neilson, and H. C. S. Wood, J. Chem. Soc. London p. 476 (1961); for this method of synthesis compare T. J. Bardos, D. B. Olsen, and T. Enkoji, J. Amer. Chem. Soc. 79, 4704 (1957).
[122a] D. E. O'Brien, L. T. Weinstock, and C. C. Cheng, Chem. and Ind. 48, 2044 (1967).

a. Synthesis of Riboflavin 5'-Phosphate (Flavin Mononucleotide, FMN)

The phosphorylation of riboflavin with phosphoryl chloride in pyridine provides a method for small-scale preparation of riboflavin 5'-phosphate. The original method of Kuhn and Rudy[123] yields mainly a cyclic phosphate, riboflavin 4',5'-phosphate, as shown by Forrest and Todd.[124] Acid hydrolysis of the cyclic ester gives riboflavin 5'-phosphate, which is identical with the natural riboflavin phosphate.

D-Riboflavin 5'-phosphate

Dichlorophosphoric acid is a more useful reagent for the phosphorylation of riboflavin than phosphorus oxychloride; FMN has been prepared by this method in quantities greater than milligrams.[125] Later on, anhydrous metaphosphoric acid and polyphosphoric acid were used as phosphorylating agents.[126]

The alcoholysis reaction of catecholic cyclic phosphate with riboflavin gives a mixture of riboflavin 5'-phosphate and riboflavin 4',5'-cyclic phosphate in a yield of 75–78%; after acid hydrolysis pure FMN can be obtained by zone electrophoresis without any loss.[127]

Newer methods are the reactions of riboflavin with phosphoric acid in the presence of trichloronitrile or with phosphodamiates.[127a]

FMN gives a crystallized monodiethyanolamine salt with a water solubility of more than 200 times that of riboflavin.

---

[123] R. Kuhn and H. Rudy, Ber. Deut. Chem. Ges. 68, 383 (1935).

[124] H. S. Forrest and A. R. Todd, J. Chem. Soc. London, p. 3295 (1950). The cyclic riboflavin 4', 5'-phosphate is identical with the "fourth flavin compound," an intermediate product of hydrolysis from flavin adenine dinucleotide (FAD), to FMN; K. Yagi and Y. Matsuoka, J. Biochem. (Tokyo) 48, 93 (1960); FMN, the flavin mononucleotide-like compound of Rhizopus oryzae, might be 3'-, 2', 5'-cylic, or 2',3'- cyclic monophosphate; S. Tachibana, J. Shiode, and S. Matsuno, J. Vitaminol (Kyoto) 9, 197 (1963).

[125] L. A. Flexser and W. G. Farkas, Chem. Ind. (London) p. 3947 (1951); U.S. Patent No. 2,610,176 (Sept. 9, 1952) [Chem. Abstr. 47, P8781a, d; P8792a (1953).

[126] M. Viscontini, C. Ebnother, and P. Karrer, Helv. Chim. Acta. 35, 457 (1952); M. Viscontini et al., Helv. Chim. Acta. 38, 15 (1955).

[127] T. Ukita and K. Nagasawa, Chem. Pharm. Bull. 7, 465 (1959).

[127a] R. V. Arternlina and V. M. Berezouski, Zh. Obshch. Khim. 36, 823 (1966); Adangazous et al., ibid. 36, 1753 (1966); cf. Index Chemicus, 22, 68249 (1966); 24, 74373 (1967).

b. Synthesis of Flavin Adenine Dinucleotide (FAD)

The first synthesis of FAD was achieved in Todd's laboratory[128] by condensation of the monosilver salt of FMN with 2',3'-isopropylidene adenosine 5'-benzyl phosphorchloridate and removal of the protective groups with an overall yield of about 7%.

After other syntheses[129, 130] the following method (Fig. 3) has been described recently.[131] After addition of ethoxyacetylene to adenosine 5'-phosphate in dimethyl sulfoxide the thus activated phosphate is reacted with riboflavin 5'-phosphate. The method avoids the formation of by-products such as riboflavin 4',5' cyclic phosphate. The yields of FAD are 10–15%.

2. BIOSYNTHESIS OF RIBOFLAVIN[132]

The biosynthetic pathways for purines, riboflavin, and pteridines are closely linked. Thus the carbon atoms of glycine are incorporated into these

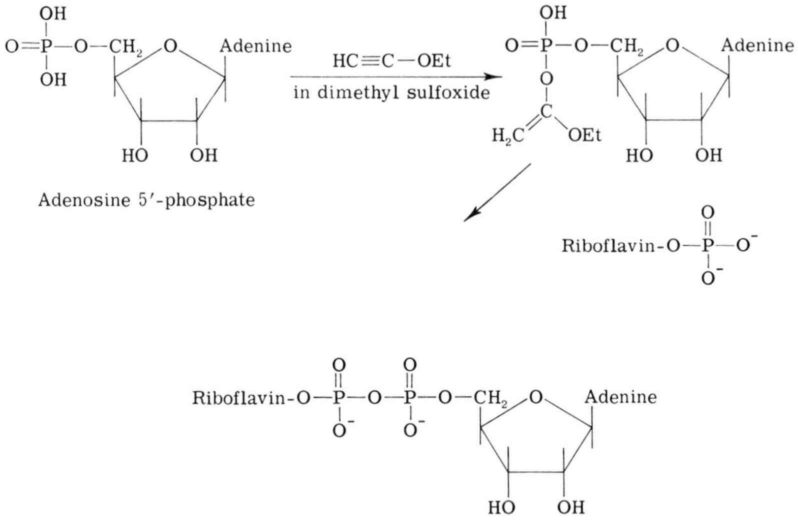

FIG. 3. Synthesis of flavin adenine ribonucleotide.

[128] S. M. H. Christie, G. W. Kenner, and A. R. Todd, *J. Chem. Soc. London* p. **46** (1954).

[129] F. M. Huennekens and G. L. Kilgour, *J. Amer. Chem. Soc.* **44**, 6716 (1955).

[130] C. Deluca and N. O. Kaplan, *Biochim. Biophys. Acta* **30**, 6 (1958).

[131] H. Wassermann and D. Cohen, *Chem. Eng. News* 47 (1962).

[132] For a recent description see G. W. E. Plaut *in* "Comprehensive Biochemistry" (M. Florkin and E. H. Stotz, eds.) Vol. 21 (1970), Elsevier Publish. Co., Amsterdam and New York.

three classes of compounds in structurally analogous positions.[133, 134] A preformed purine can be converted directly into riboflavin[135, 136] with the loss of only carbon 8 of the purine ring: other purine carbons and all the ring nitrogens[137] appear finally in the pyrimidine portion for the riboflavin molecule.

According to Masuda et al.,[138] riboflavin (IV) is formed in *Eremothecium ashbyii* from the purine (I) (9-ribitylxanthin) through the unstable 4-ribityl-amino-5-aminouracil (II) and the dioxopteridine (III) (6,7-dimethyl-8-ribityl-lumazine); this substance exhibits green fluorescence in ultraviolet light and is one of the few examples of a naturally occurring pteridine without a 2-amino group.

R = D-Ribityl

It has been synthesized by condensation of II with diacetyl[139, 140] and the same way has been suggested for the biological synthesis.[141, 142] However, unequivocal demonstration of II as an intermediate remained to be achieved.

That lumazine III alone is the precursor of riboflavin (IV) in organisms

[133] G. W. E. Plaut *Annu. Rev. Biochem.* **30**, 409 (1961).
[134] G. W. E. Plaut, *in* "Metabolic Pathways" (D. M. Greenberg, ed.), 2nd Ed., Vol. 2, pp. 673–712. Academic Press, New York, 1961.
[135] W. S. McNutt, *J. Biol. Chem.* **210**, 511 (1954).
[136] W. S. McNutt, *J. Biol. Chem.* **219**, 365 (1956).
[137] W. S. McNutt, *J. Amer. Chem. Soc.* **83**, 2303 (1961).
[138] T. Masuda *et al.*, *Pharm. Bull.* (*Japan*) **4**, 71, 217, 375 (1956); **5**, 28 136, 598 (1957).
[139] A. J. Birch and C. J. Moye, *J. Chem. Soc. London* p. 2622 (1958).
[140] G. F. Maley and G. W. E. Plaut, *J. Biol. Chem.* **234**, 641 (1959); G. F. Maley and G. W. E. Plaut, *J. Amer. Chem. Soc.* **81**, 2025 (1959); G. F. Maley and G. W. E. Plaut, *Arch. Biochem. Biophys.* **80**, 219 (1959).
[141] T. W. Goodwin and D. H. Treble, *Biochem. J.* **70**, 14P (1958).
[142] T. Masuda *et al.*, *Pharm. Bull.* (*Japan*) **6**, 291, 618 (1958); **7**, 361, 366 (1959).

such as *Eremothecium ashbyii* and *Ashbya gossypii* has been established by biochemical studies.[140] All the carbon atoms of the *o*-xylene moiety of riboflavin are derived from the lumazine III, 2 molecules of which are converted by riboflavin syntheses into one molecule of riboflavin (IV)[143, 143a] and 4-ribitylamino-5-amino-2,6-dihydroxypyrimidine.[143b] In this interesting biochemical reaction the lumazine (III) simultaneously functions as a donor and an acceptor of a C_4 unit which consists of the two methyl groups and the C atoms 6 and 7. Apparently a similar mechanism operates for riboflavin formation in plants, since Mitsuda *et al.*[144] established that the lumazine (III) alone is required as a substrate for vitamin B_2 formation by extracts from various green leaves.

The biochemical conception of riboflavin formation has been verified *in vitro* under nonenzymatic conditions later by Rowan and Wood[145] with the conversion of 6,7-dimethyl-8-ribityllumazine (III) into riboflavin (IV) *in vitro* by dissolving III in phosphate buffer at pH 7.3 and refluxing it under nitrogen for 15 hours: on cooling, riboflavin separated in 55% yield. The following mechanism of this transformation has been suggested: (1) ring opening of the pyrazine ring in the pteridine initiated by nucleophilic attack at position 7 (III → V → VI); (2) aldol condensation involving two molecules of compound VI to give a derivative (VII) of dimeric biacetyl as suggested by Birch;[146] (3) cyclization of the intermediate VII with loss of one diamino-pyrimidine portion to give riboflavin (IV).

Addition of metal ions accelerates the conversion of 6,7-dimethyl-8-ribityllumazine (III) into riboflavin in the *in vitro* system. This observation seems to be in agreement with the fact that the presence of a certain concentration of ferric or zinc ions is necessary for optimal synthesis of riboflavin by *Candida guilliermondia.*[147]

Experiments to elucidate the biogenesis of the ribityl side chain of riboflavin showed[148] that ^{14}C is mainly incorporated at position 5' with $^{14}CH_3COOH$ and at the positions 2', 3', and 4' with $CH_3{}^{14}COOH$. With glucose-6-^{14}C, radioactive carbon was introduced at the 5' position. These

[143] G. W. E. Plaut *et al., J. Biol. Chem.* **235**, PC41 (1960); **238** 2866 (1963).

[143a] T. W. Goodwin and A. A. Horton, *Nature (London)* **191**, 772 (1961).

[143b] H. Wacker, R. A. Harvey, C. W. Winestock, and G. W. E. Plaut, *J. Biol. Chem.* **239**, 3493 (1964).

[144] H. Mitsuda, F. Kawai, S. Morituka, Y. Suzuki, and Y. Nakayama, *J. Vitaminol. (Kyoto)* **7**, 128, 243, 247, (1961); **8**, 178 (1962).

[145] T. Rowan and H. C. S. Wood, *Proc. Chem. Soc. London* p. 21 (1963); *J. Chem. Soc. London* p. 452 (1968).

[146] A. J. Birch, *Proc. Chem. Soc. London* p. 11 (1962).

[147] W. H. Schopfer and H. Knüsel, *Z. Allgem. Pathol. Bakteriol.* **19**, 659 (1956); W. H. Schopfer and H. Knüsel, *Arch. Mikrobiol.* **27**, 219 (1957) [*Chem. Abstr.* **53**, 5390g (1959)]; T. Enari, *Acta Chem. Scand.* **9**, 1726 (1955).

[148] G. W. Plaut and P. L. Broberg, *J. Biol. Chem.* **219**, 131 (1956).

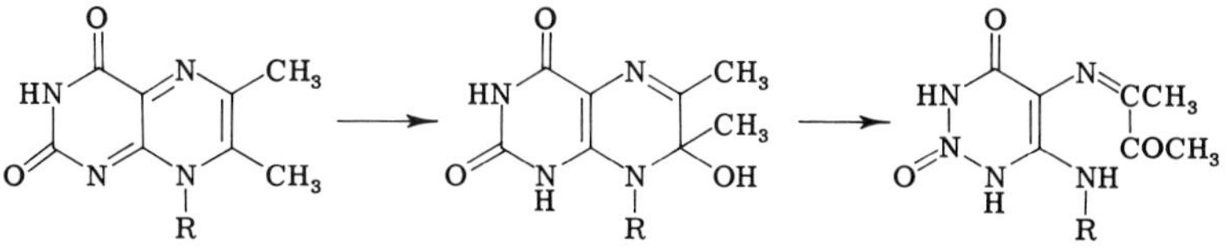

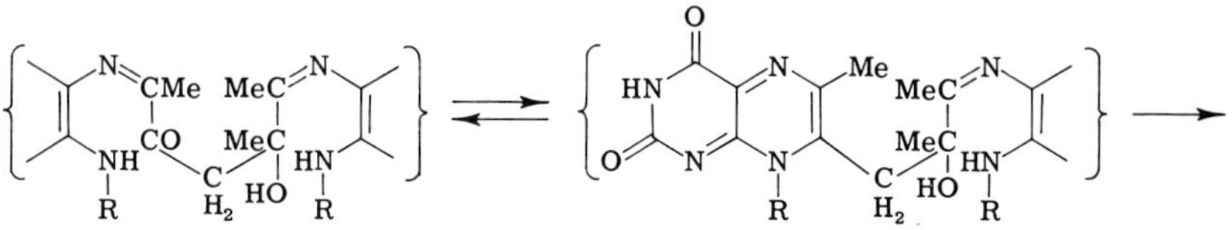

R = D-Ribityl

VII

⟶ IV (Riboflavin)

observations suggest that at least two pathways of carbohydrate metabolism, the hexose monophosphate shunt and the transaldolase transketolase system, contribute to the formation of the ribityl moiety. It is possible that a ribityl or phosphoribityl intermediate exists already at the purine level.

For the Biosynthesis of phosphorylated flavins, see McCormick et al.[148a]

3. MICROORGANISMS AS PRODUCERS OF RIBOFLAVIN.[148b]

Different natural sources have been used for the production of vitamin B_2 by fermenting microorganisms. Whey and other milk by-products have been treated with lactose-fermenting yeasts, especially *Saccharomyces fragilis*, or with *Clostridium butylicum*, several species of *Lactobacillus*, or molds, e.g., *Aspergillus niger, Aspergillus flavus, Penicillium chrysogenum*, and species of *Fusarium*.

Molasses or other carbohydrate mashes were fermented with various strains of butanol-producing *Clostridium*, especially *C. acetobutylicum*; among the bacteria, this microorganism is one of the best producers of riboflavin.

Riboflavin is formed by numerous strains of *Mycobacterium tuberculosis*. In *Mycobacterium smegmatis*, up to 3.6 mg of riboflavin is formed per 100 mg of the dried cells.[148c]

[148a] D. B. McCormick et al., Biochim. Biophys. Acta **65**, 326 (1962); D. B. McCormick et al., Biochem. Biophys. Res. Commun. **14**, 493 (1964).

[148b] For more details and references, see T. W. Goodwin, "The Biosynthesis of Vitamins and Related Compounds," Academic Press 1963, London and New York.

[148c] R. L. Mayer and M. Rodbart, Arch. Biochem. **11**, 49 (1946).

Most varieties of the yeast species *Candida* produce substantial amounts of riboflavin when glucose is used as the carbon source. *Candida guilliermondia* and *Candida flaveri* were found to produce high yields of riboflavin on a simple synthetic medium of low cost.[148d] The use of the *Candida* bacteria for commercial exploitation is very difficult because of their extremely low tolerance for iron. 2,2'-Dipyridyl has been recommended to control the iron content in fermentation media.[148e]

In 1935 Guilliermond, a French mycologist, observed that *Eremothecium ashbyii* in laboratory cultivation produced a yellow pigment which formed crystals in the threadlike cells. The microorganism originally was isolated as a pathogen for cotton plants in the Belgian Congo. The pigment has since been identified as riboflavin.

Ashbya gossypii also was found to be of value in the microbiological production of riboflavin.[148f] In shake cultures on a medium containing 4% glucose, 0.5% peptone, and 2.5% corn steep liquor solids, titers of 1000 mg/liter were obtained; animal residues such as slaughterhouse wastes (stick liquor) can replace peptone.

F. Biologically Active Isoalloxazines

Some of the more important relations between chemical constitution and biological activity of isoalloxazines chemically related to riboflavin will be discussed here.

Only slight changes in the chemical structure of riboflavin can be made without loss of vitamin B_2 activity. This fact is in agreement with the high chemical specificity of vitamins in general. In replacing the ribityl side chain by other sugar alcohols, or by alteration of substituents in the benzene ring of the isoalloxazine nucleus, derivatives can be obtained that are antagonists of riboflavin.

1. DERIVATIVES AND ISOMERS OF RIBOFLAVIN

Riboflavin tetraacetate and both the *mono-* and *diacetone riboflavin* are fully active in supporting rat growth, probably as a result of hydrolysis in the mammalian organism, but they are inactive for lactic acid bacteria.[148g] *Riboflavin 5'-phosphate* and *flavin adenine dinucleotide* not only promote growth in rats,[148h] but both are also as effective as riboflavin for growth and acid production of *Lactobacillus helveticum*.

[148d] H. Levine *et al.*, *Ind. Eng. Chem.* **42**, 1176 (1950).
[148e] R. Hickey, U.S. Patent No. 2,425,280 (Aug. 5, 1947) [*Chem. Abstr.* **41**, 6668 (1947)].
[148f] J. Wickerham, M. H. Flickinger, and R. M. Johnston, *Arch. Biochem.* **9**, 95 (1946).
[148g] R. Kuhn, H. Rudy, and F. Weygand, *Ber. Deut. Chem. Ges.* **68**, 625 (1935).
[148h] P. György, *Proc. Soc. Exp. Biol. Med.* **35**, 207 (1936).

Isoriboflavin, 5,6-dimethyl-9-(1'-ribityl) isoalloxazine is a rather weak reversible antagonist of riboflavin in the nutrition of the rat with an inhibition index[149] of about 100. It is not inhibitory for the growth of *Lactobacillus casei* and will not support it as the sole source of flavin, but it will stimulate the production of acid by this organism when suboptimal amounts of riboflavin are present.[150, 151]

It has been demonstrated[151a] that, in certain strains of rats fed with isoriboflavin, fetal development can be deranged, with production of congenital malformations.

D-*Araboflavin*, 6,7-dimethyl-9-(D-1'-arabityl)isoalloxazine, is an antagonist of riboflavin; 200 µg/day decrease the rate of growth of rats receiving 7 µg of riboflavin/day to such an extent that no growth takes place by the third week.[152]

L-*Araboflavin*, 6,7-dimethyl-9-(L-1'-arabityl)isoalloxazine,[153] showed some little stimulating activity for rats and lactic acid bacteria in the presence of suboptimal amounts of riboflavin.

The same is true for the following derivatives of this flavin: 6,7-trimethylene-9-(L-1'-arabityl-isoalloxazine, 6,7-tetramethylene-9-(L-1'-arabityl)isoalloxazine,[154] 6-methyl-7-amino-9-(L-1'-arabityl)isoalloxazine. The D-arabityl isomer of the latter substance is said to be about half as effective as riboflavin in promoting the growth of B_2-avitaminotic rats.[155]

In rats receiving 7 µg of riboflavin per day L-araboflavin in higher doses (200 µg per day) reduces growth very slightly.[152]

L-*Lyxoflavin*, 6,7-dimethyl-9-(1'-L-lyxityl)isoalloxazine,[156] is devoid of riboflavin activity in rats when tested by the standard assay, but in a certain rat assay for unidentified vitamins in liver and other source materials, as well as for *Lactobillus lactis*, L-lyxoflavin has shown growth-promoting or vitamin activity.[157]

In 1949 from 10 kg of human heart, 5 mg of a flavin, considered to be

[149] G. A. Emerson and M. Tishler, *Proc. Soc. Exp. Biol. Med.* **55**, 184 (1944).
[150] E. E. Snell, O. A. Klatt, H. W. Bruins, and W. W. Cravens, *Proc. Soc. Exp. Biol. Med.* **82**, 583 (1953).
[151] H. P. Sarett, *J. Biol. Chem.* **162**, 87 (1946).
[151a] W. Neuweiler and R. H. H. Richter, *Schweiz. Med. Wochenschr.* **91**, 67 (1961).
[152] H. von Euler and P. Karrer, *Helv. Chim. Acta* **29**, 353 (1946).
[153] P. Karrer *et al.*, *Helv. Chim. Acta* **18**, 908 (1935).
[154] R. Kuhn, H. Vetter, and W. Rzeppa, *Ber. Deut. Chem. Ges.* **70**, 1307 (1937).
[155] S. Nishida, *Chem. Abstr.* **45**, 7127, (1951); **46**, 6715 (1952).
[156] D. Heyl, E. C. Chase, F. Koniuszy, and K. Folkers, *J. Amer. Chem. Soc.* **73**, 3826 (1951).
[157] G. A. Emerson and K. Folkers, *J. Amer. Chem. Soc.* **73**, 5383 (1951); M. S. Shorb *Proc. Soc. Exp. Biol. Med.* **79**, 611 (1952); cf. however, E. E. Snell, O. A. Klatt, H. W Bruins, and W. W. Cravens, *Proc. Soc. Exp. Biol. Med.* **82**, 583 (1953).

lyxoflavin were isolated;[158] however, the natural existence of this flavin has not been definitely confirmed.[159] It is suspected that the "lyxo-flavin" preparation from heart might be a mixture of riboflavin and its anhydride formed from riboflavin phosphate in the course of the isolation procedure.[160]

2. HOMOLOGS OF RIBOFLAVIN

The 6,7-alkyl homologs of riboflavin are summarized in Table I.

It can be seen from Table I that one methyl group only, instead of two, gives a rather drastic reduction in the vitamin B_2 activity, while one ethyl group reduces it to zero and makes the molecule an antagonist of riboflavin (6-ethyl-flavin). In the methylethyl flavins the vitamin B_2 activity resembles that of the methylflavins but the animals are not able to reproduce. 6,7-Diethyl riboflavin is a competitive antagonist of riboflavin for growth in the rat. When any but very small quantities are administered to the riboflavin-deficient rat, a growth response is obtained but no survival is permitted.

When the 6 and 7 positions are not substituted, the compounds are toxic.[172a]

As a growth factor for nutrition of *L. casei* and *Bacillus lactis acidi*, the specificity of riboflavin as compared with its homologs in general is less pronounced.

5'-Deoxyriboflavin, 6,7-dimethyl-9-1'-(5'-deoxy-D-ribityl)isoalloxazine, antagonizes riboflavin in the growth of *L. casei* with an inhibition index of 150. It has weak activity under limited conditions for lymphosarcoma regression.[173]

D-*Galactoflavin*, 6,7-dimethyl-9(1'-D-dulcityl)isoalloxazine, is a reversible antagonist of riboflavin in the rat with an inhibition index[173a] of about 25. The presence of galactoflavin in the diet can accelerate the onset of riboflavin deficiency in animals on a riboflavin-free diet.[174] This flavin is inert for the chick and for *L. casei* and *L. lactis*. However, at low concentrations it stimulates acid production by *L. casei* in the presence of suboptimal quantities of riboflavin, becoming inhibitory when the ratio of galactoflavin to riboflavin becomes 500:1 or greater.[174a] The symptoms of ariboflavinosis produced by

[158] E. Sodi Pallares and H. Martínez Garza, *Arch. Biochem.* **22**, 63 (1949); E. Sodi Pallares and H. Martínez Garza, *Arch. Inst. Cardiol. Mex.* **19**, 753 (1949) [*Chem. Abstr.* **44**, 5368 (1950)].

[159] T. S. Gardner, E. Wenis, and J. Lee, *Arch. Biochem. Biophys.* **34**, 98 (1951).

[160] J. Baddiley, J. G. Buchanan and B. Carss, *J. Chem. Soc. London* p. 4058 (1957).

[172a] R. Kuhn and P. Boulanger, *Hoppe-Seyler's Z. Physiol Chem.* **241**, 233 (1936).

[173] C. H. Shunk, J. B. Lavigne, and K. Folkers, *J. Amer. Chem. Soc.* **77**, 2210 (1955).

[173a] C. A. Emerson, E. Wurtz, and O. H. Johnson, *J. Biol. Chem.* **160**, 165 (1945).

[174] L. Prosky *et al.*, *J. Biol. Chem.* **239**, 2691 (1964).

[174a] M. S. Shorb, *Proc. Soc. Exp. Biol. Med.* **79**, 611 (1952).

D-galactoflavin in man have been described.[175] In mice and rats, galacto-flavin-containing diets induce teratogenic abnormalities.[175a]

3. ANALOGS OF RIBOFLAVIN

a. Chloro Analogs

6-Methyl-7-chloroflavin. 6-Methyl-7-chloro-9-(1'-D-ribityl)isoalloxazine[120] has no effect on the riboflavin-deficient rat even when 2 mg/day are given. In the nutrition of *L. casei* it reversibly and very efficiently antagonizes ribo-flavin with an inhibition index[175b] of 59. For several clinically important microorganisms, it has been found to be inert.

6-Chloro-7-methylflavin. 6-Chloro-7-methyl-9-(1'-D-ribityl)isoalloxazine is remarkable for the response it elicits in both *L. casei* and the riboflavin-deficient rat.[176] Administered in any quantity from 3 μg to 2 mg/day, it stimulates the growth of the riboflavin-deficient rat. The growth response for 6-chloro-7-methylflavin when small quantities are given for limited periods of time is equal to that produced by half the quantity of riboflavin. However, all quantities lead to the death of the animal in spite of this growth, but the animals can be protected against the lethal effects of this flavin by the administration of adequate amounts of riboflavin. The stimulus for growth of the riboflavin-deficient rat by the 6-chloro-7-methyl analog is due to the apparent mobilization of newly available riboflavin which does not appear to be derived from displacement of bound riboflavin but to be available in part by increased utilization of the vitamin, increased intestinal synthesis of riboflavin, and increased utilization of the food the animal consumes. The healthy appearing animals die, and a severely depressed tissue content of riboflavin is observed.

In *L. casei*, it was found to be a potent, reversible antagonist of riboflavin with an inhibition index of 76. In the presence of appropriate mixtures of this analog and riboflavin, a modified form of *L. casei* emerged which could be isolated as an independent strain. This new, "modified" strain, differed from the normal or "stock" strain in that it could use either the analog or ribo-flavin as its sole source of flavin. This ability to utilize the inhibitor was due to the modified bacteria being able to phosphorylate the analog.[176a]

Dichloro-D-riboflavin, 6,7-dichloro-9-(D-1'-ribityl)isoalloxazine, the first

[175] McLane, *J. Clin. Invest.* **43**, 357 (1964); *Blood* **25**, 932 (1965).

[175a] H. Kalter and J. Warkam, *Physiol. Rev.* **39**, 69 (1959); *J. Exptl. Zool.* **136**, 531 (1957); M. M. Nelson, H. M. Evans *et al. J. Nutr.* **58**, 125 (1956).

[175b] Inhibition index $= \dfrac{\mu\text{g analog at half max. acid prod.}}{0.3\ \mu\text{g riboflavin (max. acid prod.)}} \times \dfrac{\text{mol. wt. riboflavin}}{\text{mol. wt. analog}}$

[176] J. P. Lambooy and E. E. Haley, *J. Nutr.* **72**, 169 (1960); R. D. Faulkner and J. P. Lambooy, *J. Med. Chem.* **9**, 495 (1966).

[176a] R. A. Scala and J. P. Lambooy, *Arch. Biochem. Biophys.* **78**, 10 (1958); J. P. Lambooy, *Arch. Biochem.* **117**, 120 (1966).

TABLE I

6,7-ALKYL HOMOLOGS OF RIBOFLAVIN (6,7-DIMETHYLFLAVIN)

Homolog	Vitamin B_2-activity as % of riboflavin in rats	Inhibition index as antagonist of riboflavin in rats	Nutrition of	
			Lactobac. casei	Bacillus lactis acidi
6-Methylflavin	30% (20 μg/day)[161,162]	—	Serves as the sole source of flavin; stimulates the production of about 40% of the acid produced by equivalent amounts of riboflavin.[163]	
7-Methylflavin	50–100% (10–20 μg/day)[164]	—	As above;[163] 60% activity of riboflavin	As above;[163] 80% activity of riboflavin
6-Ethylflavin	—	400[165]	3%[165]	—
7-Ethylflavin	0%. Small growth stimulus when given with suboptimal amounts of riboflavin[166]	—		—
6-Methyl-7-ethylflavin	36%. Animals grow to full adulthood but are not able to reproduce[167]	—	100% at $<26{,}6 \times 10^{-11}$ mole/liter; 90% at $>26{,}6 \times 10^{-11}$ mole/liter[168]	—

6-Ethyl-7-methylflavin	45% (10 μg/day)[168] Animals grow to full adulthood but are unable to reproduce[167]	—	As above[163, 168]	70%[163]
6,7-Diethylflavin	When any but very small quantities are administered growth is obtained but animals do not survive[170, 171]	6[169]	Serves as the sole source of riboflavin[170] 100% at $<8.22 \times 10^{-11}$ mole/liter[172]; 90% at $>8.22 \times 10^{-11}$ mole/liter	

[161] P. Karrer and F. M. Strong, *Helv. Chim. Acta* **18**, 1343 (1935).
[162] R. Kuhn, H. Vetter, and H. W. Rzeppa, *Ber. Deut. Chem. Ges.* **70**, 1302 (1937).
[163] E. E. Snell and F. M. Strong, *Enzymologia* **6**, 186 (1939).
[164] P. Karrer, H. von Euler, H. Malmberg, and K. Schöpp, *Sv. Kem. Tidskr.* **47**, 153 (1953).
[165] J. P. Lambooy and H. V. Aposhian, *J. Nutr.* **71**, 182 (1960).
[166] P. Karrer and T. H. Quibell, *Helv. Chim. Acta* **19**, 1034 (1936).
[167] J. P. Lambooy, *Biochim. Biophys. Acta* **29**, 221 (1958); J. P. Lambooy and Krin, *Proc. Fed. Amer. Soc. Exp. Biol.* **27**, 788 (art. 3221) (1968).
[168] J. P. Lambooy, *Fed. Proc. Fed. Amer. Soc. Exp. Biol.* **16**, 208 (1957); J. P. Lambooy, *J. Nutr.* **75**, 116 (1961).
[169] H. V. Aposhian, J. P. Lambooy, and M. M. Aposhian, *Fed. Proc. Fed. Amer. Soc. Exp. Biol.* **12**, 170 (1953).
[170] J. P. Lambooy and H. V. Aposhian, *J. Nutr.* **47**, 539 (1952).
[171] J. P. Lambooy, *Amer. Clin. Nutr.* **3**, 282 (1955).
[172] J. P. Lambooy, *J. Biol. Chem.* **188**, 459 (1951).

antagonist of riboflavin to be known,[177] inhibits the growth of *Staphylococcus aureus, Streptobacterium plantarum* P 32 (which do not need external riboflavin supply), *L. casei*,[177a] and *Bacillus lactis acidi*, but not of yeast. The inhibition is competitively prevented by riboflavin. The growth of *Eremothecium ashbyii* is inhibited by high doses of dichloroflavin without reduction of its riboflavin production.[178]

Dichloroflavin has an oxidation–reduction potential of $E_0 = -0.095$ V (pH 7); for riboflavin it is $E_0 = -0.185$ V (pH 7). This difference has been regarded as a cause of the inhibitory behavior of dichloroflavin; perhaps the vitamin analog cannot function like riboflavin in the oxidation–reduction reactions that are catalyzed by the riboflavin coenzymes. However, it has been demonstrated that dichloro-D-riboflavin and its 5'-phosphoric acid ester *in vitro* have no influence on the activity of enzymes which contain riboflavin-5' phosphoric acid ester as a prosthetic group, e.g., *d*-amino acid oxidase from liver and xanthine dehydrase and aldehyde dehydrase from milk, even when present in a 1000-fold excess over the yellow enzymes.[179]

Twelve other halogen-substituted flavins with various sugar chains in the 9 position have been found to be less effective as riboflavin antagonists than dichloroflavin, as tested with *Streptobacterium plantarum* P 32.[180]

Dichloro-D-sorboflavin, 6,7-dichloro-9-(1'-D-sorbityl)isoalloxazine,[101] exhibits no significant inhibition of riboflavin microbiologically and *in vivo* in rats. However, it is effective in producing regression of established lymphosarcoma implants in mice. The D-ribityl, L-arabityl, and D-dulcityl analogs show only slight, questionable inhibition.

b. Other Analogs of Riboflavin

2-Thioriboflavin,[181] which does not fluoresce, has vitamin B_2 activity similar to that of riboflavin, as shown by animal growth experiments. Its activity perhaps is due to hydrolysis to riboflavin.

2,4-Diamino-2,4-deoxyriboflavin is said to be a competitive antagonist for folic-folinic acid in the biosynthesis of deoxyribonucleic acid.[182]

[177] R. Kuhn, F. Weygand, and E. F. Möller, *Ber. Deut. Chem. Ges.* **76**, 1044 (1943).
[177a] Contradictory statements (loc. cit. 120; 150) have not been confirmed; cf. T. Wagner-Jauregg, H. Fischer, *et al. Arzneim-Forsch.* **20**, 831 (1970).
[178] W. H. Schopfer, *Int. Z. Vitaminforsch.* **20**, 116 (1948).
[179] P. Karrer and H. Ruckstuhl, *Schweiz. Akad. Med. Wiss.* **1**, 236 (1945).
[180] F. Weygand, R. Löwenfeld, and E. F. Möller, *Chem. Ber.* **84**, 101 (1951).
[181] V. M. Berezovskii and L. M. Mel'nikova, *Zh. Obshch. Khim.* **31**, 3827 (1961) [*Chem. Abstr.* **57**, 11290d (1962)].
[182] T. J. Bardos and D. B. Olsen (to Armour and Co.), U.S. Patent No. 2,867,614 (Jan. 6., 1959) [*Chem. Abstr.* **54**, 17432c (1960)]; T. J. Bardos and D. B. Olsen, *J. Amer. Chem. Soc.* **79**, 4704 (1957).

6,7-Dimethyl-9-(β-hydroxyethyl)isoalloxazine[183] is said to be a potent competitive antagonist of riboflavin, in growing rats and against *L. casei*. It was inactive by the oral route in trials in humans with leukemia and cancer. Since the substance shows poor absorption from the digestive tract, its acetate ester, which is readily absorbed, was prepared. It has antitumor activity against the Murphy–Sturm lymphosarcoma and the Walker 256 carcinoma in animals. In clinical trials on 10 patients no antitumor activity could be seen.[183a]

6-Nitro-9-(β-hydroxyethyl)isoalloxazine[184] did not show significant effects in chemotherapeutic tests.

Lumiflavin, the photolysis product of riboflavin, is either an inhibitor or a stimulator of the utilization of riboflavin or flavin adenine dinucleotide by *L. casei*, depending upon the relative amounts of lumiflavin present.[185]

c. Mode of Action of Riboflavin Analogs[186, 186a]

The particular biological behavior of these analogs is a reflection of a combination of several factors that include permeability to the cell, reactivities with flavokinase and FAD phosphorylase, and coenzymatic functions.

Those few analogs which partially serve as a sole replacer of riboflavin in a growing organism structurally resemble riboflavin to a close degree, e.g., diethylriboflavin, 6-methylriboflavin, and 2'-deoxyriboflavin. Lack of a 7-methyl substituent markedly decreases the vitamin activity of flavin, mainly because of a lessened conversion to coenzyme forms. A comparison of 6-methylriboflavin with 6-methylpyridinoriboflavin additionally suggests unpaired coenzymatic functions of the latter as accounting for its much weaker vitamin activity, as both analogs are converted to FMN analogs about equally well.

Those analogs that antagonize may act in at least three ways to bring about growth inhibition: (1) by competition with the prosthetic group of flavoenzymes; (2) by competitively inhibiting the phosphorylation of riboflavin; (3) by being enzymatically converted to an analog of riboflavin 5-phosphate or flavin adenine dinucleotide, in which form they might competitively inhibit flavoenzymes.

It has been shown that yeast flavokinase, the enzyme that catalyzes the phosphorylation of riboflavin, also phosphorylates D-araboflavin and dichloroflavin to coenzyme forms. The more positive redox potential of the coenzyme forms of dichlororiboflavin does not permit adequate coupling of

[183] H. H. Fall and H. G. Petering, *J. Amer. Chem. Soc.* **78**, 377 (1956).
[183a] M. Lane *et al.*, *J. Pharmacol. Exp. Ther.* **122**, 315 (1958).
[184] H. Hippchen, *Ber. Deut. Chem. Ges.* **80**, 263 (1947).
[185] H. P. Sarett, *J. Biol. Chem.* **162**, 87 (1946).
[186] E. B. Kearny, *J. Biol. Chem.* **194**, 747 (1952).
[186a] D. B. McCormick, C. Arsenis, and P. Hemmerich, *J. Biol. Chem.* **238**, 3095 (1963).

oxidation–reduction reactions normally served by FMN and FAD. The net result is biological antagonism, but at the stage of flavin coenzyme function rather than formation. Similar behavior is noted with dibromoflavin and diiodoriboflavin.

D-Erythroflavin is poorly phosphorylated in the flavokinase system, and the FMN analog so formed is not readily converted to an FAD analog with FAD pyrophosphorylase. However, the redox potential of its coenzyme forms are approximately the same as the coenzymes of riboflavin, and D-erythro-flavin 4'-phosphate has been found to be active with TPNH cytochrome reductase from yeast.

Isoriboflavin, galactoflavin, and sorboflavin are not phosphorylated by flavokinase, nor do they inhibit the enzymatic phosphorylation of riboflavin by flavokinase, with the exception of isoriboflavin.[186b] Galactoflavin is said to inhibit the penetration of riboflavin into cells.[186c]

Lumiflavin,[186] its 6-methyl-7-amino analog, and 2',3',4'-trideoxyribo-flavin[186a] are antagonists for the biological utilization of riboflavin. Neither of these analogs is converted to coenzyme forms, but they do inhibit the conversion of riboflavin to FMN.

d. Analogs of Riboflavin with a Nitrogen-Containing Side Chain

The phenazine analog of riboflavin 2,4-diamino-7,8-dimethyl-10-(D-ribityl)-5,10-dihydrophenazine (I)[187] antagonizes the action of vitamin B_2 in riboflavin-requiring bacteria. The dinitrophenazine derivative from which (I) (below) is prepared produces mild riboflavin deficiency in mice. Adequate amounts of riboflavin overcome the effects of the compound.

I   II

A few substances with antimalarial activity were found to inhibit the growth-promoting effect of riboflavin on microorganisms, for instance mepacrine (Atabrine) (II)[188] substituted pyrimidines,[189] and quinine, but not

[186b] D. B. McCormick, *Nature* 201, 925 (1964).

[186c] J. Tu, *et al.*, *J. Amer. Med. Assoc.* 185, 83 (1963).

[187] D. N. Wooley, *J. Biol. Chem.* 154, 31 (1944); H. P. Sarett, *J. Biol. Chem.* 162, 87 (1946).

[188] J. Madinaveitia, *Biochem. J.* 40, 373 (1946); M. Silverman and B. A. Evans, Jr., *J. Biol. Chem.* 150, 265 (1943).

[189] F. M. Curd and F. L. Rose, *J. Chem. Soc., London* p. 343, 362, 366, 370 (1946); A. R. Todd *et al.*, *J. Chem. Soc., London* p. 357 (1946).

progumil paludrine. However the structural similarity of certain antimalarials to the flavin nucleus is not correlated to their antimalarial action, nor is Atabrine (II) a specific inhibitor of flavoproteins.[190, 191]

Atabrine is an (irreversible) inhibitor of cytochrome reductase,[192] D-amino acid oxidase, and a D-lactic acid dehydrogenase of an aerobic yeast,[192a] enzymes which require flavin adenine dinucleotides for their prosthetic group. It has been shown that reversal of inhibition by FMN is not due to competition between the flavin and Atabrine for the enzyme, but the formation of a compound between the Atabrine and FMN.[191]

The acridine salt of FMN, insoluble in cold water, has been prepared;[193] it might be considered a model for a compound between FMN and Atabrine, the latter being a derivative of acridine. The acridine–FMN salt probably belongs to the same group as do the acridine salts of AMP, ADP, and ATP, prepared in 1936.[194] However, since other basic substances, like quinine and certain pyrimidines, also inhibit the growth-promoting effect of riboflavin on a microorganism, an unspecific formation of complexes or rather insoluble salts of certain basic substances with FMN has to be considered.

For the inhibition of D-amino acid oxidase activity by chlortetracycline, chloramphenicol, streptomycin, penicillin, and chlorpromazine, a complex formation of these substances with FAD in competition with the oxidase protein, has been demonstrated,[195] the basic substances being bound to the AMP part of FAD. In connection with the manifestation of ariboflavinosis as a result of the administration of the antibiotics, their direct inhibitory action on flavin enzymes should be considered. The fact that the modification of the electroencephalogram by the administration of chlorpromazine is reversed by FAD may be partly explained by the complex formation of these two compounds *in vivo*.[196] The uncoupling action of chlorpromazine and of 1,1,3-tricyano-2-amino-1-propene on oxidative phosphorylation also seems

[190] L. Hellermann, A. Lindsay, and M. Bovarnick, *J. Biol. Chem.* **163**, 553 (1946).

[191] H. C. Hemker and W. C. Hülsmann, *Biochim. Biophys. Acta* **44**, 175 (1960).

[192] E. Haas, *J. Biol. Chem.* **155**, 321 (1944).

[192a] M. Iwatsubs and F. Labeysic, *Biochim. Biophys. Acta* **59**, 614 (1962).

[193] K. Fujisawa, *J. Biochem. (Tokyo)* **45**, 359 (1958).

[194] T. Wagner-Jauregg, *Hoppe-Seyler's Z. Physiol. Chem.* **239**, 188 (1936).

[195] K. Yagi *et al.*, *Nature (London)* **177**, 891 (1956); K. Yagi *et al.*, *Biochim. Biophys. Acta* **34**, 372 (1959); **43**, 310 (1960); *The Journal of Vitaminology* **14**, 271 (1968). A. W. Lessin, *Brit. J. Pharmacol. Chemother.* **14**, 251 (1959); S. Løvtrup, *J. Neurochem.* **11**, 377 (1964).

[196] K. Yagi, T. Ozawa, M. Ando and T. Nagatsu, *J. Neurochem.* **5**, 304 (1960); **14**, 207 (1967). The mode and site of action of phenothiazines also has been discussed by S. Gabay and S. R. Harris in "Topics in Medicinal Chemistry," edited by J. L. Rabonivitz and R. M. Myerson, Vol. 3, page 57–90 (1970), Wiley-Interscience, New York, London.

to be explainable by interaction with FAD or FMN,[196a] charge-transfer forces perhaps being involved.[197]

A certain structural relation between riboflavin and Atabrine suggested the synthesis of various basically substituted isoalloxazines of the general structure (III), R' and R'' being equal or different and identical with H, CH_3, OCH_3, Cl, NO_2; and R''' equalling dialkylaminoalkyl and eventually bearing one or two hydroxyl groups or chlorine atoms (nitrogen mustards.)[184, 198–205]

III

A number of these compounds very weakly inhibit the growth of *Lactobacillus casei*.[204] 6,7-Dichloro-9-[2-bis(2-hydroxyethylaminoethyl)] isoalloxazine hydrochloride is a reversible inhibitor of riboflavin in the rat with an inhibition index of approximately 50. This flavin has its terminal hydroxyl group at a distance from the isoalloxazine nucleus comparable to that of the 5'-hydroxyl group of riboflavin.[205]

None of the compounds tested against experimental malaria possessed any activity.[198–202] 9-(β-Diethylaminoethyl)isoalloxazine hydrochloride was ineffective in mice infected with *Trypanosoma nagana*.[184]

Certain basically substituted flavins, with substitutions in positions 6 and 7 by chlorine atoms, on subcutaneous injection cause strong tissue irritation, and "flavin edema" can be produced in the paws of rats on subplantar injection of these substances.[204]

The possible relation between structure and biological activity of phenothiazines and dihydrophenothiazines has been discussed.[71b, 206]

Concluding Remarks. During the almost 40 years since riboflavin (B_2) was discovered, it has met all the criteria for a vitamin. It is a redox catalyst of universal occurrence and significance. Interesting information on its biosyn-

[196a] H. Löw, *Biochim. Biophys. Acta* **32**, 11 (1959).

[197] L. D. Wright and D. B. McCormick, *Experientia* **20**, 501 (1964).

[198] F. E. King and R. M. Acheson, *J. Chem. Soc. London* p. 681 (1946).

[199] R. R. Adams, C. A. Weisel, and H. S. Mosher, *J. Amer. Chem. Soc.* **68**, 883 (1946).

[200] H. Burkett, *J. Amer. Chem. Soc.* **69**, 2555 (1947).

[201] F. Kipnis, N. Weiner, and P. E. Spoerri, *J. Amer. Chem. Soc.* **69**, 2555 (1947).

[202] R. B. Barlow and H. R. Ing. *J. Chem. Soc. London* p. 713 (1950); p. 2225 (1951).

[203] I. Molnar, T. Wagner-Jauregg, and O. Büch, West Ger. Patent No. 1115,262 (May 5, 1958); West Ger. Patent No. 1,124,505 (May 5, 1958); West Ger. Patent No. 1,109,179 (March 18, 1959).

[204] T. Wagner-Jauregg, I. Molnar, and O. Büch, *Chemotherapia* **2**, 96 (1961).

[205] R. D. Faulkner and J. P. Lambooy, *J. Med. Chem.* **6**, 292 (1963).

[206] H. Fenner, *Arzneim.-Forsch.* **20**, 1815 (1970), *Phasmakopsychiatrie-Neuropsychoplasmakologie* **3**, 332 (1970), *Deutsche Apotheker-Ztg.* **111**, 1496 (1971). Gabay and Harris in "Topics in Meolicind" **3**, 57–189 (1970), editors: Rabinowitz and Myerson, Wiley-Interscience, New York.

thesis and catalytic functions, and its relationships to other enzyme systems important to life, has been obtained through modern methods of organic chemistry and biochemistry.

The significance of vitamin B_2 as a nutritional factor is particularly relevant to underdeveloped countries. Because of widespread malnutrition in these and other countries, more factories for the production of riboflavin are needed to satisfy the increasing demand.

Following the discovery of the sulfonamides and their antagonism to p-aminobenzoic acid (vitamin H'), great hopes were placed on the principle of antagonism in chemotherapy. They have been rewarded with folic acid, but the other vitamins, including riboflavin, have not yielded derivatives or antagonists of practical use in medicine to date. However, a few years ago, the basically substituted flavins were used for research on antiinflammatory agents; later, their chemical structures were used as a guide in the development of Prolixan 300® (azapropazon; apazone), a new antirheumatic agent of high efficacy with only minor side effects.[207] Although there are evidently no specific causal relationships between flavins and inflammation, the study of these substances, by favorable circumstances and chance, have led to a valuable therapeutic agent in this area.

Addendum: In succinate dehydrogenase (SD) and in liver and kidney monoamine-oxidase (MAO) an FAD derivative is covalently linked to the enzyme protein. SD has been hydrolyzed to give 8α- * (N-histidyl)-riboflavin ("SD-flavin"), MAO yielded 8 α-(S-cysteinyl)-riboflavin ("MAO-flavin"). The assumed structures have been confirmed by synthesis.[208] * new numbering system.

III. Industrial Preparation

THEODOR WAGNER-JAUREGG

Pure crystallized riboflavin for therapeutic purposes is made by chemical synthesis. It is difficult to indicate actual manufacturing processes, since they are held confidential. The best index for determining the methods used in the industry is the patent literature.[1]

Concerning the pentose component, methods of riboflavin synthesis without the use of D-ribose are of interest, since none of the known syntheses of D-ribose are simple and economical. Different syntheses of N-(D-ribityl)-3,4-

[207] T. Wagner-Jauregg, *Chemische Rundschau* **24**, 543 (1971); *loc. cit.*, 204; I. Molnar, T. Wagner-Jauregg, U. Jahn and G. Mixich, U.S. Patent. 3,482, 024,Dec. 2, 1969 ; loc. cit. 204.

[208] P. Hemmerich et al., FFBS Letters **3**, 37 (1969); **16**, 229 (1971).

[1] A list of patents on vitamin B_2 can be found in Kirk-Othmer's "Encyclopedia of Chemical Technology," second edition Vol. 18, p. 445–458; "The Interscience Encyclopedia." Wiley-Interscience, New York, 1968; H. Vogel and H. Knobloch, "Chemie und Technik der Vitamine," 3rd Ed., Vol. 2, Issues 1 and 2, pp. 190–214. Enke, Stuttgart, 1953.

dimethylaniline, the key intermediate in the riboflavin synthesis, have been developed which do not involve D-ribose (page 24). The introduction of the second amino group can be performed with good yield by the method of Karrer and Meerwein (page 22).

With regard to the isoalloxazine formation, different patented methods have been described: (1) requisite diamine and alloxan; (2) requisite aminoazo compound and barbituric acid;[2] (3) requisite aminoazo compound and dialluric acid in the presence of a hydrogen transfer catalyst (in this method, reduction to the diamine occurs); (4) requisite diamine and dichlorobarbituric acid. Examples have been given in the preceding section (pages 32–42).

Vitamin B_2 concentrates suitable for the enrichment of poultry and livestock feeds can be prepared more cheaply by fermentation processes (page 28). During World War II, preparation of riboflavin was started from the residues of butanol–acetone fermentation with *Clostridium acetobutylicum*.[3] Other strongly flavinogenic organisms which have been studied are the yeasts *Candida guilliermondia* and *C. flaveri*.

Currently, most of the commercial riboflavin production by aerobic fermentation is probably obtained by biosynthesis with *Eremothecium ashbyii*, in submerged culture with continuous aeration and agitation. Patents covering this process were filed by several firms,[3, 4] and conditions for the production of riboflavin by *E. ashbyii* have been reported.[5] By the use of *E. ashbyii* grown on solid media (germ rice and germ wheat), the vitamin B_2 production on an industrial scale is said to have reached a maximum at 20 mg/gm (2%).[6] In fermentations yields of 2.2 mg of riboflavin/ml have been obtained on a medium consisting of whey and skim milk (1:1) fortified with 5% sucrose.[6a]

A medium containing grain stillage from the ethanol fermentation, cerelose, and 1% peptone is excellent for the cultivation of *Ashbya gossypii* to produce yields of riboflavin as high as 15,000 μg/gm.[7] Riboflavin production for commercial

[2] M. Tishler, K. Pfister, III, R. D. Babson, K. Ladenburg, and A. J. Fleming, *J. Amer. Chem. Soc.* **69**, 1487 (1947).

[3] Commercial Solvents Corp., U.S. Patent No. 2,202,161 [*Chem. Abstr.* **34**, 6676 (1940)]; Comercial Solvents Corp., Brit. Patent No. 527,478 (April 13, 1939); *Chem. Trade J.* **113**, 26 (1943).

[4] Commerical Solvents Corp., U.S. Patent Nos. 2,483,855 (Oct. 4, 1949) [*Chem. Abstr.* **44**, 2698 (1950)] and 2,498,549 (Feb. 21, 1950) [*Chem. Abstr.* **44**, 4630 (1950)]; Hoffmann-La Roche, Inc., U.S. Patent No. 2,493,274 (Jan. 3, 1950) [*Chem. Abstr.* **44**, 2698 (1950)]; D. H. Larson (to Commercial Solvents Corp.), U.S. Patent No. 2,615,829 (Oct. 28, 1952) [*Chem. Abstr.* **47**, 834 (1953)].

[5] C. Chin, *Hakko Kogaku Zasshi* **25**, 140 (1947) [*Chem. Abstr.* **44**, 7384 (1950)].

[6] R. Takata, *Seikagaku* **20**, 130 (1948) [*Chem. Abstr.* **44**, 8063 (1950)].

[6a] H. Hendrickz and A. de Vleeschanwer, *Meded Landbouwhogesch. Opzoekingssta. Staat Gent* **20**, 229 (1955).

[7] K. L. Smiley, M. Sobolow, F. L. Austin, R. A. Rasmussen, M. B. Smith, J. M. Van Lanen, L. Stone, and C. S. Boruff, *Ind. Eng. Chem.* **43**, 1380 (1951).

preparation by fermentation using *A. gossypii* upon a pilot-plant scale has been fully described.[8] Corn steep liquor, peptone, and tankage are suitable nitrogen sources with the fermentation of nutrient mashes.[9, 10] Good yields can be obtained with a medium containing only two constituents, corn oil and corn steep liquor.[11]

The riboflavin synthesis in *A. gossypii* and *E. ashbyii* is stimulated by the addition of a lipid to the culture medium and is unaffected by the iron level of the medium employed.[12] A disadvantage of *E. ashbyii* compared with *A. gossypii* is that it readily gives rise to stable nonflavinogenic strains, which do not revert.[13] However, Hŏstáleck[14] has described a method of lyophilization, which, in his hands, preserves flavinogenicity.

For recovery of the vitamin from the fermented liquors adsorption–elution methods have been used. Another possibility is the precipitation of reduced forms of riboflavin from nutrient media by the metabolic reducing action of certain bacteria, particularly a group of generally avirulent streptococci.[14a] For instance, up to 90% of the dissolved riboflavin can be obtained as a red-orange, amorphous precipitate with *Streptococcus faecalis*, under anaerobic conditions[15] (cf. p. 7). Instead of bacterial reduction, reducing chemicals have been used, for instance, sodium dithionite ($Na_2S_2O_4 \cdot 2H_2O$) and stannous, titanous, chromous, and vanadous salts.[16] These methods make use of the fact that the various reduced forms of riboflavin are much less soluble in water than the oxidized form. The solubility in 1 ml of water is for riboflavin 100–130 μg, for verdoflavin 50 μg, for chloroflavin 20 μg, and for leucoriboflavin approximately 8 μg.[17]

In 1959, 355,000 lb of riboflavin were produced for human and animal

[8] V. F. Pfeifer, F. W. Tanner, Jr., C. Vojnovich, and D. H. Traufler, *Ind. Eng. Chem.* **42**, 1776 (1950).

[9] Merck and Co., Brit. Patent No. 640,452 (July 19, 1950) [*Chem. Abstr.* **44**, 9622 (1950)].

[10] For more information on the microbiological production of riboflavin, see the reports of D. Perlman, W. E. Brown, and S. B. Lee, *Ind. Eng. Chem.* **44**, 1996 (1952); D. Perlman, W. E. Brown, and S. B. Lee, Production of riboflavin by fermentation. *In* "Industrial Fermentations" (L. A. Underkofler and R. J. Hickey, eds.), Vol. 2. Chem. Publ. Co., New York, 1954.

[11] T. W. Goodwin, *Progr. Ind. Microbiol.* **1**, 137 (1959).

[12] H. Hendrickz and A. de Vleeschanwer, *Meded. Landbouwhogesch. Opzoekingssta. Staat Gent* **21**, 663 (1956).

[13] W. H. Schopfer and M. Guillod, *Schweiz. Z. Pathol. Bakteriol*, **8**, 521 (1945). W. H. Schopfer and M. Guillod, *Ber. Schweiz. Bot. Ges.* **56**, 700 (1946).

[14] Z. Hŏstáleck, *J. Gen. Microbiol.* **17**, 267 (1957).

[14a] G. E. Hines, Jr. (to Commercial Solvents Corp.), U.S. Patent No. 2,387,023 (Oct. 16, 1945); G. W. McMillan (to Commercial Solvents Corp.), U.S. Patent No. 2,367646 (Jan. 16, 1945) [*Chem. Abstr.* **39**, 3400 (1945)] and loc. sit. 29 (page 7).

[15] R. J. Hickey, *Arch. Biochem.* **11**, 259 (1946).

[16] G. E. Hines, Jr. (to Commercial Solvents Corp.), U.S. Patent No. 2,367,644 (Jan. 16, 1945) [*Chem. Abstr.* **39**, 3399 (1945)].

[17] S. J. Shimizu, *Hakko Kogaku Zasshi* **28**, 139 (1950) [*Chem. Abstr.* **47**, 1755 (1953)].

consumption. Crystals of riboflavin are priced today at 33 to 35 dollars per kilogram, whereas in 1938 the price was 7945 dollars a pound. The feed grade containing 4 gm of riboflavin per pound costs 16 to 17 cents.

Besides the pharmaceutical use, small amounts of vitamin B_2 are incorporated in most bread flours and breakfast foods and in nearly all poultry and hog feeds. Cattle and sheep do not require riboflavin supplements because they obtain the vitamin by bacterial synthesis in the rumen.

IV. Estimation

See Chapter 14 by W. N. Pearson, C. I. Bliss, and Paul György "The Vitamins" (Paul György and W. N. Pearson, eds.), 2nd Ed. Vol. VII, for current methods of extraction and assay of riboflavin.

V. Occurrence in Food

M. K. HORWITT

The best sources of riboflavin are milk, egg white, liver, heart, kidney, and growing leafy vegetables. Beef muscle, veal, apricot, tomato, and poultry muscle are good sources. Fish muscle, unenriched grains, and legumes, although relatively poor sources, supply important minimal amounts to the average regimen. Yeast, the richest natural source of riboflavin, is not normally a major component of nontherapeutic diets.

The primary factors to be evaluated in a consideration of the stability of riboflavin in food products are the effects of heat, light, elution, and the intracellular reactions which take place during storage.

The relative heat stability of riboflavin is a fortunate property, which favors its preservation by ordinary cooking procedures.[1] Even the addition of bicarbonate to a pH of 8.8 does not appreciably increase the loss of riboflavin during short cooking procedures.[2] The major losses which occur during home cooking or commercial canning operations are probably attributable to

---

[1] H. Levine and R. E. Remington, *J. Nutr.* **13**, 525 (1937).

[2] C. H. Johnston, L. Schauer, S. Rapaport, and H. J. Deuel, Jr., *J. Nutr.* **26**, 227 (1943).

the extraction of the vitamin by the water used in the cooking or blanching operations.[3-6] These losses are usually less than 20%, and they can be further minimized if the cooking fluids are consumed.

Losses of riboflavin due to exposure to light during cooking may prove to be an important economic loss. Cheldelin *et al.*[7] have shown large losses, up to 48%, incurred in the cooking of eggs, milk, and pork chops in uncovered dishes under conditions where there was no loss of riboflavin when cooking dishes were covered. The loss in milk[8-10] which is allowed to stand in glass containers on the consumer's doorstep may be as high as 85% after 2 hours' exposure to bright sunlight.[11] This may be compared with practically no loss of riboflavin during pasteurization procedures,[12] where light effects are minimal.

The losses of riboflavin during storage either by quick freezing[13, 14] or in sterilized containers[15-17] are relatively small.

In the absence of liver and yeast, which contain 2–4 mg of riboflavin/100 gm, the riboflavin content of the average diet is usually related to the amount of animal protein consumed. Unenriched cereal products are poor sources. Green and yellow vegetables, although relatively high in riboflavin, are not usually eaten in sufficient amounts to supply a major portion of the daily requirement. The preparation of experimental diets low in riboflavin has been discussed by Horwitt *et al.*[18]

Table I contains representative amounts of riboflavin in foodstuffs. This table is adapted from the Leichsenring and Wilson[19] short method of dietary analysis. It is based upon their compilation of data published by Watt and

[3] H. L. Mayfield and M. T. Hedrick, *J. Amer. Diet. Ass.* **25**, 1024 (1949).

[4] J. M. McIntire, B. S. Schweigert, L. M. Henderson, and C. A. Elvehjem, *J. Nutr.* **25**, 143 (1943).

[5] J. R. Wagner, F. M. Strong, and C. A. Elvehjem, *Ind. Eng. Chem.* **39**, 985 (1947).

[6] W. A. Krehl and R. W. Winters, *J. Amer. Diet. Ass.* **26**, 966 (1950).

[7] V. A. Cheldelin, A. M. Woods, and R. R. Williams, *J. Nutr.* **26**, 177 (1943).

[8] R. R. Williams and V. A. Cheldelin, *Science* **96**, 22 (1942).

[9] J. A. Ziegler, *J. Amer. Chem. Soc.* **66**, 1039 (1944).

[10] W. J. Peterson, F. M. Haig, and A. O. Shaw, *J. Amer. Chem. Soc.* **66**, 662 (1944).

[11] A. D. Holmes and C. P. Jones, *J. Nutr.* **29**, 201 (1945).

[12] A. D. Holmes, *J. Amer. Diet. Ass.* **20**, 226 (1944).

[13] B. S. Schweigert, J. M. McIntire, and C. A. Elvehjem, *J. Nutr.* **26**, 73 (1943).

[14] M. S. Rose, *J. Amer. Med. Ass.* **114**, 1356 (1940).

[15] G. Adams and S. L. Smith, *U.S. Dep. Agr. Misc. Publ.* **536**, (1944).

[16] J. F. Feaster, J. M. Jackson, D. A. Greenwood, and H. R. Kraybell, *Ind. Eng. Chem.* **38**, 87 (1946).

[17] D. S. Moschette, W. F. Hinman, and E. G. Halliday, *Ind. Eng. Chem.* **39**, 994 (1947).

[18] M. K. Horwitt, G. Sampson, O. W. Hills, and D. L. Steinberg, *J. Amer. Diet. Ass.* **25**, 591 (1949).

[19] J. M. Leichsenring and E. D. Wilson, *J. Amer. Diet. Ass.* **27**, 386 (1951).

TABLE I

RIBOFLAVIN CONTENT OF REPRESENTATIVE FOODS[a]

Food	Approximate measure	Riboflavin (mg)
Cereal products		
Refined	1 slice bread (30 gm)	
	$\frac{1}{2}$ cup cereal (20 gm)	
	3 soda crackers (20 gm)	0.02
Whole grain and enriched	1 slice bread (30 gm), $\frac{1}{2}$ cup cereal (20 gm), 2 graham crackers (20 gm)	0.04
Dairy products		
Cheese, Cheddar	1 cu. in.	0.13
Cheese, cottage	$\frac{1}{2}$ cup	0.31
Cream, light	$\frac{1}{8}$ cup	0.04
Custard	$\frac{1}{2}$ cup	0.26
Egg	1 medium	0.14
Ice cream	$\frac{1}{2}$ cup	0.15
Milk		
Buttermilk, skim	1 cup	0.43
Whole	1 cup	0.41
Desserts		
Cake, plain, chocolate	1 piece (75 gm)	0.06
Cookies, plain	2 medium	0.02
Pie crust	$\frac{1}{6}$ shell, single crust	0.04
Puddings	$\frac{1}{2}$ cup	0.22
Fish		
Cod, haddock, cooked	1 medium serving (105 gm)	0.13
Halibut, herring, whitefish	1 medium serving (75 gm)	0.06
Salmon, canned	1 medium serving ($\frac{1}{2}$ cup)	0.16
Fruits		
Banana	1 small	0.05
Cantaloupe	$\frac{1}{2}$ melon, $4\frac{1}{2}$-in. diameter	0.06
Citrus	$\frac{1}{2}$ grapefruit, 1 medium orange	0.04
Strawberry	10 large	0.16
Meat:		
Beef, lamb, veal, cooked	1 medium serving	0.17
Fowl, fried	1 medium serving	0.11
Liver, cooked	1 small serving (2 slices)	2.38
Luncheon meats, cooked	2 slices sausage, minced ham, dried beef, $\frac{1}{2}$ frankfurter (30 gm)	0.08
Pork, ham	1 medium serving, cooked	0.17

TABLE I—*Continued*

Food	Approximate measure	Riboflavin (mg)
Sweets		
Candy bar	1–2 oz. chocolate-coated bar	0.17
Molasses; sorghum	1 tablespoon	0.05
Vegetables		
Cabbage, cooked	$\frac{2}{3}$ cup	0.05
Cauliflower, cooked	$\frac{2}{3}$ cup (70 gm)	0.04
Corn, parsnips, cooked	$\frac{1}{2}$ cup corn; 1 large parsnip	0.09
Green and yellow		
Asparagus, cooked	$\frac{2}{3}$ cup	0.17[a]
Broccoli, cooked	$\frac{2}{3}$ cup	0.15[a]
Carrots, cooked	$\frac{2}{3}$ cup	0.05
Green beans, cooked	$\frac{1}{2}$ cup	0.10[a]
Leafy greens, cooked	$\frac{2}{3}$ cup spinach, turnip, kale, other greens	0.21[a]
Peas, fresh, cooked, canned	$\frac{1}{2}$ cup	0.14[a]
Sweet potato, cooked	$\frac{1}{2}$ large	0.08[a]
Potato, cooked	1 small (100 gm)	0.03
Tomato, fresh, canned or juice	$\frac{1}{2}$ cup; 1 small tomato	0.03
Other, commonly served raw	2 pieces celery; 8 slices cucumber; $\frac{1}{8}$ head lettuce	0.03

[a] Adopted from Leichsenring and Wilson (1951).
[b] For canned, reduce by one-half.

Merrill[20] and Bowes and Church.[21] The figures presented are averages, often of a wide range of analytical results, and should be regarded as working estimates which will vary with the geography, season, and method of preparation.

VI. Standardization of Activity

M. K. HORWITT

With the elucidation of the chemical nature of riboflavin, the need for a standard of activity for vitamin B_2 or G becomes less urgent. The present USP Reference Standard is a recrystallized sample of riboflavin obtainable

[20] B. K. Watt and A. L. Merrill, *U.S. Dep. Agr., Agr. Handb.* **8** (1950).
[21] A. de P. Bowes and C. F. Church, "Food Values of Portions Commonly Used," 6th Ed. College Offset Press, Philadelphia, Pennsylvania, 1946.

from the USP Reference Standard Committee. Comparisons of purified riboflavin with the older units of activity showed that one Bourquin–Sherman rat growth unit,[1] the daily addition of which will produce an average gain of 3 gm/rat/week, was equal to about 2.5 μg of riboflavin.[2, 3] von Euler[4] had proposed a unit consisting of 5 μg of riboflavin, the amount which produced an increase in weight of 0.8–1.0 gm/day in young rats. A Cornell unit[5] was defined as the growth effect on chicks equivalent to that produced by 1 gm of riboflavin.

The need for standards of biological activity continues to exist, especially in the study of derivatives of riboflavin. As an example, consider the assay of a very water-soluble riboflavin derivative prepared by Stone.[6] Fluorometric assay of the material yielded a value of 57.2% riboflavin; microbiological assay by the USP XIII revision method yielded a value of 33% riboflavin. The biological assay by the standard rat growth method indicated that riboflavin potency was almost nil.

VII. Biogenesis

M. K. HORWITT

Riboflavin is synthesized by most higher plants, yeasts, and lower fungi, and by some bacteria. The tissues of higher animals are unable to synthesize this vitamin, but the gastrointestinal tract of many of these animals harbor bacteria that may be capable of providing riboflavin for their host. The riboflavin content of the milk of cows and goats[1] is many times the amount in the feed, as the result of synthesis by organisms which inhabit the rumen of these animals.

Observations that the fecal contents of rats,[2] fowls,[3] and man[4, 5] may have more riboflavin than the food ingested have stimulated research on the

[1] A. Bourquin and H. C. Sherman, J. Amer. Chem. Soc. 53, 3501 (1931).
[2] O. A. Bessey, J. Nutr. 15, 11 (1938).
[3] H. von Euler, P. Karrer, E. Adler, and M. Malmberg, Helv. Chim. Acta 17, 1157 (1934).
[4] H. von Euler, Inst. Int. Chim. Solvay, Cons. Chem. (Rapp. Discuss.) 6, 198 (1938).
[5] L. C. Norris, H. S. Wilgus, A. T. Ringrose, V. Heiman, and G. F. Heuser, Cornell Univ Agr. Exp. Sta. Bull. 660, 3 (1936).
[6] G. B. Stone, Science 111, 283 (1950).
[1] L. W. McElroy and H. Goss, J. Nutr. 20, 527 (1940).
[2] W. H. Griffith, J. Nutr. 10, 667 (1935).
[3] W. F. Lamoureux and R. S. Schumacher, Poultry Sci. 19, 418 (1940).
[4] V. A. Najjar, G. A. Johns, G. C. Medairy, G. Fleischmann, and L. E. Holt, Jr., J. Amer. Med. Ass. 126, 357 (1944).
[5] C. W. Denko, W. E. Grundy, N. C. Wheeler, C. R. Henderson, G. H. Berryman, T. E. Friedemann, and J. B. Youmans, Arch. Biochem, 11, 109 (1946).

nutritional usefulness of intestinal synthesis. It has been common laboratory knowledge that coprophagia by rats must be avoided if nutritional deficiencies are to be produced. Whether the riboflavin formed by microorganisms is absorbed from the lower intestinal tract in significant quantities is not certain. Najjar et al.[4] have reported that there was a rise in urinary riboflavin after normal subjects were given enemas containing 20 mg of riboflavin, but Everson et al.[6] found no increase in urinary excretion of riboflavin after administering 2 mg by retention enema. The concept of low utilization of the riboflavin of intestinal bacteria is supported by studies[7] indicating the relative nonavailability of the vitamins in ingested yeast.

Although riboflavin is required as a growth factor for a large number of microorganisms,[8] most of them are able to synthesize more than their requirement. Microbiological production of riboflavin by *Clostridium acetobutylicum* has been promoted as a commercial source.[9] There have been reports on riboflavin production by the yeast *Eremothecium ashbyii*[10] and by *Candida guilliermondia*.[11, 12] Certain molds (*Ashbya gossypii*) produce and excrete so much riboflavin that yellow crystals are formed about the mycelium.[13]

An investigation of riboflavin synthesis by the bacterial flora of the human intestine has been made by Burkholder and McVeigh.[14] The organisms studied were *Escherichia coli, Proteus vulgaris, Bacterium aerogenes, Alcaligenes faecalis, Bacillus mesentericus,* and *Bacillus vulgatus. Escherichia coli*, normally a dominant organism in human intestinal flora, produced the most riboflavin. Reviews by Knight[15] and Van Lanen and Tanner[16] on growth factors in microbiology have covered other aspects of riboflavin synthesis by microorganisms.

The synthesis of riboflavin in green plants is of major importance in supplying human riboflavin requirements. The locus of this synthesis is not known, but there is apparently a higher concentration in the leaves than in the remainder of the plant.

It is apparent that the biosynthesis of riboflavin phosphate and flavin adenine dinucleotide from riboflavin is a property possessed by all living organisms which have need of this vitamin.[17, 18]

[6] G. Everson, E. Wheeler, H. Walker, and W. J. Coulfield, *J. Nutr.* **35**, 209 (1948).
[7] H. T. Parsons, A. Williamson, and M. L. Johnson, *J. Nutr.* **29**, 373 (1945).
[8] W. H. Peterson and M. S. Peterson, *Bacteriol. Rev.* **9**, 19 (1945).
[9] C. F. Arzberger, U.S. Patent No. 2,326,425 (Aug. 10, 1943).
[10] A. Raffy and M. Fontaine, *C. R. Acad. Sci.* **201**, 1005 (1937).
[11] P. R. Burkholder, *Proc. Nat. Acad. Sci. U.S.* **29**, 166 (1943).
[12] F. W. Tanner, Jr., C. Vojnovich, and J. M. Van Lanen, *Science* **101**, 180 (1945).
[13] A. Raffy, *C. R. Soc. Biol.* **126**, 875 (1937).
[14] P. R. Burkholder and I. McVeigh, *Proc. Nat. Acad. Sci. U.S.* **28**, 285 (1912).
[15] B. C. J. G. Knight, *Vitam. Horm.* (*New York*) **3**, 108 (1945).
[16] J. M. Van Lanen and F. W. Tanner, Jr., *Vitam. Horm.* (*New York*) **6**, 163 (1948).
[17] E. B. Kearney and S. Englard, *J. Biol. Chem.* **193**, 821 (1951).
[18] J. R. Klein and H. I. Kohn, *J. Biol. Chem.* **136**, 177 (1940).

The work of Plaut[19] has thrown some light on the mechanism of riboflavin biosynthesis by *Ashbya gossypii*. The addition of formate-^{14}C to flask cultures of yeast gave rise to riboflavin tagged in the c-2 position. The tracer atom from bicarbonate-^{14}C ended up in the c-4 position. ^{14}CH$_3$COOH, CH$_3$^{14}COOH, and totally labeled glucose produced riboflavin containing ^{14}C in both the side chain and *o*-xylene portions of the molecule.

VIII. Active Compounds

M. K. HORWITT

Riboflavin, riboflavin 5-phosphate,[1] and flavin adenine dinucleotide[2] are the only naturally occurring flavins that have been found to have vitamin B$_2$ activity. They are equally effective in promoting the growth of rats and *Lactobacillus casei*.

The new vitamin activity of L-lyxoflavin, the 9-L-1'-lyxityl stereoisomer of riboflavin, has been investigated. This compound has been reported as a constituent of heart muscle.[3, 4]

Synthetic derivatives of isoalloxazine which have been found to have riboflavin activities include (a) 7-methyl-9-(D-1'-ribityl)isoalloxazine[5-7]; (b) 6-methyl-9-(D-1'-ribityl)isoalloxazine[5, 7, 8]; (c) 6-ethyl-7-methyl-9-(D-1'-ribityl)isoalloxazine.[5]

These three compounds were approximately one-half as active as riboflavin in growth tests on rats. Compound (c) was almost as active as riboflavin in stimulating the growth of lactic acid bacteria,[9] but compounds (a) and (b) stimulated the bacterial growth only moderately.

Among the synthetic arabityl derivatives which have been studied are (d) 6,7-dimethyl-9-(D-1'-arabityl)isoalloxazine[10]; (e) 6,7-dimethyl-9-(L-1'-arabityl) isoalloxazine[11]; (f) 6-methyl-9-(L-1'-arabityl)isoalloxazine[8]; (g) 6,7-trime-

[19] G. W. E. Plaut, *Federation Proc.* **12**, 254 (1953).
[1] P. György, *Proc. Soc. Exp. Biol. Med.* **35**, 207 (1936).
[2] H. P. Sarett, *J. Biol. Chem.* **162**, 87 (1946).
[3] E. Sodi Pallares and H. Martinez Garza, *Arch. Biochem.* **22**, 63 (1949).
[4] T. S. Gardner, E. Wenis, and J. Lee, *Arch. Biochem.* **34**, 98 (1951).
[5] P. Karrer and T. H. Quibell, *Helv. Chim. Acta* **19**, 1034 (1936).
[6] P. Karrer, H. von Euler, M. Malmberg, and K. Schöpp, *Sv. Kem. Tidskr.* **47**, 153 (1935).
[7] P. Karrer and F. M. Strong, *Helv. Chim. Acta* **18**, 1343 (1935).
[8] R. Kuhn, H. Vetter, and H. W. Rzeppa, *Ber. Deut. Chem. Ges.* **70**, 1302 (1937).
[9] E. E. Snell and F. M. Strong, *Enzymologia* **6**, 186 (1939).
[10] H. von Euler, P. Karrer, and M. Malmberg, *Helv. Chim. Acta* **18**, 1336 (1935).
[11] P. Karrer, H. Salomon, K. Schöpp, F. Benz, and B. Becker, *Helv. Chim. Acta* **18**, 908 (1935).

thylene-9-(L-1'-arabityl)isoalloxazine[8]; (h) 6,7-tetramethylene-9-(L-1'-arabityl) isoalloxazine.[8]

D-Araboflavin (compound d) inhibits growth and increases the mortality rate[12] more than the absence of riboflavin alone. The other arabityl derivatives can sustain life in rats at a diminished growth rate if given in relatively large amounts.

Isoriboflavin [5,6-dimethyl-9-(D-1'-ribityl)isoalloxazine] is an isomer of riboflavin which, if given to rats at levels of 2 mg/day, will counteract the growth-promoting effects of 40 μg of riboflavin. It is interesting that isoriboflavin has no inhibitory effect on *Lactobacillus casei*.

Riboflavin tetraacetate[13] and both the mono- and diacetone derivatives[13] are fully active in supporting rat growth, probably owing to hydrolysis in the mammalian organism, but they are inactive for lactic acid bacteria. Replacement of the D-ribityl group by a glucosidic group[14] results in a total loss of biological activity. The monomethylol derivative[15] prepared by reacting riboflavin with formaldehyde retains about half the original activity. Riboflavin mono-, di-, tri-, and tetrasuccinates[16] vary in rat growth activity as 100, 65, 21, and 0%, respectively. Substitution of a methyl group in the 3 position[17] results in complete loss of vitamin activity.

Generally speaking, the activity of esterified derivatives of riboflavin may vary with the ability of the test organism to effect hydrolysis of the ester; the 3 position must remain unsubstituted, and substitution in the 6 or 7 position is necessary.

When the 6 and 7 positions are not substituted, the compounds are toxic.[18] A review by Woolley[19] highlighted the increased interest in the inhibitory analogs of the vitamins.

IX. Biochemical Systems

M. K. HORWITT AND L. A. WITTING

Knowledge of the close relationship between vitamins and biological oxidations may be said to date from 1932, the year in which Warburg and Christian[1] discovered the first flavoprotein. This compound, often referred to as the

[12] H. von Euler and P. Karrer, *Helv. Chim. Acta* 29, 353 (1946).
[13] R. Kuhn, H. Rudy, and F. Weygand, *Ber. Deut. Chem. Ges.* 68, 625 (1935).
[14] R. Kuhn and K. Ströbele, *Ber. Deut. Chem. Ges.* 70, 747 (1937).
[15] K. Schoen and S. M. Gordon, *Arch. Biochem.* 22, 149 (1949).
[16] M. F. Furter, G. J. Haas, and S. H. Rubin, *J. Biol. Chem.* 160, 293 (1945).
[17] R. Kuhn, K. Reinemund, F. Weygand, and R. Ströbele, *Ber. Deut. Chem. Ges.* 68, 1765 (1935).
[18] R. Kuhn and P. Boulanger, *Hoppe-Seyler's Z. Physiol. Chem.* 241, 233 (1936).
[19] D. W. Woolley, "A Study of Antimetabolites." Wiley, New York, 1952.
[1] O. Warburg and W. Christian, *Biochem. Z.* 254, 438 (1932).

"old yellow enzyme," which they obtained from the aqueous extract of bottom yeast was soon separated[2] into a protein and a yellow prosthetic group. Stern and Holiday,[3] using spectroscopic methods, found that the prosthetic group of Warburg's yellow enzyme was a derivative of alloxazine. This fact, when combined with the observations of Ellinger and Koschara,[4] Booher,[5] and Kuhn et al.[6] on the correlations between vitamin B_2 and a water-soluble yellow-green fluorescent pigment, was soon corroborated by the synthesis of riboflavin by the Kuhn[7, 8] and Karrer[9] schools. Theorell's[10] demonstration that Warburg's enzyme contained one molecule of phosphate and Kuhn, Rudy, and Weygand's[11] proof of constitution of riboflavin-5-phosphoric acid were the concluding steps in a fascinating story of the first separation, identification, and synthesis of the prosthetic group of an enzyme.

A. Coenzymes

Flavoproteins can be characterized as specific proteins that contain either flavin mononucleotide or flavin dinucleotide as prosthetic groups or coenzymes. The flavin mononucleotide (FMN) riboflavin phosphate is not in the strict sense a nucleotide, since the compound is derived from D-ribitol rather than from D-ribose.[11] The location of the phosphoric acid at the 5 position has been definitely established.[12] The enzymatic phosphorylation of ribo-flavin by an enzyme in yeast, flavokinase, has been reported by Kearney and England.[12a] The reaction may be written

$$\text{Riboflavin} + \text{ATP} \rightarrow \text{FMN} + \text{ADP}$$

Examples of flavoproteins containing FMN are Warburg's old yellow enzyme NADPH-cytochrome c reductase from yeast, L-amino acid oxidase from rat kidney, and glycolic acid oxidase from spinach.

Flavin adenine dinucleotide (FAD) is isoalloxazine adenine dinucleotide.

[2] O. Warburg and W. Christian, Biochem. Z. 266, 377 (1933).

[3] K. G. Stern and E. R. Holiday, Ber. Deut. Chem. Ges. 67B, 1104, 1442 (1934).

[4] P. Ellinger and W. Koschara, Ber. Deut. Chem. Ges. 66B, 315, 808 (1933).

[5] L. E. Booher, J. Biol. Chem. 102, 39 (1933).

[6] R. Kuhn, P. György, and T. Wagner-Jauregg, Ber. Deut. Chem. Ges. 66B, 317, 576, 1034 (1933).

[7] R. Kuhn, K. Reinemund, H. Kaltschmitt, R. Ströbele, and H. Trischmann, Naturwissenschaften 23, 260 (1935).

[8] R. Kuhn, K. Reinemund, F. Weygand, and R. Ströbele, Ber. Deut. Chem. Ges. 68B, 1765 (1935).

[9] P. Karrer, K. Schöpp, and F. Benz, Helv. Chim. Acta 18, 426 (1935).

[10] H. Theorell, Biochem. Z. 272, 155 (1934).

[11] R. Kuhn, H. Rudy, and F. Weygand, Ber. Deut. Chem. Ges. 69B, 2034 (1936).

[12] P. Karrer, P. Frei, and H. Meerwein, Helv. Chim. Acta 20, 79 (1937).

[12a] E. B. Kearney and S. England, J. Biol. Chem. 193, 821 (1951).

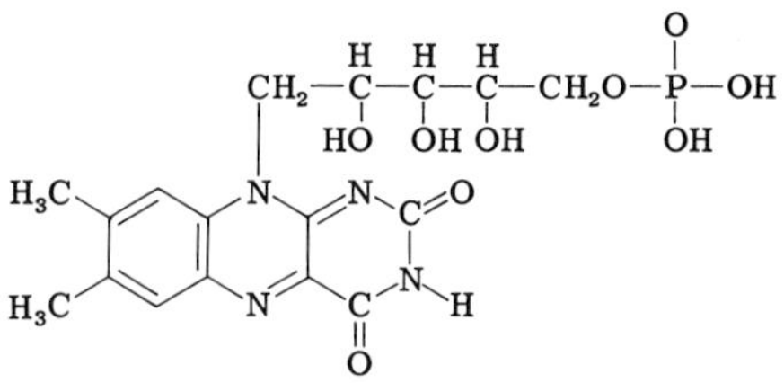

Riboflavin 5-phosphate

This coenzyme has been obtained in highly purified form[13, 13a] and its structure established by chemical synthesis.[13b,c] The dinucleotide may be visualized as a combination of FMN and adenosine monophosphate. An enzyme, FAD pyrophosphorylase,[14] has been partially purified from yeast; it catalyzes the transformation of FMN to FAD according to the scheme

$$FMN + ATP \rightarrow FAD + pyrophosphate$$

The transformation is also known to occur in human red blood cells.[15]

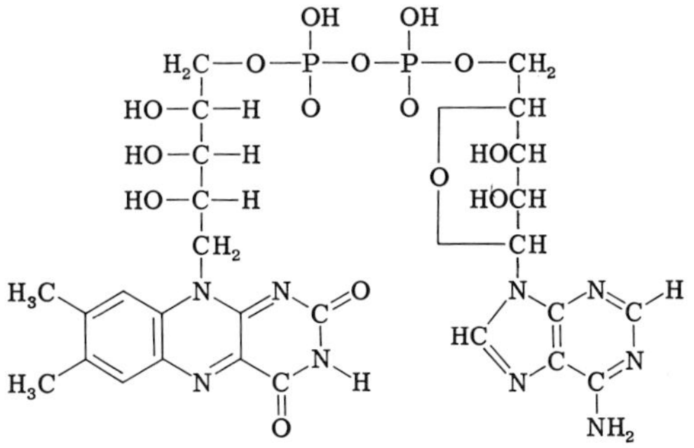

Flavin adenine dinucleotide

1. General Properties of Flavin Coenzymes

Riboflavin phosphate and flavin adenine dinucleotide resemble the parent vitamin riboflavin in many respects. They exhibit the same characteristic yellow color and yellow-green fluorescence. Reduction with hyposulfite, platinum, or H_2 will reduce riboflavin and its coenzymes to colorless compounds, which will reoxidize to their original state when shaken with air. If

[13] L. B. Whitby, *Biochem. J.* **54**, 437 (1953).

[13a] O. Walaas and E. Walaas, *Acta Chem. Scand.* **10**, 118 (1956).

[13b] S. M. H. Christie, G. W. Kenner, and A. R. Todd, *J. Chem. Soc.* **46**, (1954).

[13c] F. M. Huennekens and G. L. Kilgour, *J. Am. Chem. Soc.* **77**, 6716 (1955).

[14] A. W. Schrecker and A. Kornberg, *J. Biol. Chem.* **182**, 795 (1950).

[15] J. R. Klein and H. I. Kohn, *J. Biol. Chem.* **136**, 177 (1940).

Riboflavin-5-phosphate   Apoenzyme

reduced in strongly acidic solution, a red intermediate is formed that has the properties of a semiquinoid radical.[16] In solution they are essentially unstable. This decomposition is influenced by light, heat, and pH, riboflavin being rapidly decomposed in strongly alkaline solutions.

Riboflavin phosphate is considerably more soluble in water than free riboflavin and can be precipitated by various salts. It is hydrolyzed quite slowly in weakly alkaline solutions, quite rapidly in acid solutions, and by phosphatases such as α-glycerophosphatase. Riboflavin phosphate combines with specific proteins,[17] the apoenzymes, by attachment at the phosphoric acid group and in the case of the old yellow enzyme at the slightly acidic imino group in the 3 position.

The principal binding site of FMN appears to be the free amino groups of the apoenzyme.[17a] This may be shown by either acetylation or treatment with formaldehyde. Quenching of fluorescence appears in turn to depend on bonding of the 3 imino group of FMN to a tyrosine hydroxyl group.[17a,b]

The typical fluorescence of riboflavin is dependent upon the presence of a free 3-imino group, and neither 3-substituted riboflavin nor the enzyme systems will fluoresce. D-Amino acid oxidase, however, is fluorescent as is free FAD indicating that, in this case, the imino group is not bound to the protein.[13a]

2. RIBOFLAVIN PHOSPHATE

Banja et al.[18] obtained a yellow substance from heart muscle in 1932, which may have been the first preparation of riboflavin phosphate. However,

---

[16] E. Haas, *Biochem. Z.* **290**, 291 (1937).

[17] R. Kuhn and H. Rudy, *Ber. Deut. Chem. Ges.* **69B**, 2557 (1936).

[17a] A. P. Nygaard and H. Theorell, *Acta Chem. Scand.* **9**, 1587 (1955).

[17b] H. Theorell, *Proc. 4th Intern. Congr. Biochem., Vienna, 1958.* **8**, 167 (1959).

[18] I. Banha, A. Szent-Györgyi, and L. Vargha, *Hoppe-Seyler's Z. Physiol. Chem.* **210**, 288 (1932).

the yellow enzyme which Warburg and Christian[1] obtained from yeast in the same year was more thoroughly investigated. They purified an aqueous extract of autolyzed bottom yeast by treatment with lead subacetate, removed excess lead with phosphate, and precipitated the yellow enzyme in the form of a viscous oil at low temperature with carbon dioxide and acetone. After reprecipitation from acetone and precipitation with methanol at 0°, a dry product was obtained that could be readily dissociated into a colorless protein and a yellow prosthetic group. The latter was later proved to be riboflavin phosphate.

Theorell[19] has shown that the combination of riboflavin phosphate with the apoenzyme could be reversibly dissociated as follows: when a solution of the yellow enzyme was dialyzed against 0.02 N HCl at 0°, the dialyzate was slowly decolorized. The colored group (riboflavin phosphate) passed through the membrane, and the colorless protein remained behind. The protein was changed to a metaprotein by its contact with the dilute acid (i.e., precipitated when brought to pH 7), but when the protein was dialyzed against water to remove all traces of hydrochloric acid, 50–70% of the metaprotein was renatured. This renatured protein was now capable of recombination with the coenzyme riboflavin phosphate to produce a complex with all the properties of the original yellow enzyme.

The combination between the coenzyme and the apoenzyme[20] takes place in a stoichiometric manner as shown in Fig. 4.

The reversible dissociation procedure of Theorell, which requires several days for its completion, was replaced by a simpler method by Warburg and

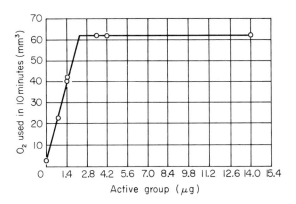

FIG. 4. Synthesis of Warburg–Christian flavoprotein. The activity of the enzyme increases as more of the prosthetic group riboflavin phosphate is added to form the original catalytically active flavoprotein. From Theorell.[20]

[19] H. Theorell, *Biochem. Z.* **275**, 344 (1934).
[20] H. Theorell, *Biochem. Z.* **278**, 263 (1935).

Christian[21] in which a good yield could be obtained in about 1 hour. To a solution of yellow enzyme, purified by electrophoresis, an equal volume of saturated ammonium sulfate was added. Sufficient 0.1 N hydrochloric acid was added to this solution at 0° to shift the pH to about 2.8. The colorless precipitate formed contained 78 % of the apoenzyme in native form while the coenzyme remained in the supernatant fluid. Resynthesis was accomplished by merely remixing the components.

3. RIBOFLAVIN ADENINE DINUCLEOTIDE

The dinucleotide is widely distributed in animal tissues and in microorganisms. It has been isolated from liver, kidney, muscles, tumor tissue, yeast,[12, 21a, 22–24, 24a] and *Neurospora.*[25]

Since riboflavin is necessary for the growth of many bacteria and is a common component of plant products, it is logical to assume that the dinucleotide is a common constituent of the cells of most living things. Yeast offers the most convenient source for preparation. Warburg and Christian[24a] extracted yeast at 75°; the filtrate was two-thirds saturated with ammonium sulfate and extracted with phenol. The phenol extracts were mixed with ether, and the dinucleotide was extracted with water. The ether was removed by evacuation, the aqueous solution was acidified with nitric acid to about pH 2, and the dinucleotide precipitated as the silver salt. The precipitate was resuspended in water and decomposed with hydrogen sulfide. The dinucleotide, which was almost completely absorbed on the silver sulfide precipitate, was eluted with dilute barium acetate. The eluates were mixed with ammonium acetate solution and concentrated to dryness *in vacuo.* By taking advantage of the fact that the barium salt of the dinucleotide is twice as soluble at 60° as at room temperature, it was possible to separate the barium salts of the dinucleotide from the barium salts of the contaminating adenine nucleotides.

The similarities of the dinucleotide to riboflavin phosphate in color, fluorescence, and reversible reduction and oxidation have been discussed (Section IX, A, 1). It is less stable than riboflavin because of its tendency to hydrolyze to riboflavin phosphate and adenylic acid. The absorption spectra of riboflavin and flavin adenine dinucleotide are given in Fig. 5.[24a]

[21] O. Warburg and W. Christian, *Biochem. Z.* **298**, 368 (1938).
[21a] O. Warburg and W. Christian, *Biochem. Z.* **298**, 150 (1938).
[22] P. Karrer, P. Frei, B. H. Ringier, and H. Bendas, *Helv. Chim. Acta* **21**, 826 (1938).
[23] O. Warburg, W. Christian, and A. Griese, *Biochem. Z.* **295**, 261 (1938).
[24] O. Warburg, W. Christian, and A. Griese, *Biochem. Z.* **297**, 417 (1938).
[24a] O. Warburg and W. Christian, *Biochem. Z.* **298**, 150 (1938).
[25] N. H. Horowitz, *J. Biol. Chem.* **154**, 141 (1944).

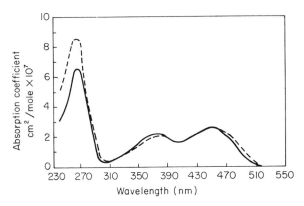

FIG. 5. Absorption spectra of riboflavin (————) and flavin adenine dinucleotide (– – – – –). From Warburg and Christian.[21a]

B. Enzymes

The flavoprotein enzymes participate in the transfer of electrons from metabolites and pyridine nucleotides to molecular oxygen. Our knowledge of the reaction mechanisms involved is inversely proportional to the complexity of this transfer. For convenience the flavoproteins will be considered under three headings: aerobic dehydrogenases, or oxidases, not containing metals, aerobic dehydrogenases containing metals, and anaerobic dehydrogenases. The following examples will illustrate the varying degrees of complexity encountered in some of the better characterized reactions.

1. SIMPLE OXIDASES

These enzymes are usually found in the cytoplasm and do not contain metals, which participate in the enzymatic reaction. They are obtained in soluble form, in most cases, by relatively mild procedures.

a. D-Amino Acid Oxidase and L-Amino Acid Oxidase

i. D-Amino Acid Oxidase. Krebs[26-28] observed that liver and kidney homogenates of a variety of animals would oxidize amino acids of both the L and D configuration. He clearly distinguished the D-amino acid oxidase from the L-amino acid oxidase in 1935.[28] Warburg and Christian[24a] showed that the prosthetic group is FAD. Negelein and Brömel[29] isolated the apoenzyme

[26] H. A. Krebs, *Z. Physiol. Chem.* **218**, 191 (1933).
[27] H. A. Krebs, *Z. Physiol. Chem.* **218**, 157 (1933).
[28] H. A. Krebs, *Biochem. J.* **29**, 1620 (1935).
[29] E. Negelein and H. Brömel, *Biochem. Z.* **300**, 225 (1939).

portion in a high degree of purity. A Japanese group[30,31] and Massey *et al.*[32] have prepared the crystalline enzyme by techniques that capitalize on the protection of the enzyme by the competitive inhibitor benzoic acid during processing. The crystalline enzyme so obtained, however, still contains benzoic acid.[33] On the basis of a molecular weight of 91,000 the enzyme contains 2 moles of FAD.

ii. L-Amino Acid Oxidase. Although L-amino acid oxidase was investigated by Krebs in 1935,[28] it was not until some time later that Blanchard *et al.*[34–36] succeeded in preparing the enzyme in a homogeneous form from rat kidneys. In contrast to the D-amino acid oxidase, the prosthetic group was found to be FMN.[35] The molecular weight has been reported to be 138,000 and the enzyme contains 2 moles of FMN. Snake venoms are an excellent source of L-amino acid oxidase. Singer and Kearney[37] isolated the enzyme from the venom of the cottonmouth moccasin and Wellner and Meister[38] obtained the crystalline enzyme from the venom of the eastern diamondback rattlesnake. From this latter source the oxidase has a molecular weight of 128–164,000 and contains 2 moles of FAD.

iii. Mechanism of Action. The oxidation of the amino acids may be described by Eqs. (1)–(3).

$$\mathrm{R\underset{H}{\overset{NH_2}{C}}CO_2H} + \mathrm{E}\begin{matrix}\mathrm{FAD}\\ \mathrm{FAD}\end{matrix} \rightarrow \mathrm{R\overset{NH}{\overset{\|}{C}}CO_2H} + \mathrm{E}\begin{matrix}\mathrm{FADH\cdot}\\ \mathrm{FADH\cdot}\end{matrix} \quad (1)$$

$$\mathrm{R\overset{NH}{\overset{\|}{C}}CO_2H} + \mathrm{H_2O} \rightarrow \mathrm{R\overset{O}{\overset{\|}{C}}CO\,H} + \mathrm{NH_3} \quad (2)$$

$$\mathrm{E}\begin{matrix}\mathrm{FADH\cdot}\\ \mathrm{FADH\cdot}\end{matrix} + \mathrm{O_2} \rightarrow \mathrm{E}\begin{matrix}\mathrm{FAD}\\ \mathrm{FAD}\end{matrix} + \mathrm{H_2O_2} \quad (3)$$

[30] H. Kubo, T. Yamano, M. Iwatsubo, H. Watari, T. Soyama, J. Shiraishi, S. Sawada, N. Kawashima, S. Mitani, and K. Ito, *Bull. Soc. Chim. Biol.* **40**, 431 (1958).

[31] H. Kubo, T. Yamano, M. Iwatsubo, H. Watari, T. Shita, and A. Isomoto, *Bull. Soc. Chim. Biol.* **42**, 569 (1960).

[32] V. Massey, G. Palmer, and R. Bennett, *Biochim. Biophys. Acta* **48**, 1 (1961).

[33] K. Yagi, T. Ozawa, and T. Ooi, *Biochim. Biophys. Acta* **77**, 20 (1963).

[34] M. Blanchard, D. E. Green, V. Nocito, and S. Ratner, *J. Biol. Chem.* **155**, 421 (1944).

[35] M. Blanchard, D. E. Green, V. Nocito, and S. Ratner, *J. Biol. Chem.* **161**, 583 (1945).

[36] M. Blanchard, D. E. Green, V. Nocito-Carroll, and S. Ratner, *J. Biol. Chem.* **163**, 137 (1946).

[37] T. P. Singer and E. B. Kearney, *Arch. Biochem. Biophys.* **29**, 190 (1950).

[38] D. Wellner and A. Meister, *J. Biol. Chem.* **235**, 2013 (1960).

In a highly purified system, devoid of catalase, the α-keto acid reacts with the peroxide formed (Eq. 4).

$$\underset{\displaystyle \text{RCCOH}_2}{\overset{\displaystyle \overset{O}{\|}}{}} + H_2O_2 \rightarrow RCO\ H + CO_2 + H_2O \tag{4}$$

Considerable evidence[20,32,39,40] suggests that free radicals occur in flavoprotein catalyzed reactions and these may be closely neighboring flavin semiquinones.

The reaction is inhibited by excess substrate[37,41,42] since the fully reduced enzyme may be formed, as in Eq. (5).

$$E\overset{\displaystyle \text{FADH·}}{\underset{\displaystyle \text{FADH·}}{}} + RCHCO_2H \rightarrow E\overset{\displaystyle \text{FADH}_2}{\underset{\displaystyle \text{FADH}_2}{}} + RCCO_2H \tag{5}$$

(with NH$_2$ and NH groups shown on the substrate/product)

This compound reacts much more slowly with oxygen than does the half-reduced form and there is some question as to the route back to FAD.

The reaction[42] may proceed either as shown in Eq. (6) or (7).

$$E\overset{\text{FADH}_2}{\underset{\text{FADH}_2}{}} \xrightarrow{O_2} E\overset{\text{FADH·}}{\underset{\text{FADH·}}{}} \xrightarrow{O_2} E\overset{\text{FAD}}{\underset{\text{FAD}}{}} \tag{6}$$

$$E\overset{\text{FADH}_2}{\underset{\text{FADH}_2}{}} \xrightarrow{O_2} E\overset{\text{FAD}}{\underset{\text{FADH}_2}{}} \xrightarrow{O_2} E\overset{\text{FAD}}{\underset{\text{FAD}}{}} \tag{7}$$

iv. Specificity of Action. With the enzyme from snake venom the reaction proceeds most rapidly[41,43,44] with the L-isomers of leucine, methionine, phenylalanine, tyrosine, and tryptophan. A number of L-α-hydroxy acids are also oxidized by this enzyme.[36] These include lactic, hydroxy butyric, hydroxy-γ-methylthiobutyric, phenyllactic, and phenylglycolic acids.

The best substrates for the D-amino acid oxidase from pig kidney are the D-isomers of alanine, methionine, proline and tyrosine followed by isoleucine, leucine, phenylalanine, serine, valine, and tryptophan. For an extensive study

[39] B. Commoner, B. B. Lippincott and J. V. Passonneau, *Proc. Nat. Acad. Sci. U.S.* **44**, 1099 (1958).
[40] H. Beinert, *J. Biol. Chem.* **225**, 465 (1957).
[41] E. A. Zeller and A. Maritz, *Helv. Chim. Acta* **27**, 1888 (1944).
[42] D. Wellner and A. Meister, *J. Biol. Chem.* **236**, 2357 (1961).
[43] A. E. Bender and H. A. Krebs, *Biochem. J.* **46**, 210 (1950).
[44] J. P. Greenstein, S. M. Birnbaum, and M. C. Otey, *J. Biol. Chem.* **204**, 307 (1953).

of specificity, the reader is referred to Bender and Krebs[43] and Greenstein et al.[44]

b. Glycolic Acid Oxidase

The flavoprotein,[45] containing FMN, may play an important role in the respiration of higher plants. It catalyzes the oxidation of glycolate to glyoxylate. The H_2O_2 formed oxidizes the glyoxylate to formate, CO_2, and H_2O.

c. Glucose Oxidase

A flavoprotein, notatin, obtained from *Penicillium notatum* was originally described as an antibiotic. The enzyme catalyzes the oxidation of glucose to glucuronic acid and bactericidal quantities of hydrogen peroxide accumulate.[46] Notatin has a molecular weight of about 150,000[47-49] and contains 2 FAD per mole. This enzyme shows a pronounced specificity for glucose[50] and has very little or no activity for about 50 other sugars tested. The product of the reaction is actually glucuronolactone, but this is readily hydrolyzed to glucuronic acid.

It is thought that the flavin semiquinone mechanism described above also applies to this enzyme.[51, 52]

d. Warburg "Old Yellow Enzyme"

The discovery, isolation, and some of the properties of the old yellow enzyme have been discussed in the sections describing the coenzyme FMN. Theorell and Akeson[53] have found that the crystalline enzyme has a molecular weight of 100–105,000 and contains 2 FMN per mole.

i. Mechanism of Action. The reaction catalyzed by this enzyme is slightly more complicated than those outlined above since an additional reactant, nicotinamide adenine dinucleotide phosphate (NADP), is involved in the oxidation.

Glucose-6-phosphate is oxidized via NADP by glucose-6-phosphate dehydrogenase (Reaction 1). The pyridine nucleotide then reacts with flavoprotein

---

[45] I. Zelitch and S. Ochoa, *J. Biol. Chem.* **201**, 707 (1953).
[46] C. E. Coulthard, R. Michaelis, W. F. Short, G. Sykes, G. E. H. Skrimshire, A. F. B. Standfast, J. H. Birkinshaw, and H. Raistrick, *Biochem. J.* **39**, 24 (1945).
[47] K. Kusai, *Ann. Rept. Sci. Works, Fac. Sci., Osaka Univ., 1960* **8**, 43 (1960).
[48] K. Kusai, I. Sekuzu, B. Hagihara, K. Okunuki, S. Yamauchi, and M. Nakai, *Biochim. Biophys. Acta* **40**, 555 (1960).
[49] R. Cecil and A. G. Ogston, *Biochem. J.* **42**, 229 (1948).
[50] K. Keilin and E. F. Hartree, *Biochem. J.* **42**, 221 (1948).
[51] R. Bentley and A. Neuberger, *Biochem. J.* **45**, 584 (1949).
[52] H. Laser, *Proc. Roy. Soc. (London)* **B140**, 230 (1952).
[53] H. Theorell and A. Akeson, *Arch. Biochem. Biophys.* **65**, 439 (1956).

$$
\begin{array}{l}
\text{H}\diagdown_{\text{C}}\diagup^{\text{OH}} \\
\quad | \\
\text{HCOH} \\
\text{(1)} \quad \text{HOCH} \qquad \text{NADP}^+ + \text{H}_2\text{O} \longrightarrow \\
\quad | \\
\text{HCOH} \\
\quad | \\
\text{CH} \\
\quad | \\
\text{CH}_2\text{OPO}_3\text{H}_2
\end{array}
\qquad
\begin{array}{l}
\text{CO}_2\text{H} \\
\quad | \\
\text{HCOH} \\
\text{HOCH} \qquad \text{NADPH} + \text{H}^+ \\
\quad | \\
\text{HCOH} \\
\quad | \\
\text{HCOH} \\
\quad | \\
\text{CH}_2\text{OPO}_3\text{H}_2
\end{array}
$$

$$
\text{(2)} \quad \text{NADPH} + \text{H}^+ + \text{E}\overset{\diagup \text{FMN}}{\diagdown_{\text{FMN}}} \longrightarrow \text{NADP}^+ + \text{E}\overset{\diagup \text{FMNH} \cdot}{\diagdown_{\text{FMNH} \cdot}}
$$

$$
\text{(3)} \quad \text{E}\overset{\diagup \text{FMNH} \cdot}{\diagdown_{\text{FMNH} \cdot}} + \text{O}_2 \longrightarrow \text{E}\overset{\diagup \text{FMN}}{\diagdown_{\text{FMN}}} + \text{H}_2\text{O}_2
$$

FMN (Reaction 2), which in turn may react with oxygen to produce hydrogen peroxide (Reaction 3). Observations on this enzyme by Haas[20] in 1937 were for a long time considered to be the only existing evidence for a free radical participation in an enzyme reaction. More recent experiments utilizing electron spin resonance have also demonstrated the formation of free radicals in the reaction between the old yellow enzyme and NADPH.[54, 55]

2. Oxidases Containing Metals

These oxidases differ from the simple oxidases discussed above in their content of metals, usually molybdenum and iron, which appear to participate in the enzymatic reaction.

a. Xanthine Oxidase–Aldehyde Oxidase

The enzymatic oxidation of hypoxanthine and xanthine to uric acid in the presence of tissue brei and oxygen was recognized by Spitzer[56] in 1899. In 1922 Morgan[57] showed that milk was a rich source of xanthine oxidase. Subsequently Corran et al.[58] found that this flavoprotein was also an aldehyde oxidase. This served to explain the prior observation of Schardinger[59] in 1902 that if formaldehyde and methylene blue were added to fresh milk in the absence of oxygen the methylene blue was rapidly decolorized.

Xanthine oxidase has been obtained in crystalline form from rabbit liver[60] and milk.[61] The aldehyde oxidase of mammalian liver closely resembles

[54] A. Ehrenberg and G. D. Ludwig, Science 127, 1177 (1958).
[55] A. Ehrenberg, Acta Chem. Scand. 14, 766 (1960).
[56] W. Spitzer, Pflügers Arch. ges. Physiol. 76, 192 (1899).
[57] E. J. Morgan, C. P. Stewart, and F .G. Hopkins, Proc. Royal Soc. (London) B94, 109 (1922).
[58] H. S. Corran, J. G. Dewan, A. H. Gordon, and D. E. Green, Biochem. J. 33, 1694 (1939).
[59] F. Schardinger, Z. Untersuch. Naher. u. Genussm. 5, 1113 (1902).
[60] V. P. Korotkoruchko, Ukrain. Brokhim Zhur. 26, 363 (1954).
[61] P. G. Avis, F. Bergel, R. C. Bray and K. V. Shooter, Nature 173, 1230 (1954).

xanthine oxidase, and it has been suggested[62] that it is a form of xanthine oxidase.

The milk enzyme has a molecular weight of about 300,000[63,64] and contains 2 moles of FAD per mole of enzyme. Both enzymes, milk xanthine oxidase and liver aldehyde oxidase, seem to contain 2 moles of FAD, 2 moles of molybdenum, and 8 moles of iron per mole of protein.

i. Mechanism of Action. While the substrate to product reaction may be written simply, we are dependent on recent electron spin resonance data[65-68] for the interpretation of changes in the enzyme and its prosthetic groups.

(1)

Xanthine   Hydrated xanthine

(2) $RCHO + H_2O \longrightarrow RCH\begin{smallmatrix}OH\\OH\end{smallmatrix} \xrightarrow{-2H} RC\begin{smallmatrix}O\\OH\end{smallmatrix}$

A very wide variety of purines and substituted purines as well as certain pyrimidines[69,70] and pteridines[71-73] may be oxidized by this enzyme. In all cases, it should be noted the reaction proceeds as a hydroxylation followed by a dehydrogenation. A similar lack of specificity is seen in the oxidation of aldehydes to the corresponding carboxylic acids. The enzyme will also slowly oxidize $NADH_2$.[64]

On the basis of electron spin resonance data, Bray[65-68] presents a complex pattern for the oxidation. Flavin semiquinone Mo^V and Fe^{III} all seem to be involved. A suggested sequence of reactants through which the electrons are transferred to oxygen has been presented.[66]

$$\text{Substrate} \rightarrow Mo^V \rightarrow FADH \rightarrow Fe^{III} \rightarrow O_2$$

3. ANAEROBIC DEHYDROGENASES

The tremendous difficulties encountered in work on the anaerobic dehydrogenases stems in large part from their position in cellular architecture. In mammalian systems they normally occur as a part of the mitochondrion

[62] R. P. Igo and B. Mackler, *Biochim. Biophys. Acta* **44**, 310 (1960).
[63] P. G. Avis, F. Bergel, R. C. Bray, D. W. F. James, and K. V. Shooter, *J. Chem. Soc.* 1212 (1956).
[64] P. G. Avis, F. Bergel, and R. C. Bray, *J. Chem. Soc.* 1219 (1956).
[65] R. C. Bray, R. Pettersson, and A. Ehrenberg, *Biochem. J.* **81**, 178 (1961).
[66] R. C. Bray, *Biochem. J.* **81**, 189 (1961).
[67] R. C. Bray and R. Pettersson, *Biochem. J.* **81**, 194 (1961).
[68] R. C. Bray, *Biochem. J.* **81**, 196 (1961).
[69] D. C. Lorz and G. H. Hitchings, *Federation Proc.* **9**, 197 (1950).
[70] S. S. Debor, *Proc. Med. Chem., Moscow*, **1**, 401 (1961).
[71] H. M. Kalckar, N. O. Kjeldgaard, and H. Klenow, *Biochim. Biophys. Acta* **5**, 575 (1950).
[72] F. Bergmann and H. Kwietney, *Biochim. Biophys. Acta* **28**, 613 (1958).
[73] F. Bergmann and H. Kwietney, *Biochim. Biophys. Acta* **33**, 29 (1959).

rather than as a soluble enzyme in the mitochondrion released on disruption. Green's group[74-76] has done considerable work on what they call electron transport particles. While only 1 % the size of the original mitochondrion, these particles qualitatively possess all the functions of the larger intact system.

The flavoproteins are closely linked physically to the other respiratory chain enzymes, the cytochromes, with which they react. In some cases the enzyme activity under study is best handled as a particulate material during the early stages of fractionation. The enzyme is then solubilized by treatment of the particulate material with phospholipase A, nonionic detergents, or certain lipid solvents. Once solubilized, a natural or an artificial hydrogen acceptor must be added to system containing the purified enzyme. Technical difficulties involved in the use of dyes for this purpose have been described by Singer.[77] The mechanism of action of the anaerobic dehydrogenases is illustrated below by some of the better characterized systems.

a. Lipoyl Dehydrogenase–Straub's Diaphorase

i. Properties. In 1939 Straub[78, 79] succeeded in separating a soluble flavoprotein from pig heart in poor yield under somewhat harsh conditions. While Straub reported the enzyme oxidized the reduced form of nicotinamide adenine dinucleotide (NADH) or NADPH, it was not until 1960 that work by Massey[80, 81] revealed that the true biological substrate was enzyme-bound lipoic acid.

Lipoyl dehydrogenase occurs as part of a macromolecular complex. The *E. coli*–pyruvate dehydrogenase[82] and α-ketoglutarate dehydrogenase,[82] pigeon breast muscle pyruvate dehydrogenase,[83, 84] and hog heart α-ketoglutarate dehydrogenase[85] complexes have molecular weights of 4.8, 2.4, and 4 and 2×10^6, respectively. The macromolecular complex contains a thiamine pyrophosphate (TPP) dependent decarboxylase, enzyme-bound lipoic acid, lipoyl dehydrogenase and, in some cases (*E. coli*–pyruvate dehydrogenase complex), a transacetylase. Treatment with urea[81, 86] or trypsin[87] has been used to disrupt these complexes.

[74] D. E. Green, R. L. Lester, and D. M. Ziegler, *Biochim. Biophys. Acta* **23**, 516 (1957).

[75] D. M. Ziegler, A. W. Linnane, D. E. Green, C. M. S. Dass, and H. Ris, *Biochim. Biophys. Acta* **28**, 524 (1958).

[76] D. E. Green, *in* "Advances in Enzymology" (F. F. Nord, ed.), Vol. 21, p. 73. Interscience Publishers, Inc., New York, 1959.

[77] T. P. Singer and E. B. Kearney, *in* "The Enzymes" (P. D. Boyer, H. Lardy, and K. Myrback eds.), Vol. 7, p. 383. Academic Press, New York, 1963.

[78] F. B. Straub, *Nature* **143**, 76 (1939).

[79] F. B. Straub, *Biochem. J.* **33**, 787 (1939).

[80] V. Massey, *Biochim. Biophys. Acta* **37**, 314 (1960).

[81] V. Massey, *Biochim. Biophys. Acta* **38**, 447 (1960).

[82] M. Koike, L. J. Reed, and W. R. Carroll, *J. Biol. Chem.* **235**, 1924 (1960).

[83] V. Jagannathan, and R. S. Schweet, *J. Biol. Chem.* **196**, 551 (1952).

[84] R. S. Schweet, B. Katchman, R. M. Bock, and V. Jagannathan, *J. Biol. Chem.* **196**, 563 (1952).

[85] D. R. Sanadi, D. M. Gibson, P. Ayengar, and M. Jacob, *J. Biol. Chem.* **218**, 505 (1956).

[86] M. Koike and L. J. Reed, *J. Biol. Chem.* **236**, PC33 (1961).

[87] R. L. Searls and D. R. Sanadi, *J. Biol. Chem.* **235**, 2485 (1960).

ii. Mechanism of Action. The oxidative decarboxylation of α-keto acids has been discussed in chapters on thiamine, niacin, and lipoic acid. According to Gunsalus[88] and Reed[89] the reaction proceeds in a manner such that the overall reaction may be written as

$$RCOCO_2H + CoASH + NAD \rightarrow CoASCOR + CO_2 + NADH$$

If the prosthetic groups of the complex are written as a unit according to Searls *et al.*,[90] the reaction proceeds as shown below according to Massey and Veeger.[91]

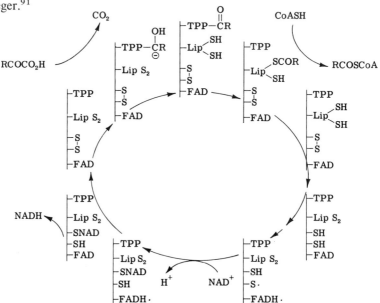

The flow of electrons toward oxygen may be represented by

Substrate → lipoic acid → FAD — NAD → flavoprotein → cytochrome → O_2

Despite the apparent complexity of the scheme presented, this is a relatively simple example of the reaction of a mitochondrial flavoprotein. No metals are involved, the intermediates on either side are simple and the formation of a high energy bond, CoASCOR, accounts for a portion of the energy derived from the oxidation. Only the enzyme sulfhydryl groups contribute a slight complexity to the reaction.

[88] I. C. Gunsalus, *Federation Proc.* **13**, 715 (1954).
[89] L. J. Reed *in* "Advances in Enzymology" (F. F. Nord, ed.), Vol. 18, p. 319. Interscience Publishers, Inc., New York, 1957.
[90] R. L. Searls, J. M. Peters, and D. R. Sanadi, *J. Biol. Chem.* **236**, 2317 (1961).
[91] V. Massey and G. Veeger, *Biochim. Biophys. Acta* **48**, 33 (1961).

b. Acyl-CoA Dehydrogenases and Electron-Transferring Flavoprotein (ETF)

i. Preparation and Properties. From his studies on ω phenyl fatty acids, Knoop[92] was led to propose a theory of stepwise degradation based on the removal of 2 carbon units. Much of our current knowledge on the subject of fatty acid oxidation comes from the Enzyme Institute of the University of Wisconsin and Lynen's Laboratory in Munich. The flavoproteins involved are readily extractable from heart mitochondrial acetone powders or from fresh mitochondria disrupted by sonication. Three acyl-CoA dehydrogenases have been obtained which differ in their chain length specificity. The first, usually referred to as butyryl dehydrogenase, acts only upon very short chain CoA esters, the second acts upon intermediate length esters, and the third upon those of somewhat longer chain length.

In general the enzymes from animal tissues or mycobacterium[93-95] appear to have a molecular weight of about 200,000 and contain 2 moles of FAD per mole. Zone electrophoresis has been used in the purification. These dehydrogenases do not contain metals except as minor contaminants. Butyryl dehydrogenase as isolated from pig or cattle tissue has a green color, but this is not caused by the presence of copper.[96] When the enzyme is reduced by substrate, reoxidation produces a normal yellow flavoprotein.[96]

ii. Mechanism of Action.

$$RCH_2CH_2\overset{\overset{O}{\|}}{C}SCoA \;+\; E\!\!\begin{array}{c}FAD\\FAD\end{array} \longrightarrow \;\;\overset{R\quad H}{\underset{H\quad C-SCoA}{C=C\diagdown O}} \;+\; E\!\!\begin{array}{c}FADH\cdot\\FADH\cdot\end{array}$$

$$E\!\!\begin{array}{c}FADH\cdot\\FADH\cdot\end{array} \;+\; ETF_{oxid} \longrightarrow \; E\!\!\begin{array}{c}FAD\\FAD\end{array} \;+\; ETF\ red$$

Certain peculiarities of the reaction should be noted. Substrate is very strongly bound by the enzyme.[97] Only those treatments which liberate the prosthetic group release the substrate. The acyl dehydrogenases are not linked directly to the cytochrome system but are closely associated with an intermediate flavoprotein described as the electron transferring flavoprotein.[98]

Crane and Beinert found that the fatty acyl-CoA dehydrogenases required

[92] F. Knoop, *Beitr. Chem. Physiol. Pathol.* **6**, 150 (1904).
[93] H. R. Mahler, *J. Biol. Chem.* **206**, 13 (1954).
[94] A. Gelbard and D. S. Goldman, *Arch. Biochim. Biophys.* **94**, 228 (1961).
[95] H. Beinert *in* "The Enzymes" (P. D. Boyer, H. Lardy, and K. Myrback, eds.), Vol. 7, p. 447. Academic Press, New York, 1963.
[96] E. P. Steyn-Parvé and H. Beinert, *J. Biol. Chem.* **233**, 853 (1958).
[97] E. P. Steyn-Parvé and H. Beinert, *J. Biol. Chem.* **233**, 843 (1958).
[98] F. L. Crane and H. Beinert, *J. Biol. Chem.* **218**, 717 (1956).

an additional flavoprotein as a linkage to most dyes used for conventional assays. This flavoprotein is readily separated from the dehydrogenases by electrophoresis.[99] With a molecular weight of about 80,000, the enzyme contains only 1 mole of FAD per mole and only trace contamination with metals. ETF from various systems seem remarkably similar. The mycobacterial ETF may be used with pig liver or cattle heart acyl dehydrogenases or vice versa.[94] Sarcosine dehydrogenase from rat liver[100, 101] also requires an ETF. Here again systems have been successfully crossed.[102] The oxidation of reduced ETF is linked to the cytochrome system, a problem much too complex for discussion here.

c. Succinic Dehydrogenase–Fumaric Reductase

i. Preparation and Properties. Our knowledge of this enzyme goes back to the work of Thunberg in 1909.[103] In animal tissue and in higher plants succinic dehydrogenase is a mitochondrial enzyme, while in yeasts and some bacteria, it is found in the corresponding respiratory particles. The fumaric reductase[104] referred to in the first edition of " The Vitamins " has since been identified as succinic dehydrogenase.[105, 106] In certain anaerobic reactions, i.e., propionic acid fermentations,[107, 108] fumarate is the sole electron acceptor, and the reductive reaction is normal to the organism.

While succinic dehydrogenase refers to only the flavoprotein, much of the work done on this reaction has utilized a multienzyme succinic dehydrogenase complex. This preparation contains the flavoprotein-to-cytochrome *c* portion of the respiratory chain. Solubilization of the enzyme was first reported by Hogeboom[109] and later by Morton.[110] Treatment with an organic solvent is apparently essential. A reasonable preparation is achieved by extraction of

[99] H. Beinert, *in* "Methods in Enzymology" (S. P. Colowick and N. O. Kaplan, eds.), Vol. 5, p. 546. Academic Press, New York, 1962.

[100] D. D. Hoskins and C. G. Mackenzie, *J. Biol. Chem.* **236**, 177 (1961).

[101] G. P. Mell and F. M. Huennekens, *Federation Proc.* **19**, 411 (1960).

[102] H. Beinert and W. R. Frisell, *J. Biol. Chem.* **237**, 2988 (1962).

[103] T. Thunberg, *Scand. Arch. Physiol.* **22**, 430 (1909).

[104] F. G. Fischer and H. Eysenbach, *Ann.* **530**, 99 (1937).

[105] T. P. Singer, E. B. Kearney and V. Massey, *in* "Advances in Enzymology" (F. F. Nord, ed.), Vol. 18, p. 65. Interscience Publishers, Inc., New York, 1957.

[106] V. Massey and T. P. Singer, *J. Biol. Chem.* **228**, 263 (1957).

[107] H. A. Barker and F. Lipmann, *Arch. Biochem. Biophys.* **4**, 361 (1944).

[108] R. Molinari and F. J. S. Lara, *Biochem. J.* **75**, 57 (1960).

[109] G. H. Hogeboom, *J. Biol. Chem.* **162**, 739 (1946).

[110] R. K. Morton, *Nature* **166**, 1092 (1950).

[111] T. P. Singer and E. B. Kearney, *Biochem. Biophys. Acta* **15**, 151 (1954).

[112] R. E. Basford, H. D. Tisdale, and D. E. Green, *Biochem. Biophys. Acta* **24**, 290 (1957).

[113] G. Rendina and T. P. Singer, *J. Biol. Chem.* **243**, 1605 (1959).

[114] R. L. Ringler, S. Minakami, and T. P. Singer, *Biochem. Biophys. Res. Comm.* **3**, 417 (1960).

[115] R. L. Ringler, *J. Biol. Chem.* **236**, 1192 (1961).

mitochondrial acetone powders with basic buffers.[111, 112] Phospholipase A, which solubilizes other dehydrogenases,[113–115] does not extract succinic dehydrogenase.

From several sources the enzyme has a molecular weight of about 200,000[116, 117] with 4 moles of non-heme Fe and 1 mole of FAD per mole. While degradation studies suggest that the prosthetic group is FAD,[118] technical difficulties arising from a peptide linkage, perhaps to the 4 position of the isoalloxazine,[119] preclude a definitive statement at present. Peptides containing the nucleotide and six or twelve amino acids have been obtained from pig or bovine heart preparations of the enzyme.[118, 120, 121] After treatment with proteolytic enzymes, the yeast enzyme responds similarly.[122]

The soluble enzyme is less stable than the complex and Hopkins *et al.*[123, 124] established the essential nature of sulfhydryl groups for activity. Materials that chelate the iron inactivate the enzyme.

ii. Mechanism of Action.

$$
\begin{array}{c}
CH_2CO_2H \\
| \\
CH_2CO_2H
\end{array}
\ + \ E\text{-}FAD_{oxid}
\qquad
\begin{array}{c}
HC\!-\!CO_2H \\
\| \\
HO_2CCH
\end{array}
\ + \ E\text{-}FAD \ red
$$

$$
E\text{-}FAD \ red \ \xrightarrow{\ cytochromes\ } \ E\text{-}FAD \ oxid
$$

Beinert and Sands[125, 126] detected the flavin semiquinone by electron paramagnetic resonance techniques. The formation of this free radical system appears to precede an $Fe^{III} \, Fe^{II}$ transition. Only a small portion of the iron in the enzyme appears to be active in this transformation.[126, 127] Chemical evidence[127–129] would seem to indicate that only 20–30%, or one Fe out of

[116] T. P. Singer, E. B. Kearney, and P. Bernath, *J. Biol. Chem.* **223**, 599 (1956).

[117] T. Y. Wang, C. L. Tsou, and Y. L. Wang, *Sci. Sinica. Peking* **5**, 73 (1956).

[118] T. P. Singer, E. B. Kearney, and V. Massey, *in* "Enzymes: Units of Biological Structure and Function" (O. H. Gaebler, ed.), p. 417. Academic Press, New York, 1956.

[119] Y. L. Wang, T. Y. Wang, C. L. Tsou, K. Y. Wu, and S. M. Chen, *Abstr. 5th Intern. Cong. Biochem., Moscow, 1961,* 103 (1961).

[120] E. B. Kearney, *J. Biol. Chem.* **235**, 865 (1960).

[121] T. Y. Wang, C. L. Tsou, and Y. L. Wang, *Sci. Sinica, Peking* **7**, 65 (1958).

[122] T. P. Singer, V. Massey, and E. B. Kearney, *Arch. Biochem. Biophys.* **69**, 405 (1957).

[123] F. G. Hopkins and E. J. Morgan, *Biochem. J.* **32**, 611 (1938).

[124] F. G. Hopkins, E. J. Morgan, and C. Lutwak-Mann, *Biochem. J.* **32**, 1829 (1938).

[125] H. Beinert and R. H. Sands, *Biochem. Biophys. Res. Comm.* **3**, 41 (1960).

[126] H. Beinert and W. Lee, *Biochem. Biophys. Res. Comm.* **5**, 40 (1961).

[127] D. E. Green, *Plenary Lecture 5th Intern. Congress Biochem., Moscow, 1961 Preprint* 176, Pergamon Press, London, 1961.

[128] D. M. Ziegler and K. A. Doeg, *Arch. Biochem. Biophys.* **97**, 41 (1962).

[129] D. M. Ziegler, *in* "Biological Structure and Function" (T. W. Goodwin and O. Lindberg, eds.), Vol. II p. 253, Academic Press, New York, 1961.

the four present in the molecule, is reduced. The involvement of a disulfide–disulfhydryl group reaction analogous to that noted above for lipoyl dehydrogenase has been suggested by Keilin and King.[130] Succinic dehydrogenase is linked to the cytochrome system. The transfer reactions taking place to this system are beyond the scope of the present chapter.

d. Other Flavoprotein Enzymes

Mention should also be made of choline dehydrogenase that forms betaine aldehyde. The molecular weight is not known, but the flavoprotein contains 1 mole of FAD and 4 moles Fe per 850,000 gm of protein.[131] Dihydroxyacetone phosphate arises from the action of α-glycerophosphate dehydrogenase. This enzyme contains 1 mole of FAD and 6 gm atoms of Fe per 2.1×10^6 gm of protein.[132] L-Galactono-γ lactone dehydrogenase produces L-ascorbic. This flavoprotein probably contains iron.[133] L-Lactate dehydrogenase contains 2 FMN and 2 protoheme groups and has 'a molecular weight of 172,000.[134] D-Lactate cytochrome reductase, on the other hand, contains 1 mole of FAD and 2–3 gm atoms of Zn per 50,000 g of protein.[135] Of the many nitrate reductases, a few seem to be metal-containing flavoproteins.[136] Pyridine nucleotide-cytochrome c reductases[137] and quinone reductases[138] are best left for the next revision of this chapter.

4. OXIDATIVE PHOSPHORYLATION

The energy made available by the oxidation of substrate is trapped by formation of ATP, hence the description oxidative phosphorylation. One ATP may arise when NADH is oxidized by FAD, while two more ATP are subsequently formed in the cytochrome system. Boyer[139] has suggested that protein-bound phosphohistidine may be the key intermediate in the generation of the high energy phosphate bond. An attractive flavin–imidazolide complex may be formulated, but experimental data are lacking at this time.

[130] D. Keilin and T. E. King, Proc. Roy. Soc. (London) B152, 163 (1960).
[131] T. Kimura and T. P. Singer, in "Methods in Enzymology" (S. P. Colowick and N. O. Kaplan, eds.), Vol. 5 p. 562. Academic Press, New York, 1962.
[132] R. L. Ringler, J. Biol. Chem. 236, 1192 (1961).
[133] L. W. Mapson and E. Breslow, Biochem. J. 68, 395 (1958).
[134] C. A. Appleby and R. K. Morton, Biochem. J. 71, 492 (1959).
[135] C. Gregolin and T. P. Singer, Biochem. Biophys. Acta 57, 410 (1962).
[136] A. Nason in "The Enzymes" (P. Boyer, H. Lardy, and K. Myrback, eds.), Vol. 7, p. 587. Academic Press, New York, 1963.
[137] Y. Hatefi in "The Enzymes" (P. Boyer, H. Lardy, and K. Myrback, eds.), Vol. 7, p. 495. Academic Press, New York, 1963.
[138] C. Martius in "The Enzymes" (P. Boyer, H. Lardy, and K. Myrback, eds.), Vol. 7, p. 517. Academic Press, New York, 1963.
[139] P. D. Boyer, Science 141, 1147 (1963).

X. Deficiency Effects

E. E. SNELL

A. In Microorganisms

Shortly after the isolation of riboflavin as a vitamin for animals, Orla-Jensen and co-workers[1] showed that the compound also was an essential growth factor for many lactic acid bacteria. This finding was rapidly confirmed,[2] and the effect of several variations in the riboflavin structure on the bacterial response was determined.[3] The response proved to be very specific, and on these grounds a microbiological assay for the vitamin was developed and proposed.[4] Both growth and acid production of lactic acid bacteria are proportional to riboflavin in the suboptimal range of concentrations.[4, 5] Riboflavin is required as a growth factor by fewer microorganisms than are most of the other vitamins;[5, 6] besides the lactic acid bacteria, however, many of the hemolytic streptococci, some propionic acid bacteria, some clostridia, and some luminescent bacteria require it. Few if any naturally occurring yeasts or other fungi have been found that require riboflavin;[5] mutants of *Neurospora crassa* that require it have, however, been obtained,[7] and all organisms so far examined that do not require preformed supplies of this vitamin synthesize it.[3, 6] Indeed, the synthesis of riboflavin by certain fungi, e. g., by *Ashbya gossypii* and related organisms, provides a commercial source for the production of this vitamin.[8]

Aside from decreased growth in the absence of sufficient supplies, few other effects of riboflavin deficiency in microorganisms have been described. From the role of this vitamin as a hydrogen carrier, it might be expected that, as in higher animals, the level of certain oxidative enzyme systems would be depressed during growth on suboptimal supplies. That this is true is shown by investigations of Doudoroff[9] with the luminescent organism *Photobacterium phosphorescens*. Cultures grown on a yeast autolyzate agar frequently

[1] S. Orla-Jensen, N. C. Otte, and A. Snog-Kjaer, *Zentralbl. Bakteriol., Parasitenk., Infektionskr.,* Abt. 2 **94**, 134 (1936).

[2] E. E. Snell, F. M. Strong, and W. H. Peterson, *Biochem. J.* **31**, 1789 (1937).

[3] E. E. Snell and F. M. Strong, *Enzymologia* **6**, 186 (1939).

[4] E. E. Snell and F. M. Strong, *Ind. Eng. Chem., Anal. Ed.* **11**, 346 (1939).

[5] E. E. Snell, *in* "Vitamin Methods" (P. Gyorgy, ed.), Vol. I. p. 327. Academic Press, New York, 1950.

[6] R. C. J. G. Knight, *Vitam. Horm. (New York)* **3**, 105 (1945).

[7] G. W. Beadle and E. L. Tatum, *Amer. J. Bot.* **32**, 678 (1945).

[8] F. W. Tanner, Jr., C. Vojnovich, and J. M. Van Lanen, *J. Bacteriol.* **58**, 737 (1949).

[9] M. Doudoroff, *Enzymologia* **5**, 239 (1938).

produced, as variants, dull or dark colonies; these luminesced more brightly when riboflavin was added. The same "dark" colonies were stimulated in growth on a riboflavin-deficient medium by additions of this vitamin. Apparently the dull variants had lost the ability to synthesize sufficient riboflavin for their needs; this was not true of the original bright colonies. In this case, amounts of riboflavin sufficient for growth of the "dull" variants were sufficient to permit maximum luminescence. That riboflavin enzymes are among those concerned in light production by such luminescent organism has been proved by Johnson and Eyring.[10]

At low concentrations, many fatty materials show a "sparing effect" on the requirement of lactic acid bacteria for riboflavin;[5] this effect, which is sometimes troublesome in microbiological assays, may possibly indicate that riboflavin participates in fat synthesis by these organisms. If the fatty material required were supplied preformed, the requirement for riboflavin might well be decreased thereby.

M. K. HORWITT

B. In Plants

Riboflavin is apparently synthesized by higher plant life,[11, 12] as evidenced by its distribution in our vegetable foods. There is no recorded evidence of riboflavin deficiency in plants.

According to Galston,[13] riboflavin determines the photooxidation of indoleacetic acid and may be regarded as a photoreceptor in light–growth reactions. Ferri[14] has emphasized the fact that the induction of the photoinactivation of indoleacetic acid is a property common to many fluorescent substances. It has been known that the photooxidation of indoleacetic acid could be determined by eosin[15] and that eosin-treated roots yielded less auxin than untreated ones.[16] It will be interesting to observe the development of this subject.

M. K. HORWITT

C. In Insects

It has been apparent for some time[17] that riboflavin is essential for many insects. Among those whose requirements have been studied are the larvae of

[10] F. H. Johnson and H. Eyring, *J. Amer. Chem. Soc.* **66**, 818 (1944).
[11] P. R. Burkholder, *Science* **97**, 562 (1943).
[12] J. Bonner, *Bot. Gaz.* (*Chicago*) **103**, 581 (1942).
[13] A. W. Galston, *Science* **111**, 619 (1950).
[14] M. G. Ferri, *Arch. Biochem.* **31**, 127 (1951).
[15] F. Skoog, *J. Cell. Comp. Physiol.* **7**, 227 (1935).
[16] P. Boysen-Jensen, *Planta* **22**, 404 (1934).
[17] R. Craig and W. M. Hoskins, *Ann. Rev. Biochem.* **9**, 617 (1940).

the flesh fly *Sarcophagia* sp.,[18] the cockroach *Blattella germanica*,[19] the larvae of the confused flour beetle *Tribolium confusum*,[20, 21] the larvae of *Drosophila*,[22] and the yellow fever mosquito *Aedes aegypti*.[23]

Fraenkel and Blewett,[24] who have made extensive studies of the nutritional requirements of beetles, have shown that riboflavin is required by *Tribolium* and *Ptinus*, but that *Lasiodermia*, *Sitodrepa*, and *Silvanus* do not need riboflavin in their diet because of the presence of intracellular symbiotic microorganisms that synthesize the vitamin.

The American cockroach *Periplaneta americana*[25] and *Tincola bisselliella*[26] accumulate much more riboflavin in the Malpighian tubes than can be accounted for by the diet.

M. K. HORWITT

D. In Animals

Riboflavin is essential for growth and normal health for all animals. Its restriction has been studied in nearly all species which are related to human economics. The primary effect of riboflavin restriction is the cessation of growth. Because it is a fundamental constituent of animal tissue, new tissue cannot be formed unless a minimum amount of riboflavin is available. It is therefore necessary not only for growth but also for tissue repair.[27] The amounts of riboflavin needed for normal growth have been discussed in the section on animal requirements. When less than these requirements is provided, a variety of pathological trends become evident. Wolbach and Bessey[28] have published an excellent review of the tissue changes in vitamin deficiencies, in which they summarized most of the studies reported prior to 1942. The large majority of the older papers on the B_2 vitamin dealt with mixed deficiencies and often described syndromes which are not seen in modern work with a " pure " deficiency of riboflavin. At present, most of our interpretations of ariboflavinosis in animals are based upon experiments which deal with the removal of all, or nearly all, of the riboflavin from the diet. The application to man of such work is limited by the fact that one rarely, if ever, observes a human deficiency syndrome due to the complete

[18] G. Di Maria, *Arch. Zool. Ital.* **25**, 469 (1938).

[19] C. M. McCay, *Physiol. Zool.* **11**, 89 (1938).

[20] G. Frobrich, *Z. Vergl. Physiol.* **27**, 336 (1939).

[21] K. Offhaus, *Z. Vergl. Physiol.* **27**, 384 (1939).

[22] E. L. Tatum, *Proc. Nat. Acad. Sci., U.S.* **25**, 490 (1939).

[23] W. Trager and Y. SubbaRow, *Biol. Bull.* **75**, 75 (1938).

[24] G. Fraenkel and M. Blewett, *J. Exp. Biol.* **20**, 28 (1943).

[25] R. L. Metcalf and R. L. Patton, *J. Cell. Comp. Physiol.* **19**, 373 (1942).

[26] R. G. Busnel and A. Drilhon, *C. R. Acad. Sci.* **216**, 213 (1943).

[27] M. K. Horwitt, O. W. Hills, C. C. Harvey, E. Liebert, and D. L. Steinberg, *J. Nutr.* **39**, 357 (1949).

[28] S. B. Wolbach and O. A. Bessey, *Physiol. Rev.* **22**, 233 (1942).

absence of dietary riboflavin. More work on the effect of longstanding suboptimal intakes of riboflavin is indicated.

1. RATS

Goldberger and Lilly[29] were apparently the first to describe symptoms of riboflavin deficiency in the rat, as a result of a study in which they attempted to produce rat pellagra. They reported a severe ophthalmia and a bilateral, symmetrical alopecia, which almost completely denuded the head, neck, and trunk. The dermatitis, which these authors also observed has since been shown to have been complicated by a pyridoxine deficiency.[30, 31] Whereas the lesions of pyridoxine deficiency are characterized by a florid dermatitis of the extremities and a swelling of the ears, the lesions of ariboflavinosis are less specific and slower to develop. An eczematous condition of the skin especially affects the nostrils and eyes. The eyelids become denuded of hair and may be stuck together with a serous exudate.

Conjunctivitis, blepharitis, corneal opacities, and vascularization of the cornea are common manifestations of rat ariboflavinosis.[32-35] The question of specificity of cataract formation, first reported in 1931 by Day et al.[36] in rats deficient in what was then known as vitamin G, has not yet been resolved. There is an apparent inverse relationship between cataract formation[37-39] and the amount of riboflavin in the diet. There also seems to be a relationship between corneal opacities and amino acid deficiencies.[40-42] In a study of the growth of the eye during riboflavin and tryptophan deficiencies, Pirie[43] note that the eye continued to grow at a normal rate, so that the deficient animals had relatively large eyes in undersized bodies.

Before the pathology of choline deficiency was recognized, there were frequent reports of hepatic injury as a consequence of riboflavin deficien-

[29] J. Goldberger and R. D. Lilly, *Pub. Health Rep.* **41**, 1025 (1926).
[30] P. György, *Nature (London)* **133**, 498 (1933).
[31] P. György, *Biochem. J.* **29**, 741 (1935).
[32] H. Chick, T. F. Macrae, and A. N. Worden, *Biochem. J.* **34**, 580 (1940).
[33] L. R. Richardson and A. G. Hogan, *M. Agr. Exp. Sta. Res. Bull.* **241** (1936).
[34] B. Sure, *J. Nutr.* **22**, 295 (1941).
[35] H. R. Street, G. R. Cowgill, and H. M. Zimmerman, *J. Nutr.* **22**, 7 (1941).
[36] P. L. Day, W. C. Langston, and C. S. O'Brien, *Amer. J. Ophthalmol.* **14**, 1005 (1931).
[37] P. L. Day, W. J. Darby, and W. C. Langston, *J. Nutr.* **13**, 389 (1937).
[38] O. A. Bessey and S. B. Wolbach, *J. Exp. Med.* **69**, 1 (1939).
[39] M. M. El-Dadr, *Chem. Ind.* **58**, 1020 (1939).
[40] P. B. Curtis, S. M. Hauge, and H. R. Kraybill, *J. Nutr.* **5**, 503 (1932).
[41] H. S. Mitchell and G. M. Cook, *Proc. Soc. Exp. Biol. Med.* **36**, 806 (1937).
[42] W. K. Hall, L. L. Bowles, V. P. Sydenstricker, and H. L. Schmidt, Jr., *J. Nutr.* **36**, 277 (1948).
[43] A. Pirie, *Brit. J. Nutr.* **2**, 14 (1948).

cy.[34, 45] It is now assumed that the fatty livers associated with deficiencies of B complex vitamins are not directly related to riboflavin depletion.[28, 46]

A variety of neuropathological changes have been reported, and it is likely that the proportions of fat, carbohydrate, and protein in the diet, as well as the severity of the riboflavin depletion, may play an important part in determining the exact nature of the pathology. Partial paralysis of the legs of the rat are produced more easily on a high fat ration.[47, 48] In its severe form this paralysis is characterized by degeneration of the myelin sheaths of the sciatic nerves, axis cylinder swelling, and fragmentation. Myelin degeneration and gliosis in the spinal cord have also been observed. Sourkes et al.[48a] have noted decreases in liver epinephrine and norepinephrine and in brain epinephrine during riboflavin deficiency, but no such changes were found in the adrenal glands or the spleen.

Histological changes in the skin have been described by Welbach and Bessey[28, 49, 50] as follows: "We find that the initial responses are in the epidermis and its appendages. The vascular engorgement, so characteristic of pyridoxine deficiency, does not occur. The epidermis as a whole shows little change other than a moderate hyperkeratosis. In some locations there is slight hyperplasia of the epidermis, particularly of the snout and sides of the head, possibly related to scratching. Sebaceous glands, including the Meibomian glands of the eyelids, become somewhat atrophic. There is an increased rate of shedding of hair which we believe to be the result of separation of the cornified anchoring cells from the epithelial sheaths. The outstanding and thus far, to us, distinctive feature of the deficiency is the effect upon regeneration of hair follicles and hair formation. In the late stage of the deficiency, regeneration of the hair follicles does not occur or is incomplete. Follicles engaged in hair formation during the establishment of the deficiency undergo atrophy and for a time continue to form imperfect hair. The atrophy is apparent in all parts of the hair follicle but is more evident in the matrix. The cuticular cells continue longest but undergo atypical cornification. Thus various degrees of retardation of hair production are found in a given area of skin; complete suppression, hair roots represented by loosely packed columns of cornified fusiform cells, and hair roots consisting of medulla with imperfectly formed cortical substance. Sharply flexed or buckled hair follicles are common, presumably occasioned by the lack of support normally afforded

[44] P. György and H. Goldblatt, J. Exp. Med. 70, 185 (1939).
[45] G. Gavin and E. W. McHenry, J. Biol. Chem. 132, 41 (1940).
[46] P. György and H. Goldblatt, J. Exp. Med. 72, 1 (1940).
[47] J. H. Shaw and P. H. Phillips, J. Nutr. 22, 345 (1941).
[48] R. W. Engel and P. H. Phillips, Proc. Soc. Exp. Biol. Med. 40, 597 (1939).
[48a] T. L. Sourkes, G. F. Murphy, and V. R. Woodford, Jr., J. Nutr. 72, 145 (1960).
[49] S. B. Wolbach, J. Amer. Med. Ass. 108, 7 (1937).
[50] S. B. Wolbach and O. A. Bessey, Science 91, 559 (1940).

by the forming hair shaft or root. In cross section, the hair roots are often oval or flat in outline. The microscopic appearances account satisfactorily for the gross appearances of the sparsely distributed hair. The gross impression of thickening of the skin may be accounted for by the persistence of many atrophic regenerated follicles because these may and often do extend to the depth of normal active follicles (i.e., to the muscle panniculus), and owing to their number, should affect the texture of the skin. In 48 hours after riboflavin therapy, there is marked restoration of normal appearances of the follicles and in 72 hours the epithelium of the follicle has assumed normal appearances The matrix cells respond first."

According to Kornberg et al.[51] rats fed a diet deficient in riboflavin developed granulocytopenia in about 5.0% of the cases and, less frequently, anemia. The granulocytopenia responded to folic acid more frequently than to riboflavin. However, the anemia observed was alleviated in more rats by riboflavin than by folic acid. There was a hyperplasia of bone marrow in the riboflavin-deficient rats which was indistinguishable from that seen in rats with folic acid deficiency. There was also an atrophy of the lymphoid tissue and no evidence of blood formation in the spleen. Further study of these observations has led to the assumption that riboflavin deficiency[52–54] can cause anemia in the rat.

The importance of riboflavin in the reproductive cycle has been quite apparent to animal breeders. Its absence from the diet of rats may result in anestrus, and if riboflavin is not restored within 10 weeks, the damage becomes irreparable.[55] Female rats bred on a deficient diet by Warkany[56, 57] gave birth to litters one-third of which had congenital skeletal malformations including shortening of the mandible, tibia, fibula, radius, and ulna, fusion of the ribs, sternal centers of ossification, fingers, and toes, and cleft palate. There were no abnormal young when riboflavin was added to the diet.[58] Nelson et al.[59] did not observe skeletal abnormalities at birth in the litters of their riboflavin-deficient rats. The principal changes which appeared in their deficient animals were retarded development of the epiphyses, progressive decrease in the width of the epiphyseal cartilage, increased hyalinization of its matrix, and calcification and separation of the epiphyseal cartilage from the marrow cavity by a thin layer of bone. Hematopoietic tissue was replaced by

[51] A. Kornberg, F. S. Daft, and W. H. Sebrell, Arch. Biochem. 8, 341 (1945).
[52] W. H. Sebrell, Federation Proc. 8, 568 (1949).
[53] C. F. Shukers and P. L. Day, J. Nutr. 25, 511 (1943).
[54] A. Kornberg, H. Tabor, and W. H. Sebrell, Amer. J. Physiol. 145, 54 (1945).
[55] K. H. Coward, B. G. E. Morgan, and L. Waller, J. Physiol. (London) 100, 423 (1942).
[56] J. Warkany and R. C. Nelson, Science 92, 383 (1940).
[57] J. Warkany, Vitam. Horm. (New York) 3, 73 (1945).
[58] J. Warkany and E. Schraffenberger, Proc. Soc. Exp. Biol. Med. 54, 92 (1943).
[59] M. M. Nelson, E. Sulon, H. Becks, and H. M. Evans, Proc. Soc. Exp. Biol. Med. 66, 631 (1947).

fat in all the rats after they had been on the deficient diet for 144 days. Multiple congenital abnormalities were reported by Nelson et al.[59a] when the vitamin deficiency was accentuated by administering the antimetabolite galactoflavin.

Riboflavin has been found to be protective to the rat against the rickettsiae of murine typhus.[60] Chronic riboflavin deficiency is often accompanied by a type of pediculosis against which riboflavin seems to have a specific effect.[61]

It has been shown that there is no appreciable loss of appetite during ribo-flavin deficiency. On the contrary, there is a relatively increased food intake during the final stages of riboflavin deficiency.[34, 62] Pair-fed control rats grew much faster than the riboflavin-depleted rats. Consequently, riboflavin has been associated with an increased economy of food utilization.

2. Dogs and Foxes

Sebrell[63, 64] was probably the first to critically evaluate the pathological state in dogs now known to be due to a deficiency of riboflavin. Among the signs noted was the characteristic "yellow liver" due to fatty infiltration. Later, during studies of canine blacktongue, it was shown that riboflavin often prevents death in animals on blacktongue-producing diets.[65–67] With inadequate riboflavin, collapse, coma, and death occurred in less than 102 days. The onset was sudden and characterized by ataxia, weakness, and loss of deep reflexes, so that the dog was unable to stand. The animal appeared fully conscious and without pain prior to final collapse, as though death were due to a cellular asphyxia brought on by a failing chemical mechanism.[28] This collapse syndrome was also noted by Street and Cowgill[68] in dogs on diets which contained not more than traces of riboflavin.

Street et al.,[35] while investigating neurological manifestations of ribo-flavin deficiency, were not able to confirm the finding of fatty degeneration of the liver in their dogs. They noted myelin degeneration in peripheral nerves and in the posterior columns of the spinal cord, becoming more extensive with the length of the period on the deficient diet. Opacities of the cornea were also noted. The suggestion of these authors that inanition was the cause of previously published reports of fatty liver cannot be reconciled with the

[59a] M. M. Nelson, E. Sulon, H. Becks, and H. M. Evans, Proc. Soc. Exp. Biol. Med. 66, 631 (1947).
[60] H. Pinkerton and O. A. Bessey, Science 89, 368 (1939).
[61] P. György, Proc. Soc. Exp. Biol. Med. 38, 383 (1938).
[62] B. Sure and M. Dichek, J. Nutr. 21, 453 (1941).
[63] W. H. Sebrell, Pub. Health Rep. 44, 2697 (1929).
[64] W. H. Sebrell, Nat. Inst. Health Bull. 162, Part 3, 23 (1933).
[65] W. H. Sebrell, D. J. Hunt, and R. H. Onstott, Pub. Health Rep. 52, 235 (1937).
[66] W. H. Sebrell, R. H. Onstott, and D. J. Hunt, Pub. Health Rep. 52, 427 (1937).
[67] W. H. Sebrell and R. H. Onstott, Pub. Health Rep. 53, 83 (1938).
[68] H. R. Street and G. R. Cowgill, Amer. J. Physiol. 125, 323 (1939).

observations of Potter *et al.*,[69] who noted no fatty liver in their inanition-control dogs, whereas their riboflavin-deficient, choline-supplemented diets produced typical friable, fatty, yellow livers. Also noted was a dry, flaky dermatitis, usually accompanied by a marked erythema on the hind legs, chest, and abdomen, and a purulent discharge from the eye, which was associated with a conjunctivitis. This was followed in a few days by vascularization of the cornea, which in several dogs went on to corneal opacification.

Anemias have been noted in riboflavin-deficient dogs,[59, 69, 70] but it remains a question whether this is a specific part of the deficiency syndrome.

The deficiency symptoms that develop in the fox closely resemble those observed in the dog. Loss of weight, muscular weakness, coma, opacity of the lens, and fatty infiltration of the liver have been reported.[71]

3. PIGS

The similarity of vitamin B_2 deficiency in the pig to human pellagra was noted by Hughes[72] in 1938, and subsequent reports highlighted the economic importance of adequate riboflavin in the diet of swine.[73, 74] Patek *et al.*[75] characterized riboflavin deficiency in the pig as a syndrome including retarded growth, corneal opacities, dermatitis, changes in the hair and hoofs, and terminal collapse associated with hypoglycemia. These pigs showed changes in the corneal epithelium, lenticular cataracts, hemorrhages of the adrenals, and lipoid degeneration of the proximal convoluted tubules of the kidneys. Mitchell *et al.*[76] did not find any cataracts or corneal changes but did note anorexia and vomiting in their riboflavin-deficient pigs. They considered the absolute and relative neutrophilic granulocyte concentrations in the blood as the most sensitive indices of riboflavin deficiency.

4. YOUNG RUMINANTS

It is generally agreed that ruminants can meet most of their requirement of B-complex vitamins by intestinal synthesis. However, during the first days after birth the rumen of the young animal has not yet reached functional capacity, and unless riboflavin is supplied to the feed of young dairy calves, definite signs of riboflavin deficiency develop. Synthetic milk diets have been devised which do not favor normal rumen function.[77] On such diets the

[69] R. L. Potter, A. E. Axelrod, and C. A. Elvehjem, *J. Nutr.* **24**, 449 (1942).
[70] H. Spector, A. R. Maass, L. Michaud, C. A. Elvehjem, and E. B. Hart, *J. Biol. Chem.* **150**, 75 (1943).
[71] A. E. Schaefer, C. K. Whitehair, and C. A. Elvehjem, *J. Nutr.* **34**, 131 (1947).
[72] E. H. Hughes, *Hilgardia* **11**, 595 (1938).
[73] E. H. Hughes, *J. Nutr.* **20**, 233 (1940).
[74] M. M. Wintrobe, *Amer. J. Physiol.* **126**, 375 (1939).
[75] A. J. Patek, Jr., J. Post, and J. Victor, *Amer. J. Physiol.* **133**, 47 (1941).
[76] H. H. Mitchell, B. C. Johnson, T. S. Hamilton and W. T. Haines, *J. Nutr.* **41**, 317 (1950).
[77] A. C. Wiese, B. C. Johnson, H. H. Mitchell, and W. B. Nevens, *J. Nutr.* **33**, 268 (1947).

dairy calf develops hyperemia of the buccal mucosa, lesions in the corners of the mouth, along the edges of the lips, and around the navel, loss of appetite, scours, excessive salivation and lacrimation, and loss of hair.[77-79] Pounden and Hibbs[80] observed that the type of ration fed to calves was a controlling factor in the development of riboflavin-producing flora and fauna[81] in the rumen.

Riboflavin deficiency has also been observed in young lambs reared on artificial diets.[82]

5. OTHER MAMMALS

Mice show effects[83, 84, 84a] quite similar to those described for rats. A histological basis for the inhibition of lengthwise growth in riboflavin-deficient animals has been suggested in studies of endochondral ossification in mice.[85]

Rhesus monkeys[86] develop a freckled type of dermatitis on face, hands, legs, and groin, and a hypochromic, normocytic anemia, both of which are improved by riboflavin administration. Fatty livers which cannot be related to inanition have also been demonstrated in these monkeys.

The similarity between periodic ophthalmia in horses during the course of which corneal vascularization and cataracts frequently occur, and riboflavin deficiency in experimental animals, has suggested a possible common etiology.[87] It has been reported[88] that riboflavin is effective in preventing the appearance of equine periodic ophthalmia but that it does not influence the course of the disease in established cases. Studies of horses on diets low in riboflavin[89] have shown a correlation between their urinary excretion and their dietary intake. Cats develop cataracts if fed only slightly less than their minimum requirement.[89a]

6. BIRDS

The economic importance of poultry raising has stimulated much excellent research on the vitamin requirements of birds. The needs of chicks and fowls

[78] R. G. Warner and T. S. Sutton, *J. Dairy Sci.* **31**, 976 (1948).

[79] G. J. Brisson and T. S. Sutton, *J. Dairy Sci.* **34**, 28 (1951).

[80] W. D. Pounden and J. W. Hibbs, *J. Dairy Sci.* **30**, 582 (1947).

[81] W. D. Pounden and J. W. Hibbs, *J. Dairy Sci.* **31**, 1041 (1948).

[82] R. W. Luecke, R. Culik, F. Thorp, Jr., L. H. Blakeslee, and R. H. Nelson, *J. Amer. Sci.* **9**, 420 (1950).

[83] S. W. Lippincott and H. P. Morris, *J. Nat. Cancer Inst.* **2**, 601 (1942).

[84] P. F. Fenton and G. R. Cowgill, *J. Nutr.* **34**, 273 (1947).

[84a] B. E. Walker and B. Crain, Jr., *Proc. Soc. Exp. Biol. Med.* **107**, 404 (1961).

[85] B. M. Levy and R. Silberberg, *Proc. Soc. Exp. Biol. Med.* **63**, 355 (1946).

[86] J. M. Cooperman, H. A. Waisman, K. B. McCall, and C. A. Elvehjem, *J. Nutr.* **30**, 45 (1945).

[87] T. C. Jones, F. D. Mauer, and T. O. Roby, *Amer. J. Vet. Res.* **6**, 67 (1945).

[88] T. C. Jones, T. O. Roby, and F. D. Maurer, *Amer. J. Vet. Res.* **7**, 403 (1946).

[89] P. B. Pearson, M. K. Sheybani, and H. Schmidt, *Arch. Biochem.* **3**, 467 (1911).

[89a] S. N. Gershoff, S. B. Andrus, and D. M. Hegsted, *J. Nutr.* **68**, 75 (1959).

for growth and egg laying have been assayed by many investigators.[90-98] During these studies peculiar pathological syndromes have been observed which not only have advanced our understanding of riboflavin deficiency but also have been of major importance in the discovery of the more recently described vitamins of the B complex.

Phillips and Engel[99] have observed in chicks specific pathology in the main peripheral nerve trunks, characterized by degenerative changes in the myelin sheaths of the nerve fibers, which was quite similar to that seen during riboflavin deficiency in rats[47] on high-fat diets. A prolonged, mild deficiency produced a characteristic "curled-toe paralysis" in chickens.[99]

Riboflavin deficiency in turkeys[96, 100, 101, 101a] produced a severe dermatitis. Hegsted and Perry[98] did not observe any characteristic gross signs of riboflavin deficiency in the duckling; the animals failed to grow and died within a week.

M. K. HORWITT

E. In Man

A syndrome resembling pellagra (*pellagra sine pellagra*) has been known for centuries, but its relationship to the diet was first recognized by Stannus in 1911.[102, 103] His findings were generally confirmed and augmented by Bahr[104] (1912 to 1914) in Ceylon, Scott[105] (1918) in Jamaica, Moore[106, 107]

[90] F. H. Bird, V. S. Asmundson, F. H. Kratzer, and S. Lepkovsky, *Poultry Sci.* **25**, 47 (1946).

[91] R. M. Bethke and P. R. Record, *Poultry Sci.* **21**, 147 (1942).

[92] W. Bolton, *J. Agr. Sci.* **34**, 198 (1944).

[93] L. F. Leloir and D. E. Green, *Federation Proc.* **5**, 144 (1946).

[94] W. W. Cravens, H. J. Almquist, R. M. Bethke, L. C. Norris and H. W. Titus, "Recommended Nutritional Allowances for Poultry." Nat. Res. Counc., Washington, D.C., 1946.

[95] H. L. Lucas, G. F. Heuser, and L. C. Norris, *Poultry Sci.* **25**, 137 (1946).

[96] T. H. Jukes, E. L. R. Stokstad, and M. Belt, *J. Nutr.* **33**, 1 (1947).

[97] J. C. Fritz, W. Archer, and D. Barker, *Poultry Sci.* **18**, 449 (1939).

[98] D. M. Hegsted and R. L. Perry, *J. Nutr.* **35**, 411 (1948).

[99] P. H. Phillips and R. W. Engel, *J. Nutr.* **16**, 451 (1938).

[100] S. Lepkovsky and T. H. Jukes, *J. Nutr.* **12**, 515 (1936).

[101] T. H. Jukes, *Poultry Sci.* **17**, 227 (1938).

[101a] T. M. Ferguson, C. H. Whiteside, C. R. Creger, M. L. Jones, R. L. Atkinson, and J. R. Couch, *Poultry Sci.* **40**, 1151 (1961).

[102] H. S. Stannus, *Trans. Roy. Soc. Trop. Med. Hyg.* **5**, 112 (1912).

[103] H. S. Stannus, *Trans. Roy. Soc. Trop. Med. Hyg.* **7**, 32 (1913).

[104] P. H. Bahr, "A Report on Researches on Sprue in Ceylon, 1912–1914." Cambridge Univ. Press, London, 1915.

[105] H. H. Scott, *Ann. Trop. Med. Parasitol.* **12**, 109 (1918).

[106] D. G. F. Moore, *West Afr. Med. J.* **4**, 46 (1930).

[107] D. G. F. Moore, *J. Trop. Med. Hyg.* **42**, 109 (1939).

(1930) in West Africa, Landor and Pallister[108] (1935) in Singapore, and Ackroyd and Krishnan[109] (1936) In South India. Yeast products were first used therapeutically by Goldberger and Tanner[110] (1925) in their classic studies on induced pellagra, and by Fitzgerald[111] (1932), who reported an outbreak in an Assam prison of ulcerations at the angles of the mouth which were benefited by 1 oz of yeast daily.

The first suggestion that two separate dietary factors might be concerned in the production of clinical pellagra came from Goldberger et al.[112] in 1918, and what appears to have been riboflavin deficiency was produced on a casein diet by Goldberger and Tanner.[110] A clear-cut separation between these two deficiency states was not made until 1938, at which time both nicotinic acid and riboflavin were available. Sebrell and Butler[113, 114] studied a group of patients on a diet low in riboflavin and nicotinic acid and showed that the manifestations of *pellagra sine pellagra* were due to riboflavin deficiency.

1. ORAL AND FACIAL LESIONS OF ARIBOFLAVINOSIS

The changes observed by Sebrell and Butler[113–115] " consisted of lesions on the lips, which began with a pallor of the mucosa in the angles of the mouth. This pallor was soon followed by maceration; and within a few days superficial linear fissures, usually bilateral, appeared exactly in the corner of the mouth. These fissures showed very little inflammatory reaction, remained moist, and became covered with a superficial yellow crust, which could be scraped off without bleeding. In some instances these linear fissures showed a tendency to extend onto the skin of the face but did not extend into the mouth."

In addition, there was a " scaly, slightly greasy, desquamative lesion on a mildly erythematous base in the nasolabial folds, on the alae nasi, in the vestibule of the nose and occasionally on the ears and around the eyelids, especially at the inner and outer canthi."

In the years subsequent to the above presentation there have been many

108 V. J. Landor and R. A. Pallister, *Trans. Roy. Soc. Trop. Med. Hyg.* **19**, 121 (1935).
109 W. R. Ackroyd and B. G. Krishnan, *Indian J. Med. Res.* **24**, 411 (1936).
110 J. Goldberger and W. F. Tanner, *Pub. Health Rep.* **40**, 54 (1925).
111 G. H. Fitzgerald, *Indian Med. Gaz.* **67**, 556 (1932).
112 J. Goldberger, G. A. Wheeler, and E. Sydenstricker, *J. Amer. Med. Ass.* **71**, 944 (1918).
113 W. H. Sebrell and R. E. Butler, *Pub. Health Rep.* **53**, 2282 (1938).
114 W. H. Sebrell and R. E. Butler, *Pub. Health Rep.* **54**, 2121 (1939).
115 W. H. Sebrell, *in* "Biological Action of the Vitamins," p. 73, Univ. of Chicago Press, Chicago, Illinois, 1942.

"confirmatory" reports stemming from clinical observations of "aribo-flavinosis."[116–125] On the other hand, the failure of several groups to dupli-cate Sebrell and Butler's results and the frequency of angular stomatitis refractory to riboflavin therapy led to some skepticism regarding the syn-drome.[126] It is now apparent that the cause of failure in those studies in which the typical picture was not produced was either the brevity of the experimental period[127] or too high a level of riboflavin in the diet.[128–130] Williams et al.[128] fed a diet containing between 0.8 and 0.9 mg/day for over 9 months, and Keys et al.[129] gave 1.0 mg for 5 months without producing any clinical changes. Horwitt et al.[130] fed a diet containing between 0.8 and 0.9 mg of riboflavin daily for over 2 years, and only one of 22 subjects showed any signs (angular stomatitis) which might be attributed to a lack of ribo-flavin. However, when these workers[131–133] reduced the riboflavin intake to 0.55 mg/day, a level only slightly higher than that used by Sebrell and Butler, incontrovertible signs of ariboflavinosis appeared in less than 6 months. Subsequent studies[134] have confirmed these observations and have indicated that the course of the development and healing of the lesions was not altered by low dietary levels of nicotinic acid (6 mg) and tryptophan (250 mg).

The oral lesions which are generally accepted to be part of the clinical picture of riboflavinosis may be summarized as follows: angular stomatitis,

[116] N. P. Sydenstricker, L. E. Geeslin, C. M. Templeton, and J. W. Weaver, J. Amer. Med. Ass. 113, 1698 (1939).

[117] P. Manson-Bahr, Lancet II, 317, 356 (1940).

[118] R. W. Vilter, S. P. Vilter, and T. D. Spies, J. Amer. Med. Ass. 112, 420 (1939).

[119] J. W. Oden, L. H. Oden, Jr., and W. H. Sebrell, Pub. Health Rep. 54, 790 (1939).

[120] T. D. Spies, W. B. Bean, and W. F. Ashe, Ann. Intern. Med. 12, 1830 (1939).

[121] T. D. Spies, R. W. Vilter, and W. F. Ashe, J. Amer. Med. Ass. 113, 931 (1939).

[122] N. Jolliffe, H. D. Fein, and L. A. Rosenblum, New Engl. J. Med. 221, 921 (1939).

[123] H. D. Kruse, V. P. Sydenstricker, W. H. Sebrell, and H. M. Cleckley, Pub. Health Rep. 55, 157 (1940).

[124] V. P. Sydenstricker, W. H. Sebrell, H. M. Cleckley, and H. D. Kruse, J. Amer. Med. Ass. 114, 2437 (1940).

[125] T. D. Spies, W. B. Bean, R. W. Vilter, and N. E. Huff, Amer. J. Med. Sci. 200, 687 (1940).

[126] M. Ellenberg and H. Pollack, J. Amer. Med. Ass. 119, 790 (1942).

[127] J. J. Boehrer, C. E. Stanford, and E. Ryan, Amer. J. Med. Sci. 205, 544 (1943).

[128] R. D. Williams, H. L. Mason, P. L. Cusick, and R. M. Wilder, J. Nutr. 25, 361 (1943).

[129] A. Keys, A. F. Hensehel, O. Mickelson, J. H. Brozek, and J. H. Crawford, J. Nutr. 27, 165 (1944).

[130] M. K. Horwitt, E. Liebert, O. Kreisler, and P. Wittman, Bull. Nat. Res. Counc. (U.S.) 116 (1948).

[131] E. A. Zeller, Advan. Enzymol. Relat. Subj. Biochem. 2, 93 (1942).

[132] O. W. Hills, E. Liebert, D. L. Steinberg, and M. K. Horwitt, Arch. Intern. Med. 87, 682 (1951).

[133] M. K. Horwitt, C. C. Harvey, O. W. Hills, and E. Liebert, J. Nutr. 41, 247 (1950).

[134] M. K. Horwitt, C. C. Harvey, W. S. Rothwell, J. L. Cutler, and D. Haffron, J. Nutr. 60, Suppl. 1 (1956).

fissures in the angles of the mouth which resemble perleche, cheilosis, involvement of the vermilion border of the lips including vertical fissuring, and crusting and desquamation of the mucous membrane. Glossitis, including the magenta tongue, may be seen, but " pure " riboflavin deficiencies have been produced[132] without such defects.

The characteristic *facial* lesions include seborrheic accumulations in the folds of the skin, especially in the nasolabial folds. Mild infections of the upper respiratory tract may initiate an inflammation of the nostrils and spread as a weeping, crusty lesion over the skin of the septum. Fissures may appear in the nasolabial folds.

2. LESIONS OF SCROTUM AND VULVA

Stannus[102, 103] was the first to record that scrotal involvement may be the initial sign of deficiency (19 of 100 cases of " pellagra "). Sydenstricker[135, 136] noted an itching dermatitis of the scrotum or vulva in patients with pellagra. Purcell[137] described a scrotal dermatitis that improved with riboflavin treatment. Mitra[138] reported a urogenital lesion among Indians which responded to riboflavin. Goldberger and Wheeler[139] showed that six of their eleven patients exhibited scrotal dermatitis before any other lesions of pellagra appeared. In a later study[132] scrotal dermatitis was the most frequently observed symptom of riboflavin deficiency; twelve of fifteen subjects had it, either mildly or severely. Typically, this began as a patchy redness associated with scaling and desquamation of the superficial epithelium of the anterior surface of the scrotum. The median commissure was uninvolved in most of the patients. The more prolonged and severe cases showed a lichenification of the involved areas. The far-advanced lesion became quite raw and extended up the shaft of the penis or to the inner aspects of the thigh. The response to treatment with 6 mg of riboflavin/day was prompt, and in two cases with severe inflamation it was dramatic. This study emphasizes the question of the role of ariboflavinosis in the development of those scrotal and vulval lesions which have been considered characteristic of pellagra. Confirmation of the peculiar identification of scrotal dermatitis and ariboflavinosis was obtained by Lane *et al.*[139a] who produced a rapid development of most of the classic signs of riboflavin deficiency in 6 male adults by feeding galactoflavin.

[135] V. P. Sydenstricker, *Amer. J. Pub. Health Nat. Health* **31**, 344 (1941).

[136] V. P. Sydenstricker, *Ann. Intern. Med.* **14**, 1499 (1941).

[137] F. M. Purcell, *Trans. Roy. Soc. Trop. Med. Hyg.* **35**, 323 (1942).

[138] K. Mitra, *Indian Med. Gaz.* **78**, 330 (1943).

[139] J. Goldberger and G. A. Wheeler, *Pub. Health Serv. Hyg. Lab. Bull.* **126**, 116 (1920).

[139a] M. Lane, C. P. Alfrey, C. E. Mengel, M. A. Doherty, and J. Doherty, *J. Clin. Invest.* **43**, 357 (1964).

3. Ocular Manifestations

In experimental animals vascularization of the cornea and involvement of the lids are early and constant findings.[36, 38, 140] In man, ocular pathology is not constant, but it may occur in a high percentage of cases. Conjunctivitis, lacrimation, and burning of the eyes have been observed as manifestations which have been cured by riboflavin by sufficient investigators to be non-controversial; corneal vascularization in human riboflavin deficiencies has not been noted so often under controlled conditions.

Spies and his associates[120, 121] were among the first to note that the ocular lesions were cured by riboflavin administration. Sydenstricker and co-workers[116] reported that photophobia was associated with conjunctivitis. Reduced visual acuity, itching, a sensation of roughness of the eyelid keratitis, and mydriasis have also been reported.[116, 124, 141–143]

Rubeosis iridis has been suggested as a manifestation of deficiency that can be cured by riboflavin.[144] Vascular networks of the iris were markedly improved after only 2 days of riboflavin supplementation.

Kruse and colleagues[123, 124] reported corneal vascularization in forty-five of forty-seven patients with riboflavin deficiency. Proliferation and engorgement of the bulbar conjunctival capillaries of the limbar plexus were considered by them to be the earliest and most common sign of ariboflavinosis. As a consequence of many controversial reports,[145–151] the significance of these observations is not clear. No evidence of corneal vascularization was noted by the Elgin group[132] despite frequent slit-lamp examinations of subjects before, during, and after experimental riboflavin deficiency.

[140] R. F. Eckardt and L. V. Johnson, *Arch. Ophthalmol.* **21**, 315 (1939).

[141] H. C. Hou, *Chin. Med. J.* **59**, 344 (1941).

[142] P. H. Pock-Steen, *Geneesk. Tijdschr. Ned. Indie* **79**, 1980 (1939).

[143] P. R. Wilkinson, *Lancet* 11. 655 (1944).

[144] H. S. Stannus, *Trans. Ophthalmol. Soc. U.K.* **62**, 65 (1942).

[145] J. B. Youmans, E. W. Patton, W. D. Robinson, and R. Kern, *Trans. Ass. Amer. Physicians* **57**, 6 pp. (1942).

[146] H. R. Sandstead, *Pub. Health Rep.* **57**, 1821 (1942).

[147] D. Vail and K. W. Ascher, *Amer. J. Ophthalmol.* **26**, 1025 (1943).

[148] F. F. Tisdall, J. F. McCreary, and H. Pearce, *Can. Med. Ass. J.* **49**, 5 (1943).

[149] J. F. McCreary, J. V. V. Nicholls, and F. F. Tisdall, *Can. Med. Ass. J.* **51**, 106 (1944).

[150] H. S. Stannus, *Brit. Med. J.* 11, 103 (1944).

[151] J. G. Scott, *J. Roy. Army Med. Corps* **82**, 133 (1944).

XI. Pharmacology and Toxicology

M. K. HORWITT

The low solubility of riboflavin may be responsible for its relative innocuousness. Unna and Greslin[1] found that oral administration of 10 gm/kg to rats and 2 gm/kg to dogs produced no toxic effects. Giving 340 mg/kg to mice intraperitoneally, which is 5000 times the therapeutic dose, or the equivalent of 20 gm/day for a man, had no apparent effect.[2-4] The rat LD_{50} for riboflavin following intraperitoneal administration was 560 mg/kg.[1] Death, which was due to kidney concretions, occurred in 2 to 5 days. Similar results were obtained by Antopol[5] after intraperitoneal administration of 125–500 mg/kg of the sodium salt. In addition, cytological changes were noted in the heart, pancreas, and pituitary gland, and the adrenals were markedly congested.

Since crystalline concretions of riboflavin were readily detectable in the ureter and bladder within a few hours after a saturated solution of riboflavin was given intravenously, Selye[6] studied bilaterally nephrectomized rats to learn more about the role of the gastrointestinal tract in the absorption and excretion of riboflavin. He noted that excess riboflavin was rapidly excreted into the small intestine, especially the duodenum. Destruction of riboflavin proceeded slowly, if at all, in an isolated loop of duodenum, but quickly in an isolated large intestine. The bile does not function in the elimination of this vitamin. If the intestinal canal and kidneys are removed, the tissues of the rat cannot destroy or eliminate any significant percentage of large doses of intravenously administered riboflavin.

The riboflavin lost in sweat under tropical conditions[7] has been considered of nutritional importance. However, the amounts which can be proved to be present in sweat are too small to be significant.[8, 9]

Riboflavin is excreted predominantly in the feces, which contain not only the part contributed by the intestinal walls but also that which is synthesized by intestinal bacteria.[10]

[1] K. Unna and J. G. Greslin, *J. Pharmacol. Exp. Ther.* **76**, 75 (1942).
[2] R. Kuhn and P. Boulanger, *Hoppe-Seyler's Z. Physiol. Chem.* **241**, 233 (1936).
[3] R. Kuhn, *Klin. Wochenschr.* **17**, 222 (1938).
[4] V. Demole, *Z. Vitaminforsch.* **7**, 138 (1938).
[5] W. Antopol, *J. Med. Soc. N. J.* **39**, 285 (1942).
[6] H. Selye, *J. Nutr.* **25**, 137 (1943).
[7] D. M. Tennent and R. H. Silber, *J. Biol. Chem.* **148**, 359 (1943).
[8] O. Mickelsen and A. Keys, *J. Biol. Chem.* **149**, 479 (1943).
[9] F. Sargent, P. F. Robinson, and R. E. Johnson, *J. Biol. Chem.* **153**, 285 (1944).
[10] C. W. Denko, W. E. Grundy, N. C. Wheeler, C. R. Henderson, G. H. Berryman, T. E. Friedemann, and J. B. Youmans, *Arch. Biochem.* **11**, 109 (1946).

Urine contains riboflavin,[11] riboflavin phosphate,[12] and a compound called uroflavin,[13] a derivative which has been reported to be more soluble and to contain more oxygen than riboflavin. The methods of analysis ordinarily used for the estimation of riboflavin in urine do not distinguish between these compounds, since they have similar fluorimetric and microbiological activities.

The amount of riboflavin in the urine will vary with the recent dietary intake and with tissue storage. Urinary excretion of riboflavin will also be affected by marked alterations in nitrogen balance.[14–16] Less is excreted in the urine, on a given intake, when tissue growth is rapid, as during convalescence after severe trauma,[17] during lactation,[18] or after administration of testosterone propionate;[19] more is excreted after severe burns or surgical procedures where protein losses indicate cellular decomposition.[20]

The riboflavin content of the blood is relatively constant[21–23] (approximately 40 μg/100 ml) when measured by microbiological techniques. However, since the ingestion of riboflavin can cause a 30% increase in the flavin adenine dinucleotide content of the red blood cell,[24] it is likely that the use of improved methods[25] will show a correlation between dietary and erythrocyte content.

Although there is no appreciable storage capacity of riboflavin in animal tissues, it is apparent that the amount can vary, since the organs of animals will lose as much as two-thirds of their original content when the animals are fed riboflavin-deficient diets.[26–28] A combined protein and riboflavin deficiency is especially effective in decreasing the riboflavin content of the

[11] A. E. Axelrod, T. D. Spies, C. A. Elvehjem, and V. Axelrod, *J. Clin. Invest.* **20**, 229 (1941).

[12] A. Emmerie, *Acta Brevio. Neer. Physiol., Pharmacol., Microbiol.* **8**, 116 (1938).

[13] W. Koschara, *Hoppe-Seyler's Z. Physiol. Chem.* **232**, 101 (1935).

[14] H. P. Sarett and W. A. Perlzweig, *J. Nutr.* **25**, 173 (1943).

[15] H. P. Sarett, J. R. Klein, and W. A. Perlzweig, *J. Nutr.* **24**, 295 (1942).

[16] H. Pollack and J. J. Bookman, *J. Lab. Clin. Med.* **38**, 561 (1951).

[17] W. A. Andrea, V. Schenker, and J. S. L. Browne, *Fed. Proc. Fed. Amer. Soc. Exp. Biol.* **5**, 3 (1946).

[18] C. Roderuck, M. N. Coryell, H. H. Williams, and I. G. Macy, *J. Nutr.* **32**, 267 (1946).

[19] W. T. Beher and O. H. Gaebler, *J. Nutr.* **41**, 447 (1950).

[20] H. Pollack and S. L. Halpern, "Therapeutic Nutrition." Nat. Res. Counc., Washington, D.C., 1951.

[21] A. E. Axelrod, T. D. Spies, and C. A. Elvehjem, *Proc. Soc. Exp. Biol. Med.* **46**, 146 (1941)

[22] F. M. Strong, R. S. Feeney, B. Moore, and H. T. Parsons, *J. Biol. Chem.* **137**, 363 (1941).

[23] M. K. Horwitt, E. Liebert, O. Kreisler, and P. Wittman, *Bull. Nat. Res. Counc. (U.S.)* **116**, 1948.

[24] J. R. Klein and H. I. Kon, *J. Biol. Chem.* **136**, 177 (1940).

[25] H. B. Burch, O. A. Bessey, and O. H. Lowry, *J. Biol. Chem.* **175**, 457 (1948).

[26] R. Kuhn, H. Kaltschmitt, and T. Wagner-Jauregg, *Hoppe-Seyler's Z. Physiol. Chem.* **232**, 36 (1935).

[27] F. Vivanco, *Naturissenschaften* **23**, 306 (1935).

[28] A. E. Axelrod, H. A. Sober, and C. A. Elvehjem, *J. Biol. Chen.* **134**, 749 (1940).

tissues of the growing rat.[29] Diets on which signs of clinical ariboflavinosis are observed are usually low in protein.

The concept of a rational pharmacology based upon antivitamins, which was pioneered by Woolley,[30] has greatly stimulated the search for riboflavin antimetabolites. Wright and Sabine[31] have shown that flavin adenine dinucleotide lowered the atabrine inhibition of tissue respiration and of D-amino acid oxidase. This, and a similar observation by Haas[32] with respect to cytochrome reductase, led Hellerman et al.[33] to quantitize the metabolic antagonisms of antimalarials like atabrine and quinine.[34, 35] The phenazine analog of riboflavin,[36] as well as isoriboflavin,[37] when fed to mice and rats produced ariboflavinosis.

The effects of riboflavin derivatives on the growth of neoplasms have been receiving increasing attention. Antopol and Unna[38] and Miller and Miller[39] have shown that large amounts of riboflavin retarded the occurrence of pathological changes in liver produced by p-dimethylaminoazobenzene. Pollack et al.[40] noted that the concentration of riboflavin was lower in tumor than in normal tissue. Severe riboflavin deficiency decreased the growth rate of carcinomas[41, 42] in mice. This could be accomplished either by riboflavin deprivation or by administering[42] isoriboflavin or galactoflavin. Diethylriboflavin[43] and 6,7-dichloro-9-(1'-D-sorbityl)isoalloxazine[44] were effective in reducing the growth of tumors in rats.

[29] J. W. Czaczkes and K. Guggenheim, J. Biol. Chem. 162, 267 (1946).

[30] D. W. Woolley, Science 100, 579 (1945).

[31] C. I. Wright and J. C. Sabine, J. Biol. Chem. 155, 315 (1944).

[32] E. Haas, J. Biol. Chem. 155, 321 (1944).

[33] L. Hellerman, A. Lindsay, and M. R. Bovarnick, J. Biol. Chem. 163, 553 (1946).

[34] J. Madinaveitia, Biochem. J. 40, 373 (1946).

[35] F. H. Johnson and I. Lewin, Science 101, 281 (1945).

[36] D. W. Woolley, J. Biol. Chem. 154, 31 (1944).

[37] G. A. Emerson and M. Tishler, Proc. Soc. Exp. Biol. Med. 55, 184 (1944).

[38] W. Anfopol and K. Unna, Cancer Res. 2 694 (1942).

[39] E. C. Miller and J. A. Miller, Cancer Res. 7, 468 (1947).

[40] M. A. Pollack, A. Taylor, J. Taylor, and R. J. Williams, Cancer Res. 2, 739 (1942).

[41] H. P. Morris and W. van B. Robertson, J. Nat. Cancer Inst. 3, 479 (1943).

[42] H. C. Stoerk and G. A. Emerson, Proc. Soc. Exp. Biol. Med. 70, 703 (1943).

[43] H. V. Aposhian and J. P. Lambooy, Proc. Soc. Exp. Biol. Med. 78, 197 (1951).

[44] F. W. Holly, E. W. Peel, R. Mozingo, and K. Folkers, J. Amer. Chem. Soc. 72, 5416 (1950).

XII. Requirements and Factors Influencing Them

M. K. HORWITT

Any statement regarding the amount of riboflavin required must be a compromise depending upon variations in the heredity, growth, environment, age, activity, and health of the organism. The synthesis of riboflavin by the host and the differences in the availability of the vitamin from diverse sources must also be considered. With all these variables it is unlikely that there will ever be complete agreement among the workers in this field. Why, for example, only three out of fourteen men on identical diets low in ribo-flavin,[1] living in the same environment for over a year, should show relatively severe signs of ariboflavinosis, and why three others in the same group should show no signs of deficiency at all, are questions which will plague the investigator for years to come. The concept of "individual susceptibility" is an excuse which covers our ignorance and confounds those responsible for statements of recommended allowances. Whether to state the requirement in terms of protein needs or caloric intake is currently debatable. Although the writer prefers the theoretical concept that ties riboflavin and protein utilization together by using the factor 0.025 times the daily protein need, it must be conceded that it is simpler to tie the riboflavin requirement to the caloric expenditure.[1a] Urinary excretion of riboflavin is markedly affected by alterations in nitrogen balance.[1b] Less is excreted when tissue growth is rapid, during lactation,[1c] or after administration of testosterone propionate.[1d]

A. Of Animals

Table III presents representative published requirements of some mammals, birds, and fish. It is apparent from the data listed that there is not any unanimity of opinion. However, if one considers the ratio of riboflavin to food intake, it can be noted that 2–3 mg of riboflavin/kg of diet seems to satisfy most of the suggested requirements. Such a figure is only of approximate value, since the protein, fat, and carbohydrate proportions of the diet will vary widely.

[1] M. K. Horwitt, O. W. Hills, C. C. Harvey, E. Liebert, and D. L. Steinberg, *J. Nutr.* **39**, 357 (1949).
[1a] F. Bro-Rasmussen, *Nutr. Abst. Rev.* **28**, 1 and 369 (1958).
[1b] J. M. Smith, S. D. C. Lu, A. Hare, E. Dick, and M. Daniels, *J. Nutr.* **69**, 85 (1959).
[1c] C. Roderuck, M. N. Coryell, H. H. Williams, and I. G. Macy, *J. Nutr.* **32**, 267 (1946).
[1d] W. T. Beher and O. H. Gaebler, *J. Nutr.* **41**, 447 (1950).

1. EFFECT OF DIETARY CONSTITUENTS

It has been shown[10, 28, 29] that the fat content of the diet has a marked effect on the riboflavin requirement of the rat. Thus, the replacement of the dextrin in a rat diet with isocaloric amounts of fat increased the amount of riboflavin needed for growth and enabled the production of more severe deficiency symptoms. Riboflavin appeared to play no part in the synthesis of fat, carbohydrate, and protein.[30, 31] Extra fat gained by rats on high-ribo-flavin diets may result from the sparing of dietary fat through more efficient utilization of dietary energy.[32] Reiser and Pearson[33] found that cottonseed oil in the diet of chicks increased the requirement of riboflavin. Rats fed a diet containing only 2% of calories as fat required half as much riboflavin as rats fed the standard 20% fat diet, and rats on the latter diet, in turn, required half as much riboflavin as those fed 40% of their calories as fat.[8]

It is not possible to vary the amount of fat in a diet without changing the relative concentration of the other constituents. The effects of high-fat, low-fat, high-protein, and low-protein diets on riboflavin requirements of the rat were studied simultaneously by Czaczkes and Guggenheim.[8] They noted that rats on low-protein diets needed at least twice as much riboflavin as animals kept on a "normal" diet. These authors believe that the different requirements for riboflavin are due to differences in the amounts of riboflavin which are synthesized in an available form.

Studies by Everson et al.[34] have stressed the importance of complete digestion in evaluating the availability of riboflavin in various foods. Working with young women, they observed that a larger proportion of riboflavin was available from ice cream than from legumes or almonds.

Large doses of ascorbic acid or Aureomycin can prevent or delay signs of riboflavin deficiency in rats. Daft and Schwarz[35] have reported that ribo-flavin-deficient rats died as expected, but that on identical diets plus 2% ascorbic acid or 20 mg/100 ml Aureomycin littermates survived.

2. EFFECT OF ENVIRONMENT

Working with rats at environmental temperatures of 90 and 68° F, Mills[7] concluded that the dietary concentration of riboflavin needed for maximum

[28] J. H. Shaw and P. H. Phillips, J. Nutr. 22, 345 (1941).

[29] G. J. Mannerling, D. Orsini, and C. A. Elvehjem, J. Nutr. 28, 141 (1944).

[30] E. W. McHenry and G. Gavin, J. Biol. Chem. 125, 653 (1938).

[31] E. W. McHenry and G. Gavin, J. Biol. Chem. 138, 471 (1941).

[32] L. Voris and H. P. Moore, J. Nutr. 25, 7 (1943).

[33] R. Reiser and P. B. Pearson, J. Nutr. 38, 247 (1949).

[34] G. Everson, E. Pearson, and R. Matteson, J. Nutr. 46, 45 (1952).

[35] F. S. Daft and K. Schwarz, Fed. Proc. Fed. Amer. Soc. Exp. Biol. 11, 200 (1952).

TABLE III
SOME REPORTED RIBOFLAVIN REQUIREMENTS

Animal	Amount	Reference
Mice	1.5 μg/gm food	2, 3
	4 μg/day	4
	0.4–0.6 mg/100 gm body wt.	5
Rat	2–3 μg/gm food	6, 7
	7.5 μg/day	8
	10 μg/day	9
	18 μg/day	10
Dog	60–100 μg/kg body wt./day	11
	100–200 μg/kg body wt./day	12
Swine	20–66 μg/kg body wt./day	13
	1.7 mg/kg feed	14
Fox	1.2–4.0 μg/gm 'iet	15
Cat	3–4/μg/gm food	15a
Horse	44 μg/kg body wt./day	16
Holstein calf	1.0 mg/kg feed	17
Monkey	25–30 μg/kg body wt./day	18
Chick	2.75–3.25 μg/gm food	19
	2.9–3.6 μg/gm food	20, 21

[2] H. P. Morris and W. B. Robertson, *J. Nat. Cancer Inst.* **3**, 479 (1943).

[3] W. C. Langston, P. L. Day, and K. W. Cosgrove, *Arch. Ophthalmol.* **10**, 508 (1933).

[4] S. W. Lippincott and H. P. Morris, *J. Nat. Cancer Inst.* **2**, 601 (1942).

[5] P. F. Fenton and G. R. Cowgill, *J. Nutr.* **34**, 273 (1947).

[6] H. C. Sherman and L. N. Ellis, *J. Biol. Chem.* **104**, 91 (1934).

[7] C. A. Mills, *Arch. Biochem.* **2**, 159 (1943).

[8] J. W. Czaczkcs and K. Guggenheim, *J. Biol. Chem.* **162**, 267 (1946).

[9] G. C. Supplee, R. C. Bender, and O. J. Kahlenberg, *J. Nutr.* **20**, 109 (1940).

[10] G. F. Mannerling, M. A. Lipton, and C. A. Elvehjem, *Proc. Soc. Exp. Biol. Med.* **46**, 100 (1941).

[11] R. L. Potter, A. E. Axelrod, and C. A. Elvehjem, *J. Nutr.* **24**, 449 (1942).

[12] H. R. Street and G. R. Cowgill, *Amer. J. Physiol.* **125**, 323 (1939).

[13] E. H. Hughes, *J. Nutr.* **20**, 233 (1940).

[14] E. H. Hughes, E. W. Crampton, N. R. Ellis, and W. J. Loeffel, "Recommended Nutrient Allowances for Swine, Report of Committee on Animal Nutrition." Nat. Res. Counc. Washington, D.C., 1944.

[15] A. E. Schaefer, C. K. Whitehair, and C. A. Elvehjem, *J. Nutr.* **34**, 131 (1947).

[15a] S. N. Gershoff, S. B. Andrus, and D. M. Hegsted, *J. Nutr.* **68**, 75 (1959).

[16] P. B. Pearson, M. K. Sheybani, and H. Schmidt, *Arch. Biochem.* **3**, 467 (1944).

[17] H. H. Draper and B. C. Johnson, *J. Nutr.* **46**, 37 (1952).

[18] J. M. Cooperman, H. A. Waisman, K. B. McCall, and C. A. Elvehjem, *J. Nutr.* **30**, 45 (1945).

[19] F. H. Bird, U. S. Asmundson, F. H. Kratzer, and S. Lepkovsky, *Poultry Sci.* **25**, 47 (1946).

[20] L. C. Norris, H. S. Wilgus, A. T. Ringrose, V. Heiman, and C. F. Heuser, *Cornell Univ. Agr. Exp. Sta. Bull.* **660**, 3 (1936).

[21] R. M. Bethke and P. R. Record, *Poultry Sci.* **21**, 147 (1942).

TABLE III—*continued*

Animal	Amount	Reference
Poult	3.25–3.75 μg/gm food	19
	3–4 μg/gm food	22, 23
Duck	3 μg/gm food	24,25
Trout	5–15 μg/gm food	26
	6–9 μg/gm food	27

growth was not altered by temperature. Mitchell *et al.*,[36] using pigs as their experimental animals, have claimed that the riboflavin requirement is greater (2.3 ppm at 42° F) at low temperatures than at high temperatures (1.2 ppm at 85° F).

3. REPRODUCTION

Barrett and Everson[37] indicated that the need for B vitamins increased rapidly as pregnancy[38] progressed in the rat. Hogan and Anderson[39] showed that a synthetic diet slightly inadequate for growth was seriously inadequate for lactation. It is reasonable to expect lactation to increase the requirement, since logically the need for mother and offspring is greater than that of the mother alone.

4. INHERENT INDIVIDUAL VARIATIONS

Those who have worked with animals in nutritional studies are acutely aware of the individual variations that will occur, even in closely inbred littermates. Fenton and Cowgill[5] have highlighted this problem by studying the riboflavin requirements of two inbred strains of mice. Mice of the C_{57} strain showed maximum growth when the diet contained 0.4 mg of riboflavin per 100 gm whereas those of the A strain required a dietary level of 0.6 mg. At a

[22] W. W. Cravens, H. J. Almquist, R. M. Bethke, L. C. Norris, and H. W. Titus, " Recommended Nutritional Allowances for Poultry." Nat. Res. Counc., Washington, D.C., 1946.

[23] T. H. Jukes, E. L. R. Stokstad, and M. Belt, *J. Nutr.* **33**, 1 (1947).

[24] J. C. Fritz, W. Archer, and D. Barker, *Poultry Sci.* **18**, 449 (1939).

[25] D. M. Hegsted and R. L. Perry, *J. Nutr.* **35**, 411 (1948).

[26] B. A. McLaren, E. Keller, D. J. O'Donnell, and C. A. Elvehjem, *Arch. Biochem.* **15**, 169 (1947).

[27] A. V. Tunison, D. R. Brockway, J. M. Maxwell, A. L. Dorr, and C. M. McCay. N. Y. State Conservation Dep. Cortland Hatchery Rep. No. 11 (1942).

[36] H. H. Mitchell, B. C. Johnson, T. S. Hamilton, and W. T. Haines, *J. Nutr.* **41**, 317 (1950).

[37] M. Barrett and G. Everson, *J. Nutr.* **45**, 493 (1951).

[38] G. Everson, E. Williams, E. Wheeler, P. Swanson, M. Spivey, and M. Eppright, *J. Nutr.* **36**, 463 (1948).

[39] A. G. Hogan and G. C. Anderson, *J. Nutr.* **36**, 437 (1948).

0.2-mg level the C_{57} mice had lowered red cell counts and less riboflavin in their muscle and liver than those of the A strain on the same diet.

5. OTHER FACTORS

There have been suggestions that the growth requirements of male and female rats are different,[32] the overall effects of riboflavin deficiency being more prominent in the male. Unlike thiamine deficiency, the lack of ribo-flavin is not associated with severe anorexia; thus, appetite is not so important a factor in riboflavin depletion studies. The interrelationships between ribo-flavin and other vitamins of the B group have been studied.[40]

B. Of Man

In the absence of experimental data on human subjects, the estimation of riboflavin requirements is based upon average dietary consumptions or upon extrapolations of data from animal experiments. Calculation of average consumption is not a satisfying procedure, since different locales will show great variations depending upon dietary habits and the availability of ribo-flavin-rich foods. Attempts to calculate man's needs from data on rat growth tend to give figures that are too high to be practical. It is therefore necessary to test vitamin requirements on man, himself.

It is logical to expect that the minimum requirements of human beings would be much more variable than for the inbred laboratory animal. That this is the case was illustrated by Horwitt et al.,[1, 41] who studied fifteen men on a diet providing 0.55 mg of riboflavin/day. Three of the men developed relatively severe dermatological lesions, nine men showed mild symptoms of ariboflavinosis, and three others had no symptoms at all.

Excretion studies which compare the amount of riboflavin intake with the amount excreted in the urine have been used for many years as a means of estimating human requirements. Much confusion has resulted from this approach because there is, as yet, no agreement upon how much riboflavin should be excreted before the intake is considered adequate.

In some of the older studies on riboflavin excretion[42-44] the diet was not considered adequate if it contained less than 2 mg of riboflavin/day. Conse-quently, urinary excretion of less than 500 μg/day were designated as deficient. More recent comparative studies on the amounts of riboflavin excreted in the urine on different levels of intake have shown that a reserve of riboflavin

[40] K. Bhagyat and P. Devi, *Biochem. J.* **45**, 32 (1949).
[41] O. W. Hills, E. Liebert, D. L. Steinberg, and M. K. Horwitt, *Arch. Intern. Med.* **87**, 682 (1951).
[42] A. Emmerie, *Nature (London)* **138**, 164 (1936).
[43] F. M. Strong, R. S. Feeney, B. Moore, and H. T. Parsons, *J. Biol. Chem.* **137**, 363 (1941).
[44] V. H. Feder, G. T. Lewis, and H. S. Alden, *J. Nutr.* **27**, 347 (1944).

cannot be maintained by men at levels of intake below 1.1 mg/day[45] on a diet containing approximately 2200 cal. Brewer et al.[46] calculated the requirement of women to be 1.3–1.5 mg/day on a diet providing 2100–2300 cal/day.

The recommended daily allowances of the Food and Nutrition Board of the National Research Council state that 1.7 mg of riboflavin is adequate for a 70-kg adult man, and 1.5 mg for a 56-kg adult woman. The assumption was made that increased work and greater than average caloric consumption do not increase the need for riboflavin. The allowances during the latter half of pregnancy and during lactation were increased to 1.8 and 2.0 mg, respectively. There is as yet no proof that more than the normal daily allowance is required during pregnancy. This problem was reviewed by Oldham et al.[47] If one estimates the total amount of riboflavin stored during the gestation period, it seems likely that an additional 0.2 mg/day should satisfy the needs for growth during pregnancy. The increased allowance for lactation makes ample provision for the amount in human milk, which contains about 0.5 mg of riboflavin/liter.

The recommended allowances for children are graduated in accordance with the growth rate at different ages. It has been recommended that children from 1 to 3 years old be allowed 0.6 mg/day, and that children 6 to 9 years old be allowed 1.2 mg/day. During the rapid period of growth from 13 to 15 years of age, it has been recommended that both girls and boys receive 1.5 mg of riboflavin/day. It is apparent that, since these allowances are adjusted for growth requirements, the actual need of an individual will vary with his or her own pattern of growth.

One of the major goals of all the research described in these sections is to determine how much riboflavin is required by man for optimum nutritional health. The techniques used may be classified under four headings: (1) observations of the repair of pathology by riboflavin administration; (2) survey studies of the nutritional status of population groups; (3) experimental production of riboflavin deficiency; and (4) evaluation of urinary excretion of riboflavin in health and disease.

Riboflavin deficiency states ordinarily noted by the clinician, whose primary obligation is to facilitate the repair of apparent pathology, do not often present adequate opportunities to assay the individual's need for riboflavin. The important contributions of these observations are in the classifications of conditions which can be healed by riboflavin, usually given in amounts far in excess of the daily requirement. Without these classifications the researcher in nutrition would not know what to look for.

Excellent examples of the population survey type of study have been

[45] M. K. Horwitt, C. C. Harvey, O. W. Hills, and E. Liebert, J. Nutr. 41, 247 (1950).
[46] W. Brewer, T. Porter, B. Ingalls, and M. A. Ohlson, J. Nutr. 32, 583 (1946).
[47] H. G. Oldham, B. B. Sheft, and T. Porter, J. Nutr. 41, 231 (1950).

described by Goldsmith[48] and by Wilkins and Sebrell.[49] Wilder[50] has summarized the extensive surveys of malnutrition in Newfoundland[51-53] to show
how the enrichment of flour benefited the population. But, although these
surveys were of great value to our understanding of the nutrition of population groups, they are difficult to interpret in terms of the requirement of the
individual.

The experimental production of riboflavin deficiency has been successful
only in these studies in which levels of 0.55 mg of riboflavin/day or less have
been fed. Those investigators who provided 0.8 mg/day to their subjects could
not produce signs of ariboflavinosis. Nevertheless, no nutritional authority
has yet suggested that 0.8 mg is adequate for optimal health. Rather, one
recommends amounts which provide somewhat more than the minimal
daily need as fortification against unknown contingencies. The concept that
riboflavin cannot be stored may not be entirely correct, since even at dietary
levels of 0.5 mg/day about 6 months must elapse before signs of ariboflavinosis appear.

One of the more important advantages of depletion studies is the opportunity provided for simultaneous investigation of urinary excretion. Since the
urinary excretion is a reflection of the dietary intake and the dietary intake is,
in the last analysis, the cause of riboflavin deficiency, it is understandable why
so much effort has been devoted to the study of riboflavin in urine.

Load tests, in which a known amount of riboflavin is administered and the
percentage excreted is determined, are useful means of estimating the degree
of saturation of the tissues. Although the usual procedure is to administer
riboflavin in the postabsorptive state and to analyze the riboflavin excreted
during the following 4 hours, a 24-hour collection may be considered a load
test if the dietary intake during that period is known. Goldsmith[54] has
reviewed the literature on the use of urinary excretion tests in the evaluation of
riboflavin nutrition. Oldham et al.[55] and Pollack and Bookman[56] have shown
that increased amounts of riboflavin are excreted by subjects in marked
negative nitrogen balance. Therefore, in those special cases where tests for

[48] G. A. Goldsmith, Fed. Proc. Fed. Amer. Soc. Exp. Biol. 4, 263 (1945).

[49] W. Wilkins and W. H. Sebrell, Fed. Proc. Fed. Amer. Soc. Exp. Biol. 4, 258 (1945).

[50] R. M. Wilder, Fed. Proc. Fed. Amer. Soc. Exp. Biol. 9, 562 (1950).

[51] G. A. Goldsmith, W. J. Darby, R. C. Steinkemp, A. S. Beam, and E. McDevitt, J. Nutr.
40, 41 (1950).

[52] J. D. Adamson, N. Jolliffe, H. D. Kruse, O. H. Lowry, P. E. Moore, B. S. Platt, W. H.
Sebrell, J. W. Tice, F. F. Tisdall, R. M. Wilder, and P. C. Zamecnik, Can. Med. Ass. J.
52, 227 (1945).

[53] W. R. Aykroyd, N. Jolliffe, O. H. Lowry, P. E. Moore, W. H. Sebrell, R. E. Shank,
F. F. Tisdall, R. M. Wilder, and P. C. Zamecnik, Can. Med. Ass. J. 60, 329 (1949).

[54] G. A. Goldsmith, Fed. Proc. Fed. Amer. Soc. Exp. Biol. 8, 553 (1949).

[55] H. Oldham, E. Lounds, and T. Porter, J. Nutr. 34, 69 (1947).

[56] H. Pollack and J. J. Bookman, J. Lab. Clin. Med. 38, 561 (1951).

TABLE IV[45]

COMPARISON OF URINARY EXCRETION WITH DAILY INTAKE OF RIBOFLAVIN. EXCEPT FOR
THOSE ON THE 0.55-MG DIET, THE DATA LISTED REPRESENT PLATEAU LEVELS WHICH
WERE REACHED IN 10 WEEKS OR LESS ON THE INTAKE DESIGNATED[a]

Number of subjects on each intake	Riboflavin intake (mg)	Duration of diet at time of analyses (weeks)[b]	Riboflavin excretion, 24 hours		Excretion during 4 hours following subcutaneous injection of 1 mg of riboflavin (μg)
			Amount (μg)	Ingested riboflavin (%)	
15	0.55	15	51 ± 11	9.3	23 ± 15[c]
11	0.75	12	73 ± 5	9.7	56 ± 34
12	0.85	15	76 ± 38	8.9	58 ± 22
28	1.1	13	97 ± 62	8.8	70 ± 35
39	1.6	100	434 ± 185	26.5	227 ± 146
12	2.15	10–78	714 ± 293	33.2	297 ± 124
13	2.55	2–44	849 ± 258	33.3	298 ± 172
13	3.55	1.5	1714 ± 300[d]	48.3[d]	373 ± 90[d]

[a] At an 0.85-mg intake or higher the figures obtained at 15 weeks remain at the same level for at least 2 years more. At a 0.75-mg intake most of the subjects remained at the level designated for 6 months, at which time they were supplemented. A few individuals who remained longer on this diet showed no further change, but whether or not their excretions would have decreased further with additional time is not known.

[b] The time of analyses for diets providing 0.75, 0.85, and 1.1 mg of riboflavin represents the first time plateau levels were obtained which were repeated during subsequent months. The results recorded for the diets providing 1.6, 2.15, and 2.55 mg are averages of voluminous data obtained during the period of time indicated.

[c] After 7 weeks.

[d] These results were obtained from the same individuals who received the 2.55-mg intake. After 62 weeks on this intake, their supplementation was further increased to provide a 3.55-mg intake. The values for the 24- and 4-hour excretion periods were obtained 1.5 and 3 weeks, respectively, after the change in supplementation.

riboflavin excretion are made on patients who are catabolizing abnormal amounts of their own tissues, the excretion data may be higher than normally expected. There is a high degree of agreement in the results of excretion studies by different laboratories of subjects on low levels of riboflavin intake,[45, 57–62] but the variations are greater when the test dose or daily

[57] C. W. Denko, W. E. Grundy, N. C. Wheeler, C. R. Henderson, G. H. Berryman, T. E. Friedemann, and J. B. Youmans, *Arch. Biochem.* 11, 109 (1946).

[58] R. D. Williams, H. L. Mason, P. L. Cusick, and R. M. Wilder, *J. Nutr.* 25, 361 (1943).

[59] A. Keys, A. F. Henschel, O. Mickelsen, J. H. Brozek, and J. H. Crawford, *J. Nutr.* 27, 165 (1944).

[60] V. A. Najjar and L. E. Holt, *Bull. Johns Hopkins Hosp.* 69, 476 (1941).

[61] H. G. Oldham, F. A. Johnston, S. C. Kleiger, and H. Hedderich-Arismandi, *J. Nutr.* 27, 435 (1944).

[62] M. V. Davis, H. G. Oldham, and L. J. Roberts, *J. Nutr.* 32, 143 (1946).

intake is more than 1 mg.[44, 63-66] Table IV presents a summary of the urinary excretions obtained by the Elgin group[45] at different levels of dietary intake.

Tucker et al.[67] studied the urinary excretions of normal men under a variety of environmental conditions to note that meals, acute starvation, hard work, heat stress, and bed rest, all of which increase nitrogen excretion, increased riboflavin excretion. Sleep slowed the rate of excretion, but diuresis, induced by water, had no effect.

[63] A. E. Axelrod, T. D. Spies, C. A. Elvehjem, and V. Axelrod, J. Clin. Invest. 20, 229 (1941).

[64] F. T. Lossy, G. A. Goldsmith, and H. P. Sarett, J. Nutr. 45, 213 (1951).

[65] C. A. Conners, R. E. Eckardt, and L. V. Johnson, Arch. Ophthalmol. 29, 956 (1943).

[66] R. E. Johnson, C. Henderson, P. F. Robinson, and F. C. Consolazio, J Nutr. 30, 89 (1945).

[67] R. G. Tucker, O. Mickelsen, and A. Keys, J. Nutr. 72, 251 (1960).

CHAPTER 15

THIAMINE

I. Nomenclature

ROBERT S. HARRIS

Accepted name:	Thiamine (U.S.A.)
	Aneurin (Brit. Pharm.)
Obsolete names:	Vitamin B_1
	Oryzamin
	Torulin
	Polyneuramin
	Vitamin F
	Antineuritic vitamin
	Antiberiberi vitamin
Empirical formula:	$C_{12}H_{17}N_4OSCl \cdot HCl$
Chemical name:	3-(4-Amino-2-methylpyrimidyl-5-methyl)-4-methyl-5-β-hydroxyethylthiazolium chloride hydrochloride

Structure:

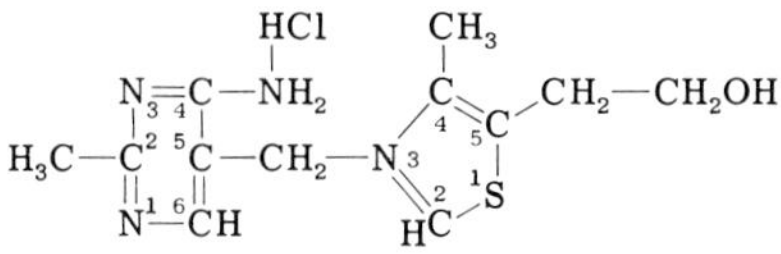

Thiamine-HCl

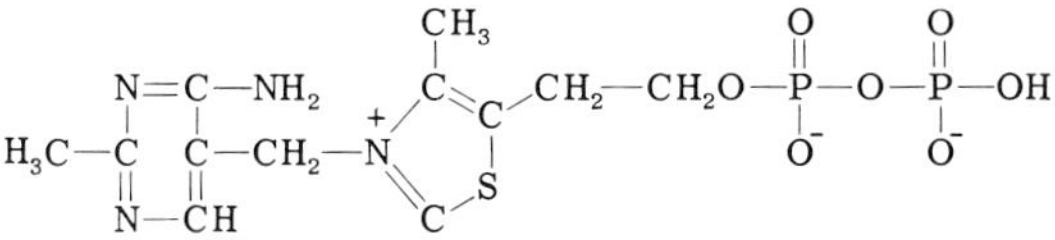

Cocarboxylase

II. Chemistry

B. C. P. JANSEN

A. Isolation

After Eijkman's discovery that polished rice was the cause of polyneuritis in birds and of beriberi in men, Grijns,[1] his successor in Batavia, was the first to state that these diseases were the result of a "partial hunger," a deficiency of some unknown substance that is present in very small quantities in the outer layers (the silverskin) of the rice. Grijns called this substance "the protective substance"; Grijns also made the first attempts to isolate this substance from an extract from the silverskin of the rice. He succeeded in getting highly active fractions, but did not obtain a pure substance. About 10 years later Casimir Funk, working in the Lister Institute in London, obtained a crystalline substance from rice polishings.[2] He coined the word "vitamine"—an amine essential for life—for it. It was proved afterwards however, that this product had no antineuritic activity, and consequently it

---

[1] l. by Prof. Dr. G. Grijns, "Researches on Vitamins 1900–1911." J. Noorduijn en Zoon, Gorinchem, 1935.)

[2] C. Funk, *J. Physiol.* (*London*) **43**, 395 (1911), "Die Vitamine." Bergmann, München and Wiesbaden, 1922.

was not the desired substance. As it was shown subsequently that several "vitamines" were not amines at all, Drummond[3] proposed that the final "e" of the name "vitamine" be dropped.

In 1926 Jansen and Donath, working in the same laboratory where Eijkman and Grijns had made their researches, obtained the crystalline substance having a great antineuritic activity.[4] They sent 40 mg of it to Eijkman, who was at that time in the Netherlands. Eijkman was able to confirm the prophylactic and curative activities of this substance against avian polyneuritis.[5] Eijkman confessed that, before he received these crystals, he had doubted if the vitamin would be a normal chemical single substance. Jansen and Donath succeeded in the isolation because they used the finding of Seidell[6] that the antineuritic substance is adsorbed by fuller's earth, and furthermore they found a fairly quick method (i.e., 10 days) for testing the antineuritic activity of the different fractions by the use of small rice birds (*Munia maja*).

About 10 years later several workers in the United States, Germany, and England improved the method of isolation and thereby obtained sufficient quantities to establish its structural formula and to find methods for its synthesis (Williams and Cline;[7] Grewe;[8] Andersag and Westphal;[9] Todd and Bergel[10]).

B. Chemical and Physical Properties

Thiamine hydrochloride crystallizes into colorless, monoclinic needles, which have a melting point of about 250°C, a characteristic smell, and a slightly bitter taste. These crystals are stable to the atmospheric oxygen. They are very soluble in water, much less so in alcohol, and insoluble in ether and other fat solvents. Thiamine chloride hydrochloride crystallizes from alcoholic aqueous solutions as the hemihydrate, $C_{12}H_{17}ON_4SCl \cdot HCl \cdot \frac{1}{2}H_2O$. Thiamine hydrochloride in water forms a strongly acid solution pH of a 5% solution about 3.5; in solution with a pH less than 5 it is fairly stable to heat and oxidation; this solution shows two absorption bands in the ultraviolet at 235 and 267 mμ.

At a pH of 5 or higher, it is destroyed by autoclaving, and at a pH of 7 or more by boiling or merely storing at room temperature.

[3] J. C. Drummond, *Biochem. J.* **14**, 660 (1920).
[4] B. C. P. Jansen and W. F. Donath, *Proc. Kon. Akad. Wetensch. Amsterdam*, **29**, 1390 (1926).
[5] C. Eijkman, *Proc. Kon. Akad Wetensch. Amsterdam*, **30**, 376 (1927).
[6] A. Seidell, *Pub. Health Rep. (US.)* **31**, 364 (1916).
[7] R. R. Williams and J. K. Cline, *J. Amer. Chem. Soc.* **58**, 1504 (1936).
[8] R. Crewe, *Hoppe-Seyler's Z. Physiol. Chem.* **242**, 89 (1936).
[9] H. Andersag and K. Westphal, *Ber. Deut. Chem. Ges.* **70**, 2035 (1937).
[10] A. R. Todd and F. Bergel, *J. Chem. Soc. London* p. 364 (1937).

By treatment with sulfite it is readily split into the pyrimidine and thiazole parts.

In a highly alkaline solution thiamine is oxidized by ferricyanide to thiochrome.

C. Constitution

The work of the above-mentioned investigators has shown that the thiamine molecule consists of a pyrimidine compound and a thiazole compound, connected by a CH_2 bridge. The structural formula of the thiamine hydrochloride is:

The elucidation of the constitution was greatly relieved by the discovery of Williams *et al.*[11] that thiamine is quantitatively split by sulfite in faintly acid solutions into the pyrimidine and the thiazole halves:

$$C_{12}H_{18}ON_4SCl_2 + Na_2SO_3 = C_6H_9N_3SO_3 + C_6H_9NSO + 2NaCl$$

D. Synthesis

The synthesis of thiamine has been performed in different ways. It is possible to synthesize the pyrimidine nucleus and the thiazole nucleus separately and afterwards to connect both parts. It is also possible to synthesize one of the nuclei with an extra side branch and afterwards to build up the other ring from this side branch.

For synthesizing the pyrimidine part, ethyl formate and β-ethoxyethylpropionate may be condensed with Na.

This product is condensed with acetamidine.

The hydroxyl group is converted into an NH_2 group by treating first with

[11] R. R. Williams, E. R. Buchman, and A. E. Ruehle, *J. Amer. Chem. Soc.* **57**, 536 (1935).

POCl$_3$ and then with NH$_3$. The ethoxy group is converted into a bromide. Thus the final product is

$$
\begin{array}{c}
\text{N}{=}\text{C}^{\displaystyle \diagup \text{NH}_2 \cdot \text{HBr}} \\
\text{CH}_3\text{C} \quad \text{C}{-}\text{CH}_2\text{Br} \\
\text{N}{-}\text{CH}
\end{array}
$$

The thiazole moiety may be synthesized in several ways (cf. Buchman;[12] Clarke and Gurin[13]). The method of Buchman consists in condensing thioformamide with bromoacetopropanol.

$$
\begin{array}{c}
\text{NH}_2 \\
\text{C}{-}\text{H} \\
\text{S}
\end{array}
\; + \; \text{CH}_3\cdot\text{CO}\cdot\text{CHBr}\cdot\text{CH}_2\cdot\text{CH}_2\text{OH} \longrightarrow
\begin{array}{c}
\text{N}{-\!-}\text{C}\cdot\text{CH}_3 \\
\text{HC} \diagdown \text{S} \diagup \text{C}\cdot\text{CH}_2\cdot\text{CH}_2\text{OH}
\end{array}
$$

By heating the hydrobromide of the pyrimidine compound with the thiazole compound, the thiamine hydrobromide is formed.

$$
\begin{array}{c}
\text{N}{=}\text{C}^{\displaystyle \diagup \text{NH}_2 \cdot \text{HBr}} \\
\text{CH}_3\cdot\text{C} \quad \text{C}\cdot\text{CH}_2\text{Br} \\
\text{N}{-}\text{CH}
\end{array}
\quad + \quad
\begin{array}{c}
\text{N}{-\!-}\text{C}\cdot\text{CH}_3 \\
\text{C} \diagdown \text{S} \diagup \text{C}\cdot\text{CH}_2\cdot\text{CH}_2\text{OH} \\
\text{H}
\end{array}
$$

$$\downarrow$$

$$
\begin{array}{c}
\text{N}{=}\text{C}^{\displaystyle \diagup \text{NH}_2 \cdot \text{HBr}} \qquad\qquad \text{Br} \\
\text{CH}_3\cdot\text{C} \quad \text{C}{-}\text{CH}_2{-\!-}\text{N}{-\!-}\text{C}\cdot\text{CH}_3 \\
\text{N}{-}\text{CH} \qquad \text{HC} \diagdown \text{S} \diagup \text{C}\cdot\text{CH}_2\cdot\text{CH}_2\text{OH}
\end{array}
$$

The bromide hydrobromide may be converted into the chloride hydrochloride by treating with AgCl or by precipitating the practically insoluble thiamine picrate and dissolving it in hydrochloric acid.

E. Specificity

The activity of thiamine seems to be very specific. Even small alterations in the molecule give inactive substances or diminish the activity 100 or 1000 times or actually produce antagonistic effects. Most instructive in this respect is the work of Emerson and Southwick.[14] They replaced the methyl group in position 2 in the pyrimidine ring of thiamine by other alkyl groups. Replacement by ethyl does not change the activity, as measured by rat experiments; replacements by propyl gives a definite reduction of the activity

[12] E. R. Buchman, *J. Amer. Chem. Soc.* **58**, 1803 (1936).
[13] H. T. Clarke and S. Gurin, *J. Amer. Chem. Soc.* **57**, 1876 (1935).
[14] G. A. Emerson and P. L. Southwick, *J. Biol. Chem.* **160**, 169 (1945).

in pigeon tests. When the methyl is changed into an *n*-butyl group, the activity is reversed. However, Schopfer[15] and Schultz,[16] some years before the work of Emerson and Southwick, had established that a thiamine having in the second position of the pyrimidine nucleus an ethyl in place of a methyl group has a greater activity than normal thiamine on *Phycomyces* and on animals. Their relative activity is expressed by the ratio of ethylthiamine to methylthiamine having the same physiological activity. This ratio for *Phycomyces* was found to be 0.83 : 1.0 (Schopfer). The ratio for the pigeon is 0.85 : 1.0 (Schultz). The discrepancies with the results of Emerson and Southwick may be due to the inaccuracy of the animal experiments.

Barton and Rogers,[17] in the book of R. J. Williams *et al.*, give a huge number of examples of the influence of modifications in the pyrimidine or in the thiazole moiety of thiamine on the biological activity of these thiamine analogs. They arrive at the following conclusion: "as a result of these tests it is evident that the thiamine molecule can undergo very little modification without extensive loss of vitamin B_1 activity."

Williams and Cline[18] were able to establish that the synthetic thiamine hydrochloride was identical with the natural in composition, ultraviolet absorption, and antineuritic potency. Eckler and Chen[19] in elaborate pharmacological studies compared the curative doses and the minimum lethal doses of natural and synthetic thiamine. This work confirmed the identity of both substances.

In several microorganisms the thiamine may be replaced by one or both of its pyrimidine and thiazole moieties.[20] Abderhalden[21] has shown that higher animals too could sustain on the thiazole + pyrimidine moieties instead of thiamine itself. One would think that this might be brought about by the phenomenon of "refection," i.e., the synthesis of thiamine by the microorganisms in the gut, as was found by Fridericia *et al.*[22] But Abderhalden and Abderhalden[23] stated that tissue extracts are capable of synthesizing thiamine from the pyrimidine and thiazole parts—only to a very small extent, however, up to about 1 % of the theoretical amount.

[15] W. H. Schopfer, *C. Rend. Seances Soc. Phys. Hist. Natur. Geneve* **58**, 64 (1941).
[16] F. Schultz, *Hoppe-Seyler's Z. Physiol. Chem.* **265**, 113 (1940).
[17] A. D. Barton and L. L. Rogers, *in* "The Biochemistry of B. Vitamins" (R. J. Williams, R. E. Eakin, E. Beerstecher, Jr., and W. Shive, eds.), pp. 684–702. Reinhold, New York, 1950.
[18] R. R. Williams and J. K. Cline, *J. Amer. Chem. Soc.* **59**, 216 (1937).
[19] C. R. Eckler and K. K. Chen, *Proc. Soc. Exp. Biol. Med.* **35**, 458 (1937).
[20] W. H. Schopfer, *Ergeb. Biol.* **16**, 1 (1939).
[21] R. Abderhalden, *Pfluegers Arch. Gesamte Physiol. Menschen Tiere* **243**, 762 (1940).
[22] L. S. Fridericia, P. Freudenthal, S. Gudjonsson, G. Johansen, and N. Schoubye, *J. Hyg.* **27**, 70 (1928).
[23] E. Abderhalden and R. Abderhalden, *Pfluegers Arch. Gesamte Physiol. Menschen Tiere* **243**, 85 (1939).

III. Industrial Preparation

H. M. WUEST

A. From Natural Sources

Low concentrates from rice bran,[1] rice polishings or yeast,[2] high concentrates from rice germs (25,000 to 30,000 units per gram, F. Hoffmann-La Roche Ltd. in Basle, Switzerland, F. Elger, A. J. Frey, and H. M. Wuest, 1935–37) and the biosynthesis of thiamine in yeast[2]) are today only forgotten precursors of the synthetic vitamin. The isolation of crystalline thiamine from natural sources[3-5] never had a chance to compete with the synthesis.

B. Synthesis

From 1935 on, three groups of scientists and industrial firms were in a dramatic race for the elucidation of the structure and the synthesis of thiamine: in this country, R. R. Williams *et al.*, later on backed by Merck and Co., Todd and Bergel in England together with Hoffmann-La Roche Ltd. in Switzerland, and Andersag and Westphal in the laboratories of I. G. Farben industrie in Elberfeld. The scientific priority without any doubt falls to Williams with his first publication of the complete synthesis in August 1936.[6] All three groups got patents for their procedures, but only Merck and Co. and Hoffmann-La Roche started manufacturing from 1937 on. A detailed history was presented at the 25th anniversary of the first synthesis of thiamine.[7]

Fifteen years ago, the details of the synthesis were of the highest interest for the pharmaceutical industry as patent rights based on the scientific findings determined the procedure followed by the two industrial groups. Today—with all the important patent claims expired—the field is open for any manufacturer and quite a number of processes now are only of historical interest.

[1] E. B. Vedder, " Beriberi," p. 405. William Wood & Co., New York, 1913.
[2] R. F. Light and C. N. Frey, U.S. Patent No. 2, 184,748 (Dec. 26, 1939).
[3] B. C. P. Jansen and W. F. Donath, *Proc. Kon. Ned. Akad. Wetensch.* **29**, 1390 (1926); *Meded. Dienst Volksgezondheid, Ned.-Indie* **16**, 186 (1926).
[4] A. Windaus, R. Tscheche, H. Ruhkopf, F. Laquer, and F. Schultz, *Nachr. Ges. Wiss. Goettingen, Math.-Phys. Kl., III* p. 207 (1932).
[5] R. R. Williams, R. E. Waterman, and J. C. Keresztesy, *J. Amer. Chem. Soc.* **56**, 1187 (1934); U.S. Patent No. 2,049,988.
[6] R. R. Williams and J. K. Cline, *J. Amer. Chem. Soc.* **58**, 1504 (1936).
[7] H. M. Wuest, *Ann. N. Y. Acad. Sci.* **98**, 385 (1962).

For practical reasons, the molecule is divided into four groups

$$
\begin{array}{c}
\text{A} \qquad\qquad \text{B} \qquad\qquad\qquad \text{C} \\[1em]
\underset{\underset{\text{N}\!-\!\!-\!\text{CH}}{\overset{\|_{1}\;|_{6}\|}{\text{H}_3\text{C}\!-\!\text{C}_2}}}{\overset{\text{N}\!\overset{}{=}\!\text{C}_{3\;4}}{}}\;\overset{\overset{\text{NH}_2\cdot\text{HCl}}{/}}{}\; {}_5\text{C}\!-\!\!-\!\!-\!\!-\!\text{CH}_2\;{}_7\!-\!\!-\! \underset{\underset{\text{Cl}\;\text{HC}\!-\!\!-\!\text{S}}{}}{\overset{\text{N3}}{}}
\end{array}
$$

Based on the established structure of thiamine, the technical synthesis has two possibilities: (1) Building up pyrimidine ring and thiazole ring separately, then connecting both by quaternization to the thiazolium ring; (2) building up the pyrimidine ring with the group CH_2-NH_2 in the 5-position, elongating this side chain, and forming the thiazolium compound by ring closure.

The theoretical possibility of closing the pyrimidine ring with an existing thiazolium ring has no technical value for obvious reasons.

Procedure (1) allows the best conditions for the ring closures—alkaline condensation for the pyrimidine and acid medium for the thiazole nucleus. The final step of quaternization goes easily and gives nearly quantitative yields.

Regarding procedure (2), the original elongation of the side chain by thioformylation of the amine $-CH_2-NH_2$ (Todd, Bergel, et al.) is now replaced by treatment of the amine with ammonia and carbon disulfide, followed by ring closure and removal of the second sulfur atom (Matsukawa and Iwatsu). In this case, the nitrogen for the thiazolium ring switches to group B which is then elongated to group D:

1. Group A, two carbon and two nitrogen atoms. Acetamidine CH_3-C $(-NH_2)=NH$ is easily obtained as its hydrochloride from acetonitrile in technical yields of 95%.[8]

2. Group B, four carbon atoms and one or two amino groups.

$$
\begin{array}{c}
\text{(4)} \;\; \text{(5)} \;\; \text{(6)} \\
\text{C} - \text{C} - \text{C} \\
| \\
\text{C} \\
\text{(7)}
\end{array}
$$

The skeleton with four carbon atoms permits quite a number of variations, and only a few will be quoted here. As originally described by Williams and Cline,[9] the synthesis of sodioformyl-β-ethoxypropionate: $EtO-CH_2-C$: $(CHONa)COOEt$ from ethyl acrylate via ethyl ethoxypropionate plus ethyl-

[8] "Organic Syntheses," Coll. Vol. 1, p. 5. Wiley, New York, 1956.
[9] R. R. Williams and J. K. Cline, J. Amer. Chem. Soc. 58, 1504 (1936).

formate does not offer the promise of a successful technical process; with radical improvements of the reaction conditions and the yields, it might lead to a feasible approach as both starting materials are so very cheap.

Todd and Bergel,[10] formylate cyanoacetic ester in acetic anhydride with ethylformate to ethoxymethylene cyanoacetic ester: CN—C:(CHOEt)COOEt; based on the abundant work of Claisen, good yields can be expected. Grewe[11] used the even more reactive malononitrile for the same reaction to form ethoxymethylene malononitrile: CN—C:(CHOEt)CN; yields of 75% are easily obtained.[12]

Ethylcyanoacetate, cyanoacetamide, and malononitrile are available in industrial quantities in this country.

3. Ring closure to the pyrimidine A + B. Normally the formyl and cyano (or carbethoxy) groups react with the free acetamidine in one step at the ring closure, with or without an alkaline condensing agent (e.g., sodium ethylate).

a. Indirect introduction of the amino group in the 4-position. The ring closure between acetamidine and sodioformyl-β-ethoxypropionate to the pyrimidine followed by treatment with phosphorus oxychloride, ammonia in ethanol, and finally hydrobromic acid in acetic acid as described by Williams and Cline[9] is straightforward and was used as a technical synthesis after improvement of some of the poor yields.

b. Direct introduction of the amino group in the 4-position. The best manner of this ring closure was first described by Grewe.[11] When alcoholic solutions of free acetamidine and ethoxymethylene malononitrile are united, the mixture solidifies at once under formation of the crystalline cyano compound.

[10] A. R. Todd and F. Bergel. *J. Chem. Soc. London* p. 364 (1937).
[11] R. Grewe, *Hoppe-Seyler's Z. Physiol. Chem.* **242**, 89 (1936).
[12] O. Diels, H. Gärtner, and R. Kaack, *Ber. Deut. Chem. Ges.* **55**, 3141 (1922).

The resulting 2-methyl-4-amino-5-cyanopyrimidine can be catalytically hydrogenated with palladium charcoal in glacial acetic acid in the presence of dry hydrogen chloride[11] or in ethanol in the presence of ammonia. In both steps, the yields are excellent.

4. Group C, five carbon atoms for the thiazole ring. The possibilities for the synthesis of the thiazole ring are nearly as numerous as those of the pyrimidine ring. Buchman[13] chlorinated α-acetobutyrolactone with sulfurylchloride to α-chloro-α-acetobutyrolactone with a very good yield (83%), followed by decarboxylation with boiling concentrated hydrochloric acid. As Stevens and Stein[14] have shown only a small part (13%) is the expected γ-chloro-γ-acetopropyl alcohol:

$$CH_3—CO—CHCl—CH_2—CH_2OH \text{ or } CH_3—C(OH)—CHCl—CH_2—CH_2—O$$

whereas 62% were isolated as an ether formed from 2 moles of alcohol minus 1 mole of water. Both compounds can be used for the synthesis of the thiazole.

An excellent decarboxylation method was found by Low and Smith,[15] who performed the reaction in glacial acetic acid with just the calculated amount of water, followed by acetylation with acetic anhydride: 93–95% of γ-chloro-γ-acetopropyl acetate is obtained.

The starting material α-aceto-γ-butyrolactone is easily obtained from sodium ethyl acetoacetate in ethanol plus ethylene oxide[16] with a yield of 60% or better.

5. Group D, nitrogen, carbon atom 2, and sulfur. Thioformamide, $NH_2—CH{=}S$, is the source most easily used for the remaining three atoms of the thiazole ring. The reaction between formamide and phosphorus pentasulfide (in ethereal solution under cooling), however, gives only medium yields[17] (45–55%), even if the crude reaction product is used for the ring closure to the thiazole.

If instead of thioformamide, compounds with a substituted amino group are used, thiazolium salts are obtained instead of thiazole. Todd et al.[18] found a simple thioformylation of 2-methyl-4-amino-5-aminomethylpyrimidine with potassium dithioformate[19] to 2-methyl-4-amino-5-thioformyi-

[13] E. R. Buchman, J. Amer. Chem. Soc. 58, 1803 (1936).

[14] J. R. Stevens and G. A. Stein, J. Amer. Chem. Soc. 62, 1045 (1940).

[15] J. A. Low and R. J. Smith, Brit. Patent No. 606,026 (Aug. 5, 1948) to Roche Products, Welwyn Garden City, England.

[16] I. L. Knunjantz, G. W. Chelintzew, and E. D. Ossetrawa, Dokl. Akad. Nauk SSSR 1, 312 (1934) [Chem. Abstr. 28, 4382 (1934)].

[17] R. Willstätter and T. Wirth, Ber. Deut. Chem. Ges. 42, 1911 (1909); S. Gabriel, Ber. Deut. Chem. Ges. 49, 1115 (1916).

[18] A. R. Todd, F. Bergel, and Karimullah, Ber. Deut. Chem. Ges. 69, 217 (1936); A. R. Todd, F. Bergel, Karimullah, and R. Keller, J. Chem. Soc. London p. 361 (1937).

[19] Levi, Atti Reale Accad. Naz. Lincei, Rend., Cl. Sci. Fis. Mat. Natur. 32, 569 (1923).

aminomethylpyrimidine; this method produced for the first 15 years about one-half of the world output of thiamine.

6. C + D, ring closure to the thiazole and thiazolium ring. Using their pure "ether" instead of the halogenated ketoalcohol, Stevens and Stein[20] obtained 70% of 4-methyl-5-β-hydroxyethylthiazole; it can be assumed that the condensation of γ-chloro-γ-acetopropylacetate with thioformamide gives still better yields.

Replacement of the unstable and rather expensive thioformamide by ammonium dithiocarbaminate (from ammonia and the cheapest organic sulfur compound carbon disulfide) leads to 2-mercapto-4-methyl-5-β-acetoxy-ethyl thiazole, as was already shown by Spiegelberg[21] in 1938. The mercapto group in 2-position can be easily replaced by hydrogen (oxidation with 30% hydrogen peroxide in acid solution) with yields of 75–87%.

It is astonishing that it was 12 years before the Spiegelberg process was used for the direct ring closure to the thiazolium compound (by Matsukawa and Iwatsu in 1950), yielding 2-mercaptothiamine and after oxidation thiamine itself; both steps give excellent yields.[22]

7. Linking the two ring systems, quaternization of the thiazole to thiazolium. This final step of the synthesis of Cline et al.[23] offers little difficulty, especially when the pyrimidine compound with bromine in the 7-position is used (e.g., 120°C in butanol for 15 minutes).

To replace the bromine ions by chlorine ions shaking with an aqueous suspension of silver chloride can be used; it seems natural, however, that the modern ion exchange resins are even more effective.

[20] J. R. Stevens and G. A. Stein, J. Amer. Chem. Soc. 62, 1046 (1940).
[21] H. Spiegelberg, Brit, Patent No. 492,637 (Sept. 23, 1938); U.S. Patent No. 2,179,984 (Nov. 14, 1939).
[22] T. Matsukawa and T. Iwatsu, U.S. Patent No. 2,592,930–31 (Apr. 15, 1952).
[23] J. K. Cline, R. R. Williams, and J. Finkelstein, J. Amer. Chem. Soc. 59, 1052 (1937).

C. Patent Situation

From 1937 on, the manufacture of thiamine on an industrial scale was dominated by the patent rights of three industrial groups: in the United States by the Williams–Buchman group (assignors to Research Corporation, New York, licensee Merck and Co., Rahway New Jersey), by Hoffmann-La Roche in Nutley, New Jersey, England, and Switzerland (based on the Todd and Bergel process), and by I. G. Farbenindustrie in Germany. However, only Merck and Co. and Roche produced thiamine in commercial quantities. The basic patent protection lasted until about 1955; by 1960 nearly all the basic patents had expired and again the patent situation is only of historical interest now.

D. Commercial Forms and Purity

Thiamine is sold commercially in the form of two salts, the chloride hydrochloride (generally quoted as hydrochloride) and the mononitrate. The hydrochloride is official in most countries (U.S. Pharmacopeia XVI, 1960, p. 751; Brit. Pharmacopoeia 1963, p. 50 ff) whereas the mononitrate is especially used in the United States (U.S.P. XVI, 1960, p. 754).

The hydrochloride is very soluble in water (1 + 1), is rather acid (1% solution pH 2.7–3.4), and contains up to 5% water (loss at 105°C for 2 hours), whereas the mononitrate is less soluble (1 + 35), nearly neutral (2% solution, pH 6.0–7.5), is not hygroscopic, and contains a maximal 1% of water (same drying conditions). It is therefore preferred in the food industry, e.g., for the fortification of flour. Its preparation is described by several patents,[24] and its pharmaceutical behavior was investigated by Macek et al.[25] and others.[26]

The U.S.P. (XVI) describes the official assay method (formation of thiochrome, p. 909), based on the comparison with the U.S.P. thiamine hydrochloride reference standard.

E. Production and Prices

The United States, England, and Switzerland are still the big producers of thiamine, and Japan must be added as a medium producer (Takeda, Osaka). The importance of the thiamine (B_1) production in the United States (Merck and Co., Inc. and Hoffmann-La Roche) is shown in the accompanying tabulation.

[24] E. W. Schoeffel (to Merck & Co., Inc.) Can. Patent No. 469,559 (Nov. 21, 1950); J. Kokura and S. Waki (to Takeda Pharm. Ind., Ltd.) Jap. Patent No. 2,778 (1955) [Chem. Abstr. 51, P 13 323b (1957)]; J. J. Lawson (to Amer. Cyanamid Co.) U.S. Patent No. 2,801, 245 (July 30, 1957); R. J. Turner and G. J. Schmitt (to Amer. Cyanamid Co.) U.S. Patent No. 2,844,579 (July 22, 1958).

[25] T. J. Macek, B. A. Feller, and E. J. Hanus, J. Amer. Pharm. Ass., Sci. Ed. 39, 365 (1950).

[26] Kee-Neng Wai, H. G. De Kay, and G. S. Banker, J. Pharm. Sci. 51, 1076 (1962).

Year	Kg	Price ($/kg)	Approximate value ($)
1937	100	—	—
1939	1,600	1000	1,600,000
1940	3,700	600	2,220,000
1951–55	100,000–120,000	145	15,000,000
1956	120,000	70	8,400,000
1960	150,000	36	5,400,000

Because the U.S. Tariff Commission has discontinued the publication of thiamine production and sales, exact figures for the United States are no longer available. Including imports from Japan of about 25 tons, the sales for 1967 may be estimated to about 200 tons with a value of about $3,000,000.

The rapid decline of the thiamine price after 1952 is illustrated by the figures tabulated below (price per kilogram of thiamine hydrochloride U.S.P. in dollars).

Year	High	Low
1952	160	135
1954	135	100
1956	80	60
1958	40	40
1960	36	36
1962	27	21
1964	16.50	15.50

The last price in 1967 was $14.00 for 1 kg of hydrochloride and $14.75 for the mononitrate. As in the case of ascorbic acid and riboflavin, thiamine is today one of the important items of the pharmaceutical industry with the smallest margin of profit.

IV. Estimation in Foods

MERTON P. LAMDEN

A. Animal Assays

The first methods used in the estimation of thiamine were animal assays. Animals that have been used are the chick, the pigeon, and the rat. These assays are based on the curative properties of thiamine for polyneuritis in the pigeon and rat, for bradycardia in the rat, and for growth or weight maintenance in these animals. Animal assays are used very little today for the routine estimation of thiamine because the cost is high and the assays are time consuming. Usually large amounts of thiamine-rich extracts are required, and the results tend to be variable, necessitating the use of large numbers of animals for precise results. The animal assays are desirable in that they are specific for thiamine and are useful in measuring the physiologically available forms of the vitamin. Furthermore, since they measure all biological forms of the vitamin, no special extractions or pretreatment of the test material are necessary as is the case with other assays. There is the possibility, however, that the physiological availability of thiamine will vary depending on the animal tested and will not be directly applicable to man.[1] For details see Kline and Daniel,[2] Coward,[3] György,[4] and Mickelsen and Yamamoto.[5]

B. Microbiological Methods

By using microbiological methods one can inexpensively assay many samples in a short time. Furthermore, these methods are exceptionally sensitive to thiamine (0.001 mμg to 1 μg) depending on the organism and are generally reproducible to better that $\pm 10\%$. Microbiological assays are used less for thiamine than for other vitamins, and less frequently than chemical methods for thiamine. A failing of several of the microbiological assays for thiamine has been a lack of specificity, in that the pyrimidine and thiazole moieties, either singly or together, have been stimulatory as have been other interfering substances. Some of the microorganisms used have been *Phycomyces blakesleeanus*, *Saccharomyces cerevisiae*, *Escherichia coli*, and *Staphylococcus aureus*, all of which are stimulated by thiamine moieties.[5]

In 1944 Sarett and Cheldelin[6] introduced the use of *Lactobacillus fermenti*, which is extremely sensitive for thiamine and is not affected by thiamine moieties. It has been considered the best bacteriological method for thiamine and has undergone improvement over the years. Deibel *et al.*[7] contend that *Lactobacillus viridescens* is more desirable than *L. fermenti* since it is not affected by pentoses, reducing agents, fructose, maltose, calcium, and heat-degradation products of glucose. Furthermore, the *L. viridescens* method is said to compare favorably with the thiochrome method with respect to comparative determinations but is more specific and convenient than the thiochrome method.[7] Baker and Sobotka[8] claim considerable success with

[1] D. Melnick and B. L. Oser, *Vitam. Horm.* (*New York*) 5, 39 (1947).
[2] O. L. Kline and E. P. Daniel, *Biol. Symp.* 12, 52 (1947) [Estimation of the Vitamins].
[3] K. H. Coward, " The Biological Standardization of Vitamins." William Wood & Co., Baltimore, Maryland, 1947.
[4] P. György, *in* "Vitamin Methods" (P. György, ed.), Vol. II, p. 45, 179, 448. Academic Press, New York, 1951.
[5] O. Mickelsen and R. S. Yamamoto, *Methods Biochem. Anal.* 6, 191 (1958).
[6] H. P. Sarett and V. H. Cheldelin, *J. Biol. Chem.* 155, 153 (1944).
[7] R. H. Deibel. J. B. Evans, and C. F. Niven, Jr., *J. Bacteriol.* 74, 818 (1957).
[8] H. Baker and H. Sobotka, *Advan. Clin. Chem.* 5, 174 (1962).

the phytoflagellate *Ochromonas malhamensis*, which is said to be highly sensitive and specific for thiamine and little affected by thiamine moieties and other interfering substances.

Schultz *et al.*[9] found that yeast fermentation is enhanced by the presence of free thiamine and utilized this fact for a quantitative method for the estimation of thiamine. This procedure has been adapted as a micromethod using the Warburg apparatus.[10] Westenbrink developed a method permitting the separate determination of about 0.5 mμg of thiamine and 0.05 mμg of cocarboxylase (TPP) in mixtures of both compounds.[11] The urinary excretion of pyramine, the pyrimidine-like component of thiamine, is considered better than thiamine as a measure of thiamine nutriture and is determined by the Caster *et al.*[12] modification of the yeast fermentation method of Schultz *et al.* A comprehensive discussion of microbiological methods is given by Mickelsen and Yamamoto.[5] Details on microbiological procedures are available from several sources.[8,13-15]

C. Chemical Methods

Presently the most widely used method for the determination of thiamine, particularly in foodstuffs and feeds, is the fluorometric thiochrome method. This is the standard method of the Association of Official Agricultural Chemists.[16] Its popularity stems from its applicability to routine determinations and its high degree of reproducibility, sensitivity, and specificity. Up to 20 assays can be carried out in 8 hours. The procedure will measure 1–20 μg of thiamine. Adaptations of this technique for microanalysis measure 2–5 mμg.[17] Thiochrome (I),

(I)

[9] A. S. Schultz, L. Atkins, and C. N. Frey, *Ind. Eng. Chem., Anal. Ed.* **14**, 35 (1942).

[10] L. Atkin, A. S. Schultz, and C. N. Frey, *J. Biol. Chem.* **129**, 471 (1939).

[11] H. G. K. Westenbrink, *Enzymologia* **8**, 97 (1940).

[12] W. O. Caster, O. Mickelsen, and A. Keys, *J. Lab. Clin. Med.* **43**, 469 (1954).

[13] E. E. Snell, *in* "Vitamin Methods" (P. György, ed.), Vol. I, p. 327. Academic Press, New York, 1950.

[14] O. L. Kline and L. Friedman, *Biol. Symp.* **12**, 65 (1947).

[15] Association of Vitamin Chemists, "Methods of Vitamin Assay," 3rd ed. Wiley (Interscience), New York, 1966.

[16] Association of Official Agricultural Chemists, "Official and Tentative Methods of Analysis," 9th Ed., p. 655. Ass. Off. Agr. Chem., Washington, D.C., 1960.

[17] H. B. Burch, O. A. Bessey, R. H. Love, and O. H. Lowry, *J. Biol. Chem.* **198**, 477 (1952).

which is characterized by a strong blue fluorescence, results from the oxidation of thiamine.[18, 19]

Whether thiamine is finally determined as thiochrome or by a colorimetric procedure, the initial steps in the determination are similar. These include extraction with dilute hydrochloric acid, sulfuric acid, or sodium acetate; hydrolysis of the phosphate esters of thiamine by phosphatase-containing preparations (thiochrome pyrophosphate, the oxidation product of thiamine pyrophosphate, is insoluble in isobutanol used for extraction of thiochrome); clarification by centrifugation or filtration; adsorption on a synthetic zeolite (Decalso); and elution of thiamine. The eluted thiamine is oxidized to thiochrome, the thiochrome extracted with isobutanol, and its fluorescence measured in a fluorometer.[5] Modifications may be warranted for urine samples of low thiamine content and for certain foodstuffs. In milk, thiamine may exist in a bound form and proteolytic digestion with papain or pepsin may be necessary to split off thiamine. Some laboratories have omitted enzyme digestion for cereals since the thiamine is largely in the free form. Omission of the adsorption step also has been suggested. A recent collaborative investigation to standardize the thiamine determination, involving 17 laboratories in 13 countries, found that adsorption of thiamine on zeolite made the procedure more precise and that enzymatic treatment of the extract and the use of an internal standard reduced the standard deviation.[20]

Prebluda and McCollum[21] devised a method using the color production of a diazotized aromatic amine (p-aminoacetophenone) with thiamine, the red compound formed being extracted with xylene or toluene. The method has been further developed by Melnick and Field[22] and is presently the most frequently used colorimetric procedure. A larger amount of thiamine (10–200 μg) is needed in the test sample than for the thiochrome procedure. The determination, while specific, is considered rather complex, laborious, and time consuming.[5] A number of modifications have been proposed for the analysis of urine and cereals. Hayden[23] claims 6-aminothymol to be an improvement over p-aminoacetophenone, particularly in the presence of carbohydrate and soluble proteins.[24]

D. Other Methods of Assay

The absorption spectrum of thiamine varies with pH; however, a peak

[18] R. A. Peters, *Nature (London)* **135**, 107 (1935).

[19] G. Barger, F. Bergel, and A. R. Todd, *Nature (London)* **136**, 259 (1935).

[20] B. Gassmann, J. Janicki, and E. Kaminski, *Int. Z. Vitaminforsch.* **33**, 1 (1963).

[21] H. J. Prebluda and E. V. McCollum, *J. Biol. Chem.* **127**, 495 (1939).

[22] D. Melnick and H. Field, *J. Biol. Chem.* **127**, 505, 515, 531 (1939).

[23] K. J. Hayden, *Analyst (London)* **82**, 61 (1957).

[24] K. J. Hayden and R. H. Elkington, *Analyst (London)* **82**, 650 (1957).

at 273 mμ is fairly constant and has been used for determining thiamine in fairly pure solutions.[25]

Increasing use is being made of paper chromatography and paper and column electrophoresis, particularly for the separation of the phosphate esters of thiamine.[5] In addition, thiamine may be determined by colorimetric measurement of its reineckate salt or by titrimetric procedures.[5] Among the enzyme assays for thiamine are the catatorulin test of the Peters group[26] using minced brain from polyneuritic pigeons, or the alkali-washed yeast method of Ochoa and Peters[27] and subsequent procedures of Goodhart and Sinclair[28] and Westenbrink.[29] A potential biological assay for the thiamine content of foodstuffs may involve transketolase activity since Brin and Owens have demonstrated a dose–response curve of erythrocyte transketolase in the rat to graded levels of thiamine in the rat diet.[30] Determination of thiamine in the presence of pyrithiamine may be accomplished by separation of the two on polyethylene powder.[31] More extensive discussion on many of these procedures is found in the treatise by Mickelsen and Yamamoto.[5]

V. Occurrence in Foods

MERTON P. LAMDEN

Thiamine has been found in most forms of life. The concentration of the vitamin in a whole organism seems to bear no relationship to size or biological phylum as exemplified in the following thiamine values in micrograms per gram for a cross section of the biological kingdom: rat, 1.7; fish, 2.9; frog, 1.4; oyster, 1.8; earthworm, 2.5; cockroach, 4.4; termite, 2.3; *Drosophila*, 4.3; dried lima bean (seed), 5.3; carrot (root), 0.38; apple (fruit), 0.96; lettuce (leaf), 0.39; Irish potato (tuber), 1.7; cauliflower (flower), 1.4; blueberry, 0.02; mushroom, 1.1; mold, 0.09; protozoan, 5.0; yeast, 8.5; bacterium, 2.2–5.5.

As with most of the vitamins of the B complex, the spread of values between the poorest and richest sources of the vitamin is not too large, being of the order of 20- to 40-fold for thiamine, compared to ascorbic

[25] J. J. Doherty, N. Cane, and F. Wokes, *J. Pharm. Pharmacol.* **7**, 1053 (1955).

[26] R. Passmore, R. A. Peters, and H. M. Sinclair, *Biochem. J.* **27**, 842 (1933).

[27] S. Ochoa and R. A. Peters, *Biochem. J.* **32**, 1501 (1938).

[28] R. S. Goodhart and H. M. Sinclair, *Biochem. J.* **33**, 1099 (1939).

[29] H. G. K. Westenbrink, *C. R. Trav. Lab. Carlsberg., Ser. Chim.* **23**, 195 (1940).

[30] M. Brin and B. A. Owens, *Fed. Proc. Fed. Amer. Soc. Exp. Biol.* **19**, 321 (1960).

[31] G. Rindi and V. Perri, *Anal. Biochem.* **5**, 179 (1963).

acid with a 100- to 2000-fold span. The ubiquity of thiamine in the plant and animal kingdoms is not surprising when one considers the functional role of thiamine in metabolism. As the coenzyme thiamine pyrophosphate, the vitamin plays a role in glycolysis and the glycolytic pathway, the citric acid cycle, and the hexose monophosphate shunt or pentose pathway. In the glycolytic pathway, which is widely distributed in animal and insect muscle, yeast, bacteria, and plants, thiamine pyrophosphate is necessary for the decarboxylation of pyruvic acid, leading to acetyl-CoA or ethanol formation depending on the tissue or organism. In the citric acid cycle, which is found in all respiring tissues of animals from protozoa to mammals, in almost all aerobic microorganisms including yeast, bacteria, and molds, and in many forms of plant material, thiamine pyrophosphate is again involved in decarboxylation, being necessary for the conversion of α-keto-glutaric acid to succinic acid. In the pentose pathway, thiamine is necessary for the action of transketolase, a carbonyl group transferring enzyme widely distributed throughout the biological kingdom.

A. Naturally Occurring Forms of Thiamine

Thiamine is found in biological materials in the free form, as the mono-, di-, and triphosphoric esters,[1, 2] and as the mono- and disulfide.[3, 4] The predominant form in animal tissues is the diphosphate or pyrophosphate,[1, 5] which exists largely as a protein complex bound to the enzyme carboxylase. It also complexes with transketolase in a not readily dissociable form.[6] Thiamine triphosphate has been found in the liver, kidney, and brain of the rat.[2] The most abundant form in plant tissue is free thiamine.[1] A derivative of thiamine, with high vitamin B_1 activity in which the thiazole ring has opened, allithiamine (I) and its propyl analog (propyl instead of allyl group) have been found in plant extracts.[7]

(I)

B. Distribution of Thiamine Pyrophosphate in Cell Fractions

The percentage distribution of thiamine pyrophosphate in cell fractions[8]

[1] G. Rindi and L. deGiuseppe, *Int. Z. Vitaminforsch.* **31**, 321 (1961).
[2] H. Greiling and L. Kiesow, *Z. Naturforsch. B* **13**, 251 (1958).
[3] K. Myrbäck, I. Vallin, and I. Magnell, *Sv. Kem. Tidskr.* **57**, 124 (1945).
[4] H. Suomalainen, S. Rihtniemi, and E. Oura, *Acta Chem. Scand.* **13**, 2131 (1959).
[5] B. Alexander, *J. Biol Chem.* **151**, 455 (1943).
[6] G. de La Haba, I. G. Leder, and E. Racker, *J. Biol. Chem.* **214**, 409 (1955).
[7] S. Yurugi, *Yakugaku Zasshi* **74**, 502 (1954).
[8] W. C. Schneider and G. H. Hogeboom, *J. Biol. Chem.* **183**, 123 (1950).

of rat liver homogenate has been determined.[9, 10] In summary, the approximate percentages for each fraction are the following: nuclear, 10%; mitochondrial, 35%; microsomal, 5%; soluble, 50%. Such a distribution seems consistent with the functional involvement of thiamine in the glycolytic and pentose pathways of the cytoplasm and the citric acid cycle of mitochondria.

C. Thiamine Distribution in Organs and Tissues of Man and Animals

There have been abundant reports and compilations on the thiamine[11, 12–15] and thiamine pyrophosphate[13] content of tissues and organs of man, dog, cat, pigeon, rabbit, rat, mouse, guinea pig, cattle, sheep, pig, fish, etc. Therefore, this discussion will attempt to summarize noteworthy findings and relationships. Values are intended to be of the proper order of magnitude rather than quotations of exact values found.

For several animals studied, including man, the organs having the highest thiamine concentration (milligrams per gram of moist tissue) were heart (2.8–7.9), kidney (2.4–5.8), liver (2.0–7.6), and brain (1.4–4.4). Lesser, but substantial, amounts are found in the spleen, lung, adrenals, and muscle.

In man, although the values for thiamine tend to be lower than for other animals, a similar pattern is seen. Outstanding is the thiamine concentration of pork muscle (8 μg/gm) compared to other pig tissue or to muscle tissue of other animals (1 μg/gm).

Because of its relationship to polyneuritis, thiamine has been studied extensively in the brain and nervous tissue of several species.[13, 16] In the peripheral nerves of warm-blooded animals, on the average, less than 0.5 μg free thiamine and not much more than 1 μg bound thiamine (phosphate esters)/gm tissue is present, whereas in the spinal cord and brain corresponding values are at least twice as much.

The blood of man contains about 9 μg/100 ml, the concentration being higher in the rat and pig and the same or somewhat lower in the ox, calf, sheep, and horse.[13] Blood cells as a group contain somewhat more thiamine

[9] G. Goethart, *Biochim. Biophys. Acta* **8**, 479 (1952).

[10] M. U. Dianzani and M. A. Dianzani Mor, *Biochim. Biophys. Acta* **24**, 564 (1957).

[11] B. K. Watt and A. L. Merrill, " Composition of Foods—Raw, Processed, Prepared." *U.S. Dep. Agr., Agr. Handb.* **8** (Revised 1963).

[12] " Studies on the Vitamin Content of Tissues II." *Tex. Univ. Publ.* **4237**, (1942).

[13] C. Long, "Biochemistry Handbook." Van Nostrand, Princeton, New Jersey, 1961.

[14] " Nutritional Data," 5th Ed., 1st Revised Printing. H. J. Heinz Co., Pittsburg, Pennsylvania, 1963.

[15] A. de P. Bowes and C. F. Church, " Food Values of Portions Commonly Used," 8th Ed. A. de P. Bowes, Philadelphia, Pennsylvania, 1956.

[16] A. von Muralt, *Vitam. Horm.* (*New York*) **5**, 93 (1947).

whereas the leukocytes in particular are in the order of seven- to eight-fold greater. Plasma,[17, 18] cerebrospinal fluid,[13] and saliva[13] contain 0–1.5 μg/100 ml. Sweat contains little thiamine.[19] Bull semen contains a considerable amount of thiamine (0.3–1.5 μg/ml).[13] Thiamine concentration in milk varies with the species: human, 0.16 μg/ml; cow, 0.42 μg/ml; and whale, 1.4 μg/ml.[13]

In a group of human normal and cancer tissues studied,[12] the cancer tissues had 71% of the thiamine level of the normal tissues; for rats the thiamine level for the cancerous tissues was 42% of the normal tissue.

D. Occurrence in Food

Foods vary in thiamine concentration in the order of 20- to 25-fold. The following list of thiamine concentrations for groups of foods represents average values (μg/100 gm) for the group. Individual values may be higher or lower but the value fairly well categorizes the group: dried beans and peas, 680; nuts and nut products, 560; whole grain cereals, 370; organ meats (liver, heart, kidney, brain), 100; flower and fruit vegetables, 70; leaf and stem vegetables, 70; root and tuber vegetables, 60; milk, 40; fruits, 30. Pork muscle is very high in thiamine, 600–800 μg/100 gm for various cuts of pork. There are several compilations giving the thiamine concentrations of specific foodstuffs.[11, 13–15, 20, 21]

The edible portion of common fish (cod, flounder, haddock, halibut, herring, yellow perch, smelts, sturgeon, white fish) contains 50–90 μg thiamine/100 gm. Mackerel and shad are higher (150 μg/100 gm) and eel is particularly high. The thiamine content of various fish tissues and organs has been presented by Love et al.[21]

Hen's eggs contain 170 μg/100 gm whole egg (70–630 μg/100 gm); all the thiamine is in the yolk (500 μg/100 gm), the variation being almost tenfold (190–1820 μg/100 gm).[13] Fish roe varies from 30–2290 μg/100 gm[13] with a value of 890 μg/100 gm given for baked shad roe.[15]

Foods that are frequently enriched, fortified, or restored to a legal standard, when one exists, are breakfast cereals, wheat white flour, degermed cornmeal, breads, macaroni, spaghetti, and milk modifiers (chocolate, malt, etc.). Interesting food materials of high thiamine content are dried brewer's yeast (1820 μg/100 gm), wheat germ (2050 μg/100 gm), tampala leaves

[17] A. P. Meiklejohn, Biochem. J. 31, 1441 (1937).
[18] H. M. Sinclair, Biochem. J. 32, 2185 (1938); Biochem. J. 33, 1816, 2027 (1939).
[19] D. M. Tennant and R. H. Silber, J. Biol. Chem. 148, 159 (1943).
[20] " The Composition of Foods." Med. Res. Counc. (Gt. Brit.), Spec. Rep. Ser. 297, (1960).
[21] R. M. Love, J. A. Lovern, and N. R. Jones, Dept. Sci. and Ind. Research (Great Britain), Food Investigation Spec. Rept. 69, (1959).

(a spinach-like vegetable) (1600 μg/100 gm), and alfalfa juice (quintal) (212 μg/100 gm).[13, 15]

E. Effect of Food Processing

The effect of agricultural practices, harvesting, handling, and processing on the thiamine content of foods is extensively covered with hundreds of references by Harris and von Loesecke.[22] Only a brief summary of findings will be attempted here.

Effects of growing season, temperature, and location of growth on the thiamine content of plants vary with the species and variety of plant grown. Light stimulates the synthesis of thiamine, and, with maturation, thiamine increases in peas, wheat, oats, and potatoes. Increased thiamine intake by pigs elevates the thiamine concentration in pork muscle. The thiamine content of muscle meats appears to be inversely related to fat content. Thiamine is stable during the storage of cereal grains of proper moisture content and undergoes only limited destruction in the commercial refrigeration of meats and vegetables. There appears to be little loss of thiamine during frozen storage of fish and vegetables. For frozen muscle meats and liver, losses are between 20 and 40% for 2–8 months' storage.

Losses during canning depend on the acidity of the food as well as on time and temperature. Retention of thiamine is high in canned fruit juices but low in most canned meats and vegetables.

Thiamine loss during the dehydration of fruits and vegetables is not considerable unless sulfite has been used. Dehydrated nonfat milk, particularly when it is prepared by low heat processes, has a fairly high retention of thiamine.

The curing of meats does not involve a large loss of thiamine whereas the salt preservation of cucumbers with subsequent desalting prior to final processing results in the loss of most of the small amount of thiamine originally present.

The milling of cereal grains removes a large proportion of their thiamine, wheat flour extraction of less than 85% resulting in a marked drop in thiamine and the degerming of corn involving a one-third loss. Parboiling of rice and drying before milling conserves the bulk of the thiamine.

Cooking processes are costly in terms of thiamine. Roasting of beef and pork involve thiamine losses of 36–53%. Pressure and steam cooking of vegetables involve considerably less loss of thiamine than boiling (about 40%). Electronic cooking destroys little thiamine in several meats. Ionizing radiation destroys 53–88% of thiamine in meats, yet, in certain poultry, fish, and vegetable samples, losses were only 5–37%.

[22] "Nutritional Evaluation of Food Processing" (R. S. Harris and H. W. von Loesecke, eds.). Wiley, New York, 1960.

F. Thiaminases and Antithiamines

A discussion of the occurrence of thiamine would not be complete without mention of the thiaminases and antithiamines which can influence the thiamine content of foods and plant and animal tissues. The subject has been reviewed by Harris,[23] Fujita,[24] Kenten,[25, 26] Jancarik,[27] and Magri.[28] Green and Evans[29] in 1940, reported that the disease Chastek paralysis produced in silver fox by feeding a diet containing 10% or more of certain raw fish was due to thiamine deficiency. Feeding cooked fish did not produce the deficiency disease. Woolley[30] and Spitzer et al.[31] found that a heat-labile principle, probably an enzyme, from an extract of carp viscera was able to inactivate a thiamine solution in vitro. Fujita in 1941 discovered the destructive effect on thiamine of certain shellfish and crustacea, which led to an extensive investigation of thiaminase.[24] There are at least two enzymes with thiaminase activity. One catalyzes an exchange reaction in which the thiazole portion of thiamine or thiamine pyrophosphate is displaced by a base with the release of hydrogen ion. The occurrence of this enzyme is limited to certain fish (largely freshwater), shellfish, and crustacea. It is not present in the tissues of land animals. It is also found in certain ferns and the cockscomb but in very few higher plants. Clams, but not oysters, are rich in thiaminase. It has been found in certain species of *Bacillus* and *Clostridium* bacteria isolated from the intestinal flora of Japanese people and has been implicated in "thiaminase disease," a beriberi-like condition with an incidence as high as 70% of the population in certain Japanese cities.[32] The natural compounds supplying base to displace the thiazole moiety of thiamine in its breakdown are not known except in the case of clams where Kupstas and Hennessey have shown that hypotaurine, $H_2NCH_2CH_2SO_2H$, is involved, giving rise to icthiamine, 4 amino-5-(2-aminoethane sulfonyl) methyl-2-methylpyrimidine.[33]

Another type of thiaminase is found largely in bacteria and hydrolytically cleaves thiamine but not thiamine pyrophosphate into its pyrimidine and thiazole components.[34, 35]

[23] R. S. Harris, in " The Enzymes " (J. B. Sumner and K. Myrbäck, eds.), 1st Ed., Vol. I, Part II, p. 1186. Academic Press, New York, 1951.

[24] A. Fujita, Advan. Enzymol. 15, 389 (1954).

[25] R. H. Kenten, Biochem. J. 67, 25 (1957).

[26] R. H. Kenten, Biochem. J. 69, 439 (1958).

[27] A. Jancarik, Vitam. Horm. (Leipzig) 7, 430 (1957).

[28] E. Magri, Acta Vitaminol. 13, 21 (1959).

[29] R. G. Green and C. A. Evans, Science 92, 154 (1940).

[30] D. W. Woolley, J. Biol. Chem. 141, 997 (1941).

[31] E. H. Spitzer, A. J. Combes, C. A. Elvehjem, and W. Wisnicky, Proc. Soc. Exp. Biol. Med. 48, 376 (1941).

[32] R. Hayashi, Nutr. Rev. 15, 65 (1957).

[33] E. E. Kupstas and D. J. Hennessey, J. Amer. Chem. Soc. 79, 5217, 5220, 5222 (1957).

[34] A. Fujita, J. Vitaminol. (Kyoto) 4, 55 (1958).

[35] K. Murata, J. Vitaminol. (Kyoto) 4, 57 (1958).

The physiological significance of thiaminase is not known. Thiaminase activity does not seem to be present in tissue until the tissue is ground. Tissue which is ground and then found to be free of thiamine may be shown to be originally high in thiamine if the thiaminase is first inactivated by subjecting the tissue to boiling buffer solution before grinding. Thiaminase has limited importance in human nutrition, being of possible consequence only in individuals whose intestinal tract harbors thiaminase-containing bacteria, or in those people who eat considerable amounts of raw clams,[36] raw fish containing thiaminase, or processed foods in which ground raw whole fish or shell fish was incorporated prior to heat treatment.

The finding by Jubb et al.[37] that thiamine deficiency was produced in cats fed canned commercial cat food containing ground whole fish, and that this deficiency appeared to be due to the destruction of thiamine by thiaminase during processing would support a recommendation that food products consisting in whole or in part of thiaminase-containing fish or shellfish should be thoroughly cooked in the whole state before it is ground or minced and incorporated with other components of the processed food.

While thiaminases have very limited occurrence in plants, much more prevalent are the thermostabile thiamine-destroying factors in the leaves, fruits, roots, and flowers of most plants.[24] Flavonoids, phenols, quinones, and catechol derivatives have thiamine-decomposing properties.[38] The heat-stable antithiamine of ferns appears to be flavonoid in nature,[39] while the active flavonoid of sweet potato leaves has been isolated and identified as isoquercitrin.[40] Plant antithiamine present in a mixture of ingested foods are not thought to destroy significant amounts of the thiamine contained therein because body temperature is too low to favor nonenzymatic destruction. However, losses of thiamine during cooking and heat-processing of foods may be partially due to the presence of heat-stable antithiamine compounds present in plant foods.[24]

VI. Standardization of Activity

MERTON P. LAMDEN

The standard for Vitamin B_1 activity is crystalline synthetic thiamine hydrochloride, the potency of the vitamin being expressed in milligrams or micrograms.

[36] D. Melnick, M. Hochberg, and B. L. Oser, J. Nutr. 30, 81 (1945).
[37] K. V. Jubb, L. Z. Saunders, and H. V. Coates, J. Comp. Pathol. Ther. 66, 217 (1956).
[38] A. Fujita, T. Okamoto, and Y. Nose, J. Vitaminol. (Osaka) 1, 108 (1955).
[39] E. Hasegawa, S. Sakamoto, K. Nagayama, and A. Fujita, J. Vitaminol. (Osaka) 2, 31 (1956).
[40] S. Sakamoto and A. Fujita, J. Vitaminol. (Osaka) 2, 39 (1956).

A great deal of the early work in assaying vitamin B_1 activity of different materials was presented in Chase–Sherman units[1] based on the growth response of the rat to graded doses of the vitamin-containing test substance. Agreement on the vitamin B_1 activity of a given test material between laboratories was not always good, largely due to differences in growth responses of the various strains of animals used, variations in the method of assay, and lack of awareness and knowledge of vitamin B complex inter-relationships.

The adoption of a specially prepared material designed to be uniform in vitamin B_1 activity, and thus suitable as a reference standard, was accomplished in 1931 by the International Conference on Vitamin Standardization of the Health Organization of the League of Nations.[2] Ten milligrams of an acid clay adsorbate of an extract from rice polishings prepared basically according to the isolation procedure of Jansen and Donath[3] was designated to have 1 International Unit (IU) of antineuritic vitamin B_1 activity. Use of the International Standard Clay resulted in gross discrepancies in vitamin assay values. With the observation that the effectiveness of the clay varied in different animal assay procedures came the disclosure of the fundamental difficulty. The extent of release of the vitamins from the clay depended on the species of animal used for assay and on the state of health of the animal. The clay was more effective for healthy animals in a protective assay than for polyneuritic animals in a curative assay. The availability of abundant supplies of crystalline synthetic thiamine hydrochloride made possible the use of this material as a uniform reference standard for vitamin B_1 activity. On the basis of many tests comparing the synthetic vitamin with the acid clay adsorbate, the Conference of Vitamin Standardization of the League of Nations in 1938 adopted crystalline synthetic thiamine hydrochloride as the International Unit (antineuritic vitamin B_1, activity of 10 mg of acid clay adsorbate) as the potency of 3 μg of synthetic thiamine hydrochloride.[4] One USP unit is equivalent to one International Unit.

For a discussion of the various animal assay units defined before and their equivalency to the International Unit and to pure thiamine, see page 169 of the monograph by Williams and Spies.[1]

[1] R. R. Williams and T. D. Spies, "Vitamin B_1 and Its Use in Medicine," p. 91. Macmillan, New York, 1938.

[2] Medical Research Council, "Vitamins: A Survey of Present Knowledge," p. 313. HM Stationery Office, London, 1932.

[3] B. C. P. Jansen and W. F. Donath, *Proc. Kon. Akad. Wetensch. Amsterdam* **29**, 1390 (1926).

[4] T. F. Macrae, *League Nat. Bull. Health Organ.* **9**, 371 (1940).

VII. Biogenesis

GENE M. BROWN

Observations concerning the nature of thiamine-requiring microorganisms allow these organisms to be divided into three groups: (a) those that will utilize either thiamine or the pyrimidine portion of thiamine; (b) those that will utilise either thiamine or the thiazole portion of the vitamin, and (c) those that require intact thiamine. These observations indicate that the biosynthesis of thiamine proceeds by the independent formation of the pyrimidine and thiazole moieties of the vitamin followed by a final step in which these two moieties are joined together to give thiamine. Organisms of group (a) (above) are those deficient in synthesizing the pyrimidine part of the vitamin; organisms of group (b) presumably cannot make the thiazole half of the molecule; and group (c) organisms would be those that are unable to carry out the final steps of thiamine synthesis from the two halves of the molecule.

A. Formation of Thiamine From Its Pyrimidine and Thiazole Moieties

A great deal of information has now been accumulated about the enzymatic reactions concerned in the formation of thiamine from its pyrimidine and thiazole moieties. The initial stimulus for this work was provided by Harris and Yavit who, in 1957,[1] reported that 2-methyl-4-amino-5-hydroxymethyl-pyrimidine (hereafter referred to as hydroxymethylpyrimidine) and 4-methyl-5-(β-hydroxyethyl)thiazole (hereafter referred to as thiazole) could be converted to thiamine by cell free extracts of baker's yeast in the presence of ATP. These workers suggested that a phosphate ester of hydroxymethyl-pyrimidine (hydroxymethylpyrimidine-P) is probably an intermediate in the reaction sequence. However, Leder[2] found that the yeast enzyme system could catalyze thiamine synthesis from hydroxymethylpyrimidine-P only when ATP was also present. Three groups of workers then independently obtained evidence that the pyrophosphate ester of hydroxymethylpyrimidine (hydroxy-methylpyrimidine-PP) is the phosphorylated form of the pyrimidine that reacts directly with the thiazole compound. Synthetic hydroxymethyl-pyrimidine-PP was prepared by Leder[3] and by Nose et al.[4] and was found to be used as substrate in place of hydroxymethylpyrimidine and ATP.

---

[1] D. L. Harris and J. Yavit, *Fed. Amer. Soc. Exp. Biol.* **16**, 192 (1957).

[2] I. G. Leder, *Fed. Amer. Soc. Exp. Biol.* **18**, 270 (1959).

[3] I. G. Leder, *Biochem. Biophys. Res. Commun.* **1**, 63 (1959).

[4] Y. Nose, K. Ueda, and T. Kawasaki, *Biochim. Biophys. Acta* **34**, 277 (1959).

Camiener and Brown[5, 6] were able to show that hydroxymethylpyrimidine-PP was formed enzymatically from ATP and hydroxymethylpyrimidine and that this enzymatic product could be used in place of the free pyrimidine and ATP for synthesis of the vitamin.

It was determined that thiamine monophosphate (thiamine-P) instead of thiamine is the primary product formed by the yeast enzyme system.[3, 6, 7] This suggested that thiazole might be phosphorylated to thiazole monophosphate (thiazole-P) prior to reacting with hydroxymethylpyrimidine-PP. Further investigations revealed that thiazole-P can be used as substrate along with hydroxymethylpyrimidine-PP to yield thiamine-P in the absence of ATP.[3, 4, 5, 7, 8] Substitution of thiazole for thiazole-P allowed no compound with thiamine activity to be formed unless ATP were also supplied. It was also established that the enzyme system was not able to phosphorylate thiamine to thiamine-P, whereas an enzyme that catalyzes the formation of thiazole-P from thiazole and ATP was detected.[5, 7]

Fractionation of the yeast extracts by Camiener and Brown[7] led to the separation of the thiamine-synthesizing enzyme system into two protein fractions, both of which were required for thiamine-P synthesis from hydroxymethylpyrimidine, thiazole, and ATP. Fraction 1 contained the enzymes necessary for the formation of hydroxymethylpyrimidine-PP, and Fraction 2 contained the enzyme that catalyzes the synthesis of thiazole-P and the enzyme responsible for the conversion of hydroxymethylpyrimidine-PP and thiazole-P to thiamine-P. Leder[9] has purified the latter enzyme some 500-fold from yeast extracts and described some of its properties.

The observations by Harris and Yavit[1] and by Leder[2] that, in the presence of ATP, thiamine synthesis proceeds at a faster rate from hydroxymethylpyrimidine-P than from hydroxymethylpyrimidine suggests that hydroxymethylpyrimidine-P may be an intermediate in the conversion of hydroxymethylpyrimidine to hydroxymethylpyrimidine-PP. Another report that appears to support this contention is the finding by Camiener and Brown[5, 6] that hydroxymethylpyrimidine-P, as well as the pyrophosphate ester, are formed enzymatically by the yeast enzyme system. Independent investigations by Lewin and Brown[10, 11] and by Kawasaki and Fujita[12, 13] confirmed this hypothesis. The former workers presented evidence for the occurrence of two

[5] G. W. Camiener and G. M. Brown, J. Amer. Chem. Soc. 81, 3800 (1959).
[6] G. W. Camiener and G. M. Brown, J. Biol. Chem. 235, 2404 (1960).
[7] G. W. Camiener and G. M. Brown, J. Biol. Chem. 235, 2411 (1960).
[8] T. Nose, K. Ueda, T. Kawasaki, A. Iwashima, and T. Fujita, J. Vitaminol. (Kyoto) 7, 98 (1962).
[9] I. G. Leder, J. Biol. Chem. 236, 3066 (1961).
[10] L. M. Lewin and G. M. Brown, Fed. Amer. Soc. Exp. Biol. 20, 447 (1961).
[11] L. M. Lewin and G. M. Brown, J. Biol. Chem. 236, 2768 (1961).
[12] T. Kawasaki and T. Fujita, Seikagaku 33, 737 (1961) Chem. Abstr. 56, 7676 (1962).
[13] T. Kawasaki and T. Fujita, Seikagaku 33, 742 (1961) Chem. Abstr. 56, 7676 (1962).

enzymes in yeast extracts, one of which catalyzed the phosphorylation of hydroxymethylpyrimidine with ATP and the second is the phosphorylation of hydroxymethylpyrimidine-P to hydroxymethylpyrimidine-PP in the presence of ATP. Fujita and his collaborators showed that ATP labeled with ^{32}P in the terminal phosphate residue yielded hydroxymethylpyrimidine-PP labeled equally with ^{32}P in both phosphate units, a fact that also indicates that two successive phosphorylations take place in the formation of hydroxymethylpyrimidine-PP.

B. Formation of Thiamine Pyrophosphate

Camiener and Brown[5, 7] discovered that yeast enzyme preparations catalyze the formation of thiamine pyrophosphate (thiamine-PP), the coenzyme form of the vitamin, from free thiamine, but not directly from thiamine-P. This observation appeared to confirm the views expressed earlier by others[14, 15, 16] that the enzymatic synthesis of thiamine-PP involves the transfer of a pyrophosphate group from ATP to thiamine in a single enzymatic step. Shimazono and co-workers[17, 18] proved that this conclusion is valid by showing that a purified enzyme from baker's yeast transferred only a pyrophosphate group from ^{32}P labeled ATP to thiamine and that thiamine-P could not be used as substrate. Thus, it seems appropriate to refer to this enzyme as "thiamine pyrophosphokinase"[17, 18] instead of the traditional "thiaminokinase."

Since thiamine-P cannot be directly phosphorylated to thiamine-PP, formulation of a biosynthetic pathway for the *de novo* formation of thiamine-PP from the pyrimidine and thiazole moieties must include an enzymatic reaction for the dephosphorylation of thiamine-P. Latham[19] has looked for a specific enzyme that might catalyze this reaction; however, none has been found. Instead, this reaction appears to be catalyzed by any one of several acid and alkaline phosphatases found in yeast.[19]

The facts that have been accumulated and that have been discussed above indicate that the conversion of hydroxymethylpyrimidine and thiazole to thiamine and thiamine-PP is accomplished by the enzymatic reactions shown in Fig. 1. The enzymes responsible for catalyzing these reactions have been named in the order in which the reactions that they catalyze are numbered

[14] H. Weil-Malherbe, *Biochem. J.* **33**, 1997 (1939).
[15] F. Leuthardt and H. Nielsen, *Helv. Chim. Acta* **35**, 1196 (1952).
[16] O. Forsander, *Commentat. Phys. Math.* **19**, 2 (1956).
[17] N. Shimazono, Y. Mano, R. Tanaka, and Y. Kaziro, *J. Biochem.* (*Tokyo*) **46**, 959 (1959).
[18] Y. Kaziro, R. Tanaka, Y. Mano, and N. Shimazono, *J. Biochem.* (*Tokyo*) **49**, 472 (1961).
[19] H. Latham, Thiamine Phosphate Phosphatases of Yeast, Masters Thesis, Mass. Inst. Technol., Cambridge, Massachusetts, 1959.

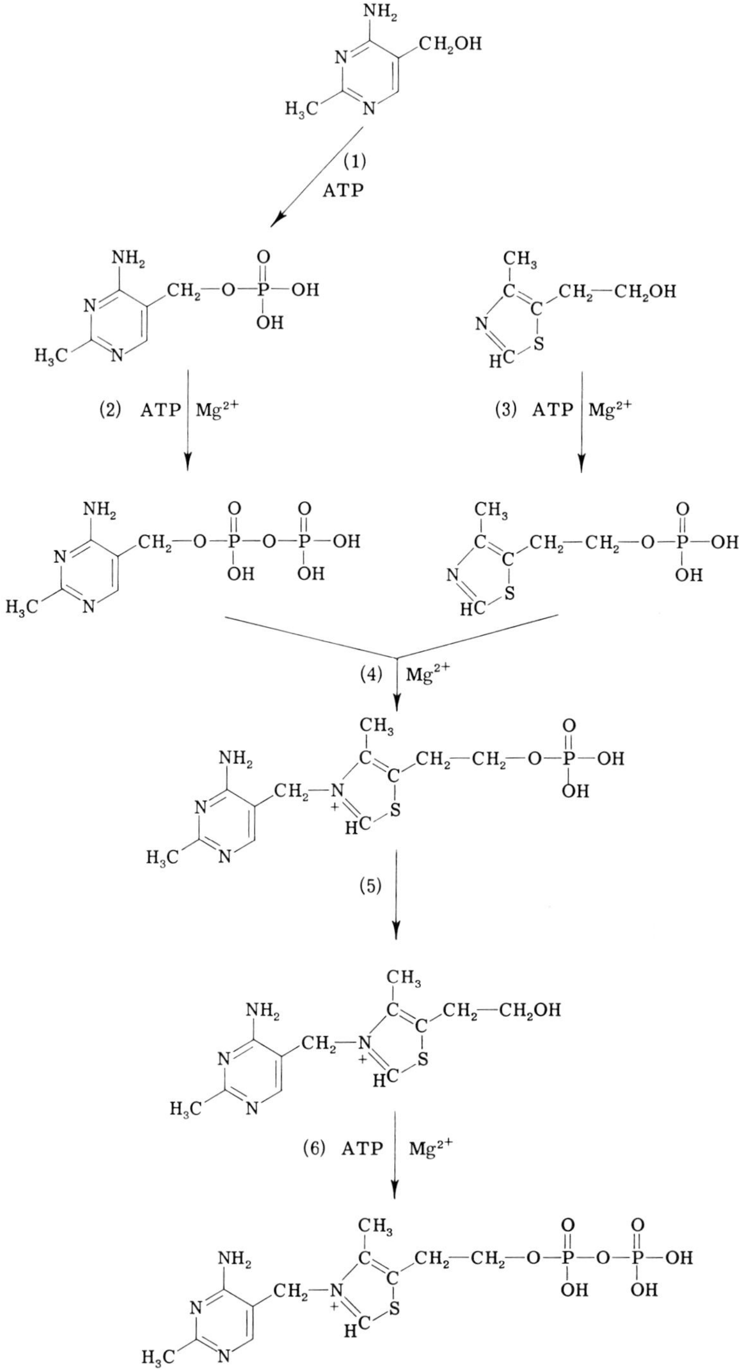

FIG. 1. Reactions involved in the enzymatic conversion of pyrimidine and thiazole to thiamine and thiamine-PP.

in the figure: hydroxymethylpyrimidine kinase,[11] hydroxymethylpyrimidine phosphokinase,[11] thiazole kinase,[7] thiamine-P synthase[7] or thiamine-P pyrophosphorylase[9] (since the reaction is reversible), phosphatase, and thiamine pyrophosphokinase.[7, 18]

C. Origin of the Pyrimidine Moiety

It has now been well established that the pyrimidine portion of thiamine is not made by the same biosynthetic pathway used for the formation of the pyrimidines of nucleic acids. This was first documented by Goldstein and Brown[20] who found that radioactivity from uracil, orotic acid, CO_2 and aspartic acid was not incorporated into thiamine by *E. coli*. Later work, to be discussed below, has confirmed this conclusion and has given some insight into the biosynthesis of this pyrimidine compound.

The first clear indication of the nature of the precursors of hydroxymethyl-pyrimidine came from reports that exogenous radioactive formate is efficiently incorporated into hydroxymethylpyrimidine by bacteria[20, 21] and yeast.[22] It has been established that in the enteric bacteria, *E. coli*[23] and *Salmonella typhimurium*,[24] carbon 2 of the pyrimidine (see Fig. 2 for number-ing system) is derived from formate, but David, *et al.*[25] have presented evi-dence that carbon 4 is derived from formate in yeast. These observations suggest that yeast and enteric bacteria make this compound by different pathways.

Other compounds that were found by Goldstein and Brown[20] to be incorporated relatively effectively into hydroxymethylpyrimidine are glycine and acetate. Johnson, *et al.*[26] reported that only C-2 of acetate is incorporated efficiently by yeast. Tomlinson[27] reported that C-2 of acetate is incorporated only into the methyl group attached to carbon 2 of the pyrimidine ring. Some doubt has arisen about the significance of the incorporation of acetate as a result of the finding by Kumaoka and Brown[23] that in *E. coli* administration of nonradioactive formate dilutes out the incorporation of acetate.

The most significant recent work has come from the studies of Newell and Tucker[28, 29, 30] who have obtained direct evidence that the formation

[20] G. A. Goldstein and G. M. Brown, *Arch. Biochem. Biophys.* **103**, 449 (1963).
[21] M. J. Pine and R. Guthrie, *J. Bacterial.* **78**, 545 (1959).
[22] S. David and B. Estramareix, *Biochim. Biophys. Acta* **42**, 562 (1960).
[23] H. Kumaoka and G. M. Brown, *Arch. Biochem. Biophys.* **122**, 378 (1967).
[24] B. Estramareix and M. Lesieur, *Biochim. Biophys. Acta* **192**, 375 (1969).
[25] S. David, B. Estramareix and H. Hirshfeld, *Biochim. Biophys. Acta* **127**, 264 (1966).
[26] D. B. Johnson, D. J. Howells and T. W. Goodwin, *Biochem. J.* **98**, 30 (1966).
[27] R. V. Tomlinson, *Biochim. Biophys. Acta* **115**, 526 (1966).
[28] P. C. Newell and R. G. Tucker, *Nature* **215**, 1384 (1967).
[29] P. C. Newell and R. G. Tucker, *Biochem. J.* **106**, 271 (1968).
[30] P. C. Newell and R. G. Tucker, *Biochem. J.* **106**, 279 (1968).

of hydroxymethylpyrimidine is closely tied to the biosynthesis of purines. Their investigations were prompted by the earlier report on the isolation of mutants of *S. typhimurium* that require both a purine and hydroxymethylpyrimidine as a result of a single mutation.[31] This suggested that purines and hydroxymethylpyrimidine are made by a common biosynthetic pathway. Newell and Tucker provided evidence for this suggestion by showing that 4-aminoimidazole ribonucleotide is a common intermediate in the biosynthesis of purines and hydroxymethylpyrimidine. Their work was made possible through their isolation of a secondary mutant that is permeable to aminoimidazole ribonucleoside. They were then able to show that this substance can satisfy both the purine and the thiamine requirement of the organism. In addition, they showed that the mutant could convert radioactive aminoimidazole ribonucleoside to hydroxymethylpyrimidine with no dilution of radioactivity. One puzzling observation made by these workers is that although methionine is required for the conversion of aminoimidazole ribonucleotide to hydroxymethylpyrimidine, no carbons of methionine are incorporated into the product. This is consistent with the earlier observation of Goldstein and Brown[20] that the methyl group of methionine is not incorporated into the pyrimidine.

The enzymic reactions involved in the transformation of aminoimidazole ribonucleotide into hydroxymethylpyrimidine remain unknown, and any speculative scheme must take into account that in enteric bacteria formate is incorporated only into carbon 2 of the pyrimidine ring. Since formate is also known to be the precursor of carbon 5 of aminoimidazole ribonucleotide, any proposed set of reactions must include the provision for carbon 5 of aminoimidazole ribonucleotide to be converted to carbon 2 of the pyrimidine. Possible general schemes are shown in Fig. 2. One possibility (Scheme 1, Fig. 2) is that the imidazole ring is ruptured between carbons 4 and 5. This would be followed by the insertion of a two-carbon unit and a methyl group and the removal of the ribose-P group. If such a scheme is correct, the source of the methyl group is puzzling since it is known not to be derived from either methionine[20, 29] or the one-carbon pool.[23] Another possibility (Scheme 2, Fig. 2) is that the imidazole ring is ruptured between N-1 and C-5, followed by the addition of three one-carbon units to provide the ring carbon 6, the hydroxymethyl group and the methyl group, and the removal of the ribose-P unit. This scheme seems less likely since three one-carbon units would be involved and it is known that none of these three carbons of the pyrimidine molecule is derived from formate. A third scheme was suggested by Newell and Tucker[30] and is shown as Scheme 3 in Fig. 2. This scheme involves the rupture of the ring between atoms 1 and 5, the

[31] M. Demerec, H. Moser, R. C. Clowes, E. L. Lahr, H. Ozeki, and W. Vielmetter, Carnegie Inst. Wash., Year Book 55, 309 (1955–1956).

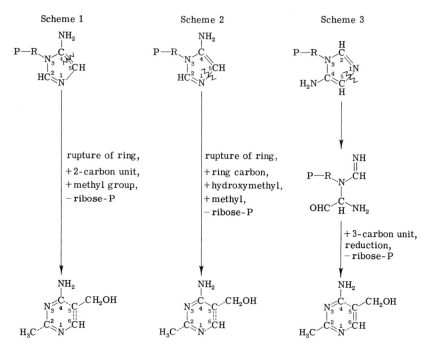

FIG. 2. Hypothetical schemes for the conversion of aminoimidazole ribonucleotide to the pyrimidine moiety of thiamine. R-P represents a ribose-5-phosphate unit.

addition of a three-carbon unit, the removal of ribose-P, and the reduction of an aldehydic group to a methyl group. In this scheme, however, carbon 5 of the imidazole ring becomes carbon 4 of the pyrimidine ring and, thus, this scheme is not consistent with the formate labeling data in enteric bacteria. It should be remembered, however, that this scheme is consistent with what has been published about labeling with formate in yeast. This scheme was proposed by Newell and Tucker before it was established that the labeling with formate in bacteria is different from that that had been reported in yeast.

Labeling experiments with (^{14}C) glycine in *S. typhimurium* have indicated that Scheme 1, Fib. 2 is more likely than Schemes 2 and 3. Extramareix and Lesieur[24] grew *S. typhimurium* in the presence of (1-^{14}C) glycine and found radioactivity exclusively in carbon 4 of the isolated pyrimidine. In a later paper Extramareix[32] showed that (2-^{14}C) glycine is incorporated exclusively into carbon 6 of pyrimidine. These observations are consistent with the splitting of the imidazole ring between carbons 4 and 5 as shown in Scheme 1. The origins of the two-carbon compound (to provide carbon 5 and the

[32] B. Estramareix, *Biochim. Biophys. Acta* **208**, 170 (1970).

hydroxymethyl group) and the methyl group attached to carbon 2 remain to be established.

Other information that possibly bears on the latter stages of the biogenesis of the pyrimidine compound comes from the work of Diorio and Lewin.[33, 34] They have isolated thiamine-requiring mutants of Neurospora that excrete 5-aminomethyl and 5-formyl derivatives of pyrimidine and have suggested that these compounds may be intermediates in the synthesis of the 5-hydroxy-methylpyrimidine.

D. Biogenesis of the Thiazole Moiety

Most of the literature on the biosynthesis of the thiazole portion of thiamine consists of speculative schemes, unsupported by data, and reports on incorporation of various radioactive compounds by microorganisms. Methionine and cysteine have most often been considered as the source of sulfur for the formation of thiazole, but data to support these possibilities have been inconclusive. Johnson et al.[26] have reported that equal quantities of ^{35}S and ^{14}C are incorporated into thiazole by yeast provided with methionine labeled with ^{35}S and ^{14}C in the methyl carbon, but the amounts incorporated were so low that the observation may not be significant. Other workers have found that the methyl of methionine is not incorporated into thiazole.[35, 36] Nakayama[37] has suggested that cysteine may provide carbons and sulfur for thiazole synthesis. This suggestion was based on his contention that certain thiazole-requiring mutants of E. coli and Neurospora crassa can utilize cysteine, 4-methylthiazole and 4-thiazolidine carboxylic acid in place of thiazole. However, serious doubts about precursor roles for these compounds have arisen as a result of the observations made by Korte, et al.[38] that 4-methyl (2-^{14}C) thiazole is not converted to thiazole by microorganisms. It has also been found by other workers that neither (^{14}C) cysteine nor (^{14}C) formate can be converted to thiazole by E. coli.[35]

Radioactive incorporation data have indicated that alanine,[26, 39] acetate (both carbons),[26, 35, 39] glycine[35, 36] and serine[36] are converted to thiazole by growing cultures of microorganisms, but the relative importance of these compounds as precursors and the details of the enzymatic steps involved in the biosynthesis of thiazole remain unknown.

[33] A. F. Diorio and L. M. Lewin, J. Biol. Chem. 243, 3999 (1968).
[34] A. F. Diorio and L. M. Lewin, J. Biol. Chem. 243, 4006 (1968).
[35] M. Julius and G. M. Brown, unpublished observations (1966).
[36] P. E. Linnett and J. Walker, Biochem. J. 109, 161 (1968).
[37] H. Nakayama, Vitamins (Kyoto) 11, 169 (1956).
[38] F. Korte, H. Weitkamp, and J. Vogel, Ann. Chem. 628, 159 (1959).
[39] R. V. Tomlinson, D. P. Kulhman, P. F. Torrence, and H. Tieckelmann, Biochim. Biophys. Acta 148, 1 (1967).

VIII. Modified Thiamines

EDWARD F. ROGERS

Hundreds of compounds embodying modifications of the thiamine molecule have been synthesized and tested as thiamine substitutes or antagonists. Recent reviews[1, 8] summarizes this work.

A. Modified Thiamines with Vitamin Activity

The structural requirements for vitamin activity are quite specific; only the 2'-ethyl and 2'-n-propyl homologs (Ia, b) are comparable in biological effects with thiamine. This specificity is not surprising as an active pseudothiamine must be convertible to a pseudothiamine pyrophosphate which can function in the various enzyme systems in which cocarboxylase normally plays a role. The situation is altered when thiamine is considered in a lesser sense than is connoted by the term "vitamin." For example, many compounds can replace thiamine as a thiaminase substrate.[2]

The modified thiamines of greatest interest in nutrition as thiamine substitutes are a class of latent thiamines which are transformed into thiamine by metabolic processes. The so-called "thiamine disulfide" of Zima and Williams[3] was the first compound synthesized with activity ascribable to its conversion *in vivo* to thiamine, presumably by the sequence III ⟶ II ⟶ I. A large number of other latent thiamines which can be represented by structure IV are now known. Like thiamine disulfide these are derivatives of the open thiol form (II) of thiamine. Hydroxyl ion attack on the 2-position of thiamine yields the thiol, *via* a carbinol base intermediate which is not shown.[4] This reversible ring opening is characteristic of thiazolium salts which are unsubstituted in the 2-position.[5]

The early observations on the disulfide were almost forgotten until the discovery of allithiamine (IV, X = SCH$_2$CH = CH$_2$, Y = H), an artifact

---

[1] E. F. Rogers, *Ann. N. Y. Acad. Sci.* 98, 412 (1962); in Methods in Enzymology (D. B. McCormick and L. B. Wright, ed.), Vol. XVIIIA, p. 245 (Academic Press, New York) (1970).

[2] A. Fujita, *Advan. Enzymol. Relat. Areas Mol. Biol.* 15, 389 (1954).

[3] O. Zima and R. R. Williams, *Ber. Deut. Chem. Ges.* 73, 941 (1940).

[4] R. R. Williams and A. E. Ruehle, *J. Amer. Chem. Soc.* 57, 1856 (1935); H. T. Clarke and S. Gurin, *J. Amer. Chem. Soc.* 57, 1876 (1935); A Watanabe and Y. Asahi, *Yakugaku Zasshi* 75, 1046 (1955).

[5] J. M. Sprague and A. H. Land, *in* "Heterocyclic Chemistry" (R. C. Elderfield, ed.), Vol. 5, p, 647, 1957.

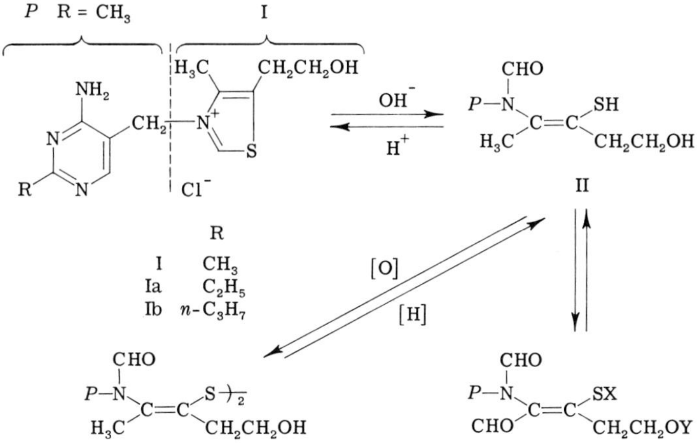

P $R = CH_3$ I

$$\underbrace{\quad}_{P\ R=CH_3} \underbrace{\quad}_{I}$$

H$_3$C CH$_2$CH$_2$OH

NH$_2$

CH$_2$—N$^+$

R

N N

Cl$^-$ S

CHO

P—N SH

H$_3$C C=C CH$_2$CH$_2$OH

II

OH$^-$ / H$^+$

	R
I	CH$_3$
Ia	C$_2$H$_5$
Ib	n-C$_3$H$_7$

[O] / [H]

CHO

P—N S$\overset{\displaystyle }{}_2$

H$_3$C C=C CH$_2$CH$_2$OH

III

CHO

P—N SX

CHO C=C CH$_2$CH$_2$OY

IV

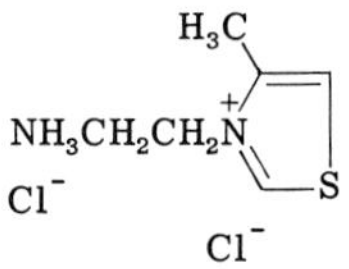

H$_3$C

NH$_3$CH$_2$CH$_2$N$^+$ S

Cl$^-$ Cl$^-$

V

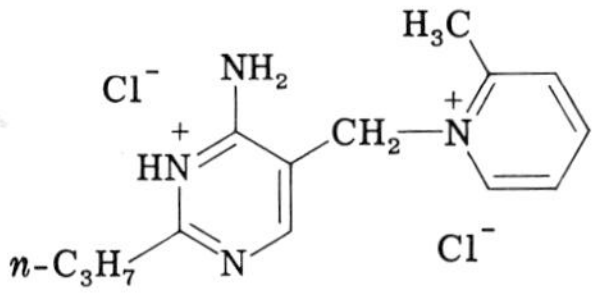

H$_3$C

Cl$^-$ NH$_2$

CH$_2$—N$^+$

HN$^+$

n-C$_3$H$_7$ N Cl$^-$

VI

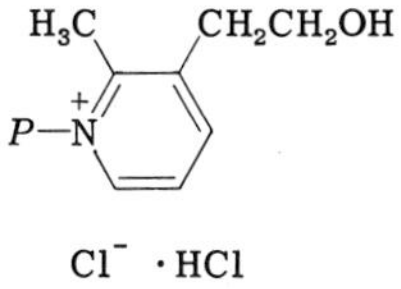

H$_3$C CH$_2$CH$_2$OH

P—N$^+$

Cl$^-$ · HCl

VI

X

CH$_2$—I

N

R N

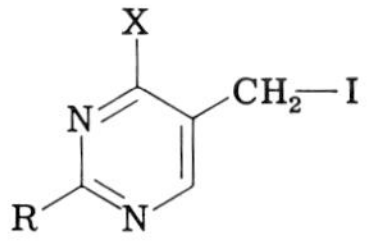

	X	R
VIIa	OH	CH$_3$
VIIb	NH$_2$	CF$_3$

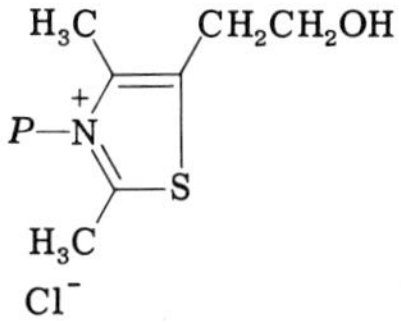

H$_3$C CH$_2$CH$_2$OH

P—N$^+$ S

H$_3$C

Cl$^-$

formed by reaction of alliin with thiamine.[6] Subsequent studies of this compound and its dihydro derivative, thiamine propyl disulfide (IV, X = $SCH_2CH_2CH_3$, Y = H), aroused interest in modified thiamines as exceptionally stable forms of the vitamin which may be better absorbed.

A large number of derivatives of the thiamine thiol have been prepared in which the sulfhydryl group is acylated, alkylated, or converted to a mixed disulfide. In many modified thiamines the hydroxyl is also acylated. Of the alkyl disulfide types similar to thiamine propyl disulfide, the tetrahydrofurfuyl and β-hydroxyethyl analogs (IV, X = $SCH_2C_4H_7O$, SCH_2CH_2OH; Y = H) are reported to be almost odorless, thus eliminating a major drawback of the propyl disulfide. O,S-Diacetylthiamine and dibenzoylthiamine (IV, X,Y = $COCH_3$; COC_6H_5) are typical acyl products. An interesting modification of mixed functionally is S-benzoylthiamine-O-phosphate (IV, X = COC_6H_5; Y = PO_3H_2).[7] Two excellent reviews of this complex field are now available.[8]

A representative modified thiamine, O,S-dibenzoylthiamine, is reported to be odorless, stable, and highly satisfactory for formulation. Absorption is proportional to dosage, and high blood thiamine levels are rapidly attained. Acitivity is variable in *in vitro* tests with bacteria and fungi. These properties agree with general chemical experience, since thiamine, a highly reactive benzyl-type quaternary in equilibrium with an appreciable fraction of free thiol form, is replaced by a nonquaternary in which the sulfhydryl and hydroxyl groups are protected by lipophilic acyl moieties hydrolyzable by liver esterases. S-Benzoylthiamine-O-phosphate lacks the lipophilic character of most modified thiamines but also is reported to be well absorbed and to produce high levels of blood cocarboxylase.

With relatively few exceptions, the latent thiamine research has been prosecuted by Japanese drug firms and cooperating groups. It is desirable that the results reported be corroborated and extended by more scientists in other countries. A matter requiring clarification is the significance of the enhanced thiamine blood levels said to be obtained with modified thiamines. There is no pathological condition attributable to thiamine malabsorption. Moreover accumulating evidence[9, 9a] indicates that thiamine transport is active, implying the possibility of a regulatory mechanism for absorption which modified thiamines may circumvent.

[6] M. Fugiwara and H. Watanabe, *Proc. Jap. Acad.* **28**, 156 (1952); T. Matsukawa and S. Yurugi, *Proc. Jap. Acad.* **28**, 146 (1952).

[7] T. Wada, H. Takagi, S. Miyazawa, Y. Susuki, and H. Minikami, *Bitamin* **22**, 342 (1961).

[8] T. Maksukawa, S. Yurugi, and Y. Oka, *Ann. N.Y. Acad. Sci.* **98**, 430 (1962); C. Kawasaki, *Vitam. Horm. (New York)* **21**, 69 (1963).

[9] H. Neujahr, *Acta Chem. Scand.* **17**, 1902 (1963); S. K. Sharma and J. H. Quastel, *Biochem. J.* **94**, 790 (1965); U. Ventura and G. Rindi, *Experientia* **21**, 645 (1965).

[9a] D. Polin, E. R. Wynosky, and C. C. Porter, *Poultry Sci.* **42**, 1057 (1963); *Proc. Soc. Exp. Biol. Med.* **114**, 273 (1963).

B. Modified Thiamines with Antivitamin Activity

Thiamine antagonists are the subject of recent reviews.[1] In general an antagonist need not resemble the substrate closely and only requires a similarity in one or more salient features to compete with some success for enzyme sites. The thiaminase inhibitors described by Sealock and Goodland[10] are a case in point. A typical active compound, 3-(2-aminoethyl)-4-methyl-thiazolium chloride hydrochloride (V), obviously simulates only the central part of the molecule close to the critical C—N bond.

Closer analogy to thiamine is noted with the large class of anticoccidial quaternaries typified by amprolium or 1-(4-amino-2-n-propyl-5-pyrimidinyl-methyl)-2-picolinium chloride hydrochloride (VI). Amprolium is employed as a prophylactic agent for coccidiosis control in broiler production.[11] The drug affects thiamine absorption and this has been suggested as the mechanism for its anticoccidial actions.[9a, 12]

The thiaminase inhibitors and anticoccidial quaternaries lack the thiamine β-hydroxyethyl group and hence cannot be phosphorylated and are unlikely to be effective in thiamine pyrophosphate-mediated reactions. The first example of cocarboxylase inhibition, observed by Buchman et al.[13] in 1940 with 4-methyl-5-(2-hydroxyethyl)-thiazole pyrophosphate (VII) was actually the first case of coenzyme inhibition. The tertiary base inhibitor approximates half of the cocarboxylase molecule.

As thiamine antagonists in the "classic" sense, that is inhibitors designed to contain a minimal variation (isostere or homolog), one may cite: pyrithiamine (VI), the first rationally designed antimetabolite, in which the thiazolium sulfur is replaced by a vinyl group;[14] oxythiamine (VIIa), in which the 4'-amino is substituted by 4'-hydroxyl;[15] 2-methylthiamine (VIII), in which the critical 2-position of thiamine is blocked by methyl[15] and 2'-trifluoromethylthiamine (VIIb), in which an isosteric replacement affects the lipophilic character and ring basicity.[16] All these inhibitors appear to function at the coenzyme level after conversion to pyrophosphates and affect a wide variety of enzymes and organisms. Pyrithiamine, long the most thoroughly studied antagonist, has lately been utilized by chemists concerned with the biochemistry of nerve tissue.

[10] R. R. Sealock and R. L. Goodland, J. Amer. Chem. Soc. 66, 507 (1944).

[11] A. C. Cuckler, M. Garzillo, C. Malanga, and E. C. McManus, Poultry Sci. 39, 1241 (1960); E. H. Peterson and J. LaBorde, Poultry Sci. 41, 207 (1962).

[12] E. F. Rogers, R. L. Clark, A. A. Pessolano, H. J. Becker, W. J. Leanza, L. H. Sarett, A. C. Cuckler, E. McManus, M. Garzillo, C. Malanga, W. H. Ott, A. M. Dickinson, and A. A. VanIderstine, J. Amer. Chem. Soc. 82, 2974 (1960).

[13] E. R. Buchman, E. Hergard, and J. Bonner, Proc. Nat. Acad. Sci. U.S. 26, 561 (1940).

[14] A. H. Tracy and R. C. Elderfield, J. Org. Chem. 6, 54 (1941); A. W. Wilson and S. A. Harris, J. Amer. Chem. Soc. 71, 2231 (1949).

[15] F. Bergel and A. R. Todd, J. Chem. Soc. London p. 1504 (1937); M. Soodak and L. R. Cerecedo, J. Amer. Chem. Soc. 66, 1988 (1944).

[16] J. A. Barone, H. Tieckelman, R. Guthrie, and J. F. Holland, J. Org. Chem. 25, 211 (1960).

IX. Biochemical Detection of Deficiency

MERTON P. LAMDEN

A. Introduction

One of the prime goals of nutritional biochemistry is to discover specific disturbances in the intermediary metabolism of body tissue arising from the deficiency of a given nutrient. For assessing nutritional deficiency in humans, this disturbance should be manifest in readily accessible material such as blood or urine. It is assumed that biochemical changes would be manifest before gross clinical signs are apparent and thus allow subclinical or borderline states of deficiency to be detected. The ultimate goal is to determine the underlying biochemical change that is directly responsible for the overt clinical signs of nutritional deficiency.

According to Arroyave,[1] who has summed up the sequence of events leading to nutritional disease and the role of biochemical tests in its assessment, such tests either measure changes in the "supply" of a nutrient or detect biochemical changes reflecting metabolic alterations consequent to nutritional effects. Such changes are considered the "biochemical nutritional pathology." An example of the first would be the level of thiamine in tissues or body fluids while an example of biochemical nutritional pathology would be the accumulation of pyruvic acid in blood or the lowering of erythrocyte transketolase activity in thiamine-deficient individuals. This would have more meaning in the detection of thiamine deficiency than a blood thiamine level since it would indicate impaired functional involvement of thiamine. Biochemical nutritional pathology would show up when the concentration of the essential nutrient in utilizable form decreases to the point where homeostatic mechanisms finally become overwhelmed, and there is interference with intermediary metabolism.

A decrease in the concentration of a given nutrient such as thiamine in body fluids may mean no more than a low intake for a variable period of time. Such a measurement would indicate the relative adequacy of intake of the given nutrient but not the existence, nature, or magnitude of nutritional disease. However, from a practical point of view, particularly for assessing the nutritional status of populations, measurement of a nutrient level such as the urinary excretion may be equally satisfactory or even more desirable.[2]

In this section a number of biochemical tests that may be useful in detecting a condition of thiamine deficiency, namely tests for blood thiamine, urinary

[1] G. Arroyave, *Fed. Proc. Fed. Amer. Soc. Exp. Biol.* **20**, 39 (1961).
[2] W. N. Pearson, *Amer. J. Clin. Nutr.* **11**, 462 (1962).

excretion of thiamine, blood levels of pyruvate and lactate, methylglyoxal, glyoxylate, and erythrocyte transketolase will be discussed briefly. For further amplification on the assessment of thiamine deficiency several references are recommended.[1-13]

B. Blood Levels of Thiamine

Goodhart and Nitzberg[14] found a definite association between the acute peripheral neuropathy of the alcohol addict and low thiamine values. Goodhart at that time (1941), and in 1962, felt that total blood thiamine values below 3.0 μg/100 ml should be regarded as indicative of a thiamine-deficiency state.[15] Their range of thiamine levels for 45 normal subjects by the fermentation method was 3.1 to 9.2 with an average of 5.4 μg/100 ml.

Rowlands and Wilkinson[16] using the Phycomyces determination obtained values of 6.5–16.5 μg/100 ml for normal subjects with values of 5 μg/100 ml or less for patients with alcoholic neuritis, nutritional neuritis, scurvy, and malnutrition.

Oldham et al.[17] studying the excretion and blood levels of young women on diets containing varying levels of thiamine, found that after 59 days on an

[3] G. Goldsmith, "Chemical Tests and Their Interpretations in Nutrition Surveys: Their Techniques and Value." Bull. Nat. Res. Counc. (U.S.) 117, 47 (1949).

[4] F. A. Robinson, "The Vitamin Co-Factors of Enzyme Systems," pp. 66–71. Pergamon, Oxford, 1966.

[5] M. Bodansky and O. Bodansky, "Biochemistry of Disease," 2nd Ed., p. 969. Macmillan, New York, 1952.

[6] O. A. Bessey, in "Methods for Evaluation of Nutritional Adequacy and Status" (H. Spector, M. S. Peterson, and T. E. Friedemann, eds.), p. 59. Advisory Board on Quartermaster Research and Development, Committee on Foods, National Research Council. Nat. Acad. Sci., Washington, D.C. 1954.

[7] W. G. Unglaub and G. A. Goldsmith, in "Methods for Evaluation of Nutritional Adequacy and Status" (H. Spector, M. S. Peterson, and T. E. Friedemann, eds.), p. 69. Advisory Board on Quartermaster Research and Development, Committee on Foods, National Research Council. Nat. Acad. Sci., Washington, D.C., 1954.

[8] R. F. Krause, in "Modern Nutrition in Health and Disease" (M. G. Wohl and R. S. Goodhart, eds.), p. 429. Lea & Febiger, Philadelphia, Pennsylvania, 1955.

[9] W. H. Sebrell, Jr., Ann. N.Y. Acad. Sci. 98, 563 (1962).

[10] I. C. Plough and E. B. Bridgforth, Pub. Health Rep. 75, 699 (1960).

[11] G. E. W. Wolstenholme and M. O'Connor, eds., "Thiamine Deficiency: Biochemical Lesions and their Clinical Significance." Ciba Found. Study Group (Pap.) 28 (1967).

[12] W. N. Pearson, Amer. J. Clin. Nutr. 20, 514 (1967).

[13] H. E. Sauberlich, Amer. J. Clin. Nutr. 20, 528 (1967).

[14] R. S. Goodhart and T. J. Nitzberg, J. Clin. Invest. 20, 625 (1941).

[15] R. S. Goodhart, in "Clinical Nutrition" (N. Jolliffe, ed.), p. 580. Harper (Hoeber), New York, 1962.

[16] E. N. Rowlands and J. F. Wilkinson, Brit. Med. J. ii, 818 (1938).

[17] H. G. Oldham, M. V. Davis, and L. V. Roberts, J. Nutr. 32, 163 (1946).

average intake of 295 µg/24 hours the average blood level dropped from 5.2 to 3.8 µg/100 ml. Although no signs of deficiency appeared, subjective symptoms were prevalent under circumstances which suggested the presence of subclinical thiamine deficiency.

Other reports relate blood level to intake.[18–20] Youmans[21] felt that while severe dietary deficiency lowered the blood level of normal individuals, increasing the intake did not increase the blood level, and Van Veen[22] attributes little significance to blood levels in detecting dietary inadequacy or assessing the requirement for thiamine compared to urinary excretion values.

Burch et al.[18] using their micromethod which includes the determination of thiamine in erythrocytes, showed there was a decrease of 20 and 30% in the thiamine level of the erythrocytes of the thiamine-deficient man and rat, respectively.

Also, Burch et al.[18] have pointed out that determinations of whole blood thiamine should take the hematocrit into consideration since the major portion of the vitamin is found in the erythrocytes and changes in whole blood thiamine concentration could be solely due to hematocrit changes.

Bessey[6] has pointed out that use of the erythrocyte thiamine level for evaluation of borderline thiamine deficiency may be warranted in the case of the rat, where the levels of thiamine and the changes due to deficiency are sufficiently great to be useful, but such is not the case for man.

Pearson in a recent paper concluded that the blood thiamine level in the human, although potentially useful, has not yet proved to be a very useful parameter of thiamine status. Similarly, Sauberlich[13] was of the opinion that blood thiamine determinations have not been entirely satisfactory and have not been particularly helpful in the evaluation of nutritional thiamine deficiencies. Cited were technical difficulties with analytical methods, the day-to-day variability in normal subjects, the minor decreases in blood thiamine levels of beriberi patients, and the considerable overlapping of such values with those of normal subjects.

On the other hand, Baker et al.[23, 24] have developed a method for blood thiamine using *Ochromonas danica*, which they feel is sensitive, specific,

[18] H. B. Burch, O. A. Bessey, R. H. Love, and O. H. Lowry, *J. Biol. Chem.* **198**, 477 (1952).

[19] R. B. Dubé, E. C. Johnson, H. Yü, and C. A. Storvick, *J. Nutr.* **48**, 307 (1952).

[20] T. E. Friedemann and T. C. Kmieciak, *J. Lab. Clin. Med.* **28**, 1262 (1943).

[21] J. B. Youmans, *Amer. J. Pub. Health* **32**, 1371 (1942); *Amer. J. Pub. Health* **33**, 58, 955 (1943); *Amer. J. Pub. Health* **34**, 368 (1944).

[22] A. G. Van Veen, *Geneesk. Tijdschr. Ned.-Indie* **80**, 1696 (1940).

[23] H. Baker, O. Frank, J. J. Fennelly, and C. M. Leevy, *Amer. J. Clin. Nutr.* **14**, 197 (1964).

[24] H. Baker, *Amer. J. Clin. Nutr.* **20**, 543 (1967).

and a more reliable diagnostic index than lactate or pyruvate blood values or transketolase levels, particularly in the case of mild thiamine deficiency or severe liver disease. Kershaw[25] found low whole blood thiamine levels in patients suffering from delirium tremens and alcoholic peripheral neuropathy and felt that whole blood vitamin levels may become of increasing value in psychiatric diagnosis.

C. Urinary Excretion of Thiamine

For many years the most frequently used laboratory aid in the detection of thiamine deficiency, and one that was considered more valuable than blood levels, was the urinary excretion test This has involved studies of the excretion of thiamine for 24 hours, or for lesser periods in conjunction with the measurement of simultaneously excreted urinary creatinine. Other methods involve the excretion of oral or injected test doses of thiamine for periods varying from 1 to 24 hours and the excretion of "pyramine," the pyrimidine half of the thiamine molecule.[26] The evaluation of vitamin adequacy by urinary excretion tests has been reviewed critically by Unglaub and Goldsmith,[7] Pearson,[12] and Sauberlich.[13]

There seems to be considerable disagreement as to the value of urinary excretion tests in the appraisal of thiamine-deficiency states of individuals, although such tests may be useful in appraising the recent thiamine intake of individuals and assessing the nutritional status of large groups. In a study of the problems of thiamine-deficiency states,[27] it has been pointed out that urinary excretion levels reflect principally the immediately preceding nutrient intake and not necessarily the body saturation. It was felt that metabolic alterations influence vitamin excretion levels and that the interpretation of vitamin load tests and their values in nutritional assessment were beset with difficulties. During a 3-year study of 36 mental patients with known intakes of thiamine, 24-hour and 4-hour urinary excretion studies were carried out after intramuscular administration of 1 mg of thiamine. It was shown that amounts of thiamine and riboflavin excreted in the urine of individuals on restricted diets were smaller than for individuals on normal diets and that the average excretion could be correlated with the extent of the depletion. However, the variation which occurred between individuals made the results of urinary analyses for thiamine and riboflavin of little diagnostic significance except to assist in the evaluation of the dietary consumption during the weeks preceding the test.[28]

[25] P. W. Kershaw, *Brit. J. Psychiat.* **113**, 387 (1967).
[26] W. O. Caster, O. Mickelsen, and A. Keys, *J. Lab. Clin. Med.* **43**, 469 (1954).
[27] C. Bhuvaneswaran and A. Sreenivasan, *Ann. N.Y. Acad. Sci.* **98**, 576 (1962).
[28] M. K. Horwitt, *Bull. Nat. Res. Counc. (U.S.)* **116**, 12 (1948).

New interest in urinary excretion tests for assessing thiamine deficiency centers around metabolites of thiamine.[12, 13, 23] At least 20 metabolites of urine have been found in rat and human urine after administration of ^{14}C-labeled thiamine.[29–31] One of the quantitatively important ones is the fluorescent metabolite pyrimidine carboxylic acid.[12] Ziporin et al.[32] measure, by a yeast coupling procedure,[33] pyrimidine and thiazole moieties of thiamine in the urine and point out that their excretion does not drop and may even increase at low thiamine intakes when thiamine itself is no longer found in the urine. The continued metabolite excretion is considered to represent thiamine metabolized by the tissues and, thus, a loss of body stores of thiamine. When intact thiamine is no longer measurable in the urine but the total excretion of thiamine metabolites exceeds the thiamine intake, a state of deficiency exists. Both Pearson[12] and Sauberlich[13] feel that further investigation of thiamine metabolites, their nature, pattern of excretion, and detection is warranted to establish their value in the assessment of thiamine deficiency.

D. Pyruvate and Lactate

As early as 1929, Kinnersley and Peters[34] demonstrated the increased lactic acid formation in thiamine-deficient pigeon brain compared to normal. In 1934 followed the suggestion by Peters and Thompson[35] that thiamine functioned as a coenzyme to pyruvic oxidase. This led to the important finding of increased blood levels of pyruvate in thiamine deficiency. Comprehensive discussions on the relation of these levels to the assessment of thiamine deficiency is to be found in the texts by Thompson and Wootton[36] and by Robinson.[4]

Robinson[4] points out that elevation of blood pyruvate cannot be used for diagnosing and evaluating thiamine deficiency without excluding many other pathological conditions in which there are elevated pyruvate levels. Thompson and Wootton[36] indicate that in severe cases of thiamine deficiency there are marked elevations of fasting pyruvate levels which do not show up in lesser degrees of thiamine deficiency. Several workers obtained more

[29] R. A. Neal and W. N. Pearson, J. Nutr. 83, 351 (1964).
[30] E. M. Baker, M. Balaghi, R. S. Pardini, and H. E. Sauberlich, Fed. Proc. Fed. Amer. Soc. Exp. Biol. 25, 245 (1966).
[31] M. Balaghi and W. N. Pearson, J, Nutr. 89, 265 (1966).
[32] Z. Z. Ziporin, W. T. Nunes, R. C. Powell, P. P. Waring, and H. E. Sauberlich, J. Nutr. 85, 287, 297 (1964).
[33] Z. Z. Ziporin, E. Beier, D. C. Holland, and E. L. Bierman, Anal. Biochem. 3, 1 (1962).
[34] H. W. Kinnersley and R. A. Peters, Biochem. J. 24, 711 (1930).
[35] R. A. Peters and R. H. S. Thompson, Biochem. J. 28, 916 (1934).
[36] R. H. S. Thompson and I. D. P. Wootton, "Biochemical Disorders in Human Disease" Ch. XIII, p. 451. Academic Press, New York, 1970.

favorable results in disclosing less severe degrees of thiamine deficiency by determining blood pyruvate after a loading dose of glucose.

Stotz and Bessey[37] found that they could detect an abnormality of pyruvate metabolism in pigeons in the early stages of thiamine deficiency and suggested the determination of the blood lactate–pyruvate ratio to minimize interference from exercise, food consumption, and anorexia in assessing thiamine nutrition.

In conjunction with a long-term controlled study in thiamine deficiency, Horwitt and Kreisler[38] developed a method which determines the combined effects of glucose ingestion and mild exercise on the blood lactic and pyruvic acid levels. The results of this method are expressed in the "carbohydrate metabolism index" (CMI).

Bessey,[6] in discussing the use of blood levels in evaluating vitamin deficiency points out the usefulness of the carbohydrate metabolism index of Horwitt and Kreisler for evaluating thiamine adequacy in the range of intake that approaches clinical manifestation of thiamine deficiency.

Brin,[39] in reporting a study of four men receiving 190 μg of thiamine/day for 42 days, found that values for the thiamine-deficient individuals by the CMI method fell well within Horwitt and Kreisler's normal range and that in his study it was difficult to evaluate an individual person on the basis of the CMI alone. Brin points out that use of the CMI is limited to persons capable of a certain amount of exercise and emphasizes the need for each laboratory to establish its own normal range of values.

New interest in blood α-keto acid levels is sparked by recent work by Buckle[40, 41] involving the use of a chromatographic procedure for the more accurate determination of blood pyruvic and α-ketoglutaric acids. Fasting levels of pyruvate were high in 3 out of 32 patients exhibiting clinical signs of thiamine deficiency and also in 9 asymptomatic patients having low dietary thiamine intakes. Pyruvate levels rose following administration of glucose. Thiamine therapy reduces blood pyruvate to normal in all patients. Results were similar for blood α-ketoglutaric acid except for a lack of response following glucose administration to asymptomatic thiamine-deficient patients.

E. Methylglyoxal

The possible role of methylglyoxal (CH_3—CO—CHO) in thiamine deficiency is once again a focus of attention. Findlay[42] found that polyneuritic

---

[37] E. Stotz and O. A. Bessey, *J. Biol. Chem.* **143**, 625 (1942).
[38] M. K. Horwitt and O. Kreisler, *J. Nutr.* **37**, 411 (1949).
[39] M. Brin, *Ann. N.Y. Acad. Sci.* **98**, 528 (1962).
[40] R. M. Buckle, *Metab. Clin. Exp.* **14**, 141 (1965).
[41] R. M. Buckle, *Proc. Roy. Soc. Med.* **60**, 48 (1967).
[42] G. M. Findlay, *Biochem. J.* **15**, 104 (1921).

pigeons had low liver glyoxalase levels which increased after thiamine administration. Vogt-Møller[43] felt that methylglyoxal accumulation due to a decreased activity of either glyoxalase or its coenzyme, glutathione, was responsible for the symptoms of beriberi. Methylglyoxal has been found in the milk of Japanese women with beriberi,[44, 45] in the urine of polyneuritic dogs,[46] in the urine and cerebrospinal fluid of infants suffering from acute toxic dyspepsia thought to be caused by thiamine deficiency,[32] and in the blood and urine of beriberi patients.[47] On the other hand, methylglyoxal has not been found in the tissues of polyneuritic pigeons.[48] The finding of methylglyoxal in thiamine-deficient rats by Salem[49, 50] and by Van Eys et al.[51] is not confirmed in the work of Liang.[52] The effusive and transient character of methylglyoxal may depend on metabolic conditions. Disagreement regarding the presence of methylglyoxal in tissues may be related to great variation in its turnover under different conditions.

Drummond[53] reported decreases in liver and blood glyoxalase activity but pointed out that since significant glyoxalase activity remained in severely deficient animals it was reasonable to conclude that pyruvaldehyde (methylglyoxal) metabolism was not an important factor in thiamine deficiency. Similarly Brum,[54] studying the metabolism of ^{14}C-labeled methylglyoxal in normal and thiamine-deficient rats, concluded that methylglyoxal is rapidly converted to $^{14}CO_2$ via pyruvate and the Krebs cycle without impairment in thiamine deficiency.

Van Eys and co-workers[51] suggested that because of lowered lactic and α-glycerophosphate dehydrogenase activities in thiamine deficiency there was an accumulation of triose phosphate which could be metabolized to methylglyoxal and then converted to D-lactic acid by the action of glyoxalase. In support of this, the authors have found D-lactic acid in both normal and thiamine-deficient animals. Both D- and L-lactic acids have been found in human urine, the D form being unaffected by exercise. Pearson[2] suggests the usefulness of a study correlating blood and urinary levels of D- and L-lactic acids in man with graded levels of thiamine intake.

[43] P. Vogt-Møller, Biochem. J. 25, 418 (1931).
[44] M. Chiba, Tohoku J. Exp. Med. 19, 486 (1932).
[45] A. Takamatsu and A. Sata, Tohoku J. Exp. Med. 23, 506 (1934).
[46] A Geiger and A. Rosenberg, Klin. Wochenschr. 12, 1258 (1933).
[47] B. S. Platt and K. G. Lu, Biochem. J. 33, 1525 (1939).
[48] R. E. Johnson, Biochem. J. 30, 31 (1936).
[49] H. M. Salem, Biochem. J. 57, 227 (1954).
[50] H. M. Salem, Arch. Biochem. 57, 20 (1955).
[51] J. Van Eys, M. A. Judge, J. Judd, W. Hill, R. C. Bozian, and S. Abrahams, J. Nutr. 76, 375 (1962).
[52] C. C. Liang, Biochem. J. 82, 429 (1962).
[53] G. I. Drummond, J. Nutr. 74, 357 (1961).
[54] V. C. Brum, J. Nutr. 91, 399 (1967).

F. Glyoxylate

A lesser known metabolic role of thiamine pyrophosphate is as a cofactor in the oxidative decarboxylation of glyoxylic acid which may arise from glycine,[54a-56] Glyoxylic acid has been found after 12–14 days in the urine of rats fed a thiamine-deficient diet, reaching a peak (about 2.7 mg/100 gm body weight/day) after 30–40 days and declining thereafter. Blood glyoxylic acid follows the same pattern, although delayed 7–8 days, reaching a peak of about 1.1 mg/100 ml of blood.[52]

Glyoxylic acid is considered highly toxic to animals[57, 58] and inhibits oxygen metabolism. Thus Liang[52] suggests that glyoxylic acid may play a significant role in the abnormal metabolism of thiamine deficiency. Liang[59] also reports a sharp rise in urinary creatine concomitant with the usual drop in body weight followed by a decrease in urinary creatine, until death, of rats on a thiamine-deficient diet. In this same study evidence is presented supporting the suggestion that glyoxylate found in the blood and urine of thiamine-deficient rats is derived from glycine liberated by excessive tissue breakdown.

Buckle[60] could not detect glyoxylic acid in the blood of normal subjects or in patients having no evidence of any nutritional, metabolic, or endocrine disorder. In 23 patients evidencing thiamine deficiency, glyoxylic acid could not be detected in 13 in whom neurological manifestations predominated, but it was detected in two of 10 patients showing fluid retention and cardiac failure predominantly. The amount of glyoxylic acid ranged from 61–286 μg/100 ml of blood. Buckle concluded that glyoxylic acid was not likely to be responsible for any of the clinical manifestations of occidental thiamine deficiency in man.

G. Transketolase Activity

In 1953 Horecker and Smyrniotis[61] and Racker et al.[62] reported thiamine pyrophosphate to be a coenzyme for transketolase in the pentose pathway of glucose metabolism. Brin et al. have demonstrated a marked depression

[54a] H. I. Nakada and L. F. Sund, J. Biol. Chem. 233, 8 (1958).

[55] S. S. Ratner, V. Nocito, and D. E. Green, J. Biol. Chem. 152, 119 (1944).

[56] S. Weinhouse and B. Friedmann, J. Biol. Chem. 191, 707 (1951).

[57] O. Adler, Arch. Exp. Pathol. Pharmakol. 37, 413 (1893).

[58] R. H. Barnes and A. Lerner, Proc. Soc. Exp. Biol. Med. 52, 216 (1943).

[59] C. C. Liang, Biochem. J. 83, 101 (1962).

[60] R. M. Buckle, Clin. Sci. 25, 207 (1963).

[61] B. L. Horecker and P. Z. Smyrniotis, J. Amer. Chem. Soc. 75, 1009 (1953).

[62] E. G. Racker, G. de La Haba, and I. G. Leder, J. Amer. Chem. Soc. 75, 1010 (1953).

in transketolase activity in rat,[63, 64] human,[65, 66] and duck erythrocytes[67] and have developed a procedure for determining transketolase in stored frozen hemolyzed erythrocytes; they have studied its value in assessing thiamine deficiency in man and animals.[68–70] The assay involves the incubation of erythrocyte hemolyzates with ribose 5-phosphate for 1 hour, after which the remaining pentose and the newly formed hexose are each measured. In addition, the percentage stimulation of hexose formation by the system involving transketolase is determined after adding thiamine pyrophosphate to each hemolysate. This further increase due to thiamine pyrophosphate (TPP) is expressed as percentage stimulation and may differentiate any lowering of transketolase activity from normal into that due to lack of coenzyme and that due to lack of the apoenzyme.

In a study of eight healthy medical students,[66] four acting as controls and four receiving only 190 μg thiamine/day for 8 weeks, transketolase activity became depressed in the thiamine-deficient group after 17 days. While hemolyzates from control individuals were stimulated less than 10% by TPP, the percentage of stimulation in the deficient group increased to 15% by the 8th day and to a maximum of 34% on the 30th day. On repletion of the deficient group with thiamine, transketolase activity returned to essentially normal levels in 24 to 48 hours and the stimulatory effect of TPP on hemolyzates disappeared. Studies by Sauberlich[2] have yielded comparable results. Brin, in a study of the effect of protein, riboflavin, and pyridoxine deficiencies on erythrocyte transketolase in rats, found them to be without effect.[71]

Dreyfus and Moniz in studies of transketolase activity in the nervous system of the rat developed a somewhat different method which has been modified for determining erythrocyte transketolase activity in fingertip blood.[72] Sedoheptulose formation is used as a measure of transketolase activity. Provision is also made for stimulating hemolyzate activity by adding TPP. Dreyfus[73] points out that in vitro addition of TPP is capable of restoring rat blood transketolase to normal levels of activity in early

[63] M. Brin, S. S. Shohet, and C. S. Davidson, Fed. Proc. Fed. Amer. Soc. Exp. Biol. 15, 224 (1956).
[64] M. Brin, S. S. Shohet, and C. S. Davidson, J. Biol. Chem. 230, 319 (1958).
[65] S. J. Wolfe, M. Brin, and C. S. Davidson, J. Clin. Invest. 37, 1476 (1958).
[66] M. Brin, Ann. N.Y. Acad. Sci. 98, 528 (1962).
[67] M. Brin, Fed. Proc. Fed. Amer. Soc. Exp. Biol. 23, 242 (1964).
[68] M. Brin, M. Tai, A. S. Ostashever, and H. Kalinsky, J. Nutr. 71, 273 (1960).
[69] M. Brin, in " The Red Cell," (C. Bishop and D. M. Surgenor, eds.), p. 451. Academic Press, New York, 1964.
[70] M. Brin, Methods Enzymol. 9, 506 (1966).
[71] M. Brin, Fed. Proc. Fed. Amer. Soc. Exp. Biol. 19, 321 (1961).
[72] P. M. Dreyfus and R. A. Moniz, Biochim. Biophys. Acta 65, 181 (1962).
[73] P. M. Dreyfus, New Engl. J. Med. 267, 596 (1962).

stages of deficiency, but, that with progressive depletion, restoration of the system declines progressively. This suggests that in progressive thiamine deficiency there may be gradual depletion of both coenzyme and apoenzyme; that is, transketolase may be an adaptive enzyme. Sie et al.[74, 75] also found a decreased ability to synthesize heptulose phosphate from ribose 5-phosphate in the tissues of thiamine-deficient rats.

The transketolase assay, including stimulation by TPP, acts as a measure of functional vitamin present in the body and should be useful in deciding within a relatively short time whether a suspected case of thiamine deficiency is in fact low in functional thiamine. Since its introduction, the transketolase assay has had increasing application in the study of experimental and clinical human thiamine deficiency and for nutritional surveys.[30, 65, 66, 73, 76–82] Its use has been critically discussed by Sauberlich[13] who expresses the opinion that, of the few tests available, erythrocyte transketolase activity measurement appears the most convenient, feasible, specific, and sensitive. Furthermore, although the erythrocyte transketolase activity procedure needs further evaluation under various dietary, population, and disease situations before final conclusions can be drawn, it is apparent that the test can be useful in the detection of marginal thiamine deficiency, as well as in certain clinical situations.

It was a major step forward in the understanding of nutritional disease when Peters[83] suggested that the acute symptoms of the central nervous system seen in thiamine-deficient pigeons were due to a block in the normal metabolism of glucose which interfered with the functioning of some groups of nerve cells. On the basis of available knowledge he felt that the "biochemical lesion" was most closely related to the oxidation of pyruvic acid. That the oxidation of pyruvic acid is the limiting factor in metabolism that eventually sparks the symptoms of thiamine deficiency is now the subject of

[74] H. G. Sie, V. N. Nigam, and W. H. Fishman, Biochim. Biophys. Acta 50, 277 (1961).
[75] H. G. Sie, Proc. Soc. Exp. Biol. Med. 113, 733 (1963).
[76] M. Brin, J. Amer. Med. Ass. 187, 762 (1964).
[77] H. E. Sauberlich and G. E. Bunce, Interdepartmental Committee on Nutrition for National Defense Nutrition Survey Oct.–Dec. 1961: Union of Burma. U.S. Govt. Printing Office, Washington, D.C., 1963.
[78] US. Army Medical Research and Nutrition Laboratory, "Annual Progress Reports." Denver, Colorado, 1960 and 1961.
[79] M. Brin, M. V. Dibble, A. Peel, E. McMullen, A. Bourquin, and N. Chen, Amer. J. Clin. Nutr. 17, 240 (1965).
[80] L. J. Embree and P. M. Dreyfus, Trans. Amer. Neurol. Ass. 88, 36 (1963).
[81] M. Akbarian, N. A. Yankopoulos, and W. H. Abelmann, Amer. J. Med. 41, 197 (1966).
[82] J. Gilroy, J. S. Meyer, R. B. Bauer, M. Vulpe, and D. Greenwood, Amer. J. Med. 40, 368 (1966).
[83] R. A. Peters, Lancet 1, 1161 (1936).

considerable controversy. The coenzyme role of thiamine pyrophosphate has been extended to α-ketoglutarate oxidase and transketolase. TPP is also implicated in the activity of glycerophosphate dehydrogenase,[84] lactic dehydrogenase,[84] and glyoxylic acid dehydrogenase.[54]

Although the decreased rate has been shown for the *in vitro* pyruvate oxidase activity of tissues from thiamine-deficient animals, it has been questioned whether the same is true in situations in which oxygen uptake and not decarboxylation for the deficient animal has been measured. Jones and de Angeli[85] have shown that thiamine-deficient rats decarboxylate as large a percentage of pyruvate to acetyl-CoA as do well-fed normal animals. Some of the unanswered questions relate to the lesser decrease in the *in vitro* oxidation of α-ketoglutarate compared to that for pyruvate in thiamine-deficient animals[86, 87] and the qualitatively and quantitatively different gross and metabolic changes brought about by thiamine deprivation *vs.* oxythiamine antagonism *vs.* pyrithiamine antagonism.[85, 88] Woolley and Merrifield[89] felt that thiamine had more than the known function of acting as the coenzyme cocarboxylase whose related enzyme activity is inhibited by oxythiamine but not by pyrithiamine; namely, a second, as yet unclarified, role in the proper functioning of the nervous system which is inhibited by pyrithiamine but not significantly antagonized by oxythiamine. The interesting work of Lofland *et al.*,[90] investigating thiamine deficiency in two different breeds of pigeons, is provocative. Although two breeds of pigeons were on the same thiamine-deficient diet, one breed showed deficiency symptoms after 2 weeks and the other after 3 weeks, yet thiamine levels in brain and liver decreased to about the same degree in each breed. In addition, increases in levels of blood pyruvate and decreases in blood transketolase and in α-ketoglutarate oxidase in brain and liver were about the same. In both breeds, brain transketolase did not seem to change as the deficiency progressed. From these findings the authors postulated that the appearance of neurological signs of thiamine deficiency were related to factors other than the decreased activity of the enzyme systems that they studied. Many of these neurological aspects of thiamine deficiency are dealt with further by E. P. Steyn-Parvé, C. J. Gubler and L. R. Johnson, M. Brin, P. Dreyfus, and J. R. Cooper and J. N. Pincus in the Ciba Foundation Study Group on thiamine deficiency.[11]

[84] J. Van Eys, *J. Nutr.* **73**, 403 (1961).
[85] J. H. Jones and E. de Angeli, *J. Nutr.* **70**, 537 (1960).
[86] R. C. Wright and E. M. Scott, *J. Biol. Chem.* **206**, 725 (1954).
[87] C. J. Gubler, *J. Biol. Chem.* **236**, 3112 (1961).
[88] M. Brin, *J. Nutr.* **78**, 179 (1962).
[89] D. W. Woolley and R. B. Merrifield, *Bull. Soc. Chim. Biol.* **36**, 1207 (1954).
[90] H. Lofland, Jr., H. O. Goodman, and T. B. Clarkson, *J. Nutr.* **79**, 188 (1963).

X. Deficiency Effects

B. C. P. JANSEN

A. In Microorganisms

Of the effects of thiamine deficiency on microorganisms, not much is known. The microorganisms that cannot synthesize thiamine can be used for the microbiological estimation of thiamine.

B. In Animals

As far back as 1892 Eykman published his results about the signs of nerve degeneration in fowls that were fed with thiamine-poor polished rice. From this work started the whole vitamin research. Thus the degeneration of the peripheral nerves was the first pathological symptom noted. Eykman stained the nerves with Marchi solution, and he thought that in the polyneuritic animals the axis of the nerves was degenerated. Half a century afterward in an extensive examination of the peripheral nerve fibers in thiamine deficiency, Swank and Prados[1] made the observation that the first neuronal histological change in thiamine-deficient pigeons is degeneration of the distal part of the axon, and changes in myelin are secondary to this and, further, that opisthotonus (the characteristic manifestation of acute thiamine deficiency in pigeons) may not be attended by any definite neurological lesions.

About 30 years after the work of Eykman, Peters in Oxford, England, was able to demonstrate that not only the peripheral nerves, but also the central nervous system was affected by a thiamine deficiency. From that work of Peters resulted a large part of our knowledge of the role thiamine plays in carbohydrate, especially in pyruvate, metabolism. It is probable that most of the pathology of thiamine deficiency is due to a disturbance in the carbohydrate metabolism. The comprehensive work of Peters and his school on the details of the biochemical action of substances causing pathological effects and in particular in trying to understand the initial changes from thiamine deficiency has led him to call these initial changes "biochemical lesions."[2] Peters studied the epistothonus signs induced in the rice-fed pigeon by thiamine deficiency. The epistothonus signs clear up very quickly when thiamine is given, and there is no detectable histological damage at this stage. It is in this sense an example of a pure "biochemical lesion."

[1] R. L. Swank and M. Prados, *Arch. Neurol. Psychiat.* **47**, 97 (1942); M. Prados and R. L. Swank, *Arch. Neurol. Psychiat.* **47**, 626 (1942).
[2] R. A. Peters, *Proc. Roy. Soc. Med.* **41**, 781 (1948).

The clinical symptoms of thiamine deficiency are connected with the metabolic disturbances. How close the connection between both is, is not precisely known. These symptoms are nearly the same in different animals. Usually there are signs of lameness, of convulsions, accompanied in pigeons with head retraction and in rats with walking in a circle, and of " biochemical lesions." Other signs are anorexia, reduction of growth or decline in weight, and emaciation. As Drummond has emphasized, many of these signs are not independent from each other. Thus the anorexia may be the cause of the decline in weight. In rats the heart rate is reduced;[3] in normal rats the rate is 500 beats/second; in severe deficiency it is not more than 250 to 300. This fact was used by Birch and Harris[3] as an indication of the severity of thiamine deficiency in rats. (In human beings just the opposite takes place; thiamine deficiency leads to tachycardia.) For an extensive investigation on the pathology of thiamine deficiency in monkeys, see, e.g., Rinehart et al.[4]

As thiamine in the form of thiamine pyrophosphate is necessary for the metabolism of pyruvate, one would expect that the amount of pyruvate in blood, and perhaps also in urine, may be increased in thiamine deficiency. Platt[5] and Platt and Lu[6] indeed found a large increase of bisulfite-binding substances, consisting mainly of pyruvic acid, in the blood of beriberi patients. Some hours after the administration of thiamine to the patients the amount of the bisulfite-binding substances dropped to normal. In animal experiments Thompson and Johnson[7] found that pigeons and rats with symptoms of acute thiamine deficiency had a high blood pyruvate level. One would be inclined to think that these symptoms of acute thiamine deficiency might be caused by a pyruvate poisoning of the animal. The work of de Jong,[8] however, makes this supposition highly improbable. De Jong devised a micromethod for determining the pyruvate level of a small drop of blood; he thus was able to execute several determinations in the course of the development of polyneuritis in the animals. In this way he proved that the symptoms of acute polyneuritis in pigeons developed before the rise of pyruvate, and the disappearance of the symptoms after the thiamine administration preceded the return of the pyruvate level to normal.

The results of this work of de Jong seem to demonstrate that the polyneuritis signs are independent of the pyruvate metabolism and, for that reason, of the catalytic action of thiamine pyrophosphate.

From the work of Loewi and of Dale we know that a chemical substance, acetylcholine, plays a role in the transmission of nerve stimuli.

[3] T. W. Birch and L. J. Harris, Biochem. J. 28, 602 (1934).

[4] J. F. Rinehart, L. D. Greenberg, and M. Friedman, Amer. J. Pathol. 23, 879 (1947).

[5] B. S. Platt, Trans. Roy. Soc. Trop. Med. Hyg. 31, 493 (1938).

[6] B. S. Platt and G. D. Lu, Biochem. J. 33, 1525 (1939).

[7] R. H. S. Thompson and J. R. Johnson, Biochem. J. 29, 694 (1935).

[8] S. de Jong, Arch. Neer. Physiol. 21, 465 (1936).

Binet and Minz[9] showed that acetylcholine not only plays a role in the transmission of the stimulus from the end of the nerve to the effective organ but that it works also in the nerves themselves. The acetylcholine content of the nerves was increased after electric stimulation. However the addition of an extract of the nonstimulated nerve to that of the stimulated nerve intensified the action of this extract or of a solution of pure acetylcholine. This points to another substance present in the extract of the stimulated nerve. The authors, considering that thiamine deficiency leads to polyneuritis, assumed that the active substance of the stimulated nerve might be this vitamin. So they compared the activity of the substance of the stimulated nerve with that of thiamine. They found that their activities in this respect were the same. They further showed that thiamine also stimulates the activity of acetylcholine in the isolated intestine of the rat and in the circulatory organ of the cat, in the absence of the eserine that inhibits the enzyme cholinesterase.

The liberation of thiamine (or a thiamine derivative) by nerve action was for the first time demonstrated by Minz.[10] Lwoff[11] had devised a highly sensitive microbiological method for the estimation of very small quantities of thiamine, using Flagellatae. With this method Minz compared the liberation of thiamine from excised resting ox nerves with that of electrically stimulated nerves. He was able to prove that the stimulated nerves delivered much more thiamine than the resting nerves (four to eight times as much). Shortly afterward these results were confirmed and extended by von Muralt. This Swiss investigator has given a review of all the work, mostly from his own laboratory, on thiamine and peripheral neurophysiology.[12] Von Muralt and his collaborators quickly froze excited nerves or resting nerves in liquid air. The frozen nerves were ground in a mortar and extracted for 10 minutes with Ringer's solution. The thiamine content of the extracts was estimated by several different methods. The extracts of the stimulated nerves were richer in thiamine than the extracts of the resting nerves. This means that thiamine in the excited nerves is in such a state that more can be extracted by Ringer's solution in 10 minutes than can be obtained from a corresponding sample of unexcited nerves. The different methods for estimating the liberated thiamine yielded on the whole practically the same results; however, the yeast ferment method of Atkin, Schultz and Frey showed much lower values for the thiamine content of both excited and resting nerves; and also the difference between excited and unexcited nerves had disappeared. It was not yet possible to give an explanation for this discrepancy. Furthermore it was

[9] L. Binet and B. Minz, *C. R. Soc. Biol.* **117**, 1027 (1934).

[10] B. Minz, *C. R. Soc. Biol.* **127**, 1251 (1938).

[11] M. Lwoff, *C. R. Soc. Biol.* **128**, 241 (1938).

[12] A. von Muralt, *Vitam. Horm.* (*New York*) **5**, 93 (1947).

difficult to draw conclusions from these experiments because Wyss and Wyss[13] in the laboratory of von Muralt found that by poisoning the nerves by monoiodoacetic acid more thiamine is obtained in the extract of resting nerves than in the extract of excited nerves. In most experiments thiamine exerts an inhibiting effect on the vagus or acethycholine action on the heart. By replacing certain groups in the thiamine molecule by other groups, the effect is mostly reduced but not abolished. It is amazing, however, that the thiamine pyrophosphate has no action at all!

From all these facts it may be assumed that thiamine or a thiamine compound plays a role in neurophysiological activity.

However, there is as yet no convincing evidence that the neurological active substance is thiamine itself or one or more derivative(s) of thiamine. Von Muralt proposes that as long as this uncertainty exists this substance be called "the second Vagusstoff," because Loewi, before he understood the exact nature of the chemical mediator in the heart, called it "Vagusstoff."

Thus we have two well-established facts concerning the pathology of thiamine in animals. The first is the activity of thiamine pyrophosphate as a coenzyme in the carbohydrate metabolism; the second is the role of thiamine or a derivative of thiamine (the "second Vagusstoff") on the neurophysiological activity. We do not yet know whether these facts are closely connected, or whether they are quite independent from each other. From the fact that the thiamine pyrophosphate lacks the neurophysiological action of thiamine it is probable that the neurophysiological activity is different from the activity on the carbohydrate metabolism.

On the other hand we know that thiamine pyrophosphate is active in the production of acetic acid which is essential to restore the active acetylcholine from the inactive choline that is formed from acetylcholine by the action of the cholinesterase.

XI. Deficiency Effects in Human Beings

B. C. P. JANSEN

In the beginning of vitamin research it was easy to compose a diet for the study of thiamine deficiency. With fowls or pigeons as experimental animals, polished rice, after being washed in running water to remove the last traces of thiamine, was a suitable diet. Polished rice, however, not only

---

[13] A. Wyss and F. Wyss, *Experientia* 1, 160 (1945).

lacks thiamine, but it also shows a shortage of many other nutrients. Therefore when other experimental animals, e.g., rats, were used, it appeared necessary to add to these other nutrients (proteins, mineral salts, nearly all other vitamins) or to compose a complete, synthetic diet.

Williams et al.,[1] in their experiments to investigate the signs of a pure thiamine deficiency in volunteers on a thiamine-poor diet, found no signs of edema in their experimental persons, whereas the natives in rice-consuming countries recognize beriberi because of the signs of edema.

Therefore, to study the effects of a pure thiamine deficiency it is necessary to provide a diet that contains all nutrients in physiological amounts, except thiamine. Since we do not yet know all the essential nutrients, it is very difficult to compose a suitable synthetic diet, not considering the cost of some nutrients! So it is better to choose a good natural diet in which only the thiamine is destroyed. In these diets the thiamine is often destroyed by autoclaving for several hours at pH 5. But by this procedure other nutrients are damaged too. A more specific way to destroy the thiamine is to treat the diet, or the thiamine-containing parts of the diet, with sulfite.[2, 3] Presumably the most specific method of destroying the thiamine would be treatment with thiaminase. Smith and Proutt[4] stated that cats fed a diet consisting exclusively of thiaminase-rich raw carp developed all the signs of the thiamine deficiency characteristic for this animal. To counteract specifically the activity of thiamine, the antithiamines, e.g., pyrithiamine or oxythiamine, can be used. Woolley[5] was able to demonstrate that at least one of the activities of pyrithiamine consists in the antagonizing of the synthesis of cocarboxylase—the active form of thiamine in carbohydrate metabolism. Woolley and White[6] state that, whereas mice fed a ration free of thiamine develop no characteristic symptoms of thiamine deficiency, the same animals, on administration of pyrithiamine, do show many of these symptoms. Therefore the best way to study the effects of uncomplicated thiamine deficiency presumably is the use of antithiamines and thiaminases, added to an otherwise optimal diet. A great difficulty is the detection of the first signs of a deficiency. This is important because beriberi is not found in Western countries, but it is possible that even here many persons suffer from a mild thiamine deficiency. Usually the excretion of thiamine in the urine per 24 hours is determined or the excretion during 3 hours after giving a measured

[1] R. D. Williams, H. L. Mason, B. F. Smith, and R. M. Wilder, Arch. Intern. Med. 69, 721 (1942).
[2] R. R. Williams, R. E. Waterman, J. C. Keresztesy, and E. R. Burchman, J. Am. Chem. Soc. 57, 536 (1935).
[3] A. S. Schultz, L. Atkin, C. N. Frey, and R. R. Williams, J. Am. Chem. Soc. 63, 632 (1941).
[4] D. C. Smith and L. M. Proutt, Proc. Soc. Exptl. Biol. Med. 56, 1 (1944).
[5] D. W. Woolley, J. Biol. Chem. 191, 42 (1951).
[6] D. W. Woolley and A. G. C. White, J. Biol. Chem. 149, 285 (1943).

dose of thiamine. Also the blood thiamine level is used as a yardstick. However, this gives only a vague indication.[7] Swank and Jasper[8] compared encephalograms of normal pigeons with those of thiamine-deficient birds. An increase in brain potentials occurred slowly in the thiamine-deficient pigeons and preceded the development of clinical signs. Shortly before the appearance of preopisthotonus the amplitude of brain potentials became three times as high as during the control period. The administration of thiamine to pigeons with preopisthotonus caused return of the brain waves to normal.

Horwitt and Kreisler,[9] from their work on patients on diets with different thiamine levels, tried to devise an index of carbohydrate metabolism, correlating the levels of glucose, lactic acid, and pyruvic acid in the blood of the patient after a measured exercise and the carbohydrate metabolism which is influenced by the thiamine intake. This carbohydrate index was thought to be an indication of the state of thiamine nutrition before any clinical signs of thiamine deficiency occurred.

Mouriquand and Coisnard[10] observed that pigeons on a thiamine-poor diet demonstrated a fall in the chronaxie of the nerves and that this fall begins before the clinical signs appear.

XII. Pharmacology and Toxicology

KLAUS R. UNNA

Thiamine has been shown to produce a variety of pharmacological effects. It should be borne in mind that these effects have been obtained in experimental animals maintained on adequate diets only on parental administration of thiamine in doses several thousand times larger than those required for optimum nutrition. These pharmacological effects in animals have no counterpart in the therapeutic use of the vitamin in man.

Death after intravenous injection of thiamine in animals is due to depression of the respiratory center.[1-4] The heart is still beating at the time of cessation

---

[7] J. E. Kirk and M. Chieffi, *J. Gerontol.* **5**, 236 (1950).

[8] R. L. Swank and H. H. Jasper, *Arch. Neurol. Psychiat.* **47**, 821 (1942).

[9] M. K. Horwitt and O. Kreisler, *J. Nutrition* **37**, 411 (1949).

[10] G. Mouriquand and J. Coisnard, *Presse Med.* **1944**, 277.

[1] H. Molitor and W. L. Sampson, *E. Merck's Jahresber.* **51**, 3 (1936).

[2] G. Hecht and H. Weese, *Klin. Wochenschr.* **16**, 414 (1937).

[3] J. A. Smith, P. P. Foa, H. R. Weinstein, A. S. Ludwig and J. M. Wertheim, *J. Pharmacol. Exp. Therap.* **93**, 294 (1948).

[4] T. J. Haley, *Proc. Soc. Exp. Biol. Med.* **68**, 153 (1948).

of the respiration. Artificial respiration enables the animals to survive otherwise lethal doses;[3] doses of thiamine resulting in concentrations of 7 to 10 mg % in the blood were fatal to dogs (under ether anesthesia), whereas blood levels of 36 mg % were tolerated when artificial respiration was provided.

Rapid intravenous injections of 5–50 mg/kg cause a transient fall in blood pressure in cats and dogs which increases with increasing dosage of thiamine. The fall in blood pressure is not influenced by atropine or antihistamines; it may be accentuated after adrenergic blockade with dibenamine.[5, 6] There is evidence that the fall in blood pressure is due to thiamine acting at several sites: on the vascular smooth muscle itself, on the vasomotor center, and on the heart. Perfusion experiments on the rabbit's ear and on various arterial areas in dogs have shown that part of the vasodilator effect obtained was due to the acidity of the highly concentrated thiamine solution. Experiments on decapitated cats in which the hypotensive effect of thiamine was markedly diminished indicate that the vasodilatation may be of central origin. A moderate decrease in heart rate following the injection of large doses of thiamine may contribute to a minor extent to the fall in blood pressure.

Thiamine has little, if any, effect on the isolated heart of the frog[1, 2, 7–9] or of the turtle.[3] Whether the bradycardia observed in dogs[3, 5, 10] is caused by an action of thiamine on the cardiac vagus or on the medullary centers remains undecided. Studies on the dog heart lung preparation[3] have failed to show any change in heart action with concentrations of thiamine far exceeding those which produced hypotension in the intact dog.

Thiamine is without effect on the isolated intestine of rats, rabbits, and guinea pigs and on the guinea pig uterus.[1, 8, 11] The claim that acetylthiamine has an acetylcholine-like effect on the gut[12] has not been confirmed.[11] In large concentrations thiamine inhibits the action of nicotine on the isolated intestine of rabbits and guinea pigs without interfering with responses to acetylcholine or epinephrine; the thiazole moiety of the vitamin, 4-methyl-5-hydroxyethylthiazole, has similar effects.[13] Thiamine also prevents the rise in blood pressure induced by nicotine.[14] It blocks transmission of nerve impulses through the superior cervical ganglion.[15]

[5] H. Mazella, *Arch. Int. Pharmacodyn.* 86, 434 (1951).
[6] S. H. Jaros, A. L. Wnuck, and E. J. de Beer, *Ann. Allergy* 10, 291 (1952).
[7] P. Kaiser, *Pfluegers Arch. Gesamte Physiol. Menschen Tiere* 242, 504 (1939).
[8] V. Erspamer, *Arch. Int. Pharmacodyn.* 63, 261 (1939).
[9] E. M. Boyd and R. W. Dingwall, *Quart. J. Pharm. Pharmacol.* 14, 209 (1941).
[10] R. Tislowitz and I. Pines, *Klin. Wochenschr.* 16, 923 (1937).
[11] R. Dufait, *Arch. Int. Pharmacodyn.* 66, 274 (1941).
[12] R. Kuhn, T. Wieland, and H. Huebschmann, *Hoppe-Seyler's Z. Physiol. Chem.* 259, 48 (1939).
[13] K. Unna and E. P. Pick, *J. Pharmacol. Exp. Ther.* 81, 294 (1944).
[14] E. P. Pick and K. Unna, *J. Pharmacol. Exp. Thec.* 87, 138 (1946),
[15] H. Mazella and N. Ferrero, *Arch. Int. Pharmacodyn.* 82, 220 (1950).

Besides its ganglionic depressant action at large doses, thiamine, in still larger doses, depresses the transmission of impulses to the skeletal muscle at the neuromuscular junction.[13, 16, 17] In accord with this curare-like action, it has been found to depress the response of the skeletal muscle to acetylcholine.[18, 19] Curarizing effects could be demonstrated in intact mammals only under artificial respiration following excessive, otherwise lethal doses of thiamine. Curare-like paralysis of the respiratory muscle is not the cause of death by intravenous injection of thiamine, since the diaphragm responds to direct and indirect electrical stimulation at the time respiration has ceased.[4] 4-Methyl-5-hydroxyethylthiazole was found to have a curare-like action similar to thiamine.[20]

Excessive doses of thiamine may produce bronchoconstriction in dogs.[21] Application of a 2 to 10% solution of thiamine directly to the motor cortex of dogs caused generalized convulsions; this effect was not obtained with either of the two moieties of the thiamine molecule.[22]

Since thiamine or a thiamine-like substance has been reported to be released together with acetylcholine on electrical stimulation of cholinergic nerves,[23, 24] numerous studies have been carried out with the object of studying a possible interdependence of the effects of thiamine and acetylcholine. Thiamine was found to potentiate the effects of acetylcholine on the leech muscle[25, 26] and on other preparations (for references, see Minz[27]). The required concentrations of thiamine were large and far beyond those found in normal tissues. Other studies on isolated organs (intestine, uterus, leech muscle, frog heart, frog rectus muscle), however, have failed to demonstrate any sensitizing effect of thiamine on the action of acetylcholine; at concentrations of 1 to 10 mg % in the nutrient solution, thiamine depressed the effects of acetylcholine.[7, 8, 11] Thus, the influence which thiamine may exert on the reactivity of the tissues to acetylcholine appears not to be sufficiently substantiated to allow general conclusions. Thiamine in large concentrations inhibits cholinesterase.[28, 29] To what extent this action may

[16] V. Demole, *Kongressber. XVI Int. Physiol. Kongr.* **11**, 19 (1938).

[17] J. A. Smith, P. P. Foa, and H. R. Weinstein, *Science* **108**, 412 (1948).

[18] C. Torda and H. G. Wolff, *Proc. Soc. Exp. Biol. Med.* **56**, 89 (1944).

[19] D. P. Sadhu, *Amer. J. Physiol.* **147**, 233 (1946).

[20] A. Smith, P. P. Foa, and H. R. Weinstein, *Amer. J. Physiol.* **155**, 469 (1948).

[21] M. Post and J. A. Smith, *Amer. J. Physiol.* **163**, 742 (1950).

[22] M. V. Dias, *Science* **105**, 211 (1947).

[23] B. Minz, *C. R. Soc. Biol.* **127**, 1251 (1938).

[24] A. von Muralt, *Nature (London)* **152**, 188 (1943).

[25] B. Minz and R. Agid, *C. R. Acad. Sci.* **205**, 576 (1937).

[26] F. von Bruecke and H. Sarkander, *Nauyn-Schmiedebergs Arch. Exp. Pathol. Pharmakol.* **195**, 218 (1940).

[27] B. Minz, "La Transmission Chimique de l'Influx Nerveux," p. 155. Flammarion, Paris, 1947.

[28] D. Glick and W. Antopol, *J. Pharmacol. Exp. Ther.* **65**, 389 (1939).

[29] W. Süllmann and H. Birkhäuser, *Schweiz. Med. Wochenschr.* **69**, 648 (1939).

be involved in some of the pharmacodynamic effects of thiamine is difficult to assess. Lacking data on the actual acetylcholine levels in the tissues of thiamine-treated animals, there is little reason to compare thiamine to such a potent cholinesterase inhibitor as eserine. Elucidation of the interdependence between acetylcholine and thiamine has already been initiated at the biochemical level; and interdependence with regard to the pharmacological effects of the vitamin has yet to receive unequivocal substantiation.

The lethal doses of thiamine by various routes of administration have been determined in a number of species.[1] On intravenous injection the lethal doses in mice were 125 mg/kg; in rats, 250 mg/kg; in rabbits, 300 mg/kg; and in dogs, 350 mg/kg. The ratios of the lethal doses on intravenous injection to those on subcutaneous and oral administration were found to be 1:6:40. These data on lethal doses in mice and rabbits have been confirmed.[2] In monkeys, intravenous administration of 200 mg/kg failed to elicit any symptoms,[1] and only 600 mg/kg caused the first toxic symptoms.[2] It is interesting to note that dogs and particularly monkeys are less sensitive than rodents. Lethal doses of thiamine mononitrate as determined in mice and rabbits were not significantly different from those of thiamine hydrochloride.[4]

On intravenous injection of 50 mg/kg daily for a period of 4 weeks, rabbits failed to show loss in weight, or other toxic manifestations. No pathological tissue changes were found on autopsy.[2] Rats have been maintained for three generations on a daily intake of 0.08 to 1.0 mg of thiamine, i.e., doses up to 100-fold of the daily requirement for the vitamin, without any untoward effects.[30] Other observations that daily subcutaneous injections of 0.1 mg of thiamine, though not affecting growth, caused impairment of lactation and cannibalism and decreased fertility in the second generation[31] can hardly be taken as evidence of thiamine toxicity, since these experiments were inadequately controlled, and the same manifestations were obtained in rats without thiamine injections on adding manganese chloride to that particular diet.[32] In the light of subsequent discovery of other nutritional factors essential for the rat, these effects were more likely due to inadequacy of the diet than to the injections of thiamine. Prolonged daily administration of 1 mg of thiamine to weanling rats maintained on a diet deficient in another B vitamin (riboflavin, pyridoxine, or pantothenic acid) failed to cause significant effects on the weight of these animals or on the manifestations of their deficiency state.[33]

The data on acute toxicity and the absence of evidence of cumulative toxicity give evidence for the very large therapeutic margin of thiamine. The ratio between the daily requirement for thiamine and its lethal dose has

[30] R. R. Williams and T. D. Spies, "Vitamin B_1 (Thiamine) and Its Use in Medicine," p. 286. Macmillan, New York, 1938.

[31] D. Perla, *Proc. Soc. Exp. Biol. Med.* **37**, 169 (1937).

[32] D. Perla and M. Sandberg, *Proc. Soc. Exp. Biol. Med.* **41**, 522 (1939).

[33] K. Unna and J. D. Clark, *Amer. J. Med. Sci.* **204**, 364 (1942).

been variously estimated at from 600 to 70,000 (depending on species and route of administration).

No toxic effects of thiamine administered by mouth have been reported in man. Parenterally, doses of 100 to 500 mg, in single and repeated injections, have been given to patients.[34-37] Toxic or other effects have not been noted on many thousands of injections by the subcutaneous, intramuscular, intraspinal, or intravenous routes in doses which in many cases were from 100 to 200 times larger than the daily maintenance dose. These excessive amounts have been well tolerated apparently without any noticeable or measurable effects on circulation, respiration, or the functions of other organ systems. A nut-like taste has been reported on injection of large amounts of thiamine; this taste sensation has been used as criterion for the measurement of circulation time by intravenous injection of 300 mg of thiamine.[37]

In relatively rare instances, thiamine has caused reactions resembling anaphylactic shock in man. Such reactions have been recorded in over 200 cases in the world literature (for extensive case references, see Jaros et al.[6]). All reactions have occurred exclusively on parenteral administration. They consist in their milder form of a feeling of burning and warmth, urticaria, weakness, restlessness, sweating, nausea, tightness of the throat and chest, dyspnea, hypotension, and tachycardia. In more severe cases the symptoms may rapidly progress to angioneurotic edema, cyanosis, pulmonary edema, hemorrhage into the gastrointestinal tract, and collapse. Five cases of sudden death following intravenous or intramuscular injection of thiamine have been reported.[38-41] The signs and symptoms of these reactions[42] are those of anaphylactic shock. Their onset follows the injection within minutes. The patient may, in milder cases, recover quickly. Treatment directed against the symptoms generally consists in injection of epinephrine, artificial respiration, and administration of oxygen and analeptics such as caffeine. The occurrence of these reactions and their severity is not related to the dose of thiamine injected, which has varied between 5 and 100 mg. The great majority of patients in which these reactions have been observed had previously tolerated parenteral injection of equal amounts of thiamine without any untoward effects. Thus, they apparently developed a hypersensitivity to thiamine. Only in rare instances[43, 44] have such reactions been observed on

[34] C. D. Aring and T. D. Spies, J. Neurol. Psychiat. 2, 335 (1939).

[35] E. L. Stern, Amer. J. Surg. 39, 495 (1938).

[36] N. Jolliffe, J. Amer. Med. Ass. 117, 1496 (1941).

[37] A. Ruskin and G. M. Decherd, Jr., Amer. J. Med. Sci. 213, 337 (1947).

[38] C. A. Mills, J. Amer. Med. Ass. 117, 1501 (1941).

[39] I. M. Reingold and F. R. Webb, J. Amer. Med. Ass. 130, 491 (1946).

[40] Fornara, cited by F. Dotti, Minerva Med. 1, 720 (1949).

[41] J. Arias, Rev. Med. Peruana 22, 160 (1951).

[42] C. C. Weigand, Geriatrics 5, 274 (1950).

[43] M. M. Mitrani, J. Allergy 15, 150 (1944).

[44] J. Seusing, Klin. Wochenschr. 29, 394 (1951).

the first known injection of thiamine. Most of the reactions have been reported to occur after four to ten or more injections.

These reactions are caused by thiamine and not by other solutes, solvents, or preservatives in the solutions which were injected, since they have occurred alike with preparations from different manufacturers and also with aqueous solutions of crystalline thiamine hydrochloride.

Since the symptomatology of these reactions is consonant with most, if not all, aspects of anaphylactic shock, the most likely explanation for the mechanism of the reactions seems to be an anaphylactic one. In many of the cases the observers have obtained immediate whealing on intradermal injection of thiamine, and, in some, positive transference of the sensitivity has been accomplished. Since the manifestations of the thiamine reactions are those known to occur with certain immunological alterations and since these patients have been shown to have such immunological alterations, it would appear reasonable to associate the two. It is conceivable that a combination of thiamine with protein develops which is antigenic to the host. The evidence is, at present, not conclusive, and the anaphylactogenic properties of thiamine require further investigation. If thiamine is an obligatory whealing agent,[45] positive intradermal tests may not be valid proof of individual sensitivity. Attempts to sensitize rabbits by massive and repeated injections of thiamine have failed.[46]

Positive patch tests obtained in individuals with these reactions do not present immunological evidence for the immediate anaphylactic type of reaction. They rather indicate the existence of the delayed eczematous type of hypersensitivity which would be the immunological substrate for the contact dermatitis type of reaction. In persons handling pharmaceutical preparations of thiamine, occurrence of contact dermatitis on the hands and forearms has been observed.[47]

Recently, on the basis of the similarity of hypotensive effects of thiamine, acetylcholine, and histamine on intravenous injection in dogs, the suggestion has been made[6, 48] that overdoses of thiamine may cause an accumulation of acetylcholine in excessive quantities in tissues which in turn may be responsible for the occurrence of the untoward reactions observed in man. Such an explanation lacks experimental evidence: the sudden onset of these reactions, lack of correlation to dose administered, limitation to parenteral injection, the manifestations comprising the entire spectrum of anaphylactic signs and symptoms, and other facts militate against such an assumption.

[45] F. Kalz, *J. Invest. Dermatol.* **5**, 135 (1942).
[46] T. J. Haley and A. M. Flesher, *Science* **104**, 567 (1946).
[47] F. C. Combes and J. Groopman, *Arch. Dermatol. Syphilol.* **61**, 858 (1950).
[48] S. H. Jaros, *Ann. Allergy* **9**, 133 (1951).

XIII. Requirements of Animals

B. C. P. JANSEN

The animal body is unable to store thiamine to any large extent. An adult human body does not contain more than about 30 mg of thiamine. Because the body continually loses thiamine in the urine, feces, and perspiration, it needs a constant supply.

It is difficult to find an exact criterion for measuring the requirement of an animal. The growth curve of young animals is most frequently used as a criterion. However, a drawback is that the curve indicating the influence of the thiamine content of the diet on the growth of the animal is an asymptotic one. Thus it is difficult to fix the maximum (or "normal") growth. Other methods used are the influence of the diet on the thiamine content of the blood or on normal or abnormal metabolism, i.e., on the pyruvic acid content of the blood.

Because a thiamine deficiency produces anorexia, Cowgill[1] used the "normal appetite" as a criterion.

Furthermore it is assumed that a certain (minimum) amount of thiamine is essential to keep an animal alive, to promote normal growth, and to protect it from polyneuritis. On the other hand, the work of Rasmussen *et al.*[2] and of Foster *et al.*[3] clearly demonstrated that mice are more resistant —or, as Schneider[4] puts it, less susceptible—to a certain strain of poliomyelitis virus if the thiamine content of the diet is reduced to an amount below the content that is required in other respects. Therefore it seems that a diet which may be considered thiamine deficient gives these animals better protection against poliomyelitis.

It is obvious that a great many factors exert influence on the requirement of thiamine in animals. The factors studied in the greatest detail are:

1. Size of the animal
2. Composition of the diet
3. Physical state of the animal (hyperthyroidism, pregnancy, lactation, fever, age, etc.)
4. Climate (temperature)
5. Intestinal microflora

[1] G. R. Cowgill, "The Vitamin B Requirement of Man." Yale Univ. Press, New Haven, Connecticut, 1934.

[2] A. F. Rasmussen, H. A. Waisman, C. A. Elvehjem, and P. F. Clark, *J. Infec. Dis.* **74**, 41 (1944).

[3] C. Foster, J. H. Jones, W. Henle, and F. Dorfman, *J. Exp. Med.* **80**, 257 (1944).

[4] H. A. Schneider, *Vitam. Horm.* (*New York*) **4**, 35 (1946).

6. Individual genetic factors

7. Performance of muscular work

(1) Size of the Animal. We know that the rate of the metabolism of an animal depends upon its body surface. Thus we expect that the requirement of thiamine, an agent in carbohydrate metabolism, will also depend on the surface area of the body. Cowgill, in studying the thiamine requirements of mice, rats, pigeons, dogs, and human beings, found that their requirement is proportional to their weight.

As the metabolism is connected with the amount of calories an animal consumes per day, it is probably better not to indicate the amount of thiamine an animal needs per day but to record the thiamine *content* of the food (or, still better, the relation between thiamine and carbohydrate intake: see below).

For the thiamine requirements of different kinds of animals, see: for the growing rat, Brown and Sturtevant;[5] for the guinea pig, Mannering;[6] for the mouse, Morris;[7] for chicks, Bird;[8] and for pigeons, Bird.[9]

(2) Composition of the Diet. Thiamine plays a role in carbohydrate metabolism. Thus, in the first place, the thiamine requirement depends on the carbohydrate content of the diet. More than two decades ago Evans and Lepkovsky[10] found the "thiamine-sparing" action of fats. Several other authors confirmed this action.

Proteins[11] and alcohol[12, 13] also have a thiamine-sparing action. These components of the diet may depress the thiamine requirement practically to zero. The most probable deduction from this fact is that thiamine is probably not involved in the enzyme system necessary for the metabolism of fats, etc. This was confirmed by the work of de Caro and Rindi.[14] These authors produced a state of athiaminosis in rats by feeding them a thiamine-deficient diet, demonstrated by a rise in the pyruvic acid level of their blood. Addition of fat to the diet reduced the pyruvic acid level to normal.

Part of the thiamine-sparing action probably is caused not only by the reduction of carbohydrates in the diet, but also by microbiol syntheses of thiamine in the gut.

We may mention here also the presence of antithiamines or of thiaminase, each of which increases the requirement for thiamine.

[5] R. A. Brown and M. Sturtevant, *Vitam. Horm.* (*New York*) 7, 176 (1949).

[6] G. J. Mannering, *Vitam. Horm.* (*New York*) 7, 207 (1949).

[7] H. P. Morris, *Vitam. Horm.* (*New York*) 5, 176 (1947).

[8] H. R. Bird, *Vitam. Horm.* (*New York*) 5, 166 (1947).

[9] H. R. Bird, *Vitam. Horm.* (*New York*) 5, 169 (1947).

[10] H. M. Evans and S. Lepkovsky, *Science* 68, 298 (1928); *J. Biol. Chem.* 83, 269 (1929).

[11] W. J. Dann, *Fed. Proc. Fed. Amer. Soc. Exp. Biol.* 4, 153 (1945).

[12] J. V. Lowry, W. H. Sebrell, F. S. Daft, and L. L. Ashburn, *J. Nutr.* 24, 73 (1942).

[13] W. W. Westerfeld and E. A. Doisy, Jr., *J. Nutr.* 30, 127 (1945).

[14] L. de Caro and G. Rindi, *Nature* (*London*) 167, 114 (1951).

(3) Physical State of the Animal. As thyroxine regulates the (basal) metabolism, it is to be expected that hyperthyroidism or the feeding of extra doses of thyroxine will increase the requirements of thiamine. The work of several investigators has confirmed this supposition (e.g., Himwich et al.;[15] Cowgill and Palmieri;[16] Drill and Sherwood;[17] Peters and Rossiter[18]). A review of this work is given by Drill.[19]

It is obvious also that pregnancy, in particular during the latter half, and lactation increase the requirements of thiamine. There are reports that the thiamine requirement of a rat successfully nursing a litter is five times as large as normal (Evans and Burr;[20] Sure;[21] Sure and Walker[22]).

Mills et al.[23] have demonstrated that the thiamine requirement of rats per gram of diet increases greatly with old age. The most probable explanation for this fact is the supposition that the efficiency of thiamine utilization is diminished.

Gerrits[24] observed that 38 infants, 0 to $2\frac{1}{2}$ months of age, never excrete thiamine in the urine, independent of their nutrition. Hamil et al.,[25] working with an improved method for the determination of thiamine, also found low values for the thiamine in the urine during the first days of life. In this respect it is interesting that the thiamine pyrophosphate content of the blood of newborn infants is much higher than the content of the blood of adults.[25a]

(4) The Climate (Temperature). Kline et al.[26] stated that by raising the environmental temperature from 78° to 90°F the thiamine requirement of the rat is decreased.

Hegsted and McPhee[27] later found that on lowering of the environmental temperature the thiamine requirement of rats increased considerably. At 78°F, the requirement of adult rats amounted to 164 to 168 γ of thiamine per 1000 nonfat calories; at 55°F, the figures were 191 to 203 γ.

[15] H. E. Himwich, W. Goldfarb, and G. R. Cowgill, Amer. J. Physiol. 99, 689 (1932).

[16] G. R. Cowgill and M. L. Palmieri, Amer. J. Physiol. 105, 146 (1933).

[17] V. A. Drill and C. R. Sherwood, Amer. J. Physiol. 124, 683 (1938).

[18] R. A. Peters and R. J. Rossiter, Biochem. J. 33, 1140 (1939).

[19] V. A. Drill, Physiol. Rev. 23, 355 (1943).

[20] H. M. Evans and G. O. Burr, J. Biol. Chem. 76, 263 (1928).

[21] B. Sure, J. Biol. Chem. 76, 685 (1928).

[22] B. Sure and D. J. Walker, J. Biol. Chem. 91, 69 (1930).

[23] C. A. Mills, E. Cottingham, and E. Taylor, Arch. Biochem. 9, 221 (1946).

[24] W. B. J. Gerrits, Thesis, Amsterdam Noord-Hollandsche Uitgever Maatschappij, 1940.

[25] B. M. Hamil, M. N. Corvell, C. Roderuck, M. Kaucher, E. Z. Moyer, M. E. Harris, and H. H. Williams, Amer. J. Dis. Child. 74, 434 (1947).

[25a] E.E. Florÿn, and H. Strengers, Acta Physiol. Pharmacol. Neer. 2, 100 (1951).

[26] O. L. Kline, L. Friedman, and E. M. Nelson, J. Nutr. 29, 35, (1945).

[27] D. M. Hegsted and G. S. McPhee, J. Nutr. 41, 127 (1950).

This is in agreement with the results of the work of Ershoff,[28] who found that rats could survive on a thiamine-deficient diet for an average of 64.7 days at 23°C (about 74°F), whereas on the same diet the average surviving time was only 27.6 days at 2°C (approximately 36°F).

Furthermore Sarett and Perlzweig[29] demonstrated that with a thiamine-rich diet the tissues laid down by rats at 91°F were twice as rich in thiamine as the tissues from rats given the same diet at 75°F.

On the other hand Mills[30, 31] found that rats require twice as much thiamine at 91° as at 65°F. He explains this by the heavy perspiration at the higher temperature. In experiments on chicks. Mills et al.[32] were able to establish the fact that the thiamine content of the diet required for protecting the animals from polyneuritis was three times as high at 90° as at 70°F. Mills[33] points out that 2 to 3 weeks are required for metabolic adaptation to heat, and he believes that the neglect of this fact may explain the different results of Kline et al.

Edison et al.[34] from their experiments came to the conclusion that the thiamine requirements for the growth of rats in a tropical environment (90°F and 70% relative humidity) were not greater and may be less than in temperate conditions (72°F and 50% relative humidity).

Considering these conflicting results, it is obvious that other factors also change at different temperatures, so that it is not a simple problem to find the sole influence of the temperature. Kline et al.[26] tried to eliminate the influence of different levels of food intake at different temperatures by giving the thiamine-free diet and the additional thiamine separately.

Not so much from the sum total of all these results but more from *a priori* reasoning an optimal temperature for a minimum thiamine requirement probably will be found; above and below this temperature the requirement will be higher. However, it is to be expected that this optimum temperature will not be a fixed one but will also depend on other factors, e.g., on humidity. At all events there seems to be a great difference in thiamine requirement at varying temperatures.

(5) Intestinal Microflora. Several of the B vitamins are synthesized by microorganisms in the gut, some of them to such an extent that this synthesis may replace the intake by food.

In some cases this is also true for thiamine. Thus as far back as 1915

[28] B. H. Ershoff, *Arch. Biochem.* **28**, 299 (1950).
[29] H. P. Sarett and W. A. Perlzweig, *J. Nutr.* **26**, 611 (1943).
[30] C. A. Mills, *Amer. J. Physiol.* **133**, 515 (1941).
[31] C. A. Mills, *Proc. Soc. Exp. Biol. Med.* **54**, 265 (1943).
[32] C. A. Mills, E. Cottingham, and E. Taylor, *Amer. J. Physiol.* **149**, 376 (1947).
[33] C. A. Mills, *Nutr. Rev.* **4**, 95 (1946).
[34] A. O. Edison, R. H. Silber, and D. M. Tennent, *Amer. J. Physiol.* **144**, 643 (1945).

Theiler *et al.*[35] demonstrated that ruminants may be sustained on a thiamine-deficient food: the thiamine is produced by the flora of the rumen.

Fridericia *et al.*[36] found that rats that normally need the thiamine from their food can produce sufficient thiamine in their intestines, if the diet contains a large amount of fresh potato starch. They called this phenomenon "refection."

Under normal circumstances, however, all nonruminant higher animals depend on their diets for their supply of thiamine. Apparently no one has yet undertaken the experiments to feed animals on a carbohydrate-free diet to see whether those animals and also the next generation can normally live a whole lifetime without thiamine. However, Dann[37] was able to maintain rats for more than a year (about half the lifetime of a rat) on a thiamine-free, carbohydrate-free synthetic diet. It is possible that the refection—the production of thiamine by microorganisms in the gut—in this case is sufficient to produce enough thiamine for protein and fat metabolism.

(6) Individual Genetic Factors. Practically all initial research on nutrient requirements has been performed with large groups of animals or human beings.

Ancel Keys, in his carefully conducted experiments with healthy volunteers who were maintained for several months under strictly controlled conditions, observed that one "normal" person may excrete two or even three times as much thiamine as another "normal" person on exactly the same diet (Mickelsen *et al.*[38]). These volunteers were all "normal" young men with no history, signs, or symptoms of nutritional, digestive, or metabolic peculiarities. Again, Williams[39] stressed the fact that individual requirements may differ widely. Thus the need for thiamine in man may vary from 0.5 to 1.5 mg. daily. Therefore it is possible that the quantity contained in a certain nutrient, which is sufficient for the average person or animal, may be too low for some individuals, depending on their genetic makeup. Williams coined the term "genetotropic diseases" for diseases that are caused by a genetically larger requirement of a nutrient in a certain individual.[39] Everyone experimenting with animals knows that even in largely inbred rats individual requirements are widely different. Therefore it is important to work with groups of at least eight to ten, but preferably with even larger groups of animals, to obtain reliable average results for the requirements of animals. Light and Cracas[40] determined the thiamine requirements of different strains

[35] A. Theiler, H. H. Green, and P. R. Viljoen, *S. Afr. Dir. Vet. Res. Resp.* p. 3 (1951).
[36] L. S. Fridericia, P. Freudenthal, S. Gudjonsson, G. Johansen, and N. Schoubye, *J. Hyg.* 27, 70 (1928).
[37] W. J. Dann, *Fed. Proc. Fed. Amer. Soc. Exp. Biol.* 4, 153 (1945).
[38] O. Mickelsen, W. O. Caster, and A. Keys, *J. Biol. Chem.* 168, 415 (1947).
[39] R. J. Williams, L. J. Berryand, and E. Beerstecher, Jr., *Arch. Biochem.* 23, 275 (1949).
[40] R. F. Light and L. J. Cracas, *Science* 87, 90 (1938).

of white rats; one strain needed twice the amount of thiamine as another strain to obtain the same growth rate.

(7) Performance of Muscular Work. We know that thiamine is essential for carbohydrate metabolism. Therefore animals doing heavy muscular work should require more thiamine than those at rest. Of course this holds true only if carbohydrates are metabolized. Otherwise thiamine requirements are not increased during heavy work. This has been demonstrated by a series of experiments by Gruber and Ruys.[41] They compared the thiamine pyrophosphate contents in breast muscle, heart, and liver of carrier pigeons that had performed an uninterrupted flight of about 140 miles with the corresponding contents of resting pigeons. Considering the work expenditure and the available carbohydrates in the bodies of the pigeons, Gruber and Ruys calculated that at least 80% of the calories for the flight must have come from fat metabolism, and only a very small percentage was supplied by carbohydrates. In accordance with these facts, the thiamine content of the organs proved not to have been decreased by the heavy work expenditure during the flight.

Taking into account all these factors that influence the thiamine requirement (and there are several others on which research has been scanty or nil), it is clear that it is impossible to state precisely the daily required amount for a certain animal. Even so it is possible to indicate a certain quantity for the requirement per 100 grams of diet containing at least 60% of carbohydrates. This content is about 100 to 150 γ. There is a surprising agreement between different investigators for different kinds of animals: for pigeons,[42] for rats,[43] for chicks,[44, 45] and even for man.[46]

As with other nutrients, life is possible at different levels of thiamine intake. To find out the optimal intake, Byerrum and Flokstra[47] determined the thiamine and the thiamine pyrophosphate content of liver, muscle, and brain of rats fed on different levels of thiamine. As the level of thiamine was increased up to 200 γ/100 gm of food, the thiamine pyrophosphate increased; beyond that level no further increase was found. Normal growth took place even on 100 γ of thiamine/100 gm of food. Therefore for maximal cocarboxylase content of these tissues twice the amount is required as is needed for normal growth. We cannot tell whether this maximal intake of thiamine has any advantage for the animal or not.

[41] M. Gruber and C. A. J. Ruys, *Acta Physiol. Pharmacol. Neer.* 2, 106 (1951).
[42] R. L. Swank and O. A. Bessey, *J. Nutr.* 22, 77 (1941).
[43] G. C. Supplee, R. C. Bender, and O. J. Kahlenberg, *J. Nutr.* 20, 109 (1940).
[44] A. Arnold and C. A. Elvehjem, *J. Nutr.* 15, 403 (1938).
[45] T. H. Jukes and H. Heitman, Jr., *J. Nutr.* 19, 21 (1940).
[46] Recommended Daily Dietary Allowances, *Nutr. Rev.* 6, 319 (1948).
[47] R. U. Byerrum and J. H. Flokstra, *J. Nutr.* 43, 17 (1951).

XIV. Requirements of Man

W. H. SEBRELL, JR.

The principal factors influencing thiamine requirements are the carbohydrate and the calorie intake. The requirement for thiamine is reduced when fat forms a large part of the diet, but for practical purposes the thiamine need may be based on the total calorie intake.

An early appraisal of the thiamine requirements of man was made by Cowgill[1] in 1934. This appraisal was based on an analysis of dietary data in the literature in relation to the occurrence of beriberi. On the basis of these data the minimum intake of thiamine necessary to prevent beriberi is not less than 0.28 mg/1000 cal (60-kg man on 2500 cal) or a total per day of 0.7 mg.

Elsom et al[1a] in a study on women volunteers concluded that 0.65 mg/day was the minimum intake necessary to maintain health.

Melnick,[2] using saturation tests, reported that adults required 0.35 mg/1000 cal or 0.875 mg/day on a 2500 cal diet.

Williams et al.[3] found that an intake of 0.22 mg of thiamine/1000 cal caused a slow depletion of tissue reserves, and with an intake of 0.45 mg/1000 cal there was a slight depletion of cocarboxylase.

Keys et al.[4] studied the performance of normal young men on controlled thiamine intakes and found that for a period of 10 to 12 weeks no benefit of any kind was observed with intakes of more than 0.23 mg of thiamine/1000 cal (intake 3050 ± 200 cal/day).

In 1944 Holt[5] critically reviewed the studies of experimental thiamine deficiency by Williams, Elsom, Keys, and Najjar and their collaborators and reinterpreted the data to conclude that the minimum thiamine requirement of an adult man on a diet of natural foods lies between 0.17 and 0.23 mg/1000 cal. He concludes that a range of intake between 0.24 mg and 0.44 mg/1000 cal appears to protect against thiamine deficiency.

Oldham et al.[6] found no change in blood thiamine levels with intakes above 0.2 mg/1000 cal.

[1] G. R. Cowgill, " The Vitamin B Requirement in Man." Yale Univ. Press, New Haven, Connecticut, 1934.
[1a] K. O'S Elsom, J. G. Rheinhold, J. T. L. Nicholson, and C. Chornoch, *Amer. J. Med. Sci.* **203**, 569 (1942).
[2] D. Melnick, *J. Nutr.* **24**, 139 (1942).
[3] R. D. Williams, H. L. Mason, and R. M. Wilder, *J. Nutr.* **25**, 71 (1943).
[4] A. Keys, A. F. Henschel, O. Mickelsen, and J. M. Brozek, *J. Nutr.* **26**, 399 (1943).
[5] L. E. Holt, Jr., *Fed. Proc. Fed. Amer. Soc. Exp. Biol.* **3**, 171 (1944).
[6] H. G. Oldham, M. V. Davis, and L. J. Roberts, *J. Nutr.* **32**, 163 (1944).

Foltz et al.,[7] using four medical students under observation in a hospital, found that a daily intake of 0.2 mg/1000 cal resulted in deficiency symptoms within 8 weeks. It is their opinion that the minimum daily requirement of thiamine for young adult men is from 0.33 to 0.45 mg/1000 cal.

Keys et al.[8] in further studies on men with restricted intake of the B vitamins found that an intake of 0.185 mg of thiamine/1000 cal (daily intake 3300 cal) was slightly less than entirely adequate.

Glickman et al.[9] found a daily intake of 0.4 mg/1000 cal entirely adequate.

In an attempt to resolve some of the differences of opinion concerning the minimum human requirement for thiamine, a study was conducted by Horwitt et al.[10] under the auspices of the National Research Council. These investigations showed that 0.4 mg of thiamine (0.18 mg/1000 cal) was below the minimal requirement of relatively inactive men on 2200 cal daily.

On the basis of all the evidence available, therefore, the opinion of the National Research Council[11] that the minimal thiamine requirement for adults is 0.23 mg or more/1000 cal is well founded. On this basis and in order to allow a suitable factor of safety for individual variation, differences in type of diet, and variations in body stores, which are never large and easily depleted by various stresses, an intake of 0.5 mg of thiamine/1000 cal is recommended by the National Research Council as a safe allowance for adults at ordinary low levels of calorie intake.

The thiamine requirement of the infant on a calorie basis is similar to that of the adult. Knott et al.[12] concluded that young infants have a minimum thiamine requirement of approximately 0.2 mg daily, which can just be met if its mother's milk contains 20 γ or more of thiamine/100 ml. They suggest that 0.4 mg of thiamine/kg may be a practical standard for the ordinary needs of the young infant. The average thiamine content of human milk was found to be about 0.15 mg/liter. A more critical analysis showed 0.2 mg/liter in a group of women whose infants were receiving no other milk in contrast to an average of 0.09 mg/liter in the milk of women whose infants required supplementary feeding.

Holt et al.[13] found the thiamine requirement of seven infants to vary

[7] E. E. Foltz, C. J. Barborka, and A. C. Ivy, Gastroenterology 2, 323 (1944).

[8] A. Keys, A. Henschel, H. L. Taylor, O. Mickelsen, and J. Brozek, Amer. J. Physiol. 144, 5 (1945).

[9] N. Glickman, R. W. Keeton, H. H. Mitchell, and M. K. Fahnestock, Amer. J. Physiol. 146, 538 (1946).

[10] M. K. Horwitt, E. Liebert, O. Kreisler, and P. Wittman, Bull. Nat. Res. Counc. (U.S.) 116 (1948).

[11] Recommended Dietary Allowances, Nat. Res. Counc. (U.S.), Reprint Circ. Ser. 129 (1948).

[12] E. M. Knott, S. C. Kleiger, F. W. Scheutz, and G. Collins, J. Pediat. 22, 43 (1943).

[13] L. E. Holt, Jr., R. L. Nemir, S. E. Snyderman, A. A. Albanese, K. C. Ketron, L. P. Guy, and R. Carretero, J. Nutr. 37, 53 (1949).

between 0.14 mg and 0.20 mg/day on the basis of a urinary excretion test. With an average thiamine content of cow's milk of 0.35 to 0.4 mg/liter, an infant weighing 7 kg is calculated to receive at least 0.3 mg of thiamine a day, but this makes no allowance for destruction by heat in pasteurization or sterilization. The margin of safety is, therefore, regarded as small by Holt and co-workers in the case of either sterilized milk or breast milk, since the latter contains roughly only half as much thiamine as cow's milk.

The meager data available on the thiamine requirement in pregnancy and lactation[14-16] indicate that in relation to calories the requirement may be considered to be in the same proportion as for infants and adult men.

[14] H. Oldham, B. B. Sheft, and T. Porter, *Fed. Proc. Fed. Amer. Soc. Exp. Biol.* **6**, 416 (1947).
[15] M. Kaucher, E. Z. Moyer, A. J. Richards, H. H. Williams, A. L. Wertz, and I. G. Macy, *Amer. J. Dis. Child.* **70**, 142 (1945).
[16] C. Roderick, H. H. Williams, and I. G. Macy, *J. Nutr.* **32**, 249 (1946).

CHAPTER 16

TOCOPHEROLS

I. Nomenclature and Formulas

ROBERT S. HARRIS

Accepted names: Vitamin E
Tocopherols
Obsolete names: Factors "X"
Antisterility vitamin
Empirical formulas: α-Tocopherol: $C_{29}H_{50}O_2$
β-Tocopherol: $C_{28}H_{48}O_2$

γ-Tocopherol: $C_{28}H_{48}O_2$
δ-Tocopherol: $C_{27}H_{46}O_2$

Chemical names: α-Tocopherol: 5,7,8-trimethyltocol, or 2,5,7,8-tetra-methyl-2-(4′ 8′ 12′-trimethyldecyl)-6-chromanol

β-Tocopherol: 5,8-dimethyltocol, or 2,5,8-trimethyl-2-(4′,8′,12′-trimethyldecyl)-6-chromanol

γ-Tocopherol: 7,8-dimethyltocol or 2,7,8-trimethyl-2-(4′,8′,12′-trimethyldecyl)-6-chromanol

δ-Tocopherol: 8-methyltocol or 2,8-dimethyl-2-(4′,8′, 12′-trimethyldecyl)-6-chromanol

Structures:

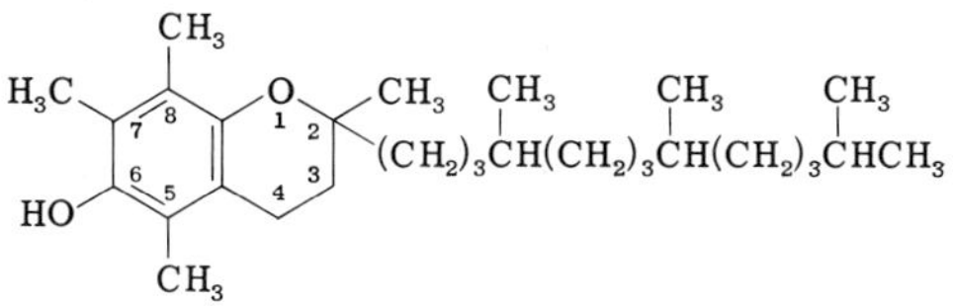

α-Tocopherol

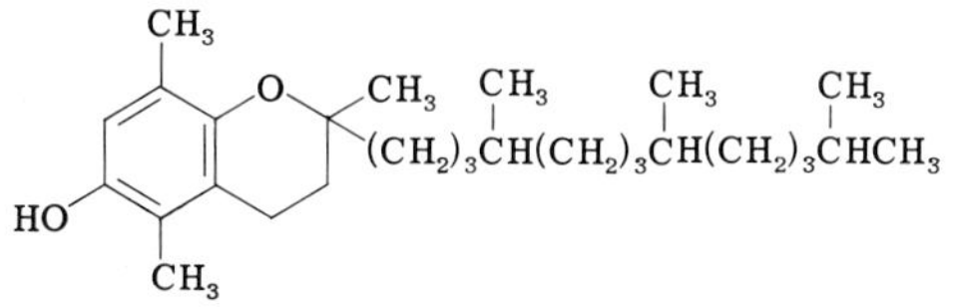

β-Tocopherol

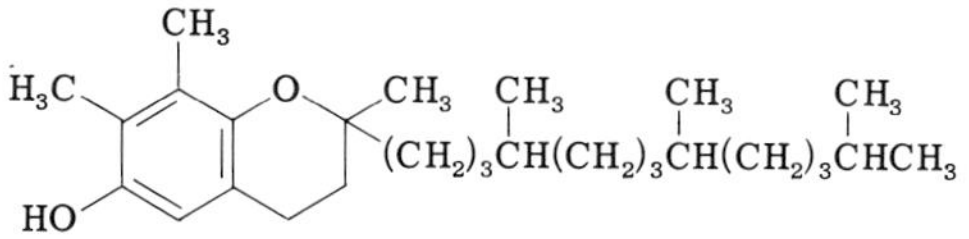

γ-Tocopherol

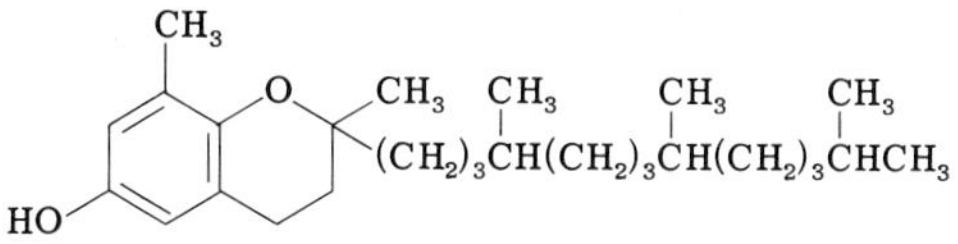

δ-Tocopherol

II. Chemistry

P. SCHUDEL, H. MAYER, AND O. ISLER

A. Introduction

A factor required in animal nutrition as a dietary constituent necessary for normal reproduction, first recognized by the teams of Evans,[1] Sure, and Mattill in the early 1920's was named vitamin E. The multiple nature of the vitamin began to unfold in 1936, when Evans et al.[2] succeeded in isolating from wheat germ oil two compounds with vitamin E activity, for which they proposed the names α-tocopherol[2] and β-tocopherol.[3, 4] Soon afterward a third active factor, γ-tocopherol,[4] was found in cottonseed oil, and in 1947 a fourth tocopherol, named δ-tocopherol, was isolated from soybean oil[5] (see Table I). In the ensuing years the investigation of several vegetable oils disclosed the existence of four tocotrienols, α-,[6] β-,[7] γ-,[6] and δ-tocotrienol[6, 8] (see Table II), so that today a total of four tocopherols and four tocotrienols are known to occur in nature.

Detailed accounts of the distribution and occurrence of tocopherols were compiled by Deuel,[9] Schmid and Haber,[10] Knobloch,[11] Dicks,[12] and Bunnell et al.[13] The chemical work on vitamin E has been summarized by

[1] H. M. Evans, *Vitam. Horm. (New York)* **20**, 379 (1962), summarizes the early history of vitamin E.

[2] H. M. Evans, O. H. Emerson, and G. A. Emerson, *J. Biol. Chem.* **113**, 319 (1936).

[3] The name "tocopherol" is derived from the Greek *tokos* (offspring), *pherein* (to bear), and *ol*, to signify a phenolic hydroxy group.[1]

[4] O. H. Emerson, G. A. Emerson, A. Mohammad, and H. M. Evans, *J. Biol. Chem.* **122** 99 (1937).

[5] M. H. Stern, C. D. Robeson, L. Weisler, and J. G. Baxter, *J. Amer. Chem. Soc.* **69**, 869 (1947).

[6] J. F. Pennock, F. W. Hemming, and J. D. Kerr, *Biochem. Biophys. Res. Commun.* **17**, 542 (1964).

[7] J. Green, P. Mamalis, S. Marcinkiewicz, and D. McHale, *Chem. Ind. (London)* p. 73 (1960).

[8] K. J. Whittle, P. J. Dunphy, and J. F. Pennock, *Biochem. J.* **100**, 138 (1966).

[9] H. J. Deuel, Jr., "The Lipids, Their Chemistry and Biochemistry," Vol. I, Ch. IX, p. 793 and Vol. III, Ch. XI, p. 683. Wiley (Interscience), New York, 1951 and 1957.

[10] H. Schmid and G. Haber, *in* "Handbuch der physiologisch- und pathologisch-chemischen Analyse-Hoppe-Seyler/Thierfelder" (K. Lang, E. Lehnartz, and G. Siebert, eds.), Vol. IV/2, p. 1005. Springer, Berlin, 1960.

[11] E. Knobloch, *in* "Vitamine" (J. Fragner, ed.), Vol. 2, p. 1584. Fischer, Jena, 1965.

[12] M. W. Dicks, *Wyo. Agr. Exp. Sta., Bull.* **435** (1965).

[13] R. H. Bunnell, J. Keating, and A. Quaresimo, *J. Agr. Food Chem.* **16**, 659 (1968).

Karrer,[14] John,[15, 16] Smith,[17] Rosenberg,[18] Vogel-Knobloch,[19] Mattill,[20] and Harris and Embree.[21] More recent reviews were given by Campbell,[22] Wagner and Folkers[23, 24] Deuel,[9] Isler et al.,[25] Dean,[26] Dyke,[27] Weichet and Knobloch,[28] Isler and Montavon,[29] Rüegg et al.,[30] Gutmann and Isler,[31] and Morton.[32] The biochemistry of vitamin E has been reviewed by Goodwin,[33] Schreiber and Koštir,[34] and Bersin.[35]

The nomenclature recommended by the IUPAC-IUB Commission on Biochemical Nomenclature[36] will be used throughout this review.

[14] P. Karrer, Helv. Chim. Acta 22, 334 (1939).

[15] W. John, Angew. Chem. 52, 413 (1939).

[16] W. John, Naturwissenschaften 26, 449 (1938).

[17] L. I. Smith, Chem. Rev. 27, 287 (1940).

[18] H. R. Rosenberg, "Chemistry and Physiology of the Vitamins," p. 435. Wiley (Interscience), New York, 1945.

[19] H. Vogel and H. Knobloch, "Chemie und Technik der Vitamine," Vol. I, p. 231. Enke, Stuttgart, 1950.

[20] H. A. Mattill, in "The Vitamins" (W. H. Sebrell and R. S. Harris, eds.), Vol. III, Ch. 17, p. 481. Academic Press, New York, 1954.

[21] P. L. Harris and N. D. Embree, in "Encyclopedia of Chemical Technology" (R. E. Kirk and D. F. Othmer, eds.), Vol. 14, p. 849. Wiley (Interscience), New York, 1955.

[22] N. Campbell, in "Chemistry of Carbon Compounds" (E. H. Rodd, ed.), Vol. IV, p. 929. Elsevier, Amsterdam, 1959.

[23] A. F. Wagner and K. Folkers, in "Medicinal Chemistry" (A. Burger, ed.). Wiley (Interscience), New York, 1960.

[24] A. F. Wagner and K. Folkers, "Vitamins and Coenzymes," p. 363. Wiley (Interscience), New York, 1964.

[25] O. Isler, P. Schudel, H. Mayer, J. Würsch, and R. Rüegg, Vitam. Horm. (New York) 20, 389 (1962).

[26] F. M. Dean, "Naturally Occurring Oxygen Ring Compounds," p. 234. Butterworths, London and Washington, D.C., 1963.

[27] S. F. Dyke, "The Chemistry of the Vitamins," p. 256. Wiley (Interscience), New York, 1965.

[28] J. Weichet and E. Knobloch, in "Vitamine" (J. Fragner, ed.), Vol. 2, p. 1530. Fischer, Jena, 1965.

[29] O. Isler and M. Montavon, Bull. Soc. Chim. Fr. p. 2403 (1965).

[30] R. Rüegg, H. Mayer, P. Schudel, U. Schwieter, R. Tamm, and O. Isler, Wiss. Veroeff. Deut. Ges. Ernaehrung 16, 14 (1967).

[31] H. Gutmann and O. Isler, in "Ullmanns Encyklopädie der technischen Chemie," 3rd Ed. (W. Foerst, ed.), Vol. 18, p. 241. Urban & Schwarzenberg, Munich, 1967.

[32] R. A. Morton, Wiss. Veroeff. Deut. Ges. Ernaehrung 16, 1 (1967).

[33] T. W. Goodwin, "The Biosynthesis of Vitamins and Related Compounds," Ch. 15, p. 320. Academic Press, New York, 1963.

[34] V. Schreiber and J. Koštiř, in "Vitamine" (G. Fragner, ed.), Vol. 2, p. 1589. Fischer, Jena, 1965.

[35] T. Bersin, "Biochemie der Vitamine," p. 211. Akad. Verlagsges., Frankfurt a. M., 1966.

[36] IUPAC-IUB Commission on Biochemical Nomenclature, Biochim. Biophys. Acta 107, 1 (1965).

B. Occurrence

The various tocopherols are found almost exclusively in plants and only to a minimal degree in animal tissues, in which α-tocopherol seems to prevail.[37] They are present in highest concentration (0.1–0.3%) in wheat germ, corn, cottonseed, sunflower seed, rapeseed, and soybean oils, in which they occur in unesterified form. Olive, coconut, and peanut oils, however, are extremely low in tocopherols. Lettuce and alfalfa again contain considerable amounts of them, while bananas and oranges are poor in vitamin E.

The tocopherol distribution in cereal grains and seed oils falls into two rather distinct patterns.[38] The more common one in higher plants—the α,γ,δ-pattern—is found in the important seed oils such as soybean, linseed, peanut, and cottonseed oil whereas in the staple cereals wheat, barley, and rye—more important for human nutrition—not only α- and β-tocopherols, but also α- and β-tocotrienols are encountered. An interesting picture is presented by palm oil, which contains all four tocotrienols and α-tocopherol.[6] In rice α- and γ-tocotrienols as well as α-tocopherol and smaller amounts of β-tocopherol and β-tocotrienol are found.[6, 39] Rubber latex from *Hevea brasiliensis* has recently been discovered to be a rich source for free and esterified α-, γ-, and δ-tocotrienols.[8, 40]

C. Isolation

The isolation of the vitamin E factors from various natural sources can be achieved along the main lines described herein.

Extraction of the substrates with organic, lipophilic solvents (such as ether, petroleum ether, benzene, and chloroform), evaporation of the solvent, saponification of the residue (e.g. with 20% alcoholic potassium hydroxide at about 30° in the absence of oxygen), and extraction with organic solvents yields the unsaponifiable matter, 90% of which consists of sterols. These can be separated by chromatographic procedures or by fractional crystallization from suitable solvents, such as alcohols, pentane, acetone. Purification of the unsaponifiable matter can also be done by partition between different solvents, such as methanol–petroleum ether, whereby the vitamin goes into the latter. The remaining oily tocopherol concentrate is purified by molecular distillation or, again, by chromatographic procedures. The vitamins E are also obtained in improved yields directly from wheat germ oils by chroma-

[37] H. Kubin and H. Fink, *Fette, Seifen, Anstrichm.* **63**, 280 (1961).

[38] J. Green, *in* "Enzyme Chemistry of Phenolic Compounds" (J. B. Pridham, ed.), Ch. 5, p. 47. Macmillan (Pergamon), New York, 1962.

[39] J. Green and S. Marcinkiewicz, *Nature (London)* **177**, 86 (1956).

[40] P. J. Dunphy, K. J. Whittle, J. F. Pennock, and R. A. Morton, *Nature (London)* **207**, 521 (1965).

tography on alumina.[41] The separation of the several tocopherols from one another is achieved by chromatography or by fractional crystallization of some of their derivatives, such as their allophanates or p-phenylazobenzoates. Experimental procedures for the isolation of the tocopherols and tocotrienols are listed in Tables I and II; for detailed procedures, see the corresponding references cited in the tables.

D. Structure

The tocopherols found in nature belong to two distinct series of compounds, all of them derivatives of chroman-6-ol. The first series derives from tocol (see Table I), which bears a saturated isoprenoid C_{16}-side chain, whereas the members of the second series (see Table II) are derivatives of tocotrienol having a triply unsaturated side chain. The term "tocol" for 2-methyl-2-(4′,8′,12′-trimethyltridecyl)chroman-6-ol was proposed by Karrer and Fritzsche[42] in 1938. The trivial name "tocotrienol" for 2-methyl-2-(4′,8′,12′-trimethyltrideca-3′,7′,11′-trienyl)chroman-6-ol which is the triunsaturated analog of tocol was introduced by Bunyan et al.,[43] and the members of the new series were designated as methylated tocotrienols.

A new nomenclature has been suggested recently by Pennock et al.[6] and accepted by the IUPAC-IUB Commission on Biochemical Nomenclature.[36] Accordingly, the Greek letters used hitherto for the tocotrienol series (ζ_1, ζ_2, ε, and η) should be dropped and these compounds be referred to as a-, β-, γ-, and δ-tocotrienols related to α-, β-, γ-, and δ-tocopherols. Thus α-tocopherol is 5,7,8-trimethyltocol, β-tocopherol is 5,8-dimethyltocol, α-tocotrienol is 5,7,8-trimethyltocotrienol, β-tocotrienol is 5,8-dimethyltocotrienol, etc. (see Tables I and II). In the tocols, the saturated side chain together with the carbon atoms 2, 3, and 4 and the methyl group at C-2 of the chroman moiety represent the carbon skeleton of phytol, which in the tocotrienols appears unsaturated at the positions 3′, 7′, and 11′.[44] Within one series the members differ from one another only in the number and position of the methyl groups attached to the aromatic ring.

Tocopherol and tocotrienol structures shown in Tables I and II were established by degradative studies together with various unequivocal syntheses achieved by several teams in different laboratories, during the years 1937–1964. Fernholz[45] was the first to propose the correct structure of α-tocopherol in 1938. His reasoning was based, among other things, on the isolation of

[41] A. R. Moss and J. C. Drummond, *Biochem. J.* **32**, 1953 (1938).
[42] P. Karrer and H. Fritzsche, *Helv. Chim. Acta* **21**, 1234 (1938).
[43] J. Bunyan, D. McHale, J. Green, and S. Marcinkiewicz, *Brit. J. Nutr.* **15**, 253 (1961).
[44] The numbering system of the tocopherol side chain was first proposed by P. Karrer, H. Koenig, B. H. Ringier, and H. Salomon, *Helv. Chim. Acta* **22**, 1139 (1939).
[45] E. Fernholz, *J. Amer. Chem. Soc.* **60**, 700 (1938).

TABLE I
THE TOCOPHEROLS

-Tocopherol	-Tocol	R_1	R_2	R_3	Isolation[a]	Structure determination[a]	Synthesis[a]
α-	5,7,8-Trimethyl-	CH₃	CH₃	CH₃	a_1	a_2–a_{11}, a_{14}–a_{17}	a_{11}–a_{14}, a_{16}, a_{18}–a_{47}
β-	5,8-Dimethyl-	CH₃	H	CH₃	b_1	a_4, a_7–a_{10}, b_2–b_4	b_5, b_6
γ-	7,8-Dimethyl-	H	CH₃	CH₃	b_1	b_2, b_3, b_8	b_5, b_6
δ-	8-Methyl-	H	H	CH₃	c_1	c_1	b_7, c_1–c_6
—	5,7-Dimethyl-	CH₃	CH₃	H	d_1	d_1, d_2	a_{20}, b_6
—	7-Methyl-	H	CH₃	H	e_1	e_1	b_7, c_2, c_5, c_6, e_2
—	5-Methyl-	CH₃	H	H	Not yet found in nature		b_7, c_5, c_6, f_1
—	Tocol	H	H	H			c_3, d_2, g_1, g_2

[a] References for Tables I and II.

a_1 H. M. Evans, O. H. Emerson, and G. A. Emerson, *J. Biol. Chem.* **113**, 319 (1936).

a_2 C. S. McArthur and E. M. Watson, *Science* **86**, 35 (1937).

a_3 E. Fernholz, *J. Amer. Chem. Soc.* **59**, 1154 (1937).

a_4 F. Bergel, A. R. Todd, and T. S. Work, *J. Chem. Soc., London* p. 253 (1938).

a_5 O. H. Emerson, *Science* **88**, 40 (1938).

a_6 E. Fernholz, *J. Amer. Chem. Soc.* **60**, 700 (1938).

a_7 W. John, E. Dietzel, and P. Günther, *Hoppe-Seyler's Z. Physiol. Chem.* **252**, 208 (1938).

a_8 W. John, *Hoppe-Seyler's Z. Physiol. Chem.* **252**, 222 (1938).

a₉ W. John, E. Dietzel, P. Günther, and W. Emte, *Naturwissenschaften* **26**, 366 (1938).

a₁₀ P. Karrer, H. Salomon, and H. Fritzsche, *Helv. Chim. Acta* **21**, 309 (1938).

a₁₁ P. Karrer, H. Fritzsche, B. H. Ringier, and H. Salomon, *Helv. Chim. Acta* **21**, 520 (1938).

a₁₂ O. Isler, cited in ref. a₁₁.

a₁₃ O. Isler, *Mitt. Naturforsch. Ges. Schaffhausen* **18**, 323 (1942–1943).

a₁₄ P. Karrer, H. Fritzsche, B. H. Ringier and H. Salomon, *Helv. Chim. Acta* **21**, 820 (1938).

a₁₅ P. Karrer, R. Escher, H. Fritzsche, H. Keller, B. H. Ringier, and H. Salomon, *Helv. Chim. Acta* **21**, 939 (1938).

a₁₆ L. I. Smith, H. E. Ungnade, and W. W. Prichard, *Science* **88**, 37 (1938).

a₁₇ H. Mayer, P. Schudel, R. Rüegg, and O. Isler, *Helv. Chim. Acta* **46**, 963 (1963).

a₁₈ F. Bergel, A. Jacob, A. R. Todd, and T. S. Work, *Nature (London)* **142**, 36 (1938).

a₁₉ F. Bergel, A. M. Copping, A. Jacob, A. R. Todd, and T. S. Work, *J. Chem. Soc., London* p. 1382 (1938).

a₂₀ L. F. Fieser, M. Tishler, and N. L. Wendler, *J. Amer. Chem. Soc.* **62**, 2861 (1940).

a₂₁ W. John and H. Pini, *Hoppe-Seyler's Z. Physiol. Chem.* **273**, 225 (1942).

a₂₂ P. Karrer and O. Isler, U.S. Patent No. 2 411 967 (1938); see *Chem. Abstr.* **41**, 1715ᶜ (1947).

a₂₃ P. Karrer and B. H. Ringier, *Helv. Chim. Acta* **22**, 610 (1939).

a₂₄ P. Karrer, R. G. Legler, and G. Schwab, *Helv. Chim. Acta* **23**, 1132 (1940).

a₂₅ O. Isler, *Mitt. Naturforsch. Ges. Schaffhausen* **18**, 321 (1942–1943).

a₂₆ P. Karrer and O. Isler, U.S. Patent No. 2 411 969 (1941); see *Chem. Abstr.* **41**, 1713ⁱ (1947).

a₂₇ J. A. Aeschlimann, U.S. Patent No. 2 307 010 (1943); see *Chem. Abstr.* **37**, 3567ᵇ (1943).

a₂₈ M. E. Maurit, G. V. Smirnova, E. A. Parfenov, I. K. Sarycheva, and N. A. Preobrazhenskii, *Dokl. Akad. Nauk SSSR* **140**, 1330 (1961); see *Chem. Abstr.* **56**, 8672ᶠ (1962).

a₂₉ J. D. Surmatis and J. Weber, U.S. Patent No. 2 723 278 (1955); see *Chem. Abstr.* **50**, 10794ᵉ (1956).

a₃₀ K. Nakajima and S. Kitamura, Jap. Patent No. 5334 (1967); see *Chem. Abstr.* **67**, 90673ᵃ (1967).

a₃₁ H. Mayer, P. Schudel, R. Rüegg, and O. Isler, *Chimia* **16**, 367 (1962).

a₃₂ H. Mayer, P. Schudel, R. Rüegg, and O. Isler, *Helv. Chim. Acta* **46**, 650 (1963).

a₃₃ L. I. Smith and H. E. Ungnade, *J. Org. Chem.* **4**, 298 (1939).

a₃₄ L. I. Smith, H. E. Ungnade, H. H. Hoehn, and S. Wawzonek, *J. Org. Chem.* **4**, 311 (1939).

a₃₅ L. I. Smith, H. E. Ungnade, J. R. Stevens, and C. C. Christman, *J. Amer. Chem. Soc.* **61**, 2615 (1939).

a₃₆ F. von Werder, U.S. Patent No. 2 230 659 (1941); see *Chem. Abstr.* **35**, 3270³ (1941).

a₃₇ O. Ehrmann, Ger. Patent No. 1 015 446 (1957); see *Chem. Abstr.* **54**, 578ᵇ (1960).

a₃₈ K. Nakagawa and S. Muraki, Jap. Patent No. 11993 (1963); see *Derwent No.* 8529 (1963).

a₃₉ K. Kakagawa, Jap. Patent No. 18338 (1966); see *Derwent No.* 23701 (1966).

TABLE I—*continued*

a_{40} L. I. Smith and H. C. Miller, *J. Amer. Chem. Soc.* **64**, 440 (1942).

a_{41} L. I. Smith and J. A. Sprung, *J. Amer. Chem. Soc.* **65**, 1276 (1943).

a_{42} J. Weichet and J. Hodrová, *Collect. Czech. Chem. Commun.* **22**, 595 (1957).

a_{43} L. Blahá and J. Hodrová, *Collect. Czech. Chem. Commun.* **24**, 2023 (1959).

a_{44} M. Matsui and S. Kitamura, *Agr. Biol. Chem.* **39**, 978 (1965).

a_{45} I. A. Miller and H. C. S. Wood, *Chem. Commun.* p. 40 (1965).

a_{46} T. Ichakawa and T. Kato, Jap. Patent No. 11064 (1967); see *Chem. Abstr.* **67**, 10003^e (1967).

a_{47} T. Ichakawa and T. Kato, Jap. Patent No. 11065 (1967); see *Chem. Abstr.* **67**, 10001^e (1967).

b_1 O. H. Emerson, G. A. Emerson, A. Mohammad, and H. M. Evans, *J. Biol. Chem.* **122**, 99 (1937).

b_2 O. H. Emerson, *J. Amer. Chem. Soc.* **60**, 1741 (1938).

b_3 O. Isler, H. Mayer, J. Metzger, R. Rüegg, and P. Schudel, *Angew. Chem.* **75**, 1030 (1963).

b_4 W. John, *Hoppe-Seyler's Z. Physiol. Chem.* **250**, 11 (1937).

b_5 A. Jacob, M. Steiger, A. R. Todd, and T. S. Work, *J. Chem. Soc., London* p. 542 (1939).

b_6 P. Karrer and H. Fritzsche, *Helv. Chim. Acta.* **21**, 1234 (1938).

b_7 P. Karrer and H. Fritzsche, *Helv. Chim. Acta.* **22**, 260 (1939).

b_8 O. H. Emerson and L. I. Smith, *J. Amer. Chem. Soc.* **62**, 1869 (1940).

c_1 M. H. Stern, C. D. Robeson, K. Weisler, and J. G. Baxter, *J. Amer. Chem. Soc.* **69**, 869 (1947).

c_2 J. Green, D. McHale, P. Mamalis, and S. Marcinkiewicz, *J. Chem. Soc., London* p. 3374 (1959).

c_3 A. Jacob, F. K. Sutcliffe, and A. R. Todd, *J. Chem. Soc., London* p. 327 (1940).

c_4 P. Karrer and P. C. Dutta, *Helv. Chim. Acta.* **31**, 2080 (1948).

c_5 S. Marcinkiewicz, D. McHale, P. Mamalis, and J. Green, *J. Chem. Soc., London* p. 3377 (1959).

c_6 P. Mamalis, J. Green, S. Marcinkiewicz, and D. McHale, *J. Chem. Soc., London* p. 3350 (1959).

d_1 J. Green, S. Marcinkiewicz, and P. R. Watt, *J. Sci. Food Agr.* **6**, 274 (1955).

d_2 J. Green, D. McHale, S. Marcinkiewicz, P. Mamalis, and P. R. Watt, *J. Chem. Soc., London* p. 3362 (1959).

e_1 J. Green and S. Marcinkiewicz, *Nature (London)* **177**, 86 (1956).

e_2 D. McHale, P. Mamalis, J. Green, and S. Marcinkiewicz, *J. Chem. Soc., London* p. 1600 (1958).

f_1 D. McHale, P. Mamalis, S. Marcinkiewicz, and J. Green, *J. Chem. Soc., London* p. 3358 (1959).

g₁ H. K. Pendse and P. Karrer, *Helv. Chim. Acta* **40**, 1837 (1957).
g₂ P. Mamalis, D. McHale, J. Green, and S. Marcinkiewicz, *J. Chem. Soc., London* p. 1850 (1958).

h₁ J. F. Pennock, F. W. Hemming, and J. D. Kerr, *Biochem. Biophys. Res. Commun.* **17**, 542 (1964).
h₂ P. J. Dunphy, K. J. Whittle, J. F. Pennock, and R. A. Morton, *Nature (London)* **207**, 521 (1965).
h₃ J. Green, P. Mamalis, S. Marcinkiewicz, and D. McHale, *Chem. Ind. (London)* p. 73 (1960).
h₄ P. Schudel, H. Mayer, J. Metzger, R. Rüegg, and O. Isler, *Helv. Chim. Acta* **46**, 2517 (1963).

i₁ D. McHale, J. Green, S. Marcinkiewicz, J. Feeney, and L. H. Sutcliffe, *J. Chem. Soc., London* p. 784 (1963).
i₂ H. Mayer, J. Metzger, and O. Isler, *Helv. Chim. Acta* **50**, 1376 (1967).
i₃ R. L. Coop and J. F. Pennock, 1964, cited in ref. h₁.

TABLE II
THE TOCOTRIENOLS

-Tocotrienol		R_1	R_2	R_3	Isolation[a]	Structure determination[a]	Synthesis[a]
α-	5,7,8-Trimethyl-	CH_3	CH_3	CH_3	d_1, d_2, h_1, h_2	d_2, b_3, h_3, h_4	b_3, h_4
β-	5,8-Dimethyl-	CH_3	H	CH_3	h_3, i_1	b_3, h_3, h_4	b_3, h_4
γ-	7,8-Dimethyl-	H	CH_3	CH_3	h_1, h_2	h_1, i_2	i_2, i_3
δ-	8-Methyl-	H	H	CH_3	h_1, h_2	h_1	
—	Tocotrienol	H	H	H	Not yet found in nature		

[a] References:: see footnote *a*, Table I.

durohydroquinone after pyrolysis (see Section E, 7) and on the structures of the chromic acid oxidation products of α-tocopherol (see Section E, 1). A first synthesis of α-tocopherol through condensation of trimethylhydroquinone with phytyl bromide was published by Karrer et al.[46] in the same year. Intensive work, especially in the laboratories of John, Smith, and Emerson,[47] provided proof of the presence of the chroman nucleus and excluded the proposed coumaran structure[48] of α-tocopherol. The structure and synthesis of β-tocopherol became also known in 1938, and the structure of γ-tocopherol was elucidated by Emerson and Smith[49] in 1940. The isolation and structure of δ-tocopherol were not reported until 1947 by Stern et al.[5]

During the years 1955–1963, Green and his colleagues made an important extension to knowledge when they discovered and chemically elaborated the naturally occurring tocotrienols, which are related to the tocopherols but which have three unsaturated isoprenoid groups in the side chain (see Table II). Green et al.[50] originally encountered in bran oil a new tocopherol, ζ-tocopherol (later designated ζ_1-tocopherol to differentiate it from ζ_2-tocopherol from rice[7]). In 1959, Green et al.[51] proved that the ζ_1-tocopherol from wheat bran and palm oil was 5,7,8-trimethyltocotrienol (now designated α-tocotrienol). Thus on hydrogenation it yielded α-tocopherol and also was identical with synthetic 5,7,8-trimethyltocotrienol. The ζ_2-tocopherol from rice was identified as 5,7-dimethyltocol.[51]

In 1952 Brown[52] observed an unidentified spot during paper chromatic analysis of the tocopherol fraction of wheat germ oil which was named ε-tocopherol and identified as 5-methyltocol.[53] Later, however, Green et al.[7] demonstrated that ε-tocopherol of wheat has the structure of 5,8-dimethyltocotrienol (now named β-tocotrienol). Thus ε-tocopherol on hydrogenation yielded β-tocopherol, by chloromethylation or hydroxymethylation followed by reduction was converted into α-tocotrienol and also proved to be identical with synthetic 5,8-dimethyltocotrienol.[54]

The structures of γ- and δ-tocotrienols have only recently been elucidated by Pennock and collaborators.[6, 8] When investigating palm oil and rubber

[46] P. Karrer, H. Fritzsche, B. H. Ringier, and H. Salomon, Helv. Chim. Acta 21, 520 (1938).
[47] For references see Table I.
[48] P. Karrer, H. Salomon, and H. Fritzsche, Helv. Chim. Acta 21, 309 (1938).
[49] O. H. Emerson and L. I. Smith, J. Amer. Chem. Soc. 62, 1869 (1940).
[50] J. Green, S. Marcinkiewicz, and P. R. Watt, J. Sci. Food Agr. 6, 274 (1955).
[51] J. Green, D. McHale, S. Marcinkiewicz, P. Mamalis, and P. R. Watt, J. Chem. Soc., London p. 3362 (1959).
[52] F. Brown, Biochem. J. 51, 237, 523 (1952).
[53] D. W. Eggitt and L. D. Ward, J. Sci. Food Agr. 4, 569 (1953).
[54] P. Schudel, H. Mayer, J. Metzger, R. Rüegg, and O. Isler, Helv. Chim. Acta 46, 2517 (1963).

latex from *Hevea brasiliensis* these authors isolated two new compounds which resembled γ- and δ-tocopherol, respectively, but which could be separated by two-dimensional thin-layer chromatography from all the tocopherols and tocotrienols hitherto known. Indeed they were converted to γ- and δ-tocopherol on hydrogenation. The γ-tocopherol like compound proved to be identical with synthetic 7,8-dimethyl tocotrienol, whereas the second unknown gave β-tocotrienol on hydroxymethylation followed by reduction.

Pennock et al.[6] also claimed that at present there is no evidence for the existence of 5,7-dimethyltocol (ζ_2-tocopherol)[51] and 7-methyltocol (η-tocopherol)[39] in nature: ζ_2- and η-tocopherol from rice and palm oil turned out to be α- and γ-tocotrienol, respectively.

Detailed information about structure determinations and syntheses of the tocopherols and tocotrienols will be found under the respective references cited in Tables I and II.

1. STEREOCHEMISTRY

Only recently it was proved by Mayer et al.[55] that natural α-tocopherol from vegetable oils has the 2R,4'R,8'R-configuration. The 2R-configuration of β-tocopherol, of α- and β-tocotrienol from wheat bran, and of γ-tocotrienol from rubber latex of *Hevea brasiliensis* is also established.[56, 57] The same holds for γ-tocopherol from vegetable oils.[56, 58] If one considers that many of the tocopherols occur together in the same plant[9] and therefore probably have a very close biogenesis,[6, 38] then it seems most likely that all the naturally occurring tocols exhibit the 2R,4'R,8'R-configuration. The three tocotrienols, α- and β-tocotrienol from wheat bran and γ-tocotrienol from latex, are definitely 2R,3'-*trans*,7'-*trans*-configurated, as was recently shown by Isler and co-workers.[54, 56, 57]

Regarding the specification of stereoisomeric tocopherols, the literature presents a situation which is often very confusing. For instance, the designation dl-α-tocopherol introduced by Karrer et al.[46, 59, 60] has been applied to synthetic specimens obtained both from natural, optically active[61] and from synthetic, totally racemic[59, 61] phytol. Since natural phytol has been shown

[55] H. Mayer, P. Schudel, R. Rüegg, and O. Isler, *Helv. Chim. Acta* **46**, 963 (1963).
[56] O. Isler, H. Mayer, J. Metzger, R. Rüegg, and P. Schudel, *Angew. Chem.* **75**, 1030 (1963).
[57] H. Mayer, J. Metzger, and O. Isler, *Helv. Chim. Acta* **50**, 1376 (1967).
[58] P. Schudel, unpublished observations (1962).
[59] P. Karrer and B. H. Ringier, *Helv. Chim. Acta* **22**, 610 (1939).
[60] P. Karrer, H. Fritzsche, B. H. Ringier, and H. Salomon, *Helv. Chim. Acta* **21**, 820 (1938).
[61] P. Karrer, H. Koenig, B. H. Ringier, and H. Salomon, *Helv. Chim. Acta* **22**, 1139 (1939).

TABLE III
TOCOPHEROL STEREOISOMERS

Specifications	Stereoformulas

D[a,b,c];(+)[d]

(2D, 4'D, 8'D)[e]

(2R, 4'R, 8'R)[d,g,h]

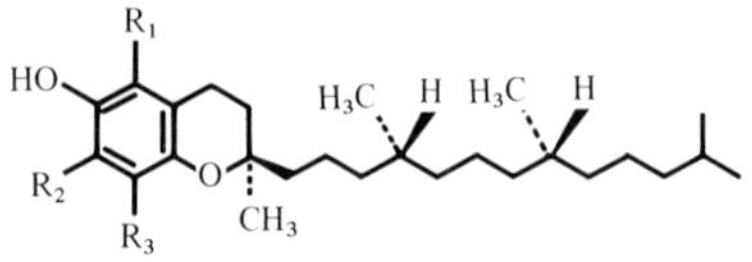

L[b,e,i]

(2L, 4'D, 8'D)[e,j]

(2S, 4'R, 8'R)[g,k]

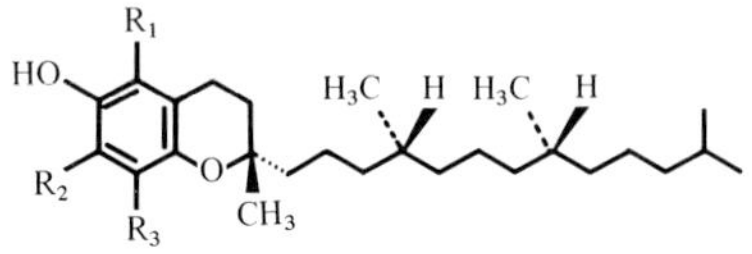

DL[b,l,m]

[C*2-d,1;C*4'8'-d][n]

(2DL, 4'D, 8'D)[e,j]

(2RS, 4'R, 8'R)[g,o]

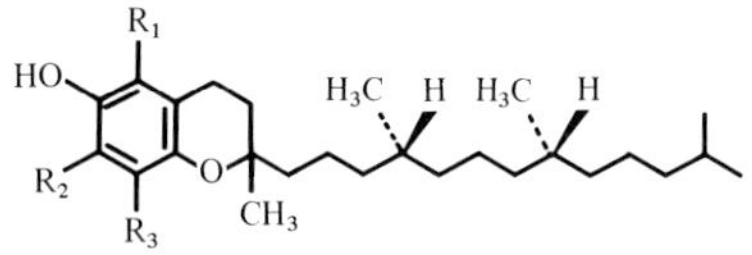

DL[b,p,q]

[C*2-d,1;C*4', 8'-d,1][n]

(2DL, 4'DL, 8'DL)[j]

(2RS, 4'RS, 8'RS)[o]

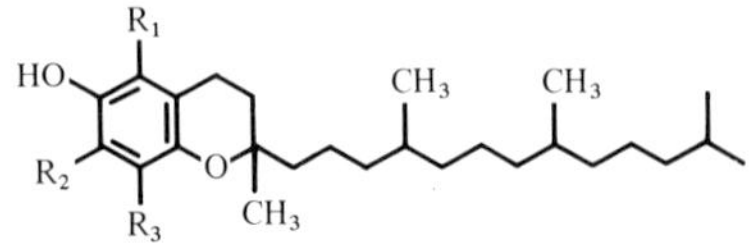

(2RS, 3'-$trans$, 7'-$trans$)[r,s]

(racemic, all-$trans$)

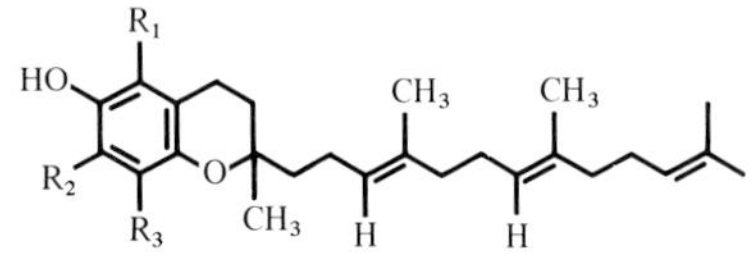

(2R, 3'-$trans$, 7'-$trans$)[s,t]

(2R, all-$trans$)

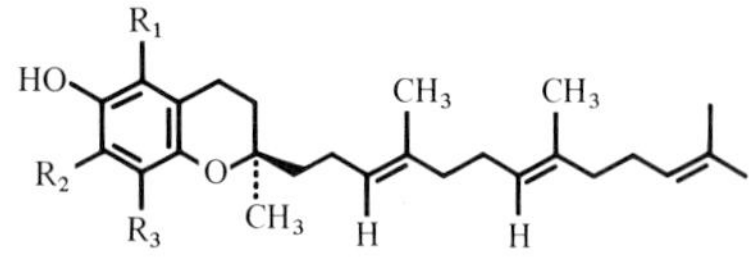

[a] L. Weisler, J. G. Baxter, and M. I. Ludwig, *J. Amer. Chem. Soc.* **67**, 1230 (1945).

[b] H. Weiser, G. Brubacher, and O. Wiss, *Science* **140**, 80 (1963).

[c] "National Formulary," 12th Ed. Mack Printing Co., Easton, Pennsylvania, 1965.

[d] IUPAC-IUB Commission on Biochemical Nomenclature, *Biochim. Biophys. Acta* **107**, 1 (1965).

[e] C. D. Robeson and D. R. Nelan, *J. Amer. Chem. Soc.* **84**, 3196 (1962).

[f] H. Mayer, P. Schudel, R. Rüegg, and O. Isler, *Chimia* **16**, 367 (1962).

[g] P. Schudel, H. Mayer, J. Metzger, R. Rüegg, and O. Isler, *Helv. Chim. Acta* **46**, 333 (1963).

[h] H. Mayer, P. Schudel, R. Rüegg, and O. Isler, *Helv. Chim. Acta* **46**, 963 (1963).

to possess the $7R,11R$-configuration,[62-64] α-tocopherol from natural phytol must be a mixture of two epimers, not of two enantiomers, whereas with racemic phytol a total of eight diastereomeric α-tocopherols must be considered. This essential point has already been discussed in detail by John and Pini,[65] but unfortunately not enough attention has been paid to it in the literature. Furthermore, the specification d- (e.g., d-α-, d-β-, d-γ-, etc.) tocopherol for a natural specimen is based on the positive optical rotation of the samples in *ethanol* solution.[66] The sign of rotation is strictly solvent dependent, since negative optical rotations are observed in *benzene* solution for, e.g., α- and γ-tocopherol[66] (see also Section F, 7). Further confusion arose by the designation of the recently prepared[26, 67-72] α-tocopherol with

[62] J. W. K. Burrell, L. M. Jackman, and B. C. L. Weedon, *Proc. Chem. Soc., London* p. 263 (1959).

[63] J. W. K. Burrell, R. F. Garwood, L. M. Jackman, E. Oskay, and B. C. L. Weedon, *J. Chem. Soc., London* p. 2144 (1966).

[64] P. Crabbe, C. Djerassi, E. J. Eisenbraun, and S. Liu, *Proc. Chem. Soc., London* p. 264 (1959).

[65] W. John and H. Pini, *Hoppe-Seyler's Z. Physiol. Chem.* 273, 225 (1942).

[66] J. G. Baxter, C. D. Robeson, J. D. Taylor, and R. W. Lehman, *J. Amer. Chem. Soc.* 65, 918 (1943).

[67] C. D. Robeson and D. R. Nelan, *J. Amer. Chem. Soc.* 84, 3196 (1962).

[68] S. R. Ames, M. I. Ludwig, D. R. Nelan, and C. D. Robeson, *Biochemistry* 2, 188 (1963).

[69] H. Mayer, P. Schudel, R. Rüegg and O. Isler, *Chimia* 16, 367 (1962).

[70] P. Schudel, H. Mayer, R. Rüegg, and O. Isler, *Chimia* 16, 368 (1962).

[71] P. Schudel, H. Mayer, J. Metzger, R. Rüegg, and O. Isler, *Helv. Chim. Acta* 46, 333 (1963).

[72] H. Mayer, P. Schudel, R. Rüegg, and O. Isler, *Helv. Chim. Acta* 46, 650 (1963).

[i] R. S. Harris, *Compr. Biochem.* 9, 187 (1963).

[j] S. R. Ames, M. I. Ludwig, D. R. Neland, and C. D. Robeson, *Biochemistry* 2, 188 (1963).

[k] H. Mayer, P. Schudel, R. Rüegg, and O. Isler, *Helv. Chim. Acta* 46, 650 (1963).

[l] P. Karrer, H. Fritzsche, B. H. Ringier, and H. Salomon, *Helv. Chim. Acta* 21, 520 (1938).

[m] P. Karrer, H. Fritzsche, B. H. Ringier, and H. Salomon, *Helv. Chim. Acta* 21, 820 (1938).

[n] P. Karrer and H. Rentschler, *Helv. Chim. Acta* 26, 1750 (1943).

[o] O. Isler, P. Schudel, H. Mayer, J. Würsch, and R. Rüegg, *Vitam. Horm. (New York)* 20, 389 (1962).

[p] P. Karrer and B. H. Ringier, *Helv. Chim. Acta* 22, 610 (1939).

[q] O. Wiss, R. H. Bunnell, and U. Gloor, *Vitam. Horm. (New York)* 20, 441 (1962).

[r] P. Schudel, H. Mayer, J. Metzger, R. Rüegg, and O. Isler, *Helv. Chim. Acta* 46, 2517 (1963).

[s] H. Mayer, J. Metzger, and O. Isler, *Helv. Chim. Acta* 50, 1376 (1967).

[t] O. Isler, H. Mayer, J. Metzger, R. Rüegg, and P. Schudel, *Angew. Chem.* 75, 1030 (1963).

unnatural configuration at C-2 which exhibits a small but definite positive optical rotation in *ethanol* solution. In order to clarify this situation, Karrer and Rentschler[73] later tried to give a definite description of the stereoisomers in question by specifying every asymmetric carbon atom involved. More recent papers on tocopherols use the capital letter prefixes *R* and *S*[74] or D and L for known absolute configurations. The small letters *d* and *l* or the signs (+) and (−) stand for known contributions to optical rotation of the molecule or of different asymmetric centers therein, but not for absolute configuration. The combinations *dl*, DL, or *RS* specify racemic centers. For the unequivocal designation of all tocopherol and tocotrienol stereoisomers, however, the *RS*-specification of absolute configuration according to the convention of Cahn *et al.*[74] should be used. The several different tocopherol and tocotrienol specifications together with their corresponding stereoformulas are listed in Table III.

E. Reactions

The chemical properties of the tocopherol molecule are mainly determined (a) by the free phenolic hydroxyl group, which can be acylated, etherified, or phosphorylated; (b) by the presence of a free position in the aromatic ring (except in α-tocopherol and α-tocotrienol) which is open to nitrosation, chloromethylation, or hydroxymethylation, etc.; and (c) by the fact that it represents essentially a monoether of a hydroquinone which is easily oxidized.

In the following sections the chemical transformations of tocopherols under the influence of oxidative reagents and heat will be summarized. Acylation,[66, 75] etherification,[76] and phosphorylation[77] of their phenolic hydroxyl group as well as nitrosation[51, 78, 79] and coupling with diazotized *p*-nitroaniline[80] of the free position in their aromatic ring will not be mentioned separately, whereas the chloromethylation and hydroxymethylation of tocopherols will be dealt with in Section G, 4, f.

1. CHROMIC ACID OXIDATION

Chromic acid in acetic acid degrades α-tocopherol to give, with retention

[73] P. Karrer and H. Rentschler, *Helv. Chim. Acta* **26**, 1750 (1943).

[74] R. S. Cahn, C. K. Ingold, and V. Prelog, *Experientia* **12**, 81 (1956); *Angew. Chem.* **78**, 413 (1966), introduced a general system for the specification of asymmetric configuration, which because of its universal applicability in organic chemistry tends to displace the original more or less restricted " DL-system."

[75] V. Demole, O. Isler, B. H. Ringier, H. Salomon, and P. Karrer, *Helv. Chim. Acta* **22** 65 (1939).

[76] H. S. Olcott and H. A. Matill, *J. Biol. Chem.* **104**, 423 (1934).

[77] P. Karrer and G. Bussmann, *Helv. Chim. Acta* **23**, 1137 (1940).

[78] J. Green and S. Marcinkiewicz, *Analyst (London)* **84**, No. 998, 297–303 (1959); S. Marcinkiewicz and J. Green. *Analyst (London)* **84**, No. 998, 304 (1959).

[79] M. L. Quaife, *J. Biol. Chem.* **175**, 605 (1948).

[80] M. L. Quaife, *J. Amer. Chem. Soc.* **66**, 308 (1944).

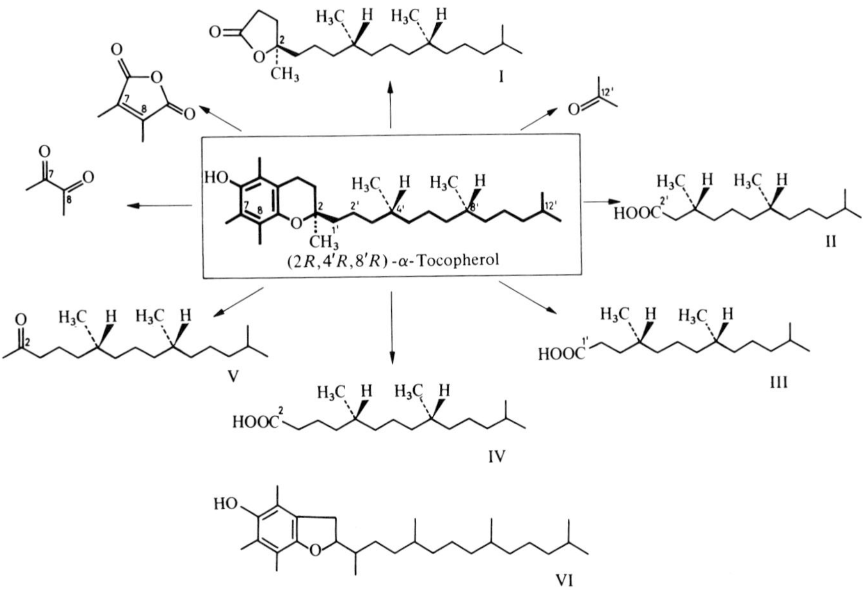

$O=$ ... H_3C H H_3C H

CH_3 I

$(2R,4'R,8'R)$-α-Tocopherol

II

III

IV

V

VI

FIG. 1. Chromic acid oxidation of α-tocopherol.

of absolute configuration, the C_{21}-lactone I,[45, 55] the C_{15}-,[55] C_{16}-,[45, 55] and C_{17}-acids[55] II, III, and IV in a proportion of about $1:8:1.2$,[55] along with the neutral C_{18}-ketone V,[45] diacetyl,[45] dimethylmaleic anhydride,[45] and acetone[45] (Fig. 1). Similar chromic acid degradations of β-[81] and γ-tocopherol[49, 81] as well as tocol[51] are also reported.

The correct structural formula of α-tocopherol was suggested by Fernholz in 1938 mainly on the basis of chromic acid and thermal degradation studies (see Section E, 7). The alternative coumaran structure VI[46, 48] had to be abandoned mainly because of two facts:

1. The γ-lactone I is also formed by $KMnO_4$ oxidation in neutral medium,[82] thus excluding acid rearrangements.

2. The α-tocopherolquinone XII (see Section E, 3) obtained from α-tocopherol by auric chloride or ferric chloride oxidation and the bis-p-bromobenzoate of the corresponding hydroquinone resisted Oppenauer and chromium trioxide oxidations, respectively, thus showing that the aliphatic hydroxyl group is tertiary, not secondary.[83, 84] Hence it was concluded that α-tocopherol possesses a chroman, not a coumaran structure.

[81] O. H. Emerson, J. Amer. Chem. Soc. 60, 1741 (1938).

[82] O. H. Emerson, Science 88, 40 (1938).

[83] P. Karrer, R. Escher, H. Fritzsche, B. H. Keller, B. H. Ringier, and H. Salomon, Helv. Chim. Acta 21, 939 (1938).

[84] W. John, E. Dietzel, P. Günther, and W. Emte, Z. Naturforsch. 26, 366 (1938).

Chromic acid oxidation was also used for the elucidation of vitamin E stereochemistry.

Mayer et al.[55] correlated the asymmetry of natural α-tocopherol with phytol (known to have the $7R,11R$-configuration[62–64]) and with $(-)$-linalool, which is R-configurated.[85] The $4'R,8'R$-configuration of natural α-tocopherol derives from the fact that the C_{18}-ketone V, the C_{16}-methyl ester VII, the C_{15}-aldehyde VIII and the meso-hydrocarbon IX, prepared from vitamin E by the transformations indicated in Fig. 2, are identical in every respect with the corresponding substances obtained from natural $(7R,11R)$-phytol. The $2R$-configuration follows from the comparison of the molecular rotation of the lactone I with that of the γ-lactone XB obtained from (R)-$(-)$-linalool. This was furthermore confirmed by the total synthesis[72] of natural α-tocopherol (see Section G, 4, d) starting from the positive rotating formylchroman XIA. The absolute configuration of the latter followed from its transformation to the γ-lactone XA, which is enantiomeric to the γ-lactone XB.

2. Nitric Acid Oxidation

Another oxidative degradation of tocopherols involves their reaction with nitric acid[85–87] (or silver nitrate[87–89]) in boiling ethanol. Detailed studies[87, 90] performed especially by John and Emte[87] showed that α-tocopherol is oxidized successively to α-tocopherolquinone XII, α-tocored XIII, the yellow para-quinone XIV (which could also be obtained by prolonged treatment of α-tocored XIII with nitric acid[87]), and finally to a fourth product, for which Frampton et al.[91] suggested the structure of α-tocopurple XV (Fig. 3). Similar transformations were observed with β-tocopherol.[66, 87] γ-Tocopherol and 7-methyltocol have also been converted to the red o-quinone XIII by silver nitrate or nitric acid oxidation.[39, 66]

3. Ferric Chloride Oxidation

Treatment of α-tocopherol with ferric chloride at room temperature in the presence of water gives α-tocopherolquinone XII[88, 89, 92] which is also

[85] R. H. Conforth, J. W. Cornforth, and V. Prelog, Justus Liebigs Ann. Chem. 634, 197 (1960).

[86] M. Further and R. E. Meyer, Helv. Chim. Acta 22, 240 (1939).

[87] W. John and W. Emte, Hoppe-Seyler's Z. Physiol. Chem. 268, 85 (1940).

[88] W. John, Hoppe-Seyler's Z. Physiol. Chem. 252, 222 (1938).

[89] W. John, E. Dietzel, and W. Emte, Hoppe-Seyler's Z. Physiol. Chem. 257, 173 (1939).

[90] L. I. Smith, W. B. Irwin, and H. E. Ungnade, J. Amer. Chem. Soc. 61, 2424 (1939).

[91] V. L. Frampton, W. A. Skinner, P. Cambour, and P. S. Bailey, J. Amer. Chem. Soc. 82, 4632 (1960).

[92] V. L. Frampton, W. A. Skinner, and P. S. Bailey, Science 116, 34 (1954).

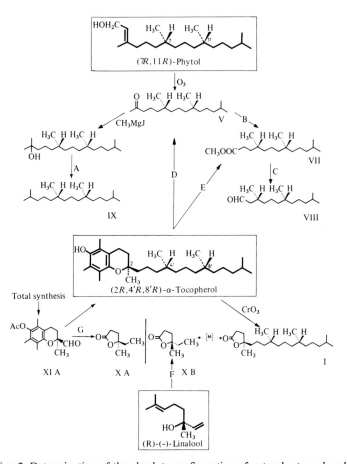

FIG. 2. Determination of the absolute configuration of natural α-tocopherol.

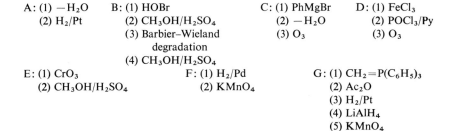

A: (1) −H₂O   B: (1) HOBr   C: (1) PhMgBr   D: (1) FeCl₃
   (2) H₂/Pt   (2) CH₃OH/H₂SO₄   (2) −H₂O   (2) POCl₃/Py
               (3) Barbier–Wieland   (3) O₃   (3) O₃
                   degradation
               (4) CH₃OH/H₂SO₄

E: (1) CrO₃   F: (1) H₂/Pd   G: (1) CH₂=P(C₆H₅)₃
   (2) CH₃OH/H₂SO₄   (2) KMnO₄   (2) Ac₂O
                                            (3) H₂/Pt
                                            (4) LiAlH₄
                                            (5) KMnO₄

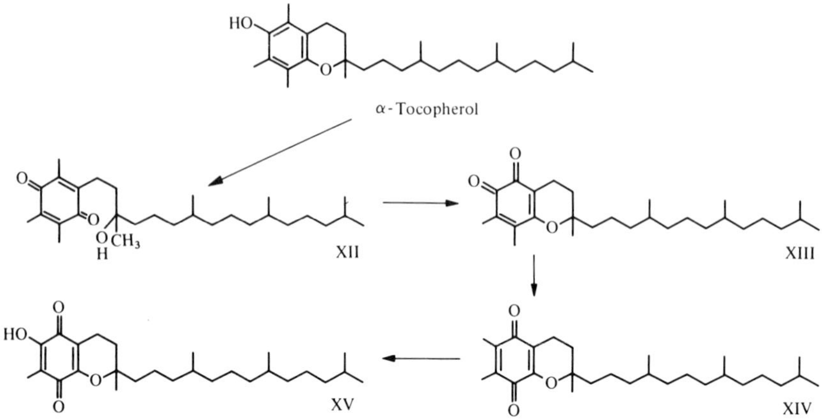

FIG. 3. Nitric acid oxidation of α-tocopherol.

formed by auric chloride,[93] ceric sulfate,[94] silver nitrate,[88, 89, 95] or nitric acid oxidations (see Section E, 2). α-Tocored XIII and α-tocopurple XV (Fig. 3) were obtained[91, 96] additionally when the oxidation was carried out at 50°C. Ferric chloride with 2,2'-bipyridyl in absolute ethanol, however, gives rise to the so-called α-tocopheroxide XVI ($R = C_2H_5$)[97-99] (Fig. 4), which is readily reduced back to α-tocopherol by ascorbic acid or is converted to α-tocopherolquinone XII by dilute mineral acid. α-Tocopheroxide has also been prepared by benzoyl peroxide oxidation of α-tocopherol in ethanol solution. In the presence of methanol, isopropanol, 1-butanol, 1-octanol, etc., the corresponding acetals XVI ($R = CH_3$, $CH(CH_3)_2$, $n\text{-}C_4H_9$, $n\text{-}C_8H_{17}$, etc.) were obtained.[100] This supports the supposition that the highly labile quinone hemiacetal XVII recently prepared[101, 102] by oxidation of α-tocopherol with tetrachloro-o-quinone or N-bromosuccinimide in buffered aqueous acetonitrile represents an intermediate in the generation of α-tocopherolquinone XII. Consistent therewith is also the fact[71] that during ferric chloride oxidation, the three centers of asymmetry retain their absolute

[93] P. Karrer and A. Geiger, Helv. Chim. Acta. 23, 455 (1940).
[94] M. Kofler, P. F. Sommer, H. R. Bolliger, B. Schmidli, and M. Vecchi, Vitam. Horm. (New York) 20, 407 (1962).
[95] W. John and W. Emte, Hoppe-Seyer's Z. Physiol. Chem. 261, 24 (1938).
[96] V. L. Frampton, W. A. Skinner, and P. S. Bailey, J. Amer. Chem. Soc. 76, 282 (1954).
[97] C. Martius and H. Eilingsfeld, Justus Liebigs Ann. Chem. 607, 159 (1957).
[98] P. D. Boyer, J. Amer. Chem. Soc. 73, 733 (1951).
[99] W. H. Harrison, J. E. Gander, E. R. Blakley, and P. D. Boyer, Biochim. Biophys. Acta 21, 150 (1956).
[100] C. T. Goodhue and H. A. Risley, Biochemistry 4, 854 (1965).
[101] W. Dürckheimer and L. A. Cohen, Biochem. Biophys. Res. Commun. 9, 262 (1962).
[102] W. Dürckheimer and L. A. Cohen, J. Amer. Chem. Soc. 86, 4388 (1964).

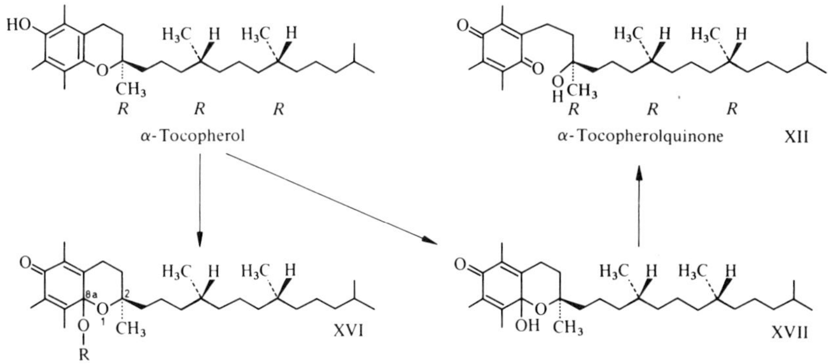

FIG. 4. Ferric chloride oxidation of α-tocopherol.

configuration. This gave the key for the preparation of $(2S,4'R,8'R)$-α-tocopherol[71] with unnatural configuration at C-2, starting from the natural $2R,4'R,8'R$-epimer (see Fig. 9, Section E, 8).

4. ALKALINE FERRICYANIDE OXIDATION

The alkaline ferricyanide oxidation of α-tocopherol attracted the attention of several chemists mainly because of its possible relation to vitamin E metabolism[103, 104] and because of the interesting fact that the optical rotation of the reaction product allows the determination of the absolute configuration at C-2 of the oxidized α-tocopherol, independently of the stereochemistry at C-4' and C-8'. $[\alpha]_D = +26°$ is the average value of the potassium ferricyanide oxidation product of $(2R)$-α-tocopherol,[69, 105, 106] $[\alpha]_D = -26°$ that of the $(2S)$-α-tocopherol,[69, 72, 106] and $[\alpha]_D = 0°$ that of the $(2RS)$-α-tocopherol[105, 106] (see also Table VIII).

Among the variety of oxidation products, the dimeric keto ether of structure XVIII[70, 104, 106, 107] is the main one. A trimer of structure XIX [104, 108, 109] which appears to be a metabolite of α-tocopherol,[104, 110] and traces of α-tocopherolquinone XII[106] were also detected (Fig. 5).

[103] H. H. Draper, A. S. Csallany, and S. N. Shah, *Biochim. Biophys. Acta* **59**, 527 (1962).
[104] W. A. Skinner and P. Alaupovic, *J. Org. Chem.* **28**, 2854 (1963).
[105] D. R. Nelan and C. D. Robeson, *Nature (London)* **193**, 477 (1962).
[106] P. Schudel, H. Mayer, J. Metzger, R. Rüegg, and O. Isler, *Helv. Chim. Acta* **46**, 935 (1963).
[107] D. R. Nelan and C. D. Robeson, *J. Amer. Chem. Soc.* **84**, 2963 (1962).
[108] W. A. Skinner and P. Alaupovic, *Science* **140**, 803 (1963).
[109] W. A. Skinner and R. M. Parkhurst, *J. Org. Chem.* **29**, 3601 (1964).
[110] H. H. Draper, A. S. Csallany, and M. Chiu, *Fed. Proc. Fed. Amer. Soc. Exp. Biol.* **25**, 242 (1966).

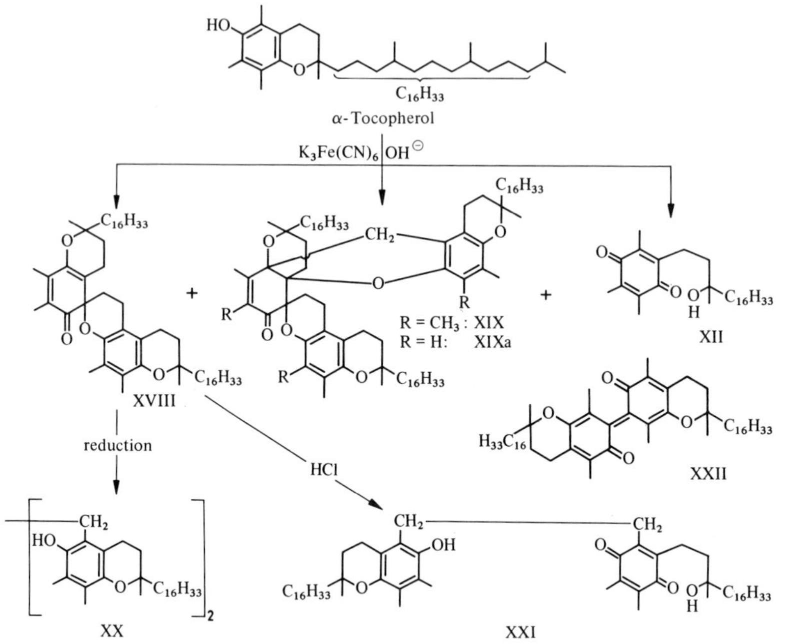

FIG. 5. Alkaline ferricyanide oxidation of α-tocopherol.

Catalytic,[106] ascorbic acid,[107] or lithium aluminum hydride[103, 111] reduction of the keto ether XVIII yields "bi-α-tocopheryl" XX,[106–108] whereas treatment with hydrogen chloride leads to the dimeric compound XXI.[107]

Recently, a dimeric metabolite of α-tocopherol which is claimed to possess structure XXII has been isolated from mammalian liver and synthesized by oxidation of the vitamin with alkaline $K_3Fe(CN)_6$.[111, 112] However, this compound has been shown by McHale and Green[113] to be identical with the already known dimer XVIII and moreover seems to be an artifact of isolation.[114]

5. FREE RADICAL OXIDATION AND IRRADIATION

When treated with benzoyl peroxide, α-tocopherol yields α-tocopherol-quinone XII[115] (Fig. 4) and a benzoate possessing the structure XXIIa[116, 117]

[111] A. S. Csallany and H. H. Draper, J. Biol. Chem. 238, 2912 (1963).
[112] A. S. Csallany and H. H. Draper, J. Biol. Chem. 239, 574 (1963).
[113] D. McHale and J. Green, Chem. Ind. (London) p. 366 (1964).
[114] U. Gloor, F. Weber, and O. Wiss, Wiss. Veroeff. Deut. Ges. Ernaehrung 16, 66 (1967).
[115] G. E. Inglett and H. A. Mattill, J. Amer. Chem. Soc. 77, 6552 (1955).
[116] C. T. Goodhue and H. A. Risley, Biochem. Biophys. Res. Commun. 17, 549 (1964).
[117] W. A. Skinner and R. M. Parkhurst, J. Org. Chem. 31, 1248 (1965).

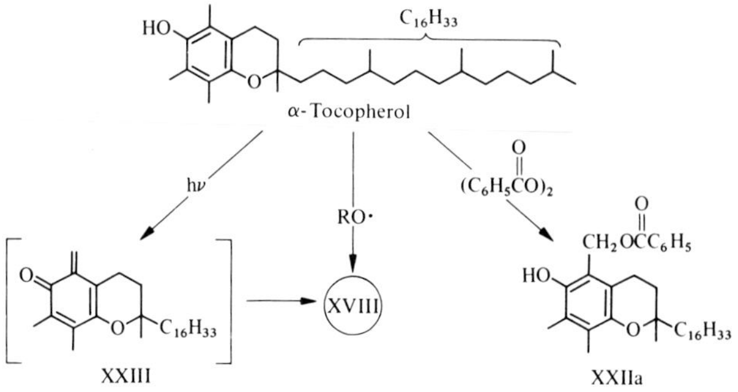

FIG. 6. Free radical oxidation of α-tocopherol.

(Fig. 6). By using primary or secondary alcohols as solvents in this reaction a series of 8a-alkoxy-α-tocopherones XVI (see Fig. 4) were obtained.[100] γ-Tocopherol under similar conditions is transformed to α-tocored[115] XIII (Fig. 3).

Tri-*tert*-butylphenoxy radical,[101] however, oxidizes α-tocopherol to the dimeric keto ether XVIII (Fig. 5), which is also obtainable by alkaline ferricyanide oxidation (see Section E, 4). When α-tocopherol is treated with azodiisobutyronitrile dimer XX (Fig. 5) is formed.[118] It is reported[119] that irradiation of α-tocopherol in isooctane solution gives rise mainly to a product of structure XXIII (Fig. 6), which, however, from its physicochemical data rather seems to have structure XVIII (Fig. 5), which may originate from dimerization[106] of XXIII.

6. REACTIONS WITH BENZOQUINONES

Tocopheryl acetates XXIV (Fig. 7) are dehydrogenated with dichloro-dicyano-benzoquinone[120] in boiling toluene to give the corresponding 3,4-dehydro derivatives XXV. This reaction was found[106] during the structure elucidation of one of the alkaline ferricyanide oxidation products of α-tocopherol. Treatment of α-tocopherol itself with benzoquinone in boiling benzene produces "bi-α-tocopheryl" XX[121, 121a] (Fig. 5), the spirodimer XVIII[121a] and the trimer XIX[121a]. β-Tocopherol gives rise to dimers XXVI and XXVIa and to trimer XIXa,[121a] whereas γ-tocopherol furnishes two dimers of structure XXVIb[121, 121a] and XXVIc, respectively. Similarly, the dimer XXVIe is

[118] W. A. Skinner, *Biochem. Biophys. Res. Commun.* 15, 469 (1964).
[119] F. W. Knapp and A. L. Tappel, *J. Amer. Oil Chem. Soc.* 38, 151 (1961).
[120] F. Hoffmann-La Roche & Co., Ltd., Belg. Patent 635 999 (1962); see *Derwent* No. 11438 (1962).
[121] D. McHale and J. Green, *Chem. Ind. (London)* p. 982 (1963).
[121a] J. L. G. Nilsson, G. D. Daves, Jr., and K. Folkers, *Acta Chem. Scand.* 22, 207 (1968).

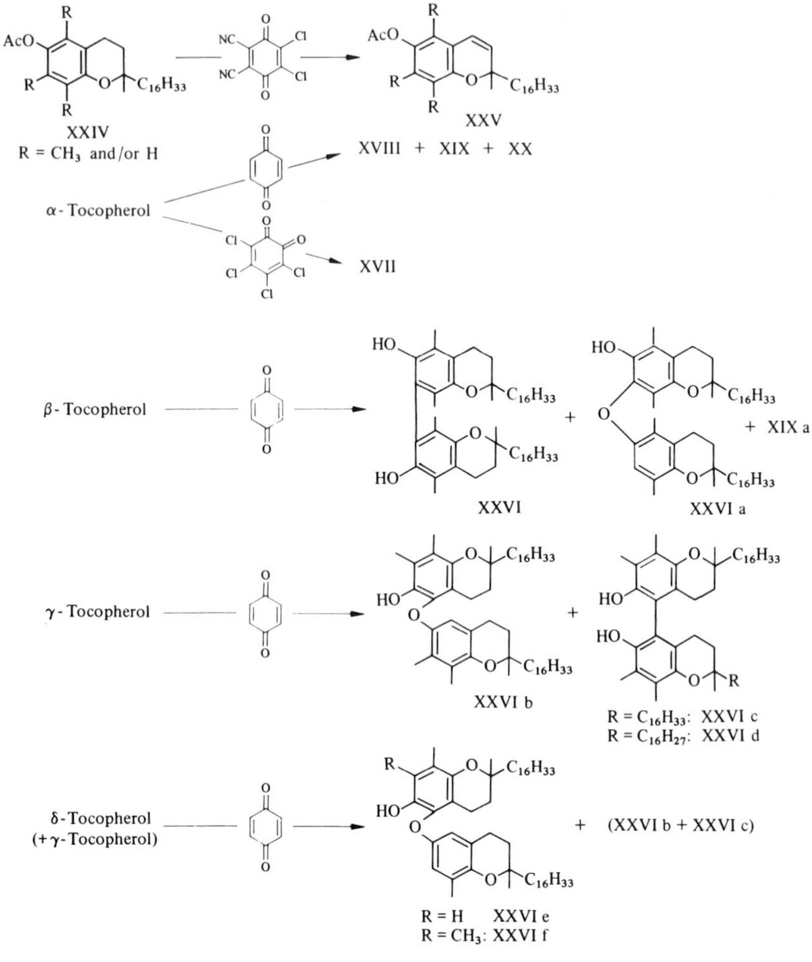

FIG. 7. Reactions of tocopherols with benzoquinones.

obtained from δ-tocopherol. Mixed dimers are formed by codimerization of various tocopherols, e.g., XXVIf in addition to XXVIb and XXVIc from an equimolar mixture of γ- and δ-tocopherol.[121a] Dimers XXVIb and XXVIc and mixed dimers XXVIf and 5-(γ-tocotrienyl)-γ-tocopherol XXVId have recently been isolated from fresh corn oil,[121b] but it has not been defined yet whether these compounds are normal metabolites or artifacts of isolation. Mechanisms of oxidation and dimerization of tocopherols have been discussed in detail.[121a] In aqueous media α-tocopherol is converted by tetrachloro-o-quinone to the quinone hemiacetal XVII[101] (Fig. 4), as already mentioned in Section E, 3.

[121b] J. L. G. Nilsson, G. D. Daves, Jr., and K. Folkers, *Acta Chem. Scand.* **22,** 200 (1968).

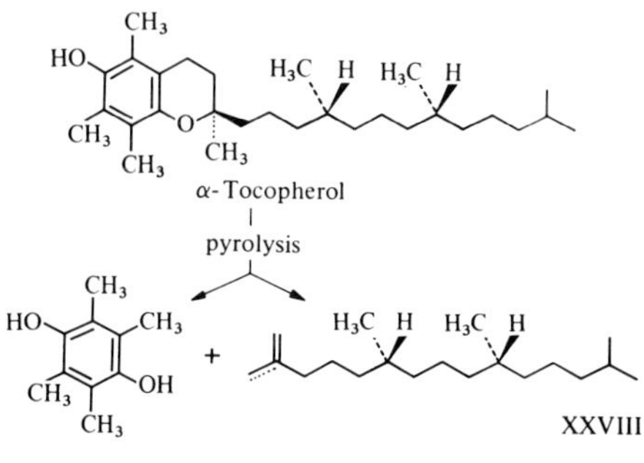

FIG. 8. Pyrolysis of α-tocopherol.

7. PYROLYSIS

The thermal decomposition of α-tocopherol to give the hydroquinone XXVII (Fig. 8) and unsaturated hydrocarbons, was first described by Fernholz.[45, 122] Recently[55] it could be shown by gas chromatographic analysis that pyrolysis mainly yields the C_{19}-hydrocarbons XXVIII (Fig. 8), besides at least nine further components in minor quantities. Catalytic reduction of the olefinic hydrocarbons obtained from natural $(2R,4'R,8'R)$-α-tocopherol yielded the *meso*-configurated, saturated C_{19}-hydrocarbon IX (Fig. 2), which played an important role in the determination of the absolute configuration of natural $(7R,11R)$-phytol[62, 63] and the α-tocopherol side chain.[55] The substitution pattern of the hydroquinone (or quinone,[123] if selenium is present) is in direct relation to the arrangement of the methyl groups on the aromatic ring of the tocopherol pyrolysed. β-[124, 125] and γ-tocopherol[81] yield trimethylhydroquinone, whereas δ-tocopherol[5] is degraded to 2,6-dimethylhydroquinone.

In some relation to the pyrolysis reaction stands the heating of α- or β-tocopherol with hydrogen iodide in acetic acid under pressure[126] giving 2,3,5-trimethylphenol and 2,5-dimethylphenol, respectively.

8. TRANSFORMATIONS OF α-TOCOPHEROLQUINONE

The descriptions of vitamin E chemistry would not be complete if one were to omit the transformations of α-tocopherolquinone, the main oxidation product of α-tocopherol.

[122] E. Fernholz, *J. Amer. Chem. Soc.* **59**, 1154 (1937).
[123] C. S. McArthur and E. M. Watson, *Science* **86**, 35 (1937).
[124] F. Bergel, A. R. Todd, and T. S. Work, *J. Chem. Soc., London* p. 253 (1938).
[125] W. John, *Hoppe-Seyler's Z. Physiol. Chem.* **250**, 11 (1937).
[126] W. John, E. Dietzel, and P. Günther, *Hoppe-Seyler's Z. Physiol. Chem.* **252**, 208 (1938).

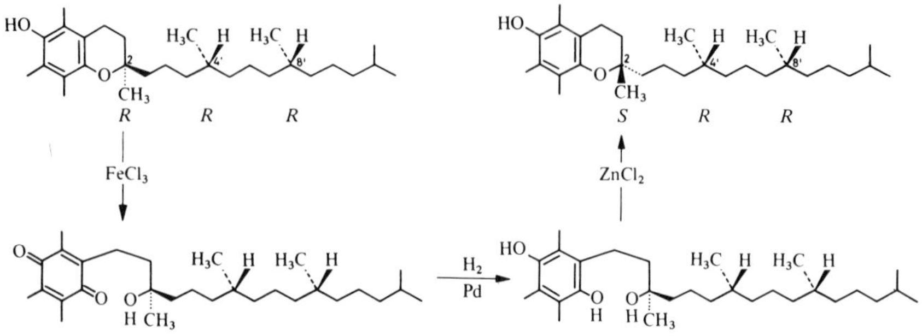

FIG. 9. Inversion of configuration at C-2 of α-tocopherol.

The preservation of absolute configurations of the three centers of asymmetry during ferric chloride oxidation of α-tocopherol to α-tocopherolquinone XII (Fig. 9) gave the basis for the preparation of α-tocopherol with unnatural configuration at C-2. Catalytic[71, 89] (or ascorbic acid[127]) reduction of α-tocopherolquinone XII obtained from natural (2R,4′R,8′R)-α-tocopherol transforms it, with retention of configuration, to the corresponding hydroquinone XXIX which after treatment with Lewis acids (e.g., $ZnCl_2$) leads to a diastereomeric α-tocopherol mixture. This contains, besides 20% of the natural compound, predominantly (80%) the 2S-epimer, with inverted configuration at C-2[71] (Fig. 9).

Some further transformations of α-tocopherolquinone XII are summarized in Fig. 10. Reductive acetylation transforms XII into the diacetate XXX,[128] which is converted by acetyl chloride to the chloride XXXI, also obtainable by addition of hydrogen chloride to the olefinic diacetate XXXII. The latter is made from trimethylphytylbenzoquinone XXXIII, which is best prepared by synthesis[129] (see Section G, 4, a).

An interesting aspect is the fact that the reductive transformation of the quinones XII or XXXIII (Fig. 10) into α-tocopherol (usually achieved through catalytic reduction followed by acid treatment[25, 65, 89, 127, 128]) can also be realized[26, 58, 130] with strong acids or Lewis acids in protic and aprotic solvents, respectively (e.g., H_2SO_4 in methanol or BF_3 in petroleum ether). Interestingly, these cyclizations proved to be highly stereospecific. Thus (3′R,7′R,11′R)-α-tocopherolquinone on treatment with concentrated sulfuric acid in methanol gave (2R,4′R,8′R)-α-tocopherol with complete

[127] W. H. Harrison, J. E. Gander, E. R. Blakley, and P. D. Boyer, *Biochim. Biophys. Acta* **21**, 150 (1956).
[128] M. Tishler and N. L. Wendler, *J. Amer. Chem. Soc.* **63**, 1532 (1941).
[129] L. F. Fieser, M. Tishler, and N. L. Wendler, *J. Amer. Chem. Soc.* **62**, 2861 (1940).
[130] A. Issidorides, *J. Amer. Chem. Soc.* **73**, 5146 (1951).

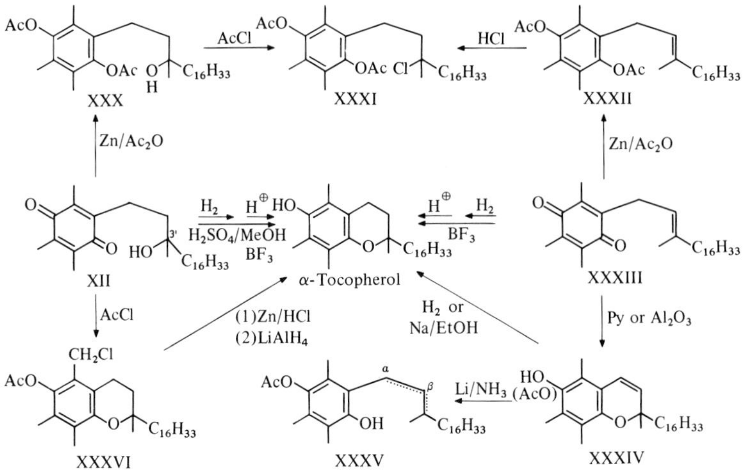

FIG. 10. Transformations of α-tocopherolquinone and trimethylphytylbenzoquinone.

retention of configuration at C-3'.[131] Similarly, cyclization of $(3'R,7'R,11'R)$-α-tocopherolquinone with 1-butanethiol and acetic acid[132] also proceeds with virtually complete retention of configuration.[131]

On treatment with acetyl chloride at room temperature, α-tocopherolquinone XII is converted into 5-chloromethyl-γ-tocopheryl acetate XXXVI[58] which can easily be reduced to α-tocopherol. When starting with $(3'R,7'R, 11'R)$-α-tocopherolquinone 87% retention of configuration is observed.[131] This transformation stands in close analogy to the corresponding reactions in the ubiquinone (coenzyme Q) and phylloquinone series[133, 134] and may be of interest in connection with biochemical transformations involving oxidative phosphorylation.

The elegant conversion of trimethylphytylbenzoquinone XXXIII into 3,4-dehydro-α-tocopherol XXXIV, a reaction found by Links[135] and further developed by McHale and Green[136] and Linn et al.[137] in the ubiquinone

[131] H. Mayer, W. Vetter, J. Metzger, R. Rüegg, and O. Isler, Helv. Chim. Acta 50, 1168 (1967).
[132] M. A. Oxman and L. A. Cohen, Biochim. Biophys. Acta 113, 412 (1966).
[133] A. F. Wagner, A. Lusi, C. H. Shunk, B. O. Linn, D. E. Wolf, C. H. Hofmann, R. E. Erickson, B. Arison, N. R. Trenner, and K. Folkers, J. Amer. Chem. Soc. 85, 1534 (1963).
[134] R. E. Erickson, A. F. Wagner, and K. Folkers, J. Amer. Chem. Soc. 85, 1535 (1963).
[135] J. Links, Biochim. Biophys. Acta 38, 193 (1960); J. Links and O. Tol, Biochim. Biophys. Acta 73, 349 (1963).
[136] D. McHale and J. Green, Chem. Ind. (London) p. 1867 (1962).
[137] B. O. Linn, C. H. Shunk, E. L. Wong, and K. Folkers, J. Amer. Chem. Soc. 85, 239 (1963).

series, is realized by treatment with boiling pyridine or aluminum oxide[58] at room temperature. It represents, in the case of geranylgeranyl-trimethyl-(or dimethyl)-benzoquinone a key step in the synthesis of α-, β-, and γ-tocotrienol[54, 57] (see Section G, 4, a).

The reduction of chromenols (e.g., XXXIV) to the corresponding chromanols (e.g., α-tocopherol) proceeds easily with catalytically activated hydrogen or with sodium in boiling ethanol.[54] The latter procedure was especially used for the conversion of 3,4-dehydrotocotrienols to tocotrienols[54] (see Section G, 4, a). Reduction of the acetate of 3,4-dehydro-α-tocopherol XXXIV with lithium in ammonia, however, splits the chromene nucleus and leads to a mixture of the α,β- and β,γ-unsaturated hydroquinone monoacetates XXXV.[58]

F. Physicochemical Properties

The tocopherols are pale yellow, viscous oils at room temperature, some of which crystallize at lower temperatures. The melting points of natural α-tocopherol (2.5–3.5°C),[138] of natural γ-tocopherol (−3° to −2°C)[138] and of synthetic 5,7-dimethyltocol (−4°C)[139] have been determined. The tocopherols are freely soluble in lipoid solvents but insoluble in water. They are slowly oxidized by atmospheric oxygen. In the absence of air, they are stable to heat treatment upto about 200°C. They darken gradually when exposed to light. They are not affected by sulfuric or hydrochloric acid up to about 100°C and are, in the absence of oxygen, relatively stable to alkali. Various tocopherol esters which were prepared by acylation of the free phenolic hydroxyl group[66, 75] are, however, stable to aereal oxidation and are often crystalline compounds (see Table IV).

1. ULTRAVIOLET ABSORPTION

The tocopherols exhibit a characteristic ultraviolet absorption around 295 mμ (chromanol-chromophore) in ethanol solution (see Table V and Fig. 11). Acylation of their phenolic hydroxyl group gives rise to a shift of the absorption to shorter wavelengths (276–285 mμ), the extinction being reduced ($E_{1\,cm}^{1\%}$ = 36–55).[66]

The ultraviolet absorption of 5- and 7-methyltocol and of 5,7-dimethyltocol has been listed by McHale et al.[139]

2. INFRARED ABSORPTION

Although the infrared spectra of the tocopherols are similar in overall appearance, characteristic differences are nevertheless found in the wave

[138] C. D. Robeson, J. Amer. Chem. Soc. 65, 1660 (1943).
[139] D. McHale, P. Mamalis, J. Green, and S. Marcinkiewicz, J. Chem. Soc., London p. 1600 (1958).

TABLE IV
MELTING POINTS OF CRYSTALLINE ESTERS OF NATURAL α-TOCOPHEROL

α-Tocopherol ester	M.p. (°C)	α-Tocopherol ester	M.p. (°C)
Acetate	26.5–27.5[a]	p-Phenylazobenzoate	62–65[d]
Acid succinate	76–77[b]	p-Nitrophenylurethane	129–131[e]
Palmitate	42–43[b]	2,4-Dinitrobenzoate	86–87[f]
p-Aminobenzoate	161.5–163[c]	Nicotinate	35–40[g]
Allophanate	157–158[b]	3,4-Dihydroxycinnamate	151–152[h]

[a] C. D. Robeson, *J. Amer. Chem. Soc.* **64**, 1487 (1942).
[b] J. G. Baxter, C. D. Robeson, J. D. Taylor, and R. W. Lehman, *J. Amer. Chem. Soc.* **65**, 918 (1943).
[c] H. Mayer, unpublished observations (1962).
[d] P. Schudel, H. Mayer, J. Metzger, R. Rüegg, and O. Isler, *Helv. Chim. Acta* **46**, 333 (1963).
[e] O. H. Emerson, G. A. Emerson, A. Mohammad, and H. M. Evans, *J. Biol. Chem.* **122**, 99 (1937).
[f] P. Karrer, H. Fritzsche, B. H. Ringier, and H. Salomon, *Helv. Chim. Acta* **21**, 520 (1938).
[g] T. Matsuura and T. Fujita, Jap. Patent No. 24968/64 (1961); see *Derwent* No. 14609 (1964).
[h] Fujisawa Pharm. Co., Ltd., Neth. Patent No. 6 414 867 (1963); see *Derwent* No. 17328 (1965).

TABLE V
UV ABSORPTION MAXIMA OF THE TOCOPHEROLS AND TOCOTRIENOLS IN ETHANOL SOLUTION

Compound	λ_{max} (mμ)	$E_{1\,cm}^{1\%}$
Tocopherol		
α-	292	75.8[a]
β-	296	89.4[a]
γ-	298	91.4[a]
δ-	298	87.3[a]
Tocotrienol		
α-	292.5,[b] 290[c]	91,[b] 77.2[c]
β-	294	87.3,[a] 85.5[c]
γ-	296	90.5[d]
δ-	297	88.1[e]

[a] P. W. R. Eggit and F. W. Norris, *J. Sci. Food Agr.* **6**, 689 (1955).
[b] J. Green, S. Marcinkiewicz, and P. R. Watt *J. Sci. Food Agr.* **6**, 274 (1955).
[c] P. Schudel, H. Mayer, J. Metzger, R. Rüegg, and O. Isler, *Helv. Chim. Acta* **46**, 2517 (1963).
[d] H. Mayer, J. Metzger, and O. Isler, *Helv. Chim. Acta* **50**, 1376 (1967).
[e] K. J. Whittle, P. J. Dunphy, and J. F. Pennock, *Biochem. J.* **100**, 138 (1966).

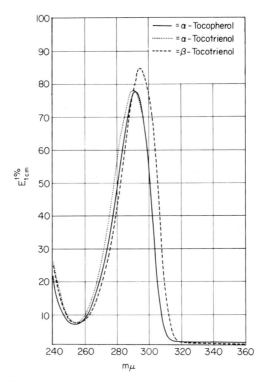

FIG. 11. Ultraviolet absorption spectra of α-tocopherol, α-tocotrienol, and β-tocotrienol.

number of certain absorption bands. Besides the common absorption bands in the OH (2.8–3 μ) and CH (3.4–3.5 μ) stretching regions, a further, typical band near 8.6 μ which seems to be characteristic of a 2-substituted chromanol-type structure,[51] is always encountered (Fig. 12). The infrared spectra of various tocopherols were discussed in greater detail by Rosenkrantz[140] and Green et al.[51]

3. NUCLEAR MAGNETIC RESONANCE

The nuclear magnetic resonance spectrum of the tocopherols allows their characterization as trimethyl-, dimethyl-, or monomethyltocol or -tocotrienol derivatives. The absence (presence) of olefinic hydrogen resonances near 5 τ and presence (absence) of a doublet near 9.1 τ characterizes the tocol (tocotrienol) structure, whereas the ratio of the integrated bands near 3.6 τ (aromatic hydrogen) and 7.9 τ (methyl-H on the benzene ring) classifies it as a tri-, di-, or monomethyl derivative (Fig. 13).

[140] H. Rosenkrantz, *J. Biol. Chem.* **173**, 439 (1948).

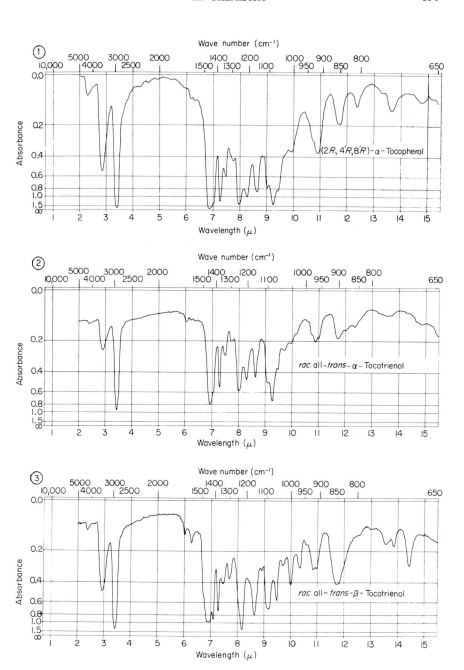

FIG. 12. Infrared spectra of (2R,4'R,8'R)-α-tocopherol, *rac.* all-*trans*-α-tocotrienol and *rac.* all-*trans*-β-tocotrienol.

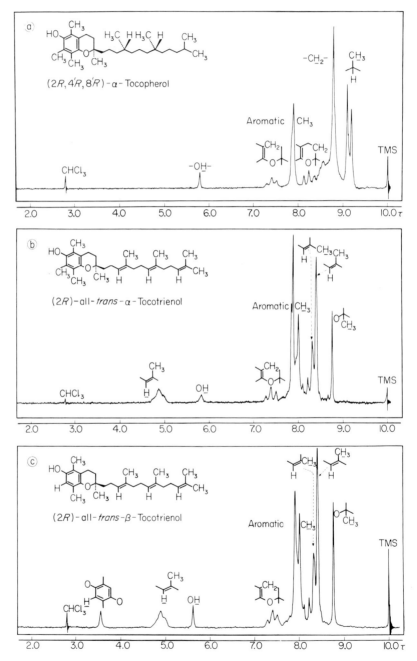

FIG. 13. Nuclear magnetic resonance spectra (60 Mc/sec; CDCl₃) of (a) (2R,4′R,8′R)-α-tocopherol, (b) (2R)-all-*trans*-α-tocotrienol, and (c) (2R)-all-*trans*-β-tocotrienol.

The ultraviolet, infrared, and nuclear magnetic resonance (NMR) spectra of α-tocopherol and of α- and β-tocotrienol are reproduced in Figs. 11–13. The corresponding spectra and spectral data, respectively, of the other tocopherols, of γ- and δ-tocotrienol, of 5,7-dimethyl- and of 7-methyltocol have been listed by Kofler et al.,[94] Whittle et al.,[8] and Mayer et al.[57]

A novel approach for the differentiation of tocopherols and tocotrienols by NMR spectroscopy has recently been reported.[141]

4. MASS SPECTROMETRY

Mass spectrometry has recently been successfully applied in the vitamin E field to establish unambiguously the molecular weight and the length and degree of unsaturation of isoprenoid side chains and to aid in mechanistic investigations based on [18]O tracer techniques.[131] Mass spectra of α-tocopheryl acetate[131] and of γ-tocotrienol, plastochromanol-8, and plastochromenol-8[57] have been recorded.

5. X-RAY DIFFRACTION PATTERN

X-Ray diffraction has been used for the differentiation of α-tocopherol diastereoisomers.[71, 72] The p-phenylazobenzoates of (2R,4'R,8'R)- and (2S,4'R,8'R)-α-tocopherol showed different characteristic patterns, whereas no difference was observed between the p-phenylazobenzoates of (2R,4'RS, 8'RS)- and (2S,4'RS,8'RS)-α-tocopherol. The identical patterns of the latter were, however, found to be distinct from those of both (2R,4'R,8'R)- and (2S,4'R,8'R)-α-tocopheryl p-phenylazobenzoates.

6. CHROMATOGRAPHIC BEHAVIOR

The tocopherols may also be characterized by their chromatographic behavior. Under clearly defined experimental conditions characteristic relative retention values in gas chromatograms and R_f values in paper and thin-layer chromatograms are observed.[94] The o-substituents of the phenolic hydroxyl group apparently determine to a certain extent the migration rates of the tocopherols in normal and reversed phase chromatography. This is reflected in the sequence: trimethyl-, dimethyl-, monomethyltocol with diminishing relative retention values in gas chromatograms on a 5% Apiezon N column (reversed phase) or diminishing R_f values in thin-layer chromatograms (normal phase) (see Table VI). Further chromatographic details are given by Kofler et al.,[94] Green et al.,[50, 78] Wilson et al.,[142] Ishikawa and

[141] H. Finegold and H. T. Slover, J. Org. Chem. **32**, 2557 (1967).
[142] P. W. Wilson, E. Kodicek, and V. H. Booth, Biochem. J. **84**, 524 (1962).

TABLE VI

RELATIVE RETENTIONS R (5% APIEZON N COLUMN, 260°C) AND R_f VALUES
(SILICAGEL G THIN LAYER; CHLOROFORM AS SOLVENT)

Substance: Tocol	Vapor-phase chromatography,[a] relative retentions R (n-$C_{28}H_{58}$ = 1.00)	Thin-layer chromatography[a] R_f values × 100
Trimethyl-	2.34	58
5,7-Dimethyl-	1.88	49
7,8-Dimethyl-	1.76	37
5,8-Dimethyl-	1.68	35
5-Methyl-	1.50	27
7-Methyl-	1.41	32
8-Methyl-	1.25	23
Tocol	1.10	19

[a] M. Kofler, P. F. Sommer, H. R. Bolliger, B. Schmidli, and M. Vecchi, *Vitam. Horm.*
(New York) **20**, 407 (1962).

Katsui,[143] Nair and Turner,[144] Bolliger and König,[145] and Slover et al.[146]
Good separations of tocopherols and tocotrienols by two-dimensional thin-layer chromatography using a chloroform- 20% isopropyl ether/light petroleum solvent system have been reported by Pennock et al.,[6, 147] Whittle et al.,[8] and Morton.[32]

The four different cis-trans-isomers of racemic α-, β-, and γ-tocotrienol can clearly be differentiated by gas chromatography.[42, 57] It is not yet possible, however, to distinguish between the four racemic stereoisomers of α-tocopherol either by UV, IR, or NMR spectroscopy or by paper, thin-layer, or gas chromatography, because they all show the same spectral and chromatographic behavior as the natural isomer.

7. OPTICAL ACTIVITY

The pure tocopherols isolated from natural sources exhibit relatively small optical rotations. α-, β-, γ-, and δ-tocopherol are dextrorotatory in ethanol, whereas in benzene α- and γ-tocopherol are levorotatory[66, 148] (see Table

[143] S. Ishikawa and G. Katsui, *J. Vitaminol. (Kyoto)* **12**, 106 (1966).
[144] P. P. Nair and D. A. Turner, *J. Amer. Oil Chem. Soc.* **40**, 353 (1963).
[145] H. R. Bolliger and A. König, in "Dünnschichtchromatographie" (E. Stahl, ed.), p. 253. Springer, Berlin, 1967.
[146] H. T. Slover, L. M. Shelley, and T. L. Burks, *J. Amer. Oil Chem. Soc.* **44**, 161 (1967).
[147] K. J. Wittle and J. F. Pennock, *Analyst (London)* **92**, 423 (1967).
[148] M. H. Stern, C. D. Robeson, L. Weisler, and J. G. Baxter, *J. Amer. Chem. Soc.* **69**, 869 (1947).

TABLE VII

SPECIFIC ROTATIONS OF NATURAL TOCOPHEROLS[a]

Natural tocopherols	$[\alpha]^{25°}_{546.1}$	
	(C_2H_5OH)	(C_6H_6)
α-	+0.32°	−3.0°
β-	+2.9°	+0.9°
γ-	+3.2°	−2.4°
δ-	+3.4°	+1.1°

[a] J. G. Baxter, C. D. Robeson, J. D. Taylor, and R. W. Lehmann, *J. Amer. Chem. Soc.* **65**, 918 (1943).

TABLE VIII

SPECIFIC ROTATIONS OF α-TOCOPHEROL STEREOISOMERS

Stereoisomers	α-Tocopherol $[\alpha]^{25°}$ (C_2H_5OH)	α-Tocopheryl p-phenylazobenzoate $[\alpha]^{25°}_{600}$ $(CHCl_3)$	$K_3Fe(CN)_6$-oxidation product of α-tocopherol $[\alpha]^{25°}$ (isooctane)
(2R,4'R,8'R)-	+0.75°[a]	+7.07°[a]	+26.0°[a]
(2S,4'R,8'R)-	+0.19°[a]	−7.64°[a]	−25.8°[a]
(2RS,4'R,8'R)-	+0.38°[c]	0°[a]	0°[a]
(2R,4'RS,8'RS)-	—	+6.96°[b]	+25.8°[b]
(2S,4'RS,8'RS)-	−0.14°[c]	−7.47°[b]	−23.6°[b]

[a] P. Schudel, H. Mayer, J. Metzger, R. Rüegg, and O. Isler, *Helv. Chim. Acta* **46**, 333 (1963).

[b] H. Mayer, P. Schudel, R. Rüegg, and O. Isler, *Helv. Chim. Acta* **46**, 650 (1963).

[c] H. Mayer, unpublished observations (1962).

VII). Since the differences in optical rotatory power are small, differentiation is rather problematical. The same holds for α-tocopherol epimers (see Table VIII). For practical use, however, the much higher rotations of the crystalline p-phenylazobenzoates or potassium ferricyanide oxidation products (for structure see Section E, 4) of the various α-tocopherol stereoisomers are employed. From the data listed in Table VIII it follows that by means of the p-phenylazobenzoate or potassium ferricyanide oxidation product of α-tocopherol one can distinguish between the 2R- and 2S-epimer, but not between diastereomers at the centers 4' and 8'.

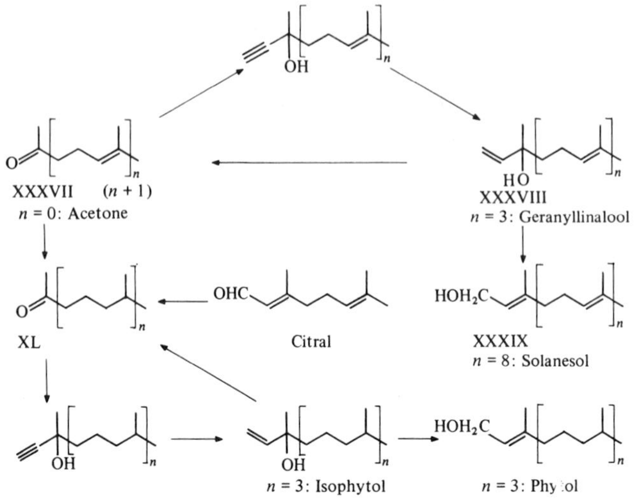

FIG. 14. Synthesis of phytol and isophytol.

G. Synthesis

1. SYNTHESIS OF ISOPRENOID CHAINS

For the synthesis of tocopherols, tocotrienols, and related compounds unsaturated terpene alcohols are required which are either extracted from natural sources (e.g., phytol[149-151] and solanesol[152]) or made by total synthesis.

The total synthesis of phytol and isophytol starting from pseudoionone and hexahydropseudoionone was first described by Fischer and Löwenberg[153] and later modified by Karrer and Ringier.[154] Today acetone and citral are employed as starting materials. Methods most widely used are outlined in Fig. 14. Condensation of the ketone XXXVII (e.g., acetone or geranylacetone; $n = 0$ or 2) with sodium acetylide in liquid ammonia followed by partial hydrogenation yields the tertiary alcohol XXXVIII which on treatment with 2-ethoxypropene[155, 156] or phosphorus tribromide and subsequent

[149] R. Willstätter and A. Stoll, "Untersuchungen über Chlorophyll." Springer, Berlin, 1913.

[150] H. Fischer and A. Oestreicher, Hoppe-Seyler's Z. Physiol. Chem. 262, 243 (1940).

[151] M. E. Wall, Ind. Eng. Chem. 41, 1465 (1949).

[152] R. L. Rowland, P. H. Latimer, and J. A. Giles, J. Amer. Chem. Soc. 78, 4680 (1956).

[153] F. G. Fischer and K. Löwenberg, Justus Liebigs Ann. Chem. 475, 183 (1929).

[154] P. Karrer and B. H. Ringier, Helv. Chim. Acta 12, 610 (1939).

[155] G. Saucy and R. Marbet, 19th Int. Cong. Pure Appl. Chem., London Abstr. A, p. 254 (1963).

[156] G. Saucy and R. Marbet, Helv. Chim. Acta 50, 2091 (1967).

acetoacetic ester synthesis[157] or by reaction with diketene and pyrolysis[158] leads to the next higher ketone XXXVII (e.g., $n = 1$ or 3). By repetition of these procedures any number of carbinols XXXVIII (e.g., geranyllinalool; $n = 3$) and ketones XXXVII can be prepared.[159] Reaction of the carbinols XXXVIII with phosphorus tribromide followed by treatment with potassium acetate and saponification gives the primary alcohols XXXIX (e.g., solanesol; $n = 8$). The unsaturated C_{18}-ketone XXXVII ($n = 3$) is hydrogenated to give the saturated ketone XL ($n = 3$). Ethynylation followed by partial hydrogenation furnishes isophytol which can easily be converted into phytol similar to the conversion XXXVIII into XXXIX. Isoprenologs of phytol and isophytol are prepared starting from appropriate saturated ketones XL. Starting with citral, the main constituent of lemon grass oil, the C_{18}-ketone XL is first synthesized[157] which is then transformed into isophytol or phytol as described.

Further syntheses have been reported by Smith and Sprung,[160] Lukeš and Zobáčová,[161] Weichet et al.,[162] Nazarov et al.,[163] Sarychewa et al.,[164] Maurit et al.,[165] Redel and Boch,[166] and Abe et al.[167]

2. SYNTHESIS OF TRIMETHYLHYDROQUINONE

Much attention has been paid to the synthesis of trimethylhydroquinone XLV as one of the components for the synthesis of α-tocopherol and numerous routes have been investigated. In the following, a survey is given of the available methods.

A commercial synthesis of trimethylhydroquinone uses 3,5-dimethylphenol XLI which is first converted into the Mannich base XLII (Fig. 15). Catalytic hydrogenation of the base gives 2,3,5-trimethylphenol XLIII[168] which on

[157] O. Isler and O. Wiss, Vitam. Horm. (New York) 17, 53 (1959).

[158] W. Kimel, N. W. Sax, S. Kaiser, G. G. Eichmann, G. O. Chase, and A. Ofner, J. Org. Chem. 23, 153 (1958).

[159] R. Rüegg, U. Gloor, A. Langemann, M. Kofler, C. von Planta, G. Ryser, and O. Isler, Helv. Chim. Acta 43, 1745 (1960).

[160] L. I. Smith and J. A. Sprung, J. Amer. Chem. Soc. 65, 1276 (1943).

[161] R. Lukeš and A. Zobáčová, Chem. Listy 51, 330 (1957).

[162] J. Weichet, L. Bláha, and J. Hodrová, Chem. Listy 51, 568 (1957).

[163] I. N. Nazarov, B. G. Gusev, and V. I. Gunor, Izv. Akad. Nauk SSSR Otd. Khim. Nauk p. 1267 (1957); see Chem. Abstr. 52, 6150ʰ (1958).

[164] I. K. Sarychewa, G. A. Vorob'eva, N. A. Kuznetsova, and N. A. Preobrazhenskii, Zh. Obshch. Khim. 28, 647 (1958); see Chem. Abstr. 52, 17320ª (1958).

[165] M. E. Maurit, G. V. Smirnova, E. A. Parfenov, I. M. Vincovskaya, and N. A. Preobrazhenskii, J. Gen. Chem. USSR 32, 2449 (1963).

[166] J. Redel and J. Boch, Fr. Patent No. 1 460 512 (1964); see Chem. Abstr. 67, 100 279ᶻ (1967).

[167] S. Abe, S. Mizuno, and K. Sato, Jap. Patent 11044 (1965); see Chem. Abstr. 67, 90965ᵈ (1967).

[168] W. T. Coldwell and T. R. Thompson, J. Amer. Chem. Soc. 61, 765 (1939).

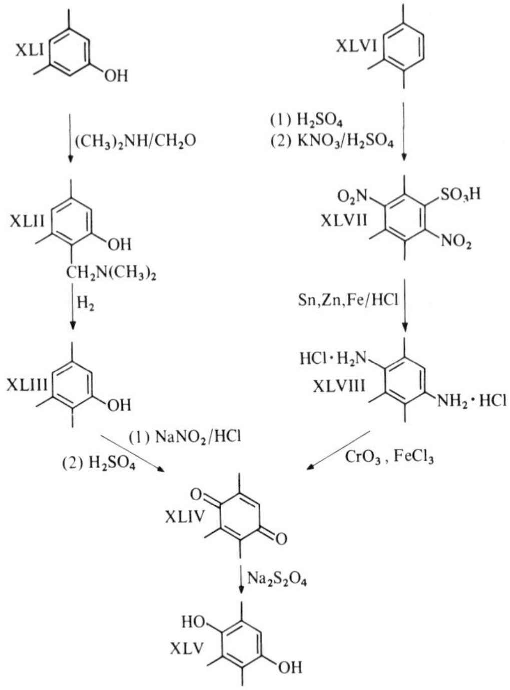

FIG. 15. Synthesis of trimethylhydroquinone.

nitrosation followed by hydrolysis leads to trimethylbenzoquinone XLIV. Reduction to trimethylhydroquinone XLV can be effected by sodium dithionite, by sulfur dioxide or catalytically.[169–172] The introduction of a second hydroxyl group into 2,3,5-trimethylphenol XLIII can also be achieved by coupling with diazotized sulfanilic acid[168, 173] or by reaction with potassium nitrosodisulfonate.[174, 175] Nitrosation has also been adapted to 2,3,5-trimethylphenol XLIII[176] which was made from 2,3-dimethylphenol through a Mannich reaction.[177]

An additional synthesis starts from 1,2,4-trimethylbenzene (pseudocumene)

[169] P. Karrer and O. Hoffmann, Helv. Chim. Acta 22, 654 (1939).

[170] H. A. Offe and W. Barkow, Chem. Ber. 80, 464 (1947).

[171] R. J. Boscott, Chem. Ind. (London) p. 201 (1955).

[172] D. Tomkuljak, I. Sausa, and B. Baranek, Czech. Patent No. 101759 (15.11.61); see Chem. Abstr. 59, 515e (1963).

[173] L. I. Smith, J. W. Opie, S. Wawzonek, and W. W. Prichard, J. Org. Chem. 4, 318 (1939).

[174] H.-J. Teuber and W. Rau, Chem. Ber. 85, 1036 (1953).

[175] I. K. Sarycheva, G. A. Serebrennikova, L. I. Mitrushkina, and N. A. Preobrazhenskii, Zh. Obshch. Khim. 31, 2190 (1961); see J. Gen. Chem. USSR 31, 2046 (1961).

[176] W. T. Sumerford and D. N. Dalton, J. Amer. Chem. Soc. 66, 1330 (1944).

[177] E. Daiwa and S. Oshiro, Jap. Patent 4617/65 (1963); see Derwent No. 16169 (1965).

XLVI (Fig. 15) which on sulfonation followed by nitration is transformed into the dinitrosulfonic acid XLVII. The acid is reduced to trimethyl-*p*-phenylenediamine XLVIII which on oxidation and subsequent reduction yields the desired trimethylhydroquinone.[178–181]

Further syntheses utilizing pseudocumene have been worked out by Hui,[182] Svishchuk *et al.*,[183] Nietzki and Schneider,[184] and Smith.[185]

Trimethylhydroquinone has also been prepared starting from 4-benzyloxyphenol[186] and methyl-substituted hydroquinones,[187] respectively, through a Mannich reaction followed by catalytic reduction. Syntheses employing mesitylene and isophorone have been published by Kraft and Tsyganova[188] and by Sarycheva *et al.*,[175] respectively. A new synthetic approach using diethyl ketone and 1-methoxybut-1-en-3-one as starting materials has been reported by Leuchs.[189]

3. SYNTHESIS OF DIMETHYL- AND MONOMETHYLHYDROQUINONES

2,5-Dimethylhydroquinone LIV is readily available from 2,5-dimethylphenol XLIX by several methods (Fig. 16). Coupling of the phenol with diazotized sulfanilic acid followed by reduction of the azo dye obtained leads to the *p*-aminophenol L which is oxidized to give 2,5-dimethylquinone LI.[173] XLIX can also be converted directly into LI by oxidation with potassium nitrosodisulfonate[174] or lead tetracetate.[190] Further convenient syntheses

[178] A. Pongratz and K. L. Zirm, *Monatsh. Chem.* **83**, 13 (1952); Austrian Patent No. 176 837 (1953).

[179] P. Bite and P. Tuzson, *Mag. Kem. Foly.* **64**, 396 (1958); see *Chem. Abstr.* **54**, 16416^i (1960).

[180] G. Leuschner and K. Pfordte, *J. Prakt. Chem.* **10**, 340 (1960).

[181] T. Mori and S. Nakanishi, Jap. Patent No. 10918 (1964); see *Chem. Abstr.* **61**, 11934^a (1964).

[182] C. K. Hui, *J. Vitaminol. (Kyoto)* **1**, 8 (1954); see *Chem. Abstr* **50**, 320^e (1956).

[183] O. A. Svishchuk, F. L. Grinberg, E. D. Basalkevich, and E. D. Overchuk, *Ukr. Khim. Zh.* **29**, 411 (1963); see *Chem. Abstr.* **59**, 6288^a (1963).

[184] R. Nietzki and J. Schneider, *Ber. Deut. Chem. Ges.* **27**, 1430 (1894).

[185] L. I. Smith, *J. Amer. Chem. Soc.* **56**, 472 (1934).

[186] W. J. Burka, J. A. Warburton, J. L. Bishop, and J. L. Bills, *J. Org. Chem.* **26**, 4669 (1961).

[187] K. Sato and S. Abe, *J. Org. Chem.* **28**, 1928 (1963); Jap. Patent Nos. 23558 and 23559 (1965); see *Chem. Abstr.* **62**, 10379^e (1965).

[188] M. Y. Kraft and A. M. Tsyganova, *Med. Prom. SSSR* **14**, 27 (1960); see *Chem. Abstr.* **55**, 6426^b (1961).

[189] D. Leuchs, Belg. Patent No. 627765 (1963); see *Chem. Abstr.* **60**, 14438^h (1964); Fr. Patent No. 1367286 (1964); see *Chem. Abstr.* **62**, 9270^f (1965); *Chem. Ber.* **98**, 1335 (1965).

[190] W. Mehlesics, E. Schinzel, H. Vilcsek, and F. Wessely, *Monatsh. Chem.* **88**, 1069 (1957).

204   16. TOCOPHEROLS

starting from 3-methylphenol LII and hydroquinone LIII, which employ the
Mannich reaction, are given by Řeřicha and Protiva[191] and by Fields et al.[192]
respectively.

The synthesis of 2,3-dimethylhydroquinone LIX employs o-xylene as
readily available starting material. Nitration followed by reduction leads to
2,3-dimethylaniline LV which is oxidized directly to 2,3-dimethylbenzo-
quinone LVI.[193] Alternatively, 2,3-dimethylphenol LVII[194] obtained from
2,3-dimethylaniline LV is coupled with diazotized sulfanilic acid and the
resulting azo dye reduced to give the aminophenol LVIII which is then
oxidized to the desired quinone LVI.[195–197] 2,3-Dimethylhydroquinone LIX
can also be conveniently prepared from hydroquinone by a Mannich reaction.[192] A synthesis starting from ethyl methyl ketone and acetoacetaldehyde
is given by Leuchs.[189]

Several procedures have been developed for the preparation of 2,6-
dimethylbenzoquinone LXII utilizing 3,5-dimethylphenol LX (Fig. 16).
Coupling with diazotized sulfanilic acid[173] or p-nitroaniline[198] followed by
reduction yields the p-aminophenol LXI which is oxidized to the quinone
LXII. Alternatively, nitrosation of 3,5-dimethylphenol LX and subsequent
reduction leads to the same p-aminophenol LXI[199] whereas nitrosation
followed by hydrolysis give 2,6-dimethylbenzoquinone LXII directly.[171, 172]
3,5-Dimethylphenol can also been converted to the quinone by oxidation with
potassium nitrosodisulfonate[174] or peracetic acid.[200]

The preparation of methylbenzoquinone LXIV is achieved starting from
2-methylphenol LXIII which can either be nitrosated[171] or oxidized with
potassium nitrosodisulfonate[174] (Fig. 16). Utilizing 3-methylphenol LXV this
is coupled with diazotized p-nitroaniline followed by reduction and oxidation.[198]

Conversion of the quinones into the corresponding hydroquinones can be
effected by zinc in acetic acid, by sodium dithionite, or catalytically.

4. SYNTHESES OF TOCOPHEROLS AND TOCOTRIENOLS

The tocopherol carbon skeleton has been built up by six different types of
approaches, schematically depicted in Fig. 17.

[191] V. Řeřicha and M. Protiva, Chem. Listy. 45, 157 (1951); see Chem. Abstr. 46, 1497ᶜ
(1952).
[192] D. L. Fields, J. B. Miller, and D. D. Reynolds, J. Org. Chem. 27, 2749 (1962).
[193] O. H. Emerson and L. I. Smith, J. Amer. Chem. Soc. 62, 141 (1940).
[194] W. M. McLamore, J. Amer. Chem. Soc. 73, 2221 (1951).
[195] R. T. Arnold and H. E. Zangg, J. Amer. Chem. Soc. 63, 1317 (1941).
[196] L. I. Smith and F. L. Austin, J. Amer. Chem. Soc. 64, 528 (1942).
[197] L. I. Smith and W. H. Tess, J. Amer. Chem. Soc. 66, 1523 (1944).
[198] L. I. Smith and W. B. Irwin, J. Amer. Chem. Soc. 63, 1036 (1941).
[199] W. R. Vaughan and G. K. Finch, J. Org. Chem. 21, 1201 (1956).
[200] D. Bryce-Smith and A. Gilbert, J. Chem. Soc., London p. 873 (1964).

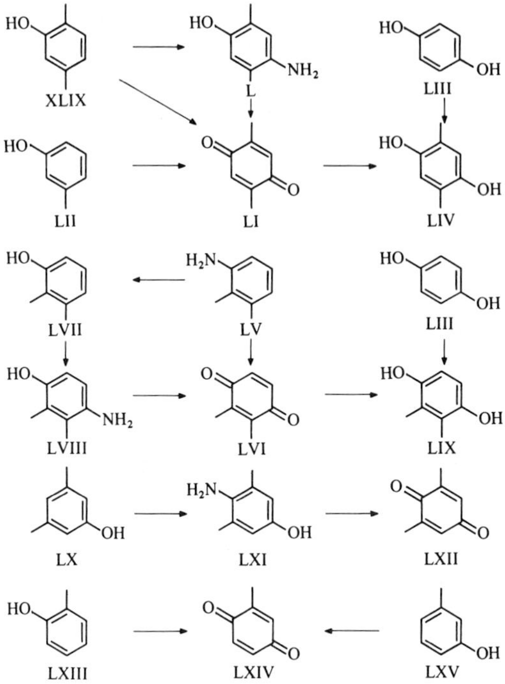

FIG. 16. Syntheses of dimethyl- and monomethylhydroquinones.

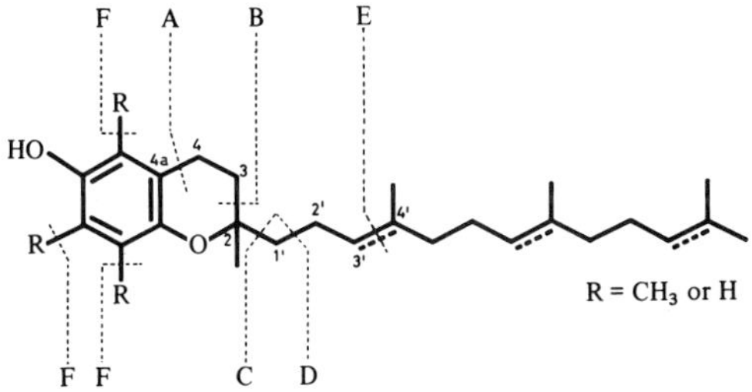

FIG. 17. Schemes of tocopherol syntheses. Scheme A. Formation of the C_4—C_{4a}-bond by condensation of an appropriate hydroquinone or a derivative thereof with phytol or a derivative thereof. Scheme B. Formation of the C_2—C_3-bond by condensation of an appropriate phenethyl derivative with the C_{18}-ketone V. Scheme C. Formation of the C_2—C_1-bond by condensation of an appropriate benzylacetone derivative with a C_{16}-component. Scheme D. Formation of the $C_{1'}$—$C_{2'}$-bond by condensation of an appropriate chromanol derivative with an isoprenoid C_{15}-component. Scheme E. Formation of the $C_{3'}$—$C_{4'}$-bond by condensation of an appropriate chromanol derivative with an isoprenoid C_{13}-component. Scheme F. Introduction of methyl groups at C_5 and (or) C_7 and (or) C_8 into tocols or tocotrienols by chloromethylation, aminomethylation, formylation, or hydroxymethylation procedures.

a. Formation of the C_4—C_{4a}-Bond (Scheme A)

The first synthesis of a vitamin E active product by condensation of trimethylhydroquinone and 1,3-dibromophytane derived from phytol has been achieved by Isler et al.[25, 201, 202] in the laboratories of F. Hoffmann-La Roche & Co. Ltd., Basle. The synthesis of (2RS,4'R,8'R)-α-tocopherol by condensation of trimethylhydroquinone with phytyl bromide was first described by Karrer et al.[46, 60] and later modified by Smith and Ungnade[203] and Karrer and Ringier.[59] Phytol was used instead of phytyl bromide by Karrer and Isler,[204] Bergel et al.,[205, 206] Smith et al.,[207] Fieser et al.,[129] von Werder,[208] Weichet and Hodrová,[209] Ehrmann,[210] and Nakagawa and Muraki.[211, 212] The team of Smith also used phytadiene[213] or 1-chlorophytan-3-ol[214] as C_{20}-component. α-Tocopherol was also synthesized using scheme A from isophytol,[209, 210, 215–218] phytyl acetate,[219] phytane-1,3-diol,[220, 221] phytenic acid,[221] or phytyl diphenyl phosphate.[222] Condensation proceeds rapidly in the presence of Lewis acid or other acidic agents,

[201] O. Isler, cited in ref. 46, p. 524.
[202] O. Isler, Mitt. Naturforsch. Ges. Schaffhausen 18, 321 (1942–1943).
[203] L. I. Smith and H. E. Ungnade, J. Org. Chem. 4, 298 (1939).
[204] P. Karrer and O. Isler, U.S. Patent No. 2 411 967 (1938); see Chem. Abstr. 41, 1713ᶜ (1947).
[205] F. Bergel, A. Jacob, A. R. Todd, and T. S. Work, Nature (London) 142, 36 (1938).
[206] F. Bergel, A. M. Copping, A. Jacob, A. R. Todd, and T. S. Work, J. Chem. Soc., London p. 1382 (1938).
[207] L. I. Smith, H. E. Ungnade, J. R. Stevens, and C. C. Christman, J. Amer. Chem. Soc. 61, 2615 (1939).
[208] F. von Werder, U. S. Patent No. 2 230 659 (1941): see Chem. Abstr. 35, 3270³ (1941).
[209] J. Weichet and J. Hodrová, Collect. Czech. Chem. Commun. 22, 595 (1957).
[210] O. Ehrmann, Ger. Patent No. 1 015 446 (1957); see Chem. Abstr. 54, 578ᵇ (1960).
[211] K. Nakagawa and S. Muraki, Jap. Patent No. 11993 (1963); see Derwent No. 8529 (1963).
[212] K. Nakagawa, Jap. Patent No. 18338 (1966); see Derwent No. 23701 (1966).
[213] L. I. Smith, H. E. Ungnade, H. H. Hoehn, and S. Wawzonek, J. Org. Chem. 4, 311 (1939).
[214] L. I. Smith and J. A. Sprung, J. Amer. Chem. Soc. 65, 1276 (1943).
[215] P. Karrer and O. Isler, U.S. Patent No. 2 411 969 (1941); see Chem. Abstr. 41, 1713ⁱ (1947).
[216] M. E. Maurit, G. V. Smirnova, E. A. Parfenov, I. K. Sarycheva, and N. A. Preobrazhenskii, Dokl. Akad. Nauk. SSSR 140, 1330 (1961); see Chem. Abstr. 56, 8672ᶠ (1962).
[217] J. D. Surmatis and J. Weber, U.S. Patent No. 2 723 278 (1955); see Chem. Abstr. 50, 10794ᵉ (1956).
[218] K. Nakajima and S. Kitmura, Jap. Patent No. 5334 (1967); see Chem Abstr. 67, 90673ᵍ (1967).
[219] J. A. Aeschlimann, U.S. Patent No. 2 307 010 (1943); see Chem. Abstr. 37, 3567ᵇ (1943).
[220] L. Bláha, J. Hodrová, and J. Weichet, Collect. Czech. Chem. Commun. 24, 2023 (1959).
[221] M. Matsui, S. Kitamura, H. Fukawa, and H. Kurihara, Jap. Patent No. 2621–2624 (1962); see Chem. Abstr. 58, 7911ᵍ (1963); Agr. Biol. Chem. 29, 978 (1965).
[222] I. A. Miller and H. C. S. Wood, Chem. Commun. p. 40 (1965).

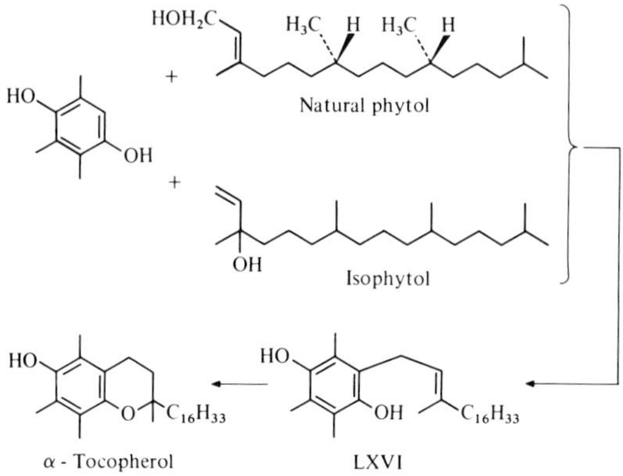

FIG. 18. Synthesis of α-tocopherol.

such as $ZnCl_2$, BF_3-etherate, P_2O_5, formic acid, acetic acid, acetic anhydride, p-toluenesulfonic acid, or sulfuric acid as catalysts. With phytol or isophytol as C_{20}-component, it becomes possible under specified experimental conditions[26, 129] to isolate the intermediate hydroquinone LXVI (Fig. 18) which can be transformed either into α-tocopherol by acid treatment or to trimethylphytylbenzoquinone XXXIII (see Fig. 10) by silver oxide oxidation.

Several unsuccessful attempts were made[25, 60, 72, 223] to separate the mixture of (2R,4′R,8′R)- and (2S,4′R,8′R)-α-tocopherol epimers (obtained from trimethylhydroquinone and natural (7R,11R)-phytol), into its two components. Only recently, however, Robeson and Nelan[67, 224] succeeded in separating the two epimers by fractional crystallization of their piperazine complex and their acetates, respectively.

The synthesis of the other (2RS,4′R,8′R)-tocopherols can be achieved following in principle the same lines as described. Difficulties, however, arise from the fact that the phytol component used may react at two or even three positions of the dimethyl- or monomethylhydroquinones required. This may be overcome in dimethyltocol syntheses by using dimethylhydroquinone monoesters, in which the free position *ortho* to the esterified hydroxyl group is deactivated (Fig. 19). 2,5-Dimethylhydroquinone monoacetate for example is the starting material of choice to synthesize (2RS,4′R,8′R)- or racemic β-tocopherol.[25] β- and γ-Tocopherols can also be prepared by condensation of 2,5- and 2,3-dimethylhydroquinone monobenzoates,[225] respectively, with phytol and $ZnCl_2$, followed by alkaline ester hydrolysis. γ-Tocopherol and 5,7-dimethyltocol are also obtained by condensation of the corresponding dimethylhydroquinones with phytol or isophytol in formic acid, followed by acid hydrolysis[25, 42] (Fig. 19).

[223] P. Karrer, A. Kugler, and H. Simon, *Helv. Chim. Acta.* **27**, 1006 (1944).
[224] D. R. Nelan, U.S. Patent No. 3 344 151 (1967).
[225] A. Jacob, M. Steiger, A. R. Todd, and T. S. Work, *J. Chem. Soc., London* p. 542 (1939).

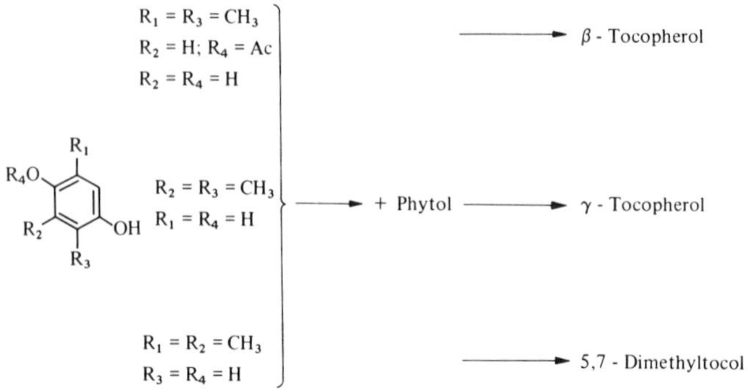

FIG. 19. Syntheses of dimethyltocols.

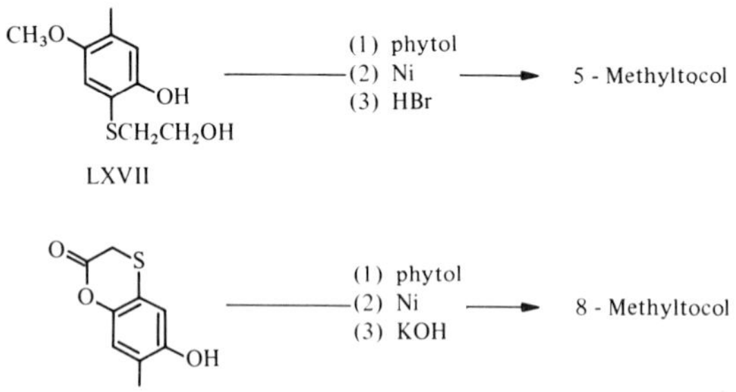

FIG. 20. Syntheses of monomethyltocols.

In the syntheses of monomethyltocols additional difficulties arise because reaction of methylhydroquinone with phytol,[226] for instance, gives a mixture of 5-, 7-, and 8-methyltocols in the ratio $1:2:1$.[227] After extensive investigations on the nucleophilic reactivity of the different positions in several methylhydroquinone derivatives Green's team[227, 228] was able to prepare 5-methyltocol,[229] free from other methyltocols, by condensation of (hydroxy-ethylthio)methylhydroquinone monomethyl ether LXVII (Fig. 20) with phytol, followed by Raney nickel desulfuration and methyl ether cleavage with hydrobromic acid. 8-Methyltocol (δ-tocopherol) was obtained from the

[226] P. Karrer and H. Fritzsche, Helv. Chim. Acta 22, 260 (1939).
[227] S. Marcinkiewicz, D. McHale, P. Mamalis, and J. Green, J. Chem. Soc., London p. 3377 (1959).
[228] P. Mamalis, J. Green, S. Marcinkiewicz, and D. McHale, J. Chem. Soc., London p. 3350 (1959).
[229] D. McHale, P. Mamalis, S. Marcinkiewicz, and J. Green, J. Chem. Soc., London p. 3358 (1959).

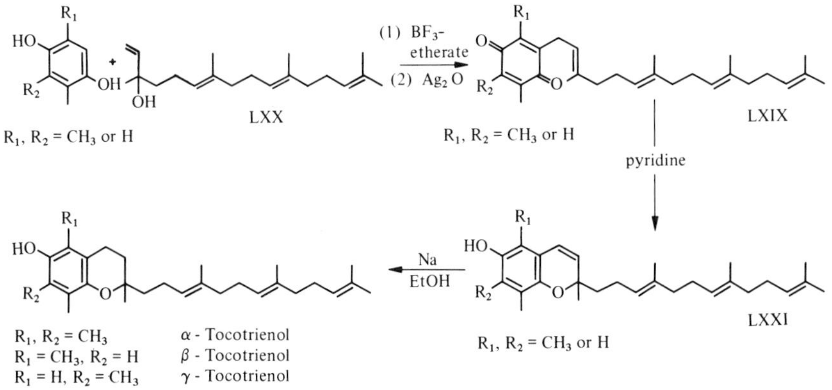

FIG. 21. Syntheses of α-, β-, and γ-tocotrienol.

benzoxathiinone LXVIII[230] or methylhydroquinone 4-monobenzoate.[228, 231] 7-Methyltocol remains the only tocopherol which has not been synthesized free from other methyltocols, using approach A under discussion.

Geranylgeranyltrimethyl(or -dimethyl)-benzoquinone LXIX (Fig. 21), analogously obtained from trimethyl(or 2,5- or 2,3-dimethyl)hydroquinone and all-*trans*-geranyllinalool LXX, are the key intermediates for the syntheses[54, 56, 57] of racemic all-*trans*-α-, β-, and γ-tocotrienol, respectively (Fig. 21). Boiling pyridine transforms these quinones into the corresponding chromenols LXXI, which are selectively reduced by sodium in boiling ethanol to give the all-*trans*-trimethyl(or dimethyl)tocotrienols, respectively.

b. Formation of the C_2—C_3-Bond (Scheme B)

It was the aim of Smith and Miller[232] in 1942 to synthesize α-tocopherol by a method not involving condensation of a phytol derivative with trimethylhydroquinone, in order to give another unambiguous proof of the chroman type structure of vitamin E. This was achieved by Grignard reaction of the phenethyl derivative LXXII with the C_{18}-ketone V (obtained from phytol) followed by hydrobromic acid treatment of the carbinol LXXIII (Fig. 22). Similarly, two further tocopherols, 7-[139] and 5-methyltocol,[229] were prepared by D. McHale *et al.* starting with the bromides LXXIV and LXXV, respectively.

c. Formation of the C_2—$C_{1'}$-Bond (Scheme C)

Another approach to synthesizing α-tocopherol was investigated by John and Pini,[65] who treated the benzylacetone derivative LXXVI (Fig. 23) with

[230] J. Green, D. McHale, P. Mamalis and S. Marcinkiewicz, *J. Chem. Soc., London* p. 3374 (1959).
[231] A. Jacob, F. K. Sutcliffe, and A. R. Todd, *J. Chem. Soc., London* p. 327 (1940).
[232] L. I. Smith and H. C. Miller, *J. Amer. Chem. Soc.* **64**, 440 (1942).

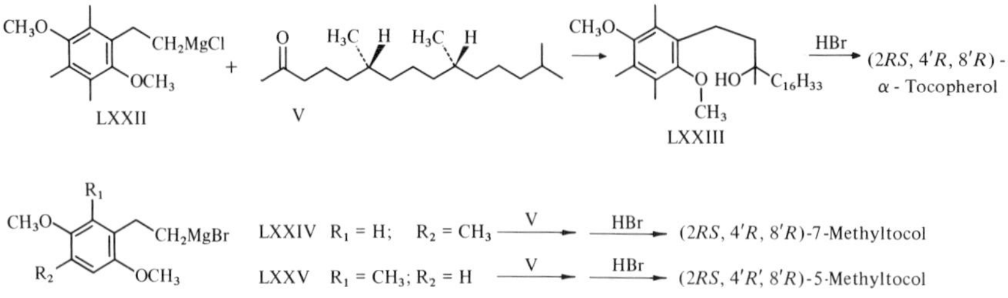

FIG. 22. Syntheses of tocopherols by scheme B.

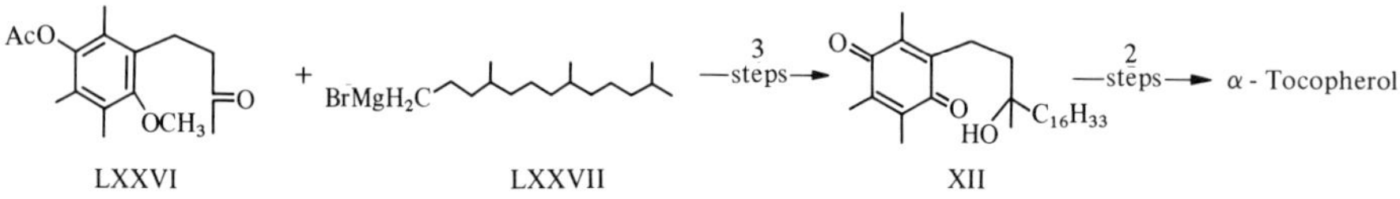

FIG. 23. Synthesis of α-tocopherol by scheme C.

the C_{16}-Grignard component LXXVII (prepared from homohexahydrofarnesol). After alkaline hydrolysis of the acetate grouping, followed by oxidation with ferric chloride, racemic α-tocopherolquinone XII was obtained. This was transferred into racemic α-tocopherol by reduction and acid cyclization (see Section E, 8).

d. Formation of the $C_{1'}$—$C_{2'}$-Bond (Scheme D)

The syntheses of tocopherols mentioned before always lead to mixtures of the 2R,4'R,8'R- and the 2S,4'R,8'R-epimers. In order to gain easy and unequivocal access to individual (2R)- and (2S)-α-tocopherol stereoisomers the following synthesis was therefore devised.[25, 69, 72]

Trimethylhydroquinone is converted in 8 steps to the propiolic acid derivative LXXVIII (Fig. 24), which is resolved into the optical antipodes by fractional crystallization of its quinine salt. The enantiomers obtained are transformed separately into the formylchromans XIA and XIB. The positive rotating enantiomer XIA [shown to have the 2S-configuration[55] by its unambiguous correlation with (R)-(−)-linalool through the γ-lactone XA, (Fig. 2)] was condensed with the R,R-configurated C_{15}-phosphonium halide LXXIX (obtained[72] from (7R,11R)-phytol) to give 1',2'-dehydro-α-tocopheryl acetate LXXXA. After catalytic hydrogenation and hydrolysis of the acetate grouping (2R,4'R,8'R)-α-tocopherol was obtained, which proved to be identical in every respect with a natural specimen from vegetable oils. This represented a total synthesis of α-tocopherol and an unequivocal proof of its 2R-configuration. Similarly, the negative rotating formylchroman XIB yielded (2S,4'R,8'R)-α-tocopherol (Fig. 24). Condensation of a racemic

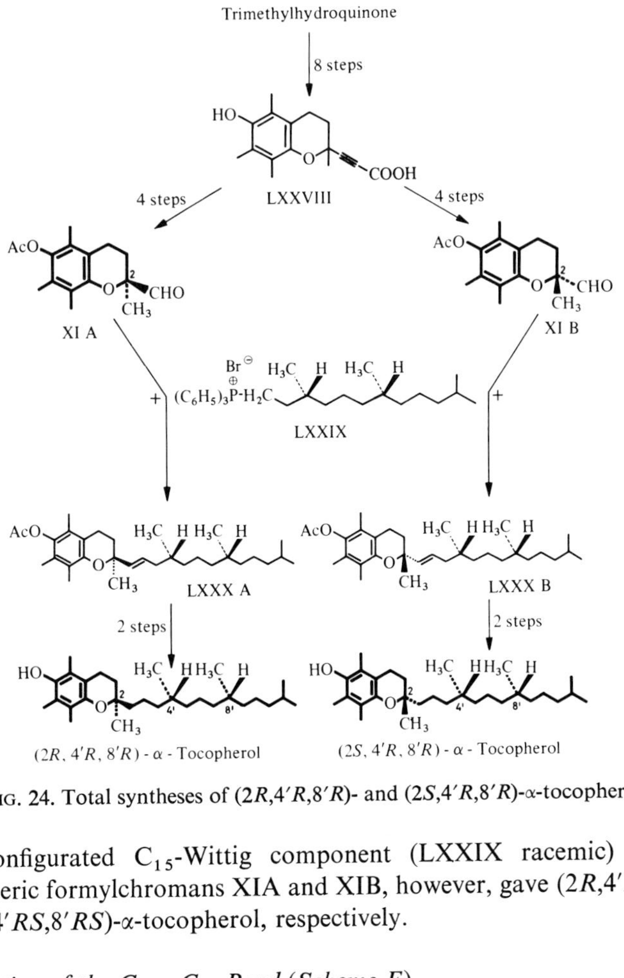

FIG. 24. Total syntheses of $(2R,4'R,8'R)$- and $(2S,4'R,8'R)$-α-tocopherol.

RS,RS-configurated C_{15}-Wittig component (LXXIX racemic) with the enantiomeric formylchromans XIA and XIB, however, gave $(2R,4'RS,8'RS)$- and $(2S,4'RS,8'RS)$-α-tocopherol, respectively.

e. Formation of the $C_{3'}$—$C_{4'}$-Bond (Scheme E)

Another synthesis of the α-tocopherol skeleton has recently been reported.[233, 234] Trimethylhydroquinone is condensed with geraniol or a geranyl halide to give tocochromanol-1 LXXXI which after acetylation and ozonolysis leads to the aldehyde LXXXII. Wittig reaction of this aldehyde with the C_{13}-phosphonium halide LXXXIII (obtained from pseudoionol) yields 5′,6′-dehydro-α-tocotrienyl acetate LXXXIV which by catalytic reduction is converted into α-tocopheryl acetate (Fig. 25).

---

[233] T. Ichakawa and T. Kato, Jap. Patent No. 11064 (1967); see *Chem. Abstr.* **67**, 10003ᵉ (1967).

[234] T. Ichakawa and T. Kato, Jap. Patent No. 11065 (1967); see *Chem. Abstr.* **67**, 10001ᶜ (1967).

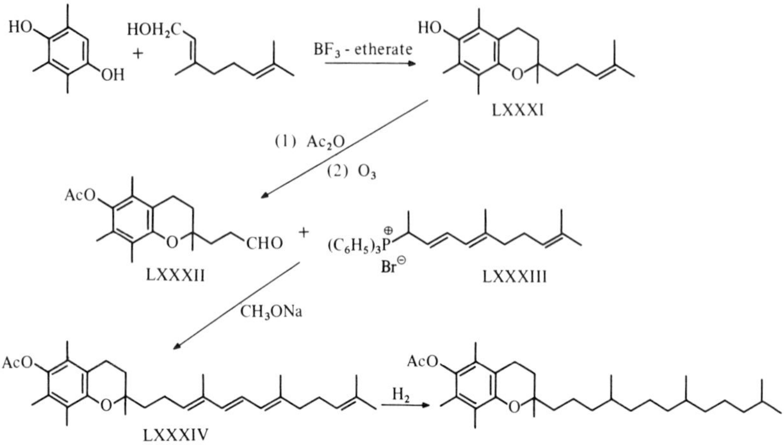

FIG. 25. Synthesis of α-tocopherol by scheme E.

f. Introduction of Methyl Groups (Scheme F)

With the successful separation[67, 224] of synthetic (2RS,4'R,8'R)-α-tocopherol into its two epimers, all the synthetic approaches described can be classified as total syntheses. The preparation of tocopherols by introduction of methyl groups into dimethyl- or monomethyl-tocols or -tocotrienols, however, represent partial syntheses inasmuch as the corresponding natural compounds are used as starting material.

Several patents describe the conversion of naturally occurring methyltocols (β-, γ-, and δ-tocopherol) into the more active α-tocopherol, in general by chloromethylation,[235–239] aminomethylation (Mannich reaction),[240] formylation,[241–243] and hydroxymethylation[244–246] procedures followed by

[235] L. Weisler and A. J. Chechak, U.S. Patent No. 2 486 542 (1949); see Chem. Abstr. 44, 2037ᶠ (1950).
[236] Eastman Kodak Company, Brit. Patent No. 791106 (1958); see Chem. Abstr. 52, 17624ⁱ (1958).
[237] K. C. D. Hickman and L. Weisler, U.S. Patent No. 2 486 540 (1949); see Chem. Abstr. 44, 1234ᶠ (1950).
[238] L. Weisler, U.S. Patent No. 2 486 539 (1949); see Chem. Abstr. 44, 2037ⁱ (1950).
[239] J. Green and S. Marcinkiewicz, Brit. Patent No. 827391 (1960); see Chem. Abstr. 54, 12502ᵈ (1960).
[240] L. Weisler, U.S. Patent 2 519 863 (1950); see Chem. Abstr. 45, 669ᶜ (1951).
[241] L. Weisler, U.S. Patent No. 2 592 628 (1952); see Chem. Abstr. 47, 1192ᵉ (1953).
[242] L. Weisler, U.S. Patent No. 2 592 630 (1952); see Chem. Abstr. 47, 1192ⁱ (1953).
[243] J. G. Baxter, U.S. Patent No. 2 592 531 (1952); see Chem. Abstr. 47, 833ⁱ (1953).
[244] L. Weisler, U.S. Patent No. 2 640 058 (1953); see Chem. Abstr. 48, 7643ᵈ (1954).
[245] Eisai Co., Ltd., Neth. Patent No. 6 411 541 (1965); see Derwent No. 17757 (1965).
[246] L. Weisler, U.S. Patent No. 2 673 858 (1954); see Chem. Abstr. 49, 5533ᶜ (1955).

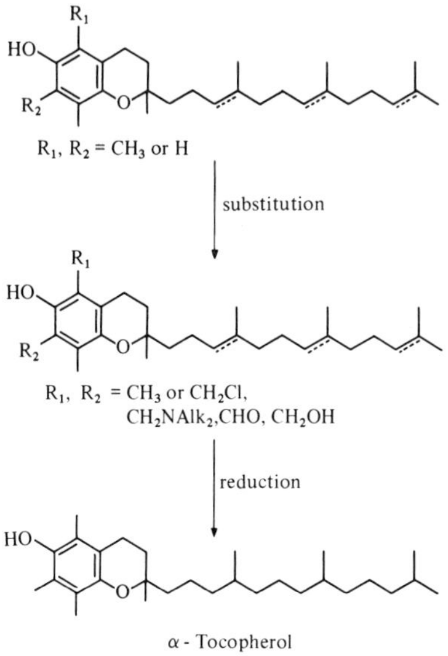

$R_1, R_2 = CH_3$ or H

substitution

$R_1, R_2 = CH_3$ or CH_2Cl,
CH_2NAlk_2, CHO, CH_2OH

reduction

α - Tocopherol

FIG. 26. Introduction of methyl groups into methyltocols and -tocotrienols.

reduction (Fig. 26). The methyltocols can also be oxidized first to the corresponding quinones (see Fig. 4) which then are chloromethylated, reduced,
and recyclized to give α-tocopherol.[247] Detailed studies on the course of
chloromethylation and hydroxymethylation reactions with different mono-
and dimethyltocols were made by Green's team[51] (Table IX). Hydroxymethylation followed by reduction has also been used to convert δ-tocotrienol into
β-tocotrienol.[8]

The transformation of natural tocols and tocotrienols into α-tocopherol
was also used[56, 57] for the determination of their stereochemistry at carbon
atom number 2, which turned out to be R-configurated. Natural β- and γ-
tocopherol from vegetable oils yielded (2R)-α-tocopherol through Mannich
reaction followed by hydrogenolysis. The 2R-configuration of the α-tocopherol obtained followed from the positive optical rotations of the corresponding potassium ferricyanide oxidation products (see Table VIII). β-
Tocotrienol was hydrogenated to β-tocopherol which was transformed into
(2R)-α-tocopherol by the procedure mentioned, whereas α-tocotrienol after
catalytic hydrogenation gave (2R)-α-tocopherol directly. γ-Tocotrienol from
latex of *Hevea brasiliensis* was first transformed into the corresponding
Mannich-base which then was hydrogenated to give (2R)-α-tocopherol (see
Fig. 26). The fact that the p-phenylazobenzoate of the α-tocopherol obtained

[247] F. J. Sevigne, U.S. Patent No. 2 998 430 (1961); see *Chem. Abstr.* **56**, 3462ᶜ (1962); U.S.
Patent No. 3 187 011 (1965); see *Chem. Abstr.* **63**, 8322ᶠ (1965).

TABLE IX

SYNTHESES OF TOCOPHEROLS BY CHLOROMETHYLATION- OR HYDROXYMETHYLATION
PROCEDURES

Starting material	Product
5-Methyltocol $\longrightarrow$	{ 5,8-Dimethyltocol[a] { 5,7,8-Trimethyltocol[a]
7-Methyltocol $\longrightarrow$	5,7-Dimethyltocol[a]
8-Methyltocol $\longrightarrow$	5,8-Dimethyltocol[a]
5,7-Dimethyltocol } 7,8-Dimethyltocotrienol } $\longrightarrow$	5,7,8-Trimethyltocol[a, b]
Tocol $\longrightarrow$	5-Methyltocol[a]
5,8-Dimethyltocotrienol $\longrightarrow$	5,7,8-Trimethyltocotrienol[a, c]

[a] J. Green, D. McHale, S. Marcinkiewicz, P. Mamalis, and P. R. Watt. *J. Chem. Soc.,*
London p. 3362 (1959).
[b] H. Mayer, J. Metzger, and O. Isler, *Helv. Chim. Acta* **50**, 1376 (1967).
[c] J. Green, P. Mamalis, S. Marcinkiewicz, and D. McHale, *Chem. Ind. (London)* p. 73
(1960).

from natural γ-tocopherol was identical in every respect (X-ray powder
diagram included) with $(2R,4'R,8'R)$-α-tocopheryl p-phenylazobenzoate
furthermore indicated the $4'R,8'R$-configuration of the former.[58]

g. Labeled Compounds

The preparation of radioactively labeled tocopherols and related compounds which are indispensable tools for the investigation of biological
function, absorption, storage, distribution, and metabolism[248] has become
possible through the various syntheses of vitamin E available today (see
Section G). Figure 27 indicates the positions and specific activities of several
stereoisomeric tocopherols, tocopheramines, and of the α-Simon-metabolite
which have been specifically labeled with radioactive carbon (^{14}C) or tritium
(^{3}H) by Dr. J. Würsch in the laboratories of F. Hoffmann-La Roche & Co.
Ltd., Basle.

H. Related Compounds

In the previous sections, the chemistry of the tocopherols has been summarized. It became evident that most of the chemical transformations observed take place only at the chroman moiety of the molecules, leaving the

[248] O. Wiss, R. H. Bunnell, and U. Gloor, *Vitam. Horm. (New York)* **20**, 441 (1962); C.
Martius, *Vitam. Horm. (New York)* **20**, 457 (1962); S. Krishnamurthy and J. G. Bieri,
J. Lipid Res. **4**, 330 (1963); U. Gloor, F. Weber, J. Würsch, and O. Wiss, *Helv. Chim.*
Acta **46**, 2457 (1963); F. Weber, U. Gloor, and O. Wiss, *Wiss. Veroeff. Deut. Ges.*
Ernaehrung **16**, 66 (1967); I. D. Desai, C. K. Perekh, and M. L. Scott, *Biochim. Biophys.*
Acta **100**, 280 (1965); U. Gloor, J. Würsch, U. Schwieter, and O. Wiss, *Helv. Chim.*
Acta **49** 2303 (1966); C. Martius, *Wiss. Veroeff. Deut. Ges. Ernaehrung* **16**, 31 (1967).

saturated aliphatic side chain intact. Therefore many of the chemical investigations in the vitamin E field were achieved in a preliminary sense with chromanols devoid of the isoprenoid side chain. 2,2,5,7,8-Pentamethylchroman-6-ol for example often served as model compound for α-tocopherol. Also the chemical properties of the lower or higher[249-251] or unbranched[252-256] side chain homologs or isoprenologs[25, 257, 258] of α-tocopherol, which have been prepared for biochemical investigations (see Fig. 28) are, for the same reason of course, similar to those of α-tocopherol. Intensive synthetic work was also devoted for the preparation (a) of tocopherols in which one of the end of chain methyl groups is replaced by a carboxyl or hydroxymethyl group;[259, 260] (b) of tocopherols in which one or two methyl groups at the aromatic ring are replaced by ethyl groups,[169, 261-263] tri- or tetramethylene rings,[264] methoxy groups,[265] or methylthio groups;[266] (c) of tocopherols with an ethyl or propyl group at C-2;[267] and (d) of tocopherols in which the phenolic hydroxyl is replaced by an amino group (e.g., α-, β-, γ-, and δ-tocopheramine)[30, 268-271] or by a mercapto group (tocopherthiols)[30], in which the chroman oxygen is replaced by a sulfur atom[272] or an NH-group (1-aza-α-tocopherol)[30] or in which both the phenolic hydroxyl and the chroman oxygen are replaced by NH_2- and NH-groups, respectively (1-aza-α-tocopheramine).[30]

Another remarkable chemical feature of the tocopherols is their interconvertibility with tocopherolquinones and 3,4-dehydrotocopherols (see

[249] W. John, P. Günther, and M. Schmeil, *Ber. Deut. Chem. Ges.* **71**, 2637 (1938); *Hoppe-Seyler's Z. Physiol. Chem.* **273**, 191 (1942).

[250] W. John and P. Günther, *Ber. Deut. Chem. Ges.* **72**, 1649 (1939).

[251] W. John and H. Herrmann, *Hoppe-Seyler's Z. Physiol. Chem.* **273**, 191 (1942).

[252] W. John and M. Schmeil, *Ber. Deut. Chem. Ges.* **71**, 2637 (1938).

[253] W. John, P. Günther, and F. H. Rathmann, *Hoppe-Seyler's Z. Physiol. Chem.* **268**, 104 (1941).

[254] W. John and F. H. Rathmann, *Ber. Deut. Chem. Ges.* **74**, 890 (1941).

[255] P. Karrer and P. Kehrer, *Helv. Chim. Acta* **25**, 29 (1942).

[256] J. Weichet and J. Hodrová, *Chem. Listy* **51**, 133 (1957).

[257] P. Karrer and K. S. Yap, *Helv. Chim. Acta* **24**, 639 (1941).

[258] P. Karrer and K. S. Yap, *Helv. Chim. Acta* **23**, 581 (1940).

[259] J. Weichet, L. Bláha and B. Kakáč, *Collect. Czech. Chem. Commun.* **31**, 2434 (1966).

[260] J. Weichet, L. Bláha, and B. Kakáč, *Collect. Czech. Chem. Commun.* **31**, 4598 (1966).

[261] L. I. Smith and W. B. Renfrow, *J. Amer. Chem. Soc.* **64**, 445 (1942).

[262] P. Karrer and O. Hoffmann, *Helv. Chim. Acta* **22**, 654 (1939).

[263] P. Karrer and R. Schläpfer, *Helv. Chim. Acta* **24**, 298 (1941).

[264] P. Karrer and A. Kuglar, *Helv. Chim. Acta* **28**, 436 (1945).

[265] P. Karrer and K. Dürr, *Helv. Chim. Acta* **32**, 1361 (1949).

[266] P. Karrer and P. C. Dutta, *Helv. Chim. Acta* **31**, 2080 (1948).

[267] P. Karrer and M. Stähelin, *Helv. Chim. Acta* **28**, 438 (1945).

[268] L. I. Smith, W. B. Renfrow, and J. W. Opie, *J. Amer. Chem. Soc.* **64**, 1082 (1942).

[269] U. Schwieter, R. Tamm, H. Weiser, and O. Wiss, *Helv. Chim. Acta* **49**, 2297 (1966).

[270] U. Gloor, J. Würsch, U. Schwieter, and O. Wiss, *Helv. Chim. Acta* **49**, 2303 (1966).

[271] J. G. Bieri and E. L. Prival, *Biochemistry* **6**, 2153 (1967).

[272] P. Karrer and P. Leiser, *Helv. Chim. Acta* **27**, 678 (1944).

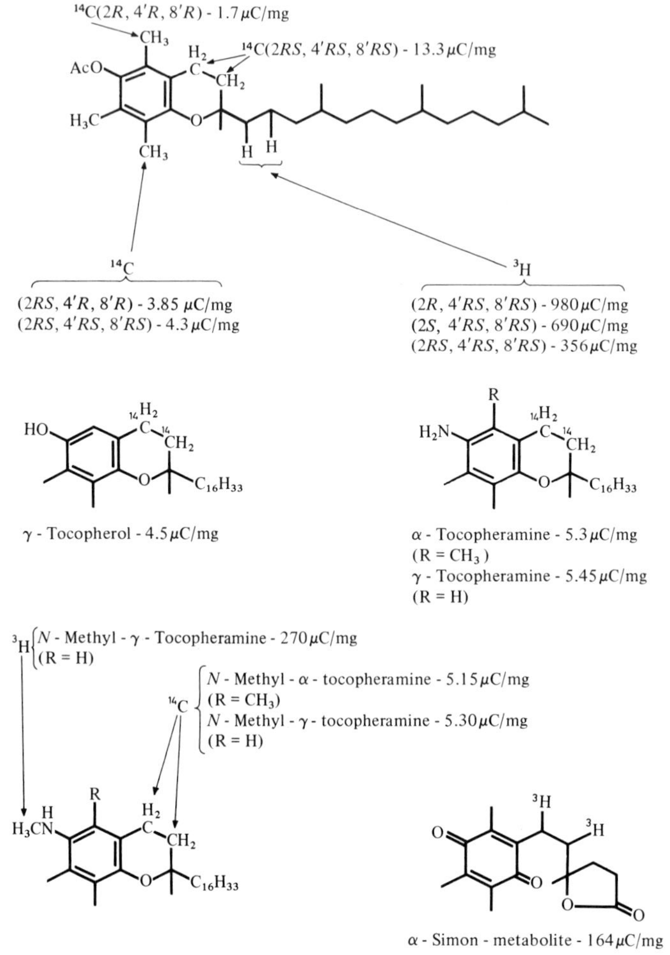

^{14}C(2R, 4'R, 8'R) - 1.7 μC/mg

^{14}C(2RS, 4'RS, 8'RS) - 13.3 μC/mg

^{14}C

(2RS, 4'R, 8'R) - 3.85 μC/mg
(2RS, 4'RS, 8'RS) - 4.3 μC/mg

^{3}H

(2R, 4'RS, 8'RS) - 980 μC/mg
(2S, 4'RS, 8'RS) - 690 μC/mg
(2RS, 4'RS, 8'RS) - 356 μC/mg

γ - Tocopherol - 4.5 μC/mg

α - Tocopheramine - 5.3 μC/mg
(R = CH$_3$)
γ - Tocopheramine - 5.45 μC/mg
(R = H)

^{3}H { N - Methyl - γ - Tocopheramine - 270 μC/mg
        (R = H)

^{14}C { N - Methyl - α - tocopheramine - 5.15 μC/mg
         (R = CH$_3$)
         N - Methyl - γ - tocopheramine - 5.30 μC/mg
         (R = H)

α - Simon - metabolite - 164 μC/mg

FIG. 27. Labeled compounds.

Fig. 10). The latter are essentially chromenols. Vitamin E therefore stands in a close chemical relationship with both the biochemically important group of isoprenoid quinones[273] (represented by phylloquinone, by the menaquinones, the ubiquinones, and the plastoquinones) and the chromenols (such as phyllochromenol, plastochromenol, and the ubichromenols) (see Fig. 28).

Related chromanols are represented by phyllochromanol (naphthotoco-

---

[273] Reviewed by O. Isler and A. Langemann, *in* "Biochemistry of Quinones" (R. A. Morton, ed.), p. 89. Academic Press, New York, 1965.

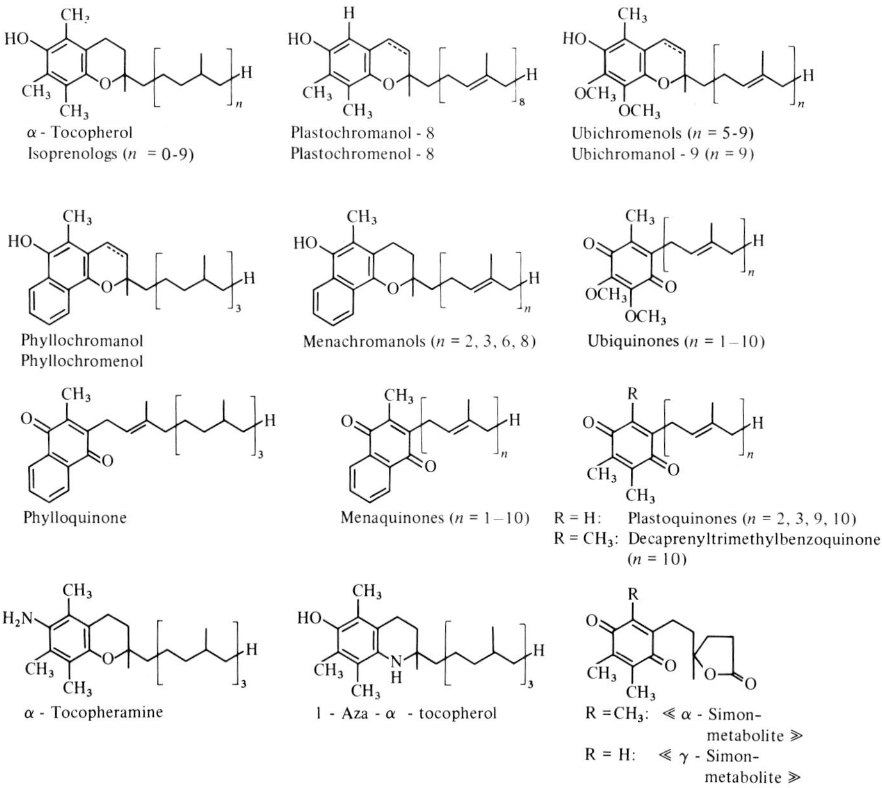

α - Tocopherol
Isoprenologs (n = 0-9)

Plastochromanol - 8
Plastochromenol - 8

Ubichromenols (n = 5-9)
Ubichromanol - 9 (n = 9)

Phyllochromanol
Phyllochromenol

Menachromanols (n = 2, 3, 6, 8)

Ubiquinones (n = 1-10)

Phylloquinone

Menaquinones (n = 1-10)

R = H: Plastoquinones (n = 2, 3, 9, 10)
R = CH₃: Decaprenyltrimethylbenzoquinone
          (n = 10)

α - Tocopheramine

1 - Aza - α - tocopherol

R = CH₃: « α - Simon-
          metabolite »
R = H: « γ - Simon-
          metabolite »

FIG. 28. Related compounds.

pherol),$^{274-276}$ by the recently synthesized menachromanols$^{277-279}$ and ubichromanol-9^{280} and by plastochromanol-8, an isoprenolog of γ-toco-trienol which has recently been isolated and synthesized$^{57, 281}$ and its stereochemistry shown to be 2R,all-*trans*.^{57}

Intensive studies of vitamin E metabolism in animals and humans led to the identification of a number of metabolites which are closely related to

^{274} T. Watanabe and A. F. Brodie, *Proc. Nat. Acad. Sci. U.S.* **56**, 940 (1966).

^{275} M. Tishler, L. F. Fieser, and N. L. Wendler, *J. Amer. Chem. Soc.* **62**, 1982 (1940).

^{276} L. H. Chem and R. D. Dallam, *Nature (London)* **198**, 386 (1963).

^{277} R. Azerad, M. O. Cyrot, and E. Lederer, *Biochem. Biophys. Res. Commun.* **27**, 249 (1967).

^{278} E. I. Kozlov and G. I. Samokhalov, *Zh. Obshch. Khim.* **36**, 2120 (1966); see *Index Chem.* **24**, 77241 (1967).

^{279} R. Powls and E. R. Redfearn, *Biochem. J.* **102**, 3C (1967).

^{280} H. W. Moore and K. Folkers, *J. Amer. Chem. Soc.* **86**, 3393 (1964).

^{281} K. J. Whittle, P. J. Dunphy, and J. F. Pennock, *Biochem. J.* **96**, 17C (1965).

α-tocopherol. Thus Simon et al.[282, 283] reported the isolation of a metabolite of α-tocopherol ("α-Simon-metabolite") which was later synthesized in its racemic[284] and optically active[285] forms. Interestingly, the same quinone has recently been found to be a metabolite of α-tocopheramine[286] and of α-tocopherolquinone[287] whereas γ-tocopherol and N-methyl-γ-tocopheramine gave the so-called "γ-Simon-metabolite"[286] (see Fig. 28). Another quinoid vitamin E metabolite, decaprenyltrimethylbenzoquinone [vitamin $E_{2(50)}$] has been postulated by Martius and Fürer,[288] and the presence in animal tissues of α-tocopherolquinone XII (see Fig. 4) was reported by several authors.[103, 289–293] The conflicting evidence about the existence of dimeric (XVIII, XXII) and trimeric (XIX) metabolites of α-tocopherol (see Fig. 5) has already been discussed in Section E, 4.

III. Industrial Preparations and Production

STANLEY R. AMES

A. d-α-Tocopherol and Its Esters

d-α-Tocopherol is the naturally occurring form of vitamin E and chemically is 2D,4'D,8'D-α-tocopherol.[1, 2, 3] This specific structure can also be prepared synthetically.[1, 4]

[282] E. J. Simon, C. S. Gross, and A. T. Milhorat, J. Biol. Chem. 221, 797 (1956).

[283] E. J. Simon, A. Eisengart, L. Sundheim, and A. T. Milhorat, J. Biol. Chem. 221, 807 (1956).

[284] J. Weichet, L. Bláha, and B. Kakáč, Collect. Czech. Chem. Commun. 24, 1689 (1959).

[285] H. Mayer, P. Schudel, R. Rüegg, and O. Isler, Helv. Chim. Acta 47, 229 (1964).

[286] U. Gloor, J. Würsch, U. Schwieter, and O. Wiss, Helv. Chim. Acta 49, 2303 (1966).

[287] H. Schmandke, Int. Z. Vitaminforsch. 35, 321 (1965).

[288] C. Martius and E. Fürer, Biochem. Z. 336, 474 (1963).

[289] R. A. Morton and W. E. J. Phillips, Biochem. J. 73, 427 (1959).

[290] P. A. Plack and J. G. Bieri, Biochim. Biophys. Acta 84, 729 (1964).

[291] F. Weber and O. Wiss, Helv. Physiol. Pharmacol. Acta 21, 131 (1963).

[292] A. Mellors and M. McC. Barnes, Brit. J. Nutr. 20, 69 (1966).

[293] A. S. Csallany, H. H. Draper, and S. N. Shah, Arch. Biochem. Biophys. 98, 142 (1962).

[1] C. D. Robeson and D. R. Nelan, J. Amer. Chem. Soc. 84, 3196 (1962).

[2] S. R. Ames, M. I. Ludwig, D. R. Nelan, and C. D. Robeson, Biochemistry 2, 188 (1963).

[3] A system of nomenclature for the stereoisomers of tocopherols and preferred trivial names has been proposed by the Committee on Nomenclature, International Union of Nutritional Sciences, see Nutr. Abstr. Rev. 40, 395 (1970), and approved by the VIII International Congress of Nutrition and by the American Institute of Nutrition, see S. R. Ames, J. Nutr. 100, 1239 (1970). The DL system is preferred to the R,S system proposed by R. S. Cahn, C. K. Ingold and V. Prelong, Experientia 12, 81 (1965).

[4] H. Mayer, P. Schudel, R. Rüegg, and O. Isler, Helv. Chim. Acta 46, 650 (1963).

1. RAW MATERIALS

Most vegetable oils contain appreciable amounts of d-α-tocopherol. Corn, cottonseed, soybean, and wheat germ oils contain from 0.02% to 0.2% vitamin E. Substantial amounts of non-α-tocopherols are also present in most vegetable oils. For example, cottonseed oil contains about 60% α- and 40% γ-tocopherols; soybean oil contains about 20% α-, 60% γ-, and 20% δ-tocopherols; and wheat germ oil contains about 60% α-, the remainder β-tocopherols.[5]

Concentrates of the vegetable oils contain predominantly the same tocopherols that were present in the original oils. The preparation of concentrates high in α-tocopherol content is of special interest since the α-form has the greatest physiological activity.

2. CONCENTRATION PROCESSES

Methods of commercial processing vary a great deal depending on the potency and quality of the desired products. Low potency concentrates of vegetable oils can be conveniently prepared by saponification, followed by extraction of the nonsaponifiables. For example, wheat germ oil concentrates representing an eightfold concentration of the tocopherols present can readily be prepared by this procedure. Alternatively, hot ethanol extraction of wheat germ followed by removal of lipids by freezing at low temperatures and removal of solvent may be employed to prepare similar concentrates.[6]

Processes involving extraction of vegetable oils with liquid propane or other hydrocarbon solvents have been described.[7-9] Details of procedures and equipment are available, but the potencies of concentrates obtained have not been revealed. Fractional extraction of vegetable oils from various solvents has also been used to obtain tocopherol concentrates.[10, 11]

Molecular distillation of vegetable oils has been extensively developed as a practical and efficient procedure for preparing tocopherol concentrates. This process involves distillation of the vegetable oil at pressures of from 1 to 10 μ and with a very short thermal exposure. The tocopherols are not destroyed under these conditions. By using molecular distillation plus saponification

[5] D. C. Herting and E.-J. E. Drury, *J. Nutr.* **81**, 335 (1963).
[6] W. D. McFarlane, U.S. Patent No. 2,497,317 (1950).
[7] N. D. Embree and N. H. Kurht, U.S. Patent No. 2,454,692 (1948).
[8] A. W. Hivson and R. Miller, U.S. Patent No. 2,508,387 (1950).
[9] W. M. Leaders and F. A. Norris, U.S. Patent No. 2,521,234 (1950).
[10] W. S. Singleton and A. E. Bailey, *Oil Soap (Chicago)* **21**, 224 (1944).
[11] C. L. Lautenschläger and F. Lindner, Can. Patent No. 480,004 (1952).

or extraction, high potency tocopherol concentrates can be readily prepared.[12-16]

The above-described procedures are suitable only for concentrating the tocopherols occurring naturally in vegetable oils and do not substantially alter the ratio of α- to non-α-tocopherols present in the raw oil. Several procedures have been described by which high potency concentrates of α-tocopherol can be prepared. Adsorption chromatography can be used to prepare relatively pure individual tocopherols.[17-20] The transformation of the mono- and dimethyltocopherols to the trimethyl-α-tocopherol by various methods has been described.[21-26] The resolution of 2DL,4'D,8'D-α-tocopherol, synthesized from natural phytol into its two epimeric forms has been investigated.[1, 4]

Tocopherol concentrates are frequently subjected to further chemical processing to convert them to other economically desirable forms. The acetate ester is very stable to atmospheric oxidation under most conditions.[27] The acid succinate ester is a solid at room temperature

3. COMMERCIAL PRODUCTS

Mixed Tocopherols Concentrate, N.F., is a type of tocopherol concentrate derived from vegetable oils. The d-α-tocopherol content is standardized at 50% of the total tocopherols with concentrations of total tocopherols ranging from 340 to 500 mg (253–372 IU)/gm. These products are clear reddish oils with a mild taste and odor and have high antioxidant activity.[28-30]

[12] K. C. D. Hickman, Chem. Eng. News 20, 1561 (1942).
[13] T. R. Olive, Chem. Met. Eng. 51, 100 (1944).
[14] W. S. Singleton and A. E. Bailey, Oil Soap (Chicago) 21, 157 (1944).
[15] J. Green and P. R. Watt, J. Sci. Food Agr. 1, 157 (1950).
[16] M. H. Stern, C. D. Robeson, L. Weisler, and J. G. Baxter, J. Amer. Chem. Soc. 69, 869 (1947).
[17] J. G. Baxter, C. D. Robeson, J. D. Taylor, and R. W. Lehman, J. Amer. Chem. Soc. 65, 918 (1943).
[18] O. Isler, Chimia 5, 249 (1951).
[19] I. G. Farbenindustrie, Ger. Patent No. 717,483 (1942).
[20] E. Lederer, Fr. Patent No. 991,170 (1951).
[21] K. C. D. Hickman and L. Weisler, U.S. Patent No. 2,486,540 (1949).
[22] L. Weisler, U.S. Patent No. 2,519,863 (1950).
[23] Vitamins Ltd., Fr. Patent No. 1,231,656 (1960).
[24] J. Green and S. Marcinkiewicz, Brit. Patent No. 827,391 (1960).
[25] J. Green and S. Marcinkiewicz, U.S. Patent No. 2,992,235 (1961).
[26] F. J. Sevigne, U.S. Patent No. 2,998,430 (1961).
[27] S. R. Ames, Poultry Sci. 35, 145 (1956).
[28] "National Formulary," 12th Ed. Mack Printing Co., Easton, Pennsylvania, (1965).
[29] Food Chemicals Codex, Nat. Acad. Sci.—Nat. Res. Counc. Publ 1143, 86, 152 (1963).
[30] P. L. Harris, in "The Vitamins" (W. H. Sebrell, Jr. and R. S. Harris, eds.), Vol. 3, p. 495. Academic Press, New York, 1954.

d-Alpha-Tocopheryl Acetate Concentrate, N.F., is standardized on the basis of its *d*-α-tocopheryl acetate content. Concentrations range from 250 to 350 mg (340–476 IU) *d*-α-tocopheryl acetate/gm oil. These products are clear yellow oils, with a mild taste and odor, are very stable to atmospheric oxidation and have no activity as antioxidants.[28–30]

d-Alpha-Tocopheryl Acetate, N.F., is pure *d*-α-tocopheryl acetate. It is a light-yellow viscous oil containing 1360 IU/gm,[28, 29] the highest rating of any commercial vitamin E product.

d-Alpha-Tocopheryl Acid Succinate, N.F., is a white granular powder, nearly odorless and tasteless, and contains 1210 IU/gm.[28, 29]

Dry forms of *d*-α-tocopheryl acetate at many different potencies are available as specialty items. Carriers such as soy grits, acacia, dextrin, gelatin, and other vegetable colloids have been utilized. The formulations involving such carriers are not used to stabilize *d*-α-tocopheryl acetate, but to offer convenience in handling, especially as supplements in the feed industry.

Wheat germ oil concentrates and other similar low potency mixtures of the various tocopherols are primarily of historical interest but are still used. They are dark brown oils, readily susceptible to oxidative destruction and have low potencies, for example, 10 IU/gm.[30]

B. Synthetic α-Tocopherols and Their Esters

1. TYPES OF SYNTHETIC α-TOCOPHEROLS

There are several types of synthetic α-tocopherols which differ in their stereoisomeric content. All-*racemic* α-tocopherol, synthesized from racemic isophytol is a mixture of the eight possible stereoisomers of α-tocopherol. All-*racemic* α-tocopherol can be termed 2*DL*,4′*DL*,8′*DL*-α-tocopherol.[2, 3] The α-tocopherol synthesized from natural phytol is a mixture of only two of the eight possible stereoisomers of α-tocopherol. This α-tocopherol can be termed 2*DL*,4′*D*,8′*D*-α-tocopherol.[2, 3] The acetate ester of this latter material was the former International Standard for vitamin E activity[31] which was discontinued in 1956.[32] Mixtures containing some of the other stereoisomers have been prepared. They are at present laboratory curiosities but the use of synthetic phytols containing an *L*-configuration at one or both of the assymetric centers may result in their commercial appearance. If prepared synthetically, all the various steroisomeric mixtures are presently termed *dl*-α-tocopherol according to the National Formulary[28] and the Food

[31] E. M. Hume, *League Nat. Bull. Health Organ.* 9, 436 (1940–1941); *Nature (London)* 148, 472 (1941); *Analyst (London)* 66, 497 (1941).

[32] World Health Organization, Expert Committee on Biological Standardization, *World Health Organ. Tech. Rep. Ser.* 127, 9, 19, (1957); *World Health Organ. Tech. Rep. Ser.* 259, 58 (1963).

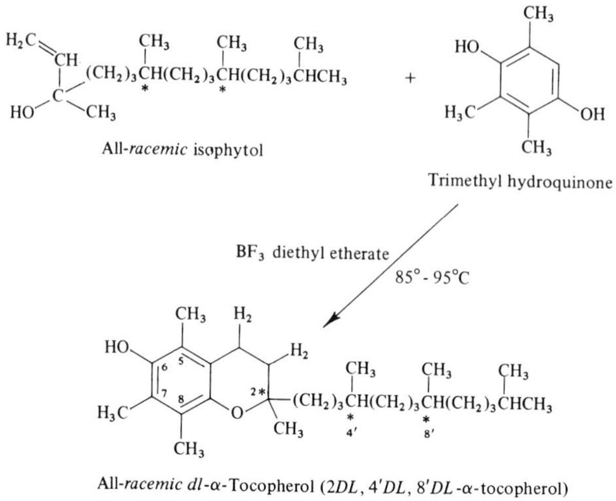

FIG. 29. Synthesis of racemic *dl*-α-tocopherol. The asterisks denote points of asymmetry giving rise to a mixture of eight optical isomers. The naturally occurring form, *d*-α-tocopherol, is structurally 2*D*,4'*D*,8'*D*-α-tocopherol.[3]

Chemicals Codex.[29] Resolution of this nomenclature problem by official bodies and commercial suppliers should be undertaken.[3]

2. Synthetic Processes

dl-α-Tocopherol (all-*racemic*) can be synthesized by condensing racemic isophytol with trimethyl hydroquinone in the presence of acidic condensing agents.[33] The condensation is reported to be carried out in excellent yield by using BF_3 diethyl etherate at 85°–95°C[34] (see Fig. 29). Synthetic phytol or phytyl halides can also be employed. These and similar reactions used commercially resemble the classic procedures announced almost simultaneously in 1938 by Karrer *et al.*[35] in Zurich, by Bergel *et al.*[36] in Manchester, and by Smith *et al.*[37] in Minnesota.

The all-*racemic* (*dl*) forms of the various dimethyl and monomethyl tocols can also be synthesized by similar procedures utilizing the corresponding di- or monomethyl hydroquinones.[33, 38] Synthesis of tocopherols other

[33] O. Isler, P. Schudel, H. Mayer, J. Würsch, and R. Rüegg, *Vitam. Horm. (New York)* **20**, 389 (1962).

[34] F. Hoffmann-LaRoche & Co., Brit. Patent No. 867,166 (1961).

[35] P. Karrer, H. Fritzsche, B. H. Ringier, and H. Salomon, *Helv. Chim. Acta* **21**, 520, 820 (1938).

[36] F. Bergel, A. Jacob, A. R. Todd, and T. S. Work, *Nature (London)* **142**, 36 (1938).

[37] L. I. Smith, H. E. Ungnade, and W. W. Prichard, *Science* **88**, 37 (1938).

[38] P. Karrer and H. Fritzsche, *Helv. Chim. Acta* **21**, 1234 (1938).

than all-*racemic-dl-α*-tocopherol has not achieved commercial importance. *dl-α*-Tocopherol can be converted to the economically important acetate ester by conventional esterification procedures.[34]

3. COMMERCIAL PRODUCTS

dl-Alpha-Tocopherol, N.F. (all-*racemic*), is a yellow, nearly odorless, clear viscous oil. It oxidizes and darkens in air and on exposure to light and contains 1100 IU/gm.[28, 29]

dl-Alpha-Tocopheryl Acetate, N.F. (all-*racemic*), is a yellow, nearly odorless, clear viscous oil and contains 1000 IU/gm.[28-30]

Dry granular or powdered forms of *dl-α*-tocopheryl acetate (all-*racemic*) at potencies of 333 mg/gm and 250 mg/gm are available as products for the pharmaceutical industry. A dry product consisting of gelatin beads is offered to the feed industry.

C. Commercial Labeling

Commercial labeling for vitamin E products in the United States, and to a considerable extent in the rest of the world, is governed by the weight-unit relationships adopted by the National Formulary[28] and the Food Chemicals Codex[29] which, taken literally from N.F. XII, are as follows:

Label claims for Tocopherol products described in this National Formulary when expressed in International Units (IU) of vitamin E are based on the following equivalents:

1 mg *dl*-Alpha-Tocopheryl Acetate = 1 International Unit
1 mg *dl*-Alpha-Tocopherol   = 1.1 International Unit
1 mg *d*-Alpha-Tocopheryl Acetate = 1.36 International Unit
1 mg *d*-Alpha-Tocopherol   = 1.49 International Unit
1 mg *d*-Alpha-Tocopheryl Acid
     Succinate   = 1.21 International Unit

However, biological potencies for the various forms of α-tocopherol are dependent on a number of factors: the response studied, the species of experimental animal, the composition of the basal diet, details of bioassay techniques and many others. There appears to be no simple relationship between the National Formulary weight/unit relationships[28] and the results for any specific bioassay. For example, the following relationships were found using the rat fetal resorption bioassay of Mason and Harris[39] modified by using the USP 14 salt mixture instead of the USP 13 salt mixture in the diet: *dl-α*-tocopheryl acetate, 1.0; *d-α*-tocopheryl acetate[2], 1.67; *d-α*-tocopheryl acid succinate[40], 1.16 and *d-α*-tocopherol[40], 1.36.

[39] K. E. Mason and P. L. Harris, *Biol. Symp.* **12**, 459 (1947).
[40] S. R. Ames and M. I. Ludwig, to be published. (1971).

D. Analytical Procedures for Production Control

Only those procedures directly applicable to high potency concentrates or pure tocopherols in various products will be discussed. The classic procedure for the analysis of vitamin E is the Emmerie and Engel reaction[41] using ferric chloride and dipyridyl. When a determination of the total tocopherol content suffices, it is the method of choice for most products containing unesterified tocopherols. Titration with cerric sulfate, originated by Kofler[42] has been adopted as official for relatively pure forms of the tocopherols by the National Formulary.[28]

If a product contains esters of tocopherol, then careful saponification before analysis for total or individual tocopherols is required. The addition of pyrogallol to the mixture to be saponified[43, 44] greatly reduces oxidation losses but does not eliminate the need for careful exclusion of air during saponification. Control assays for finished pharmaceutical products should be modified depending on the form or source of vitamin E.[45]

If tocopherols other than α-tocopherol are present, additional procedures are required to separate the mixture. The nitroso method estimates the non-α-tocopherols present and α-tocopherol can be determined by difference.[46] Column chromatography[47] and paper chromatography[48] have been recommended but are very time-consuming and not adaptable to production control.

Procedures employing either thin-layer chromatography on silica gel[49] or on alumina[50] or gas–liquid chromatography[51–53b] are applicable to production control. In time, modifications of these procedures should replace the older methods.

The various dry products containing α-tocopherol or α-tocopheryl acetate may require special procedures. Direct saponification is often applicable, but

[41] A. Emmerie and C. Engel, *Rec. Trav. Chim. Pays-Bas* **58**, 283 (1939).

[42] M. Kofler, *Helv. Chim. Acta* **30**, 1053 (1947).

[43] J. Tŏsíc and T. Moore, *Biochem. J.* **39**, 498 (1945).

[44] P. W. R. Eggitt and L. D. Ward, *J. Sci. Food Agr.* **4**, 569 (1953).

[45] R. W. Lehman, *J. Pharm. Sci.* **53**, 201 (1964).

[46] M. L. Quaife, *J. Biol. Chem.* **175**, 605 (1948).

[47] F. Bro-Rasmussen and W. Hjarde, *Acta Chem. Scand.* **11**, 34 (1957).

[48] Analytical Methods Committee, *Analyst (London)* **84**, 356 (1959).

[49] P. A. Sturm, R. M. Parkhurst, and W. A. Skinner, *Anal. Chem.* **38**, 1244 (1966).

[50] D. C. Herting and E.-J. E. Drury, *J. Chromatogr.* **30**, 502 (1967).

[51] D. A. Libby and A. J. Sheppard, *J. Ass. Offic. Agr. Chem.* **47**, 371 (1964).

[52] H. C. Pillsbury, A. J. Sheppard, and D. A. Libby, *J. Ass. Offic. Anal. Chem.* **50**, 809 (1967).

[53] P. B. Bowman and W. E. West, *J. Pharm. Sci.* **57**, 470 (1968).

[53a] F. P. Mahn, V. Viswanathan, C. Plinton, A. Menyharth and B. Z. Senkowski, *J. Pharm. Sci.* **57**, 2149 (1968).

[53b] A. J. Sheppard, W. D. Hubbard and A. R. Prosser, *J. Ass. Offic. Agr. Chem.* **52**, 442 (1969).

in some cases extraction prior to saponification is desirable. The producers of the dry products frequently recommend specific procedures, and such directions should be carefully followed.

It is now possible to differentiate physiochemically between the pure forms of natural d-α-tocopherol and all-*racemic-dl-α*-tocopherol. The oxidation of d-α-tocopherol with potassium ferricyanide under controlled conditions yields a product which exhibits an enhanced positive optical rotation.[54] Similar treatment of all-*racemic-dl-α*-tocopherol yields a product with practically no optical rotation.[1, 54] By using purified extracts, this principal has been utilized to identify and determine supplemental d- or dl-α-tocopheryl acetate in concentrates or in feeds.[55]

IV. Estimation in Foods and Food Supplements

STANLEY R. AMES

The estimation of the vitamin E content of foods and food supplements is intricate. α-Tocopherol, the active form of vitamin E, occurs in foods in a complex mixture of α- and non-α-tocopherols, tocotrienols, carotenoids, sterols, and naturally occurring and added antioxidants. The chief problem besetting the analyst is the separation of α-tocopherol from its associated contaminants.

Many values for the vitamin E levels in foods have been based on total tocopherol determinations.[1-5] Ideally, this would be an estimate of the tocopherols only, after separation from all other interfering reducing materials. Practically, however, total tocopherol values are a measure of the total reducing materials remaining after a series of purification procedures. Recently, newer methods have yielded values for the α-tocopherol content of foods and food supplements. These values too, are dependent upon the success of the purification steps employed.

[54] D. R. Nelan and C. D. Robeson, *Nature (London)* **193**, 477 (1962).
[55] F. H. Tinkler, F. V. Passero, Jr., S. R. Ames, and D. R. Nelan, *J. Ass. Offic. Anal. Chem.* **49**, 1060 (1966).
[1] R. L. Lehman, *Methods Biochem. Anal.* **2**, 153 (1955).
[2] M. W. Dicks and L. D. Matterson, *Conn., Storrs Agr. Exp. Sta., Bull.* **362**, 28 pp. (1961).
[3] A. Emmerie and C. Engel, *Z. Vitaminforsch.* **13**, 259 (1943).
[4] M. L. Quaife and P. L. Harris, *Ind. Eng. Chem. Anal. Ed.* **18**, 707 (1946).
[5] J. G. Baxter, *Biol. Symp.* **12**, 484 (1947).

A. Isolation of the Tocopherols from Natural Products

The isolation of the tocopherols from natural products has been partially accomplished by various combinations of such procedures as extraction, molecular distillation, saponification, hydrogenation, adsorption chromatography, sulfuric acid wash, and many others. None of these procedures alone has succeeded in concentrating the tocopherol in relatively pure form. The most widely used of these isolation procedures may be summarized as follows:

1. EXTRACTION

In many foods, some of the vitamin E seems to be bound up as a protein complex.[6] Thus, the more polar the solvent, the more assurance the analyst has of extracting all the vitamin E, but, simultaneously, more of the interfering materials are extracted. Thus, extraction of vitamin E with hexane is likely to be incomplete.[1] Hot ethanol will extract all the tocopherols and fat but also some phospholipids and glucosides, which further complicate the purification steps. Combinations of solvents are now employed by many investigators. The sample is initially extracted with ethanol[7] or acetone[8] followed by addition of water to the solvent extract and reextraction with hexane.

2. MOLECULAR DISTILLATION

The tocopherols along with some lipid contaminants can be quantitatively separated from triglycerides and from some high molecular weight-reducing substances by molecular distillation at about 1μ pressure.[4] However, molecular distillation involves an expensive apparatus and is relatively time consuming; the resulting distillate may contain some carotenoids and steroids. Many of the total tocopherol values cited in the literature have been obtained after concentration by this procedure.[7, 9]

3. SAPONIFICATION

Saponification is widely used to split associated trigylcerides and thus prepare a tocopherol concentrate.[1, 10-12] Tocopherols are very unstable in the presence of alkali, especially if any oxygen is present. In order to reduce

[6] O. L. Voth and R. C. Miller, *Arch. Biochem. Biophys.* **77**, 191 (1958).

[7] M. L. Quaife and P. L. Harris, *Anal. Chem.* **20**, 1221 (1948).

[8] V. H. Booth, *Analyst (London)* **84**, 464 (1959); *Analyst (London)* **88**, 627 (1963).

[9] P. L. Harris, M. L. Quaife, and W. J. Swanson, *J. Nutr.* **40**, 367 (1950).

[10] A. Emmerie, *Rec. Trav. Chim. Pays-Bas.* **59**, 246 (1940).

[11] K. T. Kjølhede, "The Chemical Determination of Tocopherol and Its Agreement with the Biological Determination of Vitamin E," 165 pp. Arnold Busck, NYT Nordisk Forlag, Copenhagen, 1943.

[12] R. W. Swick and C. A. Baumann, *Anal. Chem.* **24**, 758 (1952).

oxidative losses, various antioxidants have been employed. By using pyrogallol[13, 14] quantitative recoveries of the tocopherols have been achieved. However, the resulting nonsaponifiable fraction still contains many contaminants and must be further purified.

4. HYDROGENATION

Catalytic, low-pressure hydrogenation has been employed to eliminate carotenoids and vitamin A.[15, 16] However, other reducing materials are formed during the hydrogenation step,[17] and thus many of the reported values based on this procedure may be too high.

5. ADSORPTION CHROMATOGRAPHY

Numerous chromatographic techniques have been described, all designed to separate the tocopherols from other reducing materials.[1, 2] Success with these various techniques has varied widely from laboratory to laboratory. Strong adsorbants, while resulting in less contamination of the tocopherol concentrate may result in substantial losses, whereas a weak adsorbant frequently does not remove enough of the interfering materials. The use of milder chromatographic separations will be described subsequently.

6. SULFURIC ACID WASH

Another method for removing nontocopherol reducing materials involves treatment with sulfuric acid.[18] If the sulfuric acid is too strong (85%), substantial losses of tocopherol may result.[19] If the concentration of acid is too weak (less than 60%), not all interfering materials are removed.[1, 20] In general, a procedure involving a sulfuric acid wash cannot be recommended since it may give spurious results.

B. Total Tocopherols

Most determinations of the total tocopherol content of purified extracts of foods are based upon the Emmerie and Engel reaction,[21] which involves the reaction of the tocopherols in the extract with ferric chloride to yield

[13] J. Tŏsić and T. Moore, *Biochem. J.* **39**, 498 (1945).
[14] P. W. R. Eggitt and L. D. Ward, *J. Sci. Food Agr.* **4**, 569 (1953).
[15] M. L. Quaife and P. L. Harris, *J. Biol. Chem.* **156**, 499 (1944).
[16] M. L. Quaife and R. Biehler, *J. Biol. Chem.* **159**, 663 (1945).
[17] W. J. Pudelkiewicz and L. D. Matterson, *J. Biol. Chem.* **235**, 496 (1960).
[18] W. E. Parker and W. D. McFarlane, *Can. J. Res., Sect. B* **18**, 405 (1940).
[19] K. J. Hivon and F. W. Quackenbush, *J. Amer. Oil. Chem. Soc.* **34**, 310 (1957).
[20] D. G. Chapman and J. A. Campbell, *J. Amer. Pharm. Ass. Sci. Ed.* **40**, 252 (1951).
[21] A. Emmerie and C. Engel, *Rec. Trav. Chim. Pays-Bas* **57**, 1351 (1938).

ferrous chloride. The ferrous chloride reacts with α,α-dipyridyl to yield a red complex which is measured colorimetrically. However, these reagents will react with any reducing material still remaining in the food extract. Thus, the validity of total tocopherol values is dependent upon the success of the purification procedures employed prior to application of the nonspecific Emmerie and Engel reaction.

Other colorimetric procedures have been described for the determination of total tocopherols, but their acceptance has been limited.

C. α-Tocopherol

The goal of most analytical procedures for vitamin E has been to determine specifically the amount of α-tocopherol in the purified extract.

1. NITROSO ASSAY FOR NON-α-TOCOPHEROLS

Use of the nitroso assay[22] for the estimation of α-tocopherol was formerly widely utilized. It depends on the ability of some of the non-α-tocopherols to form colored derivatives. α-Tocopherol does not form a colored derivative and thus any unremoved reducing materials would be termed α-tocopherol. When applied to natural products and foods, the nitroso procedure often considerably overestimates the amount of α-tocopherol present.

2. PAPER CHROMATOGRAPHY

The separation of α-tocopherol from other tocopherols and other reducing substances was achieved by the use of paper chromatography employing paper impregnated with either Vaseline[23, 24] or paraffin[14, 25]. By using zinc-amine impregnated paper,[26, 27] further separation of the non-α-tocopherols was accomplished. Use of two-dimensional paper chromatography[26, 27] employing first zinc-amine and then paraffin-impregnated paper has been described in detail by the British Analytical Methods Committee.[28] A procedure employing glass-fiber paper chromatography has been described.[29] In spite of the small amounts of tocopherols used and the necessity to calibrate for losses during chromatography, paper has been extensively used for the determination of α-tocopherol in foods and other natural products.

[22] M. L. Quaife, *J. Biol. Chem.* **175**, 605 (1948).

[23] F. Brown, *Biochem. J.* **51**, 237 (1952).

[24] F. Brown, *Biochem. J.* **52**, 523 (1952).

[25] P. W. R. Eggitt and L. D. Ward, *J. Sci. Food Agr.* **4**, 176 (1953).

[26] J. Green, S. Marcinkiewicz, and P. R. Watt, *J. Sci. Food Agr.* **6**, 274 (1955).

[27] J. Green, *J. Sci. Food Agr.* **9**, 801 (1958).

[28] Analytical Methods Committee, *Analyst (London)* **84**, 356 (1959).

[29] S. J. Atlas and K. G. Pinter, *Anal. Biochem.* **17**, 258 (1966).

3. MAGNESIUM PHOSPHATE CHROMATOGRAPHY

The multiple-solvent column chromatographic procedure described by Bro-Rasmussen and Hjarde[30, 31] has been found to give good results. The lipid extract of a food is eluted through an activated dibasic magnesium phosphate column with a series of solvents containing progressively increased amounts of diethyl ether in petroleum ether. Carotenoids are eluted with 0.5 % diethyl ether, and 2.0 % diethyl ether specifically elutes the α-tocopherol and trimethyltocotrienol. Thus, the presence of trimethyltocotrienol will lead to an overestimation of α-tocopherol content, but this is not critical because trimethyltocotrienol is not widely distributed in significant amounts. The primary difficulty with this procedure is obtaining a satisfactory source of dibasic magnesium phosphate. Only by carefully checking the elution properties of each lot of activated adsorbent with a mixture of α- and γ-tocopherols can one be assured of reliable results. This procedure is more rapid than two-dimensional paper chromatography and has been used for the routine determination of α-tocopherol in foods.[32–34]

4. THIN-LAYER CHROMATOGRAPHY

The technique of thin-layer chromatography (TLC) has been successfully adapted to the separation and analysis of the tocopherols.[35–39] An extract containing the tocopherols is placed on a plate coated with a thin-layer of silica gel or alumina, developed with organic solvents and the spot of α-tocopherol is extracted and determined colorimetrically. TLC on silica gel has been used for the determination of α-tocopherol in plant tissues[40] and in vegetable oils.[41, 42] A procedure for the determination of α-tocopherol in foods has been reported using alumina CHROMAGRAM sheets[34] suitable

[30] F. Bro-Rasmussen and W. Hjarde, *Acta Chem. Scand.* **11**, 34 (1957).
[31] F. Bro-Rasmussen and W. Hjarde, *Acta Chem. Scand.* **11**, 44 (1957).
[32] D. C. Herting and E.-J. E. Drury, *J. Nutr.* **81**, 335 (1963).
[33] R. H. Bunnell, J. Keating, A. Quaresimo, and G. K. Parman, *Amer. J. Clin. Nutr.* **17**, 1 (1965).
[34] D. C. Herting and E.-J. E. Drury, *J. Chromatogr.* **30**, 502 (1967).
[35] A. Seher, *Mikrochim. Acta* **2**, 308 (1961).
[36] H. R. Bollinger, *in* "Dünnschicht-Chromatographie, ein Laboratoriumshandbuch" (E. Stahl, ed.) p. 217, Springer, Heidelberg, 1962.
[37] M. Kofler, P. F. Sommer, H. R. Bollinger, B. Schmidli, and M. Vecchi, *Vitam. Horm. (New York)* **20**, 407 (1962).
[38] H. D. Stowe, *Arch. Biochem. Biophys.* **103**, 42 (1963).
[39] J. F. Pennock, F. W. Hemming, and J. D. Kerr, *Biochem. Biophys. Res. Commun.* **17**, 542 (1946).
[40] R. A. Dilley and F. L. Crane, *Anal. Biochem.* **5**, 531 (1963).
[41] M. K. Govind Rao, S. Venkob Rao, and K. T. Achaya, *J. Sci. Food Agr.* **16**, 121 (1965).
[42] P. A. Sturm, R. M. Parkhurst, and W. A. Skinner, *Anal. Chem.* **38**, 1244 (1966).

for routine analyses. Tsen's substitution of bathophenanthroline for α,α-dipyridyl in the Emmerie and Engel reaction increased the sensitivity 2.5-fold[43] and is especially useful for the small amounts of α-tocopherol isolated from TLC plates and sheets.[34, 42]

5. GAS–LIQUID CHROMATOGRAPHY

Gas–liquid chromatographic systems for the separation of the tocopherols have been described[44, 45] and, with modifications, applied to the identification of α-tocopherol in mixtures,[37] in animal tissue extracts,[46, 47] and in some foods.[48, 49] Sterols tend to interfere in the determination and must be carefully removed.[46] Because of its speed, sensitivity, and high resolving power, this technique may ultimately find extensive application for the determination of α-tocopherol in foods and food supplements.

D. α-Tocopheryl Acetate in Food Supplements

α-Tocopheryl acetate added as a dietary supplement has been determined by saponification and analysis by methods described above. This procedure lacks specificity since the α-tocopherol present as ester cannot then be distinguished from that occurring in the unsupplemented food. In a differentia procedure developed by Ames and Tinkler,[50] a solvent extract of the food is passed through a chromatographic column containing ceric sulfate, a strong oxidizing agent. Naturally occurring reducing substances including the unesterified tocopherols are oxidized and adsorbed. The stable α-tocopheryl acetate is quantitatively eluted from the column and saponified and the α-tocopherol present determined colorimetrically. This procedure has been extended to distinguish between *d*- and *dl*-α-tocopheryl acetates in food supplements.[51]

E. Bioassays

The ultimate measure of the vitamin E activity of a food or food supplement is, of course, a bioassay. Food supplements are frequently bioassayed, but bioassays have not been extensively used to evaluate foods. The most

[43] C. C. Tsen, *Anal. Chem.* **33**, 849 (1961).
[44] P. W. Wilson, E. Kodicek, and V. H. Booth, *Biochem. J.* **84**, 524 (1962).
[45] K. K. Carroll and D. C. Herting, *J. Amer. Chem. Soc.* **41**, 473 (1964).
[46] P. P. Nair and D. A. Turner, *J. Amer. Oil Chem. Soc.* **40**, 353 (1963).
[47] J. G. Bieri and E. L. Andrews, *Iowa State J. Sci.* **38**, 3 (1963).
[48] J. Eisner, J. L. Iverson, and D. Firestone, *J. Ass. Offic. Anal. Chem.* **49**, 580 (1966).
[49] H. A. Slover, L. M. Shelley, and T. L. Burks, *J. Amer. Oil Chem. Soc.* **44**, 161 (1967).
[50] S. R. Ames and F. H. Tinkler, *J. Ass. Offic. Agr. Chem.* **45**, 425 (1962).
[51] F. H. Tinkler, F. V. Passero, Jr., S. R. Ames, and D. R. Nelan, *J. Ass. Offic. Anal. Chem.* **49**, 1060 (1966).

desirable bioassay for vitamin E activity depends on a series of sequential physiological events: intestinal absorption, blood transport, tissue storage, and ultimately biological function at the cellular level. Bioassays are of two general types depending on whether or not a true physiological response is being measured.

1. BIOASSAYS NOT BASED ON BIOLOGICAL FUNCTION

Vitamin E bioassays in which the measured response is an elevated blood or tissue level may not estimate true physiological activity. Such bioassays depend only on the extent of absorption through the intestinal wall and the relative efficiency of blood transport, and in some cases, tissue storage. Measurement of blood tocopherol levels has frequently been employed.[52-54] However, only a small portion of ingested tocopherol is present in the blood at any moment. Since this amount is determined by the relative rates of absorption and tissue deposition, blood tocopherol values do not necessarily measure vitamin E activity. The liver shows a greater increase in tocopherol level following supplementation than either blood, muscle, or fat. Bioassays based on liver storage of vitamin E[53, 55, 56] are preferred over those employing other tissues because of their greater sensitivity. Bioassays involving erythrocyte hemolysis with hydrogen peroxide[57, 58] or dialuric acid[59-61] may also be included in this group since the hemolysis response is a direct function of the plasma tocopherol level.

Under carefully controlled conditions in which the unknown material and the standard have similar chemical structures and can be administered in an identical fashion, bioassays of this type can be valuable. However, for the evaluation of the biological activities of non-α-tocopherols, stereoisomers of α-tocopherol, or other derivatives of vitamin E, bioassays based on blood plasma or liver tocopherol levels often do not reflect the true physiological activity.

[52] E. F. Week, F. J. Sevigne, and M. E. Ellis, *J. Nutr.* **46**, 353 (1952).
[53] W. J. Pudelkiewicz, L. D. Matterson, L. M. Potter, L. Webster, and E. P. Singsen, *J. Nutr.* **71**, 115 (1960).
[54] W. L. Marusich, G. Ackerman, W. C. Reese, and J. C. Bauernfeind, *J. Anim. Sci.* **27**, 58 (1968).
[55] H. R. Bolliger and M. L. Bolliger-Quaife, *Vitam. E, Atti 3rd Congr. Int. Venice, 1955* p. 30 Valdonega, Verona, 1956.
[56] R. H. Bunnell, *Poultry Sci.* **36**, 413 (1957).
[57] C. S. Rose and P. György, *Amer. J. Physiol.* **168**, 414 (1952).
[58] M. K. Horwitt, C. C. Harvey, G. D. Duncan, and W. C. Wilson, *Amer. J. Clin. Nutr.* **4**, 408 (1956).
[59] L. Friedman, W. Weiss, F. Wherry, and O. L. Kline, *J. Nutr.* **65**, 143 (1958).
[60] J. Brüggemann, K.-H. Niesar, and C. Zenta, *Int. Z. Vitaminforsch.* **33**, 180 (1963).
[61] H. Weiser, G. Brubacher, and O. Wiss, *Science* **140**, 80 (1963).

2. BIOASSAYS BASED ON BIOLOGICAL FUNCTIONS

Vitamin E bioassays in which the measured response is a change in reproduction, muscle dystrophy, or other biological function are more difficult,
but the results are more meaningful. There are several vitamin E bioassays
involving measurement of activity in reproduction. Fetal resoprtion in
rats[1, 62–64] has been extensively employed to establish the biopotencies of
the various tocopherols and their stereoisomers. Hatchability of fertile
turkey eggs[65] and testicular atrophy in male rats[66] have also been described,
but quantitative bioassays based on the responses are difficult. Carefully
controlled bioassays based on muscular dystrophy in rabbits[67] or in chicks,[68]
on creatinuria in rats,[69] and on encephalomalacia in chicks[70] have been
successfully utilized to evaluate the biological activities of non-α-tocopherols
and stereoisomers of d-α-tocopherol.

F. Chemical Assays vs. Biopotency

By means of modern analytical techniques, the α-tocopherol content of a
food or food supplement can be determined. However, this chemical value
may be very misleading in terms of effective biological activity. Many factors
tend to depress the ratio of biopotency to chemical assay. Lack of stability
of the unesterified tocopherols in the food even after ingestion will depress
this ratio. Unesterified tocopherols are markedly less effective than tocopheryl
esters in preventing fetal resorption in rats.[71] The presence of inhibitors of
intestinal absorption, such as found in alfalfa[56, 72] also depress biological
activity. Since all-*racemic* dl-α-tocopheryl acetate is less active biologically
than d-α-tocopheryl acetate,[60, 64, 68–70] foods supplemented with the dl-
form will have a lower ratio of biopotency to chemical assay than those
supplemented with the natural d-stereoisomer.

Thus, the result of chemical assay of a food or a food supplement must be
considered a maximum value in terms of biological activity. Only by careful

[62] K. E. Mason and P. L. Harris, *Biol. Symp.* **12**, 459 (1947).
[63] J. Bunyan, D. McHale, J. Green, and S. Marcinkiewicz, *Brit. J. Nutr.* **15**, 253 (1961).
[64] S. R. Ames, M. I. Ludwig, D. R. Nelan, and C. D. Robeson, *Biochemistry* **2**, 188 (1963).
[65] L. S. Jensen, M. L. Scott, G. F. Heuser, L. C. Norris, and T. S. Nelson, *Poultry Sci.*
     35, 810 (1956).
[66] L. J. Filer, R. E. Rumery, and K. E. Mason, *Conf. Biol. Antioxidants, Trans.* **1**, 67
     (1946).
[67] E. L. Hove and P. L. Harris, *J. Nutr.* **33**, 95 (1947).
[68] M. L. Scott and I. D. Desai, *J. Nutr.* **83**, 39 (1964).
[69] L. A. Witting and M. K. Horwitt, *Proc. Soc. Exp. Biol. Med.* **116**, 655 (1964).
[70] H. Dam and E. Søndergaard, *Z. Ernaehrungswiss.* **5**, 73 (1964).
[71] P. L. Harris and M. I. Ludwig, *J. Biol. Chem.* **180**, 611 (1949).
[72] G. Olson, W. J. Pudelkiewicz, and L. D. Matterson, *J. Nutr.* **90**, 199 (1966).

interpretation of all the factors involved can a valid estimate of the biologically active vitamin E content of a food or food supplement be determined.

G. AOAC Procedures

Methods for the determination of vitamin E in foods and feeds were
proposed by Ames[73] and evaluated by collaborative assay. Naturally-
occurring α-tocopherol is determined by extraction with hot ethanol,[7]
saponification,[28] isolation of α-tocopherol by TLC[34] and colorimetry.[43]
Supplemental α-tocopheryl acetate is determined by extraction, oxidative
chromatography, saponification of α-tocopheryl acetate and colorimetry of
α-tocopherol.[50] These procedures have been adopted as Official First Action
by the Association of Official Analytical Chemists.[73]

V. Occurrence in Foods

STANLEY R. AMES

The tocopherols are widely distributed in foods in an unesterified form
and occur in the highest concentration in the cereal grain oils. Various surveys[1-3] of average human diets in the United States have shown that well
over half of the daily intake of α-tocopherol results from the consumption
of various oils and fats of vegetable origin. All other food groups contribute
small but significant amounts of the tocopherols to human diets.

d-α-Tocopherol has the highest biological activity of the several tocopherols. Although attempts have been made on the basis of limited bioassay
data to include the contribution of the non-α-tocopherols in estimating the
vitamin E activity of foods,[4, 5] this contribution is minor. The role of the
non-α-tocopherols in nutrition has not been established, and this survey
will be confined to the occurrence of d-α-tocopherol in various food products.

The determination of α-tocopherol in foods and food supplements is discussed in the preceding section of this chapter. Many values for the vitamin

[73] S. R. Ames, J. Ass. Offic. Anal. Chem. 54, 1 (1971).
[1] P. L. Harris, M. L. Quaife, and W. J. Swanson, J. Nutr. 40, 367 (1950).
[2] P. L. Harris and N. D. Embree, Amer. J. Clin. Nutr. 13, 385 (1963).
[3] R. H. Bunnell, J. Keating, A. Quaresimo, and G. K. Parman, Amer. J. Clin. Nutr. 17, 1 (1965).
[4] R. J. Ward, Brit. J. Nutr. 12, 226 (1958).
[5] R. S. Harris, Vitam. Horm. (New York) 20, 603 (1962).

E content of foods have been obtained by measurement of ferric chloride-reducing substances in unpurified solvent extracts. Such values for total reducing substances, often termed "total tocopherols" or "total vitamin E," are not accurate measures of the vitamin E content. Dicks[6] has prepared a comprehensive summary of total tocopherol levels in foods and animal feeds and has cited α-tocopherol values when available. Harris, Quaife, and Swanson[1] reported on the α-tocopherol levels of many foods by using the nitroso assay to differentiate α- and non-α-tocopherols. With some exceptions, their results compare favorably with those obtained by chromatography on paper[7] or on dibasic magnesium phosphate[8] or by thin-layer chromatographic procedures.[9, 10] α-Tocopherol levels in foods cited in this survey are limited wherever possible to those obtained by reliable analytical procedures.[7-10]

A. α-Tocopherol Levels in Foods

1. VEGETABLE OILS AND FATS (TABLE X)

Because of the high levels of non-α-tocopherols in some cereal grains, the α-tocopherol levels are frequently much lower than so-called "vitamin E" levels based on total reducing substances. Vegetable oils and fats vary widely in their α-tocopherol content. Coconut and refined olive oils are poor sources (0.6–4.5 mg/100 gm) and cottonseed, safflower seed, and wheat germ oils are good sources (35–163 mg/100 gm). The comprehensive data of Herting and Drury[12] on vegetable oils and fats obtainable in the United States are generally in good agreement with data obtained by investigations in other countries. However, corn oil is an exception; British and Australian oils average about one-third of the United States oils in α-tocopherol content.

2. GRAINS AND CEREAL PRODUCTS (TABLE XI)

There is a 3-fold range in the mean α-tocopherol levels of unprocessed cereal grains, barley and oats being lowest (0.6 mg/100 gm) and United States corn, highest (1.7 mg/100 gm). However, individual samples of most grains show a 4- to 5-fold variation in α-tocopherol content. Corn samples show a wide variation in α-tocopherol content depending on country of origin. Since

[6] M. A. Dicks, Vitamin E Content of Foods and Feeds for Human and Animal Consumption. *Wyo. Agr. Exp. Sta., Bull.* **435** (1965).
[7] Analytical Methods Committee, *Analyst (London)* **84**, 356 (1959).
[8] F. Bro-Rasmussen and W. Hjarde, *Acta Chem. Scand.* **11**, 34 (1957).
[9] P. A. Sturm, R. M. Parkhurst, and W. A. Skinner, *Anal. Chem.* **38**, 1244 (1966).
[10] D. C. Herting and E.-J. E. Drury, *J. Chromatogr.* **30**, 502 (1967).
[11] M. K. Govind Rao, S. Venkob Rao, and K. T. Achaya, *J. Sci. Food Agr.* **3**, 121 (1965).
[12] D. C. Herting and E.-J. E. Drury, *J. Nutr.* **81**, 335 (1963).

TABLE X

α-Tocopherol Content of Vegetable Oils and Fats

Source of oil or fat	Type	Percent of total	α-Tocopherol		References
			Range (mg/100 gm)	Mean (mg/100 gm)	
Castor	Indian	Trace	Trace	Trace	11
Cocoa butter	Refined	9–22	1.6–3.1	2.6	12
Coconut	Refined	45–67	0–1.6	0.6	12, 13
Corn	Crude, Brit. and Austr.	4–11	4.7–10.0	6.4	14–17
	Refined, U.S.A.	24–51	14.7–23.6	18.7	12
	Refined, part hydrog., U.S.A.	30–47	16.6–17.7	17.3	12
Cottonseed	Crude and refined	36–74	10.2–54	35.8	8, 11–13, 16–19
Olive	Crude and refined	71–85	7.8–22.0	13.5	12, 20, 21
	Refined	65–100	3.0–7.2	4.5	12, 22
Palm	All types	50–60	16–40	29	1, 4, 10
Peanut	All types	24–62	7.0–36.7	15.6	10–13, 16, 21, 23
Rapeseed	All types	27–39	15.1–22.5	18.2	8, 11, 12, 16, 18
Safflower seed	All types	46–94	22.6–45.8	34.8	11, 12
Sesame	Indian	37–41	24.4–27.3	25.7	11
Soybean	All types	8–26	6.4–24.2	12.9	8, 10, 12, 13, 16, 17, 18, 20, 24
Wheat germ	All types	51–91	84.8–209.3	162.8	8, 12, 14, 16, 17, 18, 24–27

[13] R. J. Ward, Brit. J. Nutr. 12, 231 (1958).
[14] E. L. Mason and W. L. Jones, J. Sci. Food Agr. 9, 524 (1958).
[15] J. Green, J. Sci. Food Agr. 9, 801 (1958).
[16] J. Green, S. Marcinkiewicz, and P. R. Watt, J. Sci. Food Agr. 6, 274 (1955).
[17] F. Brown, Biochem. J. 52, 523 (1952).
[18] F. Bro-Rasmussen and W. Hjarde, Acta Chem. Scand. 11, 44 (1957).
[19] L. J. Machlin, Poultry Sci. 40, 1631 (1961).
[20] K. Täufel and R. Serzisko, Ernaehrungsforschung 6, 323 (1961).
[21] G. Lambertsen and O. R. Braekkan, Analyst (London) 84, 706 (1959).
[22] J. Bunyan, J. Green, P. Mamalis, and S. Marcinkiewicz, Nature (London) 179, 418 (1957).
[23] L. J. Machlin, R. S. Gordon, J. E. Marr, and C. W. Pope, J. Nutr. 76, 284 (1962).
[24] E. K. Berndorfer, Budapesti Musz. Egyet. Elelmiszer-Kem. Tansz. Kozlem. No. 1, p. 7 (1961).
[25] P. W. R. Eggitt and L. D. Ward, J. Sci. Food Agr. 6, 329 (1955).
[26] P. W. R. Eggitt and F. W. Norris, J. Sci. Food Agr. 6, 689 (1955).
[27] P. W. R. Eggitt and L. D. Ward, J. Sci. Food Agr. 4, 569 (1953).

TABLE XI

α-TOCOPHEROL CONTENT OF GRAINS AND CEREAL PRODUCTS

Food	Type	Percent of total	α-Tocopherol Range (mg/100 gm)	Mean (mg/100 gm)	References
Barley	Grain	10–21	0.17–0.92	0.61	14–16, 28, 29
	Infant Cereal	4–62	0.04–0.16	0.10	30
Corn	Seed—U.S.A.	21–30	1.3 –2.1	1.7	12
	Grain—Brit. and Austr.	4–11	0.2 –0.5	0.33	14–17, 28
	Grain—other	12–22	0.9 –2.4	1.7	12, 29
	Meal	19	0.5 –0.8	0.7	1, 3, 31
	Germ meal	—	3.8 –7.3	5.5	8, 29
	Cereal—flakes	27	0.12	0.12	3
	Hominy grits	27	0.31	0.31	3
	Frozen kernel	39–40	0.19	0.19	3
	Canned kernel	56	0.05	0.05	3
	Tortilla	—	0.24	0.2	31
Oats	Grain	13–28	0.17–0.90	0.60	14, 16, 28, 29, 32
	Rolled	—	0.22–0.28	0.24	29
	Oatmeal	18–100	0.08–2.3	0.9	3, 30
	Dry cereal—flakes	33–39	0.6 –0.9	0.75	3, 30

Rice	Brown	0.50	1.2 –1.3	1.25	1, 33
	Polished	61	0.35	0.35	1
	Dry cereal	14–100	0.03–0.49	0.19	3, 30
	Cooked white	67	0.18	0.18	3
Rye	Grain	39–41	0.74–1.65	1.2	14, 16
Wheat	Grain	20–50	0.46–1.8	1.21	10, 14, 15, 28, 29
	Bran	9–14	0.1 –4.8	1.50	14, 16, 25, 28, 29
	Germ meal	48–64	5.8 –16.3	12.5	16, 17, 25, 27, 29
	Germ	51–67	13.7 –127.6	62	8, 12, 14
	Flour—no ClO_2	14	0.22–0.38	0.31	14, 34
	Flour after ClO_2 treatment	4	0.02–0.03	0.02	14, 34
	Bread, germ enriched	—	0.69	0.69	35
	Bread whole meal	—	0.33	0.33	35
	Bread, brown	—	0.14–0.18	0.16	34, 35
	Bread, white	—	<0.01–0.02	0.01	34, 35

[28] F. Brown, *J. Sci. Food Agr.* **4**, 161 (1953).
[29] W. Hjarde, H. Lieck, and H. Soendergaard, *Acta Agr. Scand.* **12**, 125 (1962).
[30] M. W. Dicks-Bushnell and K. C. Davis, *Amer. J. Clin. Nutr.* **20**, 262 (1967).
[31] E. Kodicek, R. Braude, S. K. Kon, and K. G. Mitchell, *Brit. J. Nutr.* **13**, 363 (1959).
[32] M. Rohrlich and W. Essner, *Z. Lebensm.-Unters. Forsch.* **109**, 222 (1959).
[33] A. M. Sechi and R. Rossi-Manaresi, *J. Vitaminol. (Kyoto)* **4**, 114 (1958).
[34] T. Moore, I. M. Sharman, and L. D. Ward, *J. Sci. Food Agr.* **8**, 97 (1957).
[35] I. M. Sharman and P. J. Richards, *Brit. J. Nutr.* **14**, 85 (1960).

TABLE XII

α-TOCOPHEROL CONTENT OF MEATS, POULTRY, AND FISH

Food	Type	α-Tocopherol			References
		Per cent of total	Range (mg/100 gm)	Mean (mg/100 gm)	
Beef	Meat	>75	0.5 –0.8	0.6	1, 37
	Meat, dehydrated	—	1.1 –1.2	1.1	37
	Meat, canned	—	0.3	0.3	37
	Meat, cooked	24–59	0.13–0.37	0.25	3
	Veal, fried	21	0.05	0.05	3
	Liver	100	1.4	1.4	1
	Liver, broiled	39	0.63	0.63	3
	Tallow	—	0	0	38
Lamb	Meat	>81	0.6	0.6	1
	Meat, broiled	50	0.16	0.16	3
Pork	Meat	>89	0.40–0.63	0.5	1, 37
	Meat, cooked	27–54	0.16–0.28	0.20	3
	Bacon	>83	0.44–0.62	0.5	1, 37
	Bacon, fried	90	0.53	0.5	3
	Meat, dehydrated	—	0.93	0.9	37
	Bacon, precooked	—	0.74	0.7	37
	Meat, canned	—	0.72	0.7	37
	Bacon, canned	—	0.41	0.4	37
	Fat—lard	—	0.2 –3.0	1.7	21, 38, 39
Luncheon meat	Bologna, salami	12–16	0.06–0.11	0.09	3
	Liverwurst	51	0.35	0.35	3
Poultry	Chicken	>84	0.15–0.42	0.26	1, 37, 40

Breast, broiled	64	0.37	0.37	3
Chicken, dehydrated	—	1.15–1.16	1.2	37
Chicken, canned	—	0.26	0.3	37
Chicken, frozen fried	13–28	0.04–0.40	0.22	3
Eggs, whole	58–85	0.8 –1.2	1.1	1, 41
Egg yolk	64–70	1.6 –3.9	2.6	21, 42, 43
Eggs, cooked	32	0.46	0.46	3
Fish Haddock	>90	0.35	0.4	1
Haddock, broiled	50	0.60	0.60	3
Salmon, broiled	75	1.35	1.35	3
Herring	100	0.3 –1.6	1.1	21, 44
Cod	100	0.15–0.33	0.22	21, 36, 44
Pike	74	0.2	0.2	42
Pollock	100	0.26	0.26	44
Halibut	100	0.4 –1.3	0.9	44
Shrimp, frozen deep fried	9–32	0.6 –1.9	0.12	3
Scallops, frozen deep fried	10–18	0.60–0.71	0.66	3

[36] J. F. Pennock, R. A. Morton, and D. E. M. Lawson, *Biochem. J.* **73**, 4 (1959).
[37] M. H. Thomas and D. H. Calloway, *J. Amer. Diet. Ass.* **39**, 105 (1961).
[38] D. C. Herting and E.-J. E. Drury, *Fed. Proc. Amer. Soc. Exp. Biol.* **24**(2), 720 (1965) and unpublished observations.
[39] E. E. Edwin, A. T. Diplock, J. Bunyan, and J. Green, *Biochem. J.* **79**, 91 (1961).
[40] J. Bunyan, E. E. Edwin, A. T. Diplock, and J. Green, *Nature (London)* **190**, 637 (1951).
[41] M. Y. Dju, M. L. Quaife, and P. L. Harris, *Amer. J. Physiol.* **160**, 259 (1950).
[42] H. Kubin and H. Fink, *Fette, Seifen, Anstrichm.* **63**, 280 (1961).
[43] J. F. Pennock, G. Neiss, and H. R. Mahler, *Biochem. J.* **85**, 530 (1962).
[44] O. R. Braekkan, G. Lambertsen, and H. Myklestad, *Fiskeridir. (Norway) Skr., Ser. Teknol. Unders.* **4**(8), 1 (1963).

the α-tocopherol in wheat is concentrated principally in the germ, the vitamin E content of a wheat product will depend greatly on the amount of germ still present. Thus, a germ-enriched bread contained about 70 times as much α-tocopherol as white bread.[34, 35] Other cereal products are generally much lower in α-tocopherol than the unprocessed grain. With the exception of oats, processed breakfast cereals retain only 5–15% of their vitamin E content.

3. MEAT, POULTRY, AND FISH (TABLE XII)

Meat and poultry are moderately good sources of α-tocopherol (0.3–0.6 mg/100 gm). Eggs and liver are considerably higher (1.1–1.4 mg/100 gm). The α-tocopherol content of an animal product will depend greatly on the amount of vitamin E in the feed consumed by the animal. Fish show a seven-fold variation in α-tocopherol content, cod and pike being lowest (0.2 mg/100 gm) and salmon, highest (1.35 mg/100 gm). Ackman and Cormier[45] have recently reported data on Canadian fish.

4. DAIRY PRODUCTS AND MARGARINES (TABLE XIII)

Homogenized milk (U.S.A.) shows a sixfold range in α-tocopherol content depending on the season and reflecting wide variations in vitamin E intake in dairy feeds. Skim milk and nonfat-dry milk (reconstituted) are very low in α-tocopherol whereas butter and cheese are good sources. The α-tocopherol contents of infant formulas vary widely depending on the type of vegetable oil incorporated and the level of vitamin E supplementation. Margarines are generally good sources but vary widely in vitamin E depending on the country and reflecting the type of oil used in manufacture.

5. FRUITS AND VEGETABLES (TABLE XIV)

In general, α-tocopherol in fruits is concentrated in the skin. α-Tocopherol levels are relatively high in dark-green vegetable tissues and often very low in the colorless tissues. Thus, the α-tocopherol content of an "edible portion" of such vegetables as cabbage, cauliflower, broccoli, and celery will depend greatly on how much of the green outer leaf is discarded. Tocopherol levels tend to be lower in rapidly growing leaves and high in mature tissues. Roots and blanched vegetables are poor sources of α-tocopherol. Based on limited data, frozen and fresh vegetables have similar vitamin E levels but canned vegetables are substantially lower.

6. MISCELLANEOUS FOODS (TABLE XV)

The α-tocopherol content of miscellaneous processed food products varies widely depending on the type and amount of oil or fat incorporated in the product. For example, potato chips cooked in a vegetable oil have a far

---

[45] R. G. Ackman and M. G. Cormier, *J. Fish. Res. B. Can.* **24**, 357 (1967).

TABLE XIII

α-TOCOPHEROL CONTENT OF DAIRY PRODUCTS AND MARGARINES

Food	Type	α-Tocopherol Range	α-Tocopherol Mean	References
		mg/100 ml	mg/100 ml	
Milk, homogenized	Summer	0.077–0.082	0.079	38
	Fall	0.083–0.144	0.113	38
	Winter	0.028–0.065	0.047	38
	Spring	0.011–0.034	0.024	38
	All seasons	0.011–0.144	0.059	3, 10, 38
Milk, skim	—	0.0022–0.0049	0.0039	38, 46
Milk, nonfat dry, reconstituted	—	0.0020–0.0024	0.0021	38
Infant formulas, reconstituted				
No vegetable oil added	—	0.04	0.04	30
Vegetable oil added	—	0.21–0.30	0.23	10, 30
Vegetable oil and vitamin E supplemented	—	0.45–0.74	0.61	10, 30
		mg/100 gm	mg/100 gm	
Butter	All types	1.0–2.6	1.9	1, 3, 8, 13, 21, 47
Cheese	American	1.0	1.0	1
Other milk products	Evaporated milk	0.30	0.30	1
	Ice cream	0.06–0.37	0.26	3
	Skim milk powder	0–0.07	0.03	29
	Nonfat dry milk	0.021–0.025	0.022	38
	Buttermilk powder	0.4	0.4	29
	Whey powder	0	0	29
	Casein	0	0	31
Margarines	U.S.A.	3.3–15.8	11.6	3, 12, 13, 38
	British	0.7–5.6	2.8	13
	Scandinavian	2.0–9.0	5.0	38, 48, 49

[46] D. R. Erickson, W. L. Dunkley, and L. M. Smith, *J. Food Sci.* **29**, 269 (1964).
[47] V. Hellstrom and R. Anderson, *Var Foda* **7**, 33 (1956).
[48] V. Hellstrom and R. Anderson, *Var Foda* **18**, 9 (1956).
[49] G. Lambertsen, H. Myklestad, and O. R. Braekkan, *J. Food Sci.* **29**, 164 (1964).

TABLE XIV

α-TOCOPHEROL CONTENT OF FRUITS AND VEGETABLES

Food	Type	α-Tocopherol Range (mg/100 gm)	Mean (mg/100 gm)	References
Fruits				
Apples	Plus skin	0.3 –0.95[a]	0.5	1, 3, 50
Bananas		0.22–0.37	0.3	1, 3
Blackberry	Cultivated	0.6	0.6	50
Cherry		0.13	0.13	50
Gooseberry		0.23–0.7[a]	0.4	50
Melon		0.1 –0.14	0.12	3, 50
Pear	Plus skin	0.5	0.5	50
Raspberry		0.3	0.3	50
Rhubarb		0.2	0.2	50
Strawberry	Fresh and frozen	0.13–0.22	0.19	3, 50
Tomato		0.17–0.50[a]	0.3	1, 3, 50
Fruit juices				
Tomato	Canned	0.22	0.22	3
Citrus	Canned	0.04	0.04	3
Leafy vegetables				
Broccoli	Sprouting	1.1 –3.8[a]	2.0	50
Brussels sprouts		0.4 –2.0	1.0	50, 51
Cabbage	Edible portion	0.1 –0.7	0.2	1, 50
Cress		0.35–1.3[a]	0.7	50
Lettuce		0.05–1.0	0.5	1, 3, 50
Parsley		1.2 –2.6[a]	1.8	50
Spinach	Edible portion	1.3 –4.7[a]	2.5	50, 52
	Canned leaf	0.02	0.02	3

Asparagus				50
Beans	Fresh	<0.1 –0.6	0.1	1, 50
	Frozen green	0.09–0.11	0.1	3
	Dried navy	0.47	0.47	3
	Boston baked	0.14	0.14	3
	Canned, green	0.03	0.03	3
Carrot		0.3 –0.85[a]	0.5	1, 3, 50, 51
Cauliflower		0.01–0.3	0.15	50
Celery	Stalk	0.2 –0.38	0.3	3, 50
Cucumber	Plus skin	0.1	0.1	50
Leek		0.2 –3	1.0	50
Onion	Fresh	0.1 –0.22	0.1	1, 3, 50
	Frozen French fried	0.52–0.72	0.62	3
Mushrooms	All varieties	0.02–0.12	0.07	42, 53
Parsnip		1.0	1.0	50
Peas	Fresh	0.03–0.55	0.1	3, 15, 50
	Seed	0 –0.5	0.25	1, 15, 42
	Dried meal	1.32	1.32	31
	Frozen green	0.22–0.25	0.23	3
	Canned	0.02	0.02	3
Potato	Fresh	0.053–<0.1	0.05	3, 50
	Cooked	0.027–0.043	0.035	3
	Frozen French fried	0.12 –0.43	0.28	3
Radish		<0.03	<0.03	50
Turnip		<0.03	<0.03	50

[a] 95% Confidence limits as calculated by Booth and Bradford.[50]

[50] V. H. Booth and M. P. Bradford, *Brit. J. Nutr.* **17**, 575 (1963).

[51] V. H. Booth and M. P. Bradford, *Int. Z. Vitaminforsch.* **33**, 276 (1963).

[52] R. A. Dilley and F. L. Crane, *Anal. Biochem.* **5**, 531 (1963).

[53] A. T. Diplock, J. Green, E. E. Edwin, and J. Bunyan, *Nature (London)* **189**, 749 (1961).

TABLE XV

α-TOCOPHEROL CONTENT OF MISCELLANEOUS FOODS

Food	Type	α-Tocopherol Range (mg/100 gm)	Mean (mg/100 gm)	References
Chocolate	Unsweetened	5.3	5.3	1
Cake	Milk bar	1.1	1.1	3
	Pound	1.1	1.1	3
	Cupcake	0.14	0.14	3
Coffee	Instant	Nil	Nil	3
Cookies	Shortbread	0.46	0.46	3
	Peanut butter-oatmeal	6.0	6.0	3
Cracker	Club	0.80	0.80	3
Mayonnaise	Various	6.0–24.3	9.7	3
Nuts	Almonds	15	15	54
	Brazil nuts	6.5	6.5	54
	Chestnuts	0.5	0.5	54
	Coconuts	0.7	0.7	54
	Filberts	21	21	54
	Peanuts	4.5–7.7	6.4	1, 3, 54
	Pecans	1.5	1.5	54
	Walnuts	1.5	1.5	54
Pies	Various	2.5–3.1	2.8	3
Potato chips		2.1–6.4	4.3	1, 3
Pretzel sticks		0.15	0.15	3
Puddings	Dry	0.3–0.7	0.5	1
Yeast	Baker's and brewer's	0–0.08	0.4	1, 29, 53

[54] G. Lambertsen, H. Myklestad, and O. R. Braekkan, *J. Sci. Food Agr.* **13**, 617 (1962).

higher level of α-tocopherol than unprocessed potatoes. Various nuts show a wide variation in α-tocopherol levels.

B. Effects of Storage and Processing

α-Tocopherol is unstable in the presence of oxygen, alkalies, ultraviolet light, metal ions such as copper and iron, and especially to peroxidizing unsaturated fats. During storage and processing, foods are normally exposed to one or more of these deleterious factors. Thus, the more extensive the handling and processing, the greater the probability of large losses of α-tocopherol. Since the effects of food processing on total tocopherols in foods have been reviewed by Harris,[5] this survey will be confined to data on α-tocopherol only.

Since the vegetable oils and fats contribute over half the α-tocopherol intake of an averaged United States diet, changes in α-tocopherol levels during the refining process are of great importance. The data of Herting and Drury[12] show that refined corn oil (18.7 mg/100 gm) contains less than half as much α-tocopherol as the lipid from freshly extracted seed corn (41.9 mg/100 gm). On the other hand, the difference in α-tocopherol levels between crude and refined safflower oil was not significant. Additional data obtained by analyzing samples of the same oil before and after commercial refining are needed to resolve this important problem.

The tocopherols in grains and cereal products are unstable during storage. Kodicek et al.[31] reported retention of only 60 % of the α-tocopherol of corn after storage for 12 weeks at room temperature. Herting and Drury[12] found that ground corn lost about 6 % of its α-tocopherol content per month on storage at room temperature. Non-α-tocopherols were destroyed at an even more rapid rate.

The α-tocopherol in cereal grains is concentrated in the bran and germ. The polishing of rice results in a marked loss of α-tocopherol. Large losses of α-tocopherol occur during the milling of wheat flour.[14, 55] The production of white flour by bleaching with chlorine dioxide resulted in large losses of α-tocopherol[14, 34, 56, 57] whereas use of ascorbic acid or potassium bromate had no measurable effect.[34] The α-tocopherol content of bread made from milled or bleached flours showed similar results. Processing of most grains to produce breakfast cereals results in great losses of α-tocopherol. Fortification of bread with vitamin E to restore that lost in processing has been proposed[58] and this concept could well be extended to include processed breakfast cereals.

[55] H. M. Sinclair, Proc. Nutr. Soc. 17, 28 (1958).
[56] A. C. Frazer, J. R. Hickman, H. G. Sammons, and M. Scharratt, J. Sci. Food Agr. 7, 375 (1956).
[57] A. C. Frazer, J. R. Hickman, H. G. Sammons, and M. Scharratt, J. Sci. Food Agr. 7, 464 (1956).
[58] S. H. Rubin, Cereal Sci. Today 11, 234 (1966).

The effect of various processing conditions on the α-tocopherol content of meat products has been studied by Thomas and Calloway[37] (see Table XVI). Dehydration caused 36–45% losses of α-tocopherol in beef and chicken, but none in pork. Losses of α-tocopherol ranged from 13 to 55% due to irradiation and from 41 to 65% due to canning.

During the production of skim milk and nonfat dry milk, the bulk of the fat and thus the fat-soluble vitamins is removed. Fortification of these important foods with vitamin E in addition to vitamins A and D should be considered.

The losses of α-tocopherol during the processing of green vegetables are due mainly to discarding the tocopherol-rich undesirable or "inedible" portions. When leaves cease growing or die, the concentration of α-tocopherol increases.[50] Thus, vegetables past their prime or wilted are probably better sources of α-tocopherol than the preferred "edible" portions. α-Tocopherol losses in vegetables during boiling are negligible[51] but losses of 70–90% result in the production of canned beans, corn, and peas.

Frozen foods are an increasing component of modern diets. Frozen vegetables retain much of their vitamin E. The α-tocopherol content of frozen french fried meats and vegetables is increased due to the use of frying oils of vegetable origin but Bunnell et al.[3] have shown that the stability of α-tocopherol in such products is poor.

C. Nutritional Surveys

The relative contribution of various foods to the daily α-tocopherol intake of humans can be evaluated either for a specific diet or for an averaged diet in a specific population. Harris et al.[1] estimated the average α-tocopherol intake per capita in the United States to be about 14 mg/day of which over 50% was contributed by fats and oils. In a more recent survey, Harris and Embree[2] on the basis of per capita food consumption in the United States in 1960[59] arrived at a similar figure (15 mg d-α-tocopherol/day). Based on assays of foods as eaten, Bunnell et al.[3] calculated that an averaged American diet may supply only 7 mg of α-tocopherol/day.

About half of the calculated daily intake of α-tocopherol is derived from the "other fats and oils" group, comprised of fats and oils used in cooking, in salad oils, salad dressings, mayonnaise, and bakery products and in fish canning (see Table XVII). A diet which excludes these α-tocopherol-rich foods either by intent, or from economic pressures may contain only half as much vitamin E as an averaged human diet. Since vegetable oils are rich sources whereas animal fats are poor sources, changes within the group of visible fats can also alter drastically the daily dietary intake of α-tocopherol.

[59] "National Food Situation," No. 96, p. 19. U.S. Dept. of Agr., Economic Res. Serv., Washington, D.C., 1961.

TABLE XVI

STABILITY OF α-TOCOPHEROL IN PROCESSED MEATS[a]

Processing condition	% of α-Tocopherol remaining in			
	Bacon	Ground chuck beef	Chicken	Pork loin
Raw	(100)	(100)	(100)	(100)
Precooked	104	—	—	—
Dehydrated, raw	—	59	64	99
Dehydrated, precooked	—	54	64	—
Irradiated after enzyme inactivation	81	87	48	80
Irradiated, precooked	53	66	45	57
Canned	59	35	49	45

[a] Calculated on dry weight basis from data of Thomas and Calloway.[37]

TABLE XVII

FAT AND d-α-TOCOPHEROL IN VARIOUS FOOD GROUPS AVAILABLE FOR CONSUMPTION IN THE UNITED STATES IN 1960[a]

Source of fat	Fat (gm/day)	d-α-Tocopherol	
		Content (mg/100 gm fat)	Amount (mg/day)
Visible fats			
Butter	7.19	1.6	0.115
Lard	9.55	2.3	0.220
Margarine	9.42	10.2	0.961
Shortening	15.62	10.0	1.562
Other fats and oils	14.14	50.0	7.063
Total	55.92	—	9.921
Other food fats			
Dairy products	23.31	1.6	0.378
Eggs	5.33	10.7	0.572
Meats, etc.	52.08	1.7	0.893
Beans, peas, nuts, etc.	5.33	9.3	0.496
Fruits and vegetables	1.74	91.7	1.597
Grain products	2.23	48.9	1.092
Total	90.02	—	5.028
Totals	145.94	—	14.949

[a] Data of Harris and Embree.[2]

The calculated α-tocopherol intake for various United States diets ranged from a low of 2 mg/day for a diet consumed by pregnant women in Tennessee[60] to a high of 27 mg/day for a fattening diet.[61]

D. Summary

The α-tocopherol content of raw food is dependent on many factors—genetic, geographic, seasonal, anatomical, and many others. Handling, storage, processing, and preparation all tend to reduce the α-tocopherol originally present in the raw foodstuff. Mean values for the α-tocopherol content of an averaged foodstuff can be calculated but must be used with reservation because of the wide variation in values for individual samples. With the increasing availability of data from individual foods, the effects of dietary variation on the daily α-tocopherol intake of humans can be evaluated.

E. Addendum

Additional data on the α-tocopherol content of various foods have appeared in recent publications as follows: vegetable oils and fats[62]; grains and cereal products[62-66]; dairy products[67, 68]; and effects of storage and processing[64, 65].

VI. Standardization of Activity

G. BRUBACHER AND O. WISS

As is usual for biologically active compounds of medical interest, the League of Nations decided in 1939 to establish a standard for vitamin E.[1] For that reason, research work had been organized by the vitamin E Sub-Committee of the Accessory Food Factors Committee[2] with a view to

[60] M. E. Ferguson, E. Bridgforth, M. L. Quaife, M. P. Martin, R. O. Cannon, W. J. McGanity, J. Newbill, and W. J. Darby, *J. Nutr.* **55**, 305 (1955).

[61] M. L. Quaife, W. J. Swanson, M. Y. Dju, and P. L. Harris, *Ann. N.Y. Acad. Sci.* **52**, 300 (1949).

[62] H. T. Slover, J. Lehmann, and R. J. Valis, *J. Am. Oil Chem. Soc.* **46**, 417 (1969).

[63] R. H. Bunnell, J. P. Keating, and A. J. Quaresimo, *J. Agr. Food Chem.* **16**, 659 (1968).

[64] D. C. Herting and E.-J. E. Drury, *Agr. Food Chem.* **17**, 785 (1969).

[65] H. T. Slover, J. Lehmann, and R. J. Valis, *Cereal Chem.* **46**, 635 (1969).

[66] G. W. Grams, C. W. Blessin, and G. E. Ingelett, *J. Am. Oil Chem. Soc.* **47**, 337 (1970).

[67] D. C. Herting and E.-J. E. Drury, *Am. J. Clin. Nutr.* **22**, 147 (1969).

[68] S. K. Searles and J. G. Armstrong, *J. Dairy Sci.* **53**, 150 (1970).

[1] R. Gautier, *League Nat., Bull. Health Organ.* **12** (1), 55 (1945–1946).

[2] Lister Institute and Medical Research Council.

examining the suitability, as an international standard for vitamin E, of the synthetic racemic α-tocopheryl acetate. Seventeen research workers in Australia, Great Britain, the Netherlands, the United States, and Switzerland took part in this work. The purpose of these investigations was to determine the relation between dosage and response for vitamin E in the so-called gestation resorption sterility test (see below) and to establish the median fertility dose of synthetic racemic α-tocopheryl acetate, i.e., the dose which enables 50% of vitamin E-deficient mated female rats to produce at least one living young animal.

The results of nine laboratories, which are compiled in Table XVIII, could be statistically evaluated.[3]

From Table XVIII it can be seen that the median fertility does of synthetic racemic α-tocopheryl acetate (dl-α-tocopheryl acetate) is 0.986 mg. On the basis of these results, the Sub-committee of Vitamin E of the Accessory Food Factors Committee proposed, as biological unit, 1 mg of dl-α-tocopheryl acetate. This proposal was accepted by Sir Henry Dale, a member of the permanent Commission of Biological Standardizations of the Health Organization of the League of Nations in 1941 and confirmed by the World Health Organization (WHO) after the war. The Hampstead Institute[4] was charged with the distribution of standard samples. An oily solution of the synthetic dl-α-tocopheryl acetate was used containing 10 mg of dl-α-tocopheryl acetate of 10 IU of vitamin E (IU E)/gm of oil. In 1956, the distribution of these samples was suspended, because synthetic dl-α-tocopheryl acetate in pure form has become easily available.

Besides the convention of the WHO (1 International Unit = 1 mg of synthetic racemic dl-α-tocopheryl acetate), the following conversion factors for other vitamin E forms were accepted in the National Formulary of the American Pharmaceutical Association, 11th Edition[5]:

1 mg of d-α-tocopheryl acetate	= 1	International Unit
1 mg of dl-α-tocopherol	= 1.1	International Unit
1 mg of d-α-tocopheryl acetate	= 1.36	International Unit
1 mg of d-α-tocopherol	= 1.49	International Unit

A stabilized gelatin beadlet containing dl-α-tocopheryl acetate (on the basis of 1 mg = 1 IU) was selected by the Animal Nutrition Research Council (ANRC) as standard for animal nutrition.[6]

The gestation resorption sterility test, as it was used to establish the international standard of vitamin E, has been described by Bliss and György.[7]

---

[3] E. M. Hume, Nature (London) 148, 472 (1943).

[4] National Institute for Medical Research, Hampstead, London, N.W. 3.

[5] "National Formulary," Vol. XI, p. 459. Amer. Pharm. Ass., Washington D.C., 1960.

[6] Anonymous, Feedstuffs 34, 34 (1962).

[7] C. I. Bliss and P. György, in "The Animal Vitamin Assay—Vitamin Methods" (P. György ed.) Vol. II, p. 136. Academic Press, New York, 1951.

TABLE XVIII

BIOLOGICAL ACTIVITY OF *dl*-α-TOCOPHEROL IN THE GESTATION RESORPTION STERILITY
TEST

Trial number	Number of rats used	Median fertility dose (mgm)	Limits of error 95%
1	83	0.56	86–117
2	40	0.55	82–123
	42	0.66	85–118
3	91	0.66	72–139
4	68	0.72	58–172
5	48	0.84	85–117
6	79	1.13	88–114
	50	1.14	82–123
7	78	1.36	87–116
8	52	1.50	85–117
	52	1.05	90–112
9	58	1.71	84–119
	Total 689	Mean 0.986	78–128

This test is based on the fact that vitamin E-deficient mated female rats are
not able to produce a litter. The response of a vitamin E dose administered
during the first part of the pregnancy can be measured by counting the
number of rats giving birth to at least one living animal (all or none type). A
second manner to evaluate the response is to determine the ratio between the
total amount of implantations after mating and the total amount of living
fetus at birth (graded type). Results obtained with these two methods are
compared by Mason.[8] In a third manner of evaluation described by Gottlieb
et al.,[9] the maximum weight gain of mated females during pregnancy is
measured. Results achieved with these different types of biological evaluation
may vary to a certain extent. With the " all-or-none " type of assay, Gottlieb
et al.[9] found for *dl*-α-tocopherol 100%, whereas Harris and Ludwig[10] only
62% of the theoretically expected value.

Another disadvantage of the gestation resorption sterility test is its long
duration, which does not apply to the hemolysis test developed by György
and Rose.[11] Usually, the test is performed according to the technique of
Friedman *et al.*[12] The hemolysis test is based on the fact that the erythrocytes

[8] K. E. Mason, *J. Nutr.* **23**, 59 (1942).
[9] H. Gottlieb, F. W. Quackenbusch, and H. Steenbock, *J. Nutr.* **25**, 433 (1941).
[10] P. L. Harris and M. I. Ludwig, *J. Biol. Chem.* **180**, 611 (1949).
[11] P. György and C. S. Rose, *Science* **108**, 716 (1948).
[12] L. Friedman, W. Weiss, F. Wherry, and O. L. Kline, *J. Nutr.* **65**, 143 (1958).

TABLE XIX
BIOLOGICAL ACTIVITY OF d-α-TOCOPHERYL ACETATE

Activity	1 mg of d-α-tocopheryl acetate corresponds to
Gestation resorption sterility, rats[a]	1.36 International Unit
Hemolysis, rats[b]	1.47 International Unit
Plasma tocopherol, chicken[c]	1.36 International Unit
Liver tocopherol, chicken[c]	1.34 International Unit

[a] P. L. Harris and M. I. Ludwig, *J. Biol. Chem.* **179**, 1111 (1949).
[b] L. Friedman, W. Weiss, F. Wherry, and O. L. Kline, *J. Nutr.* **65**, 143 (1958).
[c] W. J. Pudielkiewicz, L. D. Matterson, L. M. Potter, L. Webster, and E. P. Singsen, *J. Nutr.* **71**, 115 (1960).

of vitamin E-depleted rats show an increased tendency to be hemolyzed by oxidizing agents, such as hydrogen peroxide and dialuric acid, compared with normal rats. After administration of vitamin E to the depleted rats, the grade of return to normal values of hemolysis is measured. The test can be performed in a very short time and has a good precision.

In a third test, the normalization of creatinuria in vitamin E-deficient rabbits is used as measure for the vitamin E activity of unknown compounds.[13]

There are, in addition to these three tests, in which a physiological or biochemical response of vitamin E in vitamin E-depleted animals is measured, many other tests based on the measurement of vitamin E concentration in blood or liver.[14-16] With these tests, the absorption rather than the full biological activity is measured. However, generally, they give similar results to the tests mentioned above. Table XIX contains a comparison of results which were obtained with d-α-tocopheryl acetate in different tests and which are in good agreement.

[13] E. L. Hove and P. L. Harris, *J. Nutr.* **33**, 95 (1947).
[14] E. F. Week, F. J. Sevigne, and M. E. Ellis, *J. Nutr.* **46**, 353 (1952).
[15] W. J. Pudielkiewicz, L. D. Matterson, L. M. Potter, L. Webster, and E. P. Singsen, *J. Nutr.* **71**, 115 (1960).
[16] G. Brubacher and H. Weiser, in "Wissenschaftliche Veröffentlichungen der Deutschen Gesellschaft für Ernährung" Vol. **16** Tocopherole, pp. 50–66. Dr. Dietrich Steinkopff Verlag, Darmstadt, 1967.

VII. Biogenesis

J. GREEN

Although the tocopherols appear to be universal constituents of all green plants and at least some lower forms of plant life and their biogenesis must present several interesting problems, comparatively little is known about their mode of origin. With the present revival of interest in the nature and function of chloroplastal and extra-chloroplastal lipids, however, it is to be expected that this position will be rectified in the near future. One of the most striking facts about the presence of tocopherols in plants is that whereas the growing, photosynthesizing organism contains mainly, and sometimes entirely, α-tocopherol, resting and dormant parts, such as seeds and fruits, nearly always contain non-α-tocopherols, usually in predominant amounts.[1] The change from one pattern to another is linked to the phases of the life cycle and may reflect subtle and important metabolic differences.

The biosynthesis of α-tocopherol in green plants begins with the first appearance of chlorophyll-containing leaves. This is accompanied by a diminution, and usually disappearance, of the non-α-tocopherols of the seed, although the latter persist well into the free-growing period, as in wheat, barley, and the pea.[1] In the maize plant, however, the predominant γ-tocopherol of the seed does not disappear during growth, and this tocopherol, together with much larger amounts of α-tocopherol, is synthesized through the later stages of the life cycle. In all these plants, as the processes of fructification and seed-formation begin, α-tocopherol synthesis tapers off, and synthesis of the non-α-tocopherols once again becomes predominant, although the latter are rarely found in the leaves and stems, even up to withering. Quantitative studies[1] suggest that α-tocopherol can be formed by two processes, either directly from intermediary precursors or indirectly by methylation of already formed non-α-tocopherols. Conversion of the latter and, in the maize plant, even overall total synthesis of α-tocopherol from available precursors, takes place by light-independent reactions and does not require the presence of chlorophyll or, presumably of preformed phytol. The substantial quantities of tocopherols found in mushrooms[2] and yeasts[3] confirm this view. Zacharowa[4] had already, in 1954, reported a dark synthesis of

[1] J. Green, *J. Sci. Food. Agr.* **9**, 801 (1958).
[2] H. Kubin and H. Fink, *Fette, Seifen, Anstrichm.* **63**, 280 (1961).
[3] A. T. Diplock, J. Green, E. E. Edwin, and J. Bunyan, *Nature (London)* **189**, 749 (1961).
[4] M. P. Zacharowa, *Tr. WNIWI* **5**, 159 (1954).

tocopherol in pea and barley seedlings. Baszynski[5] has confirmed these findings and has shown that increased synthesis of α-tocopherol can be obtained by supplementing 2-day-old pea seedlings with methionine in the presence of ATP at pH 6.6. A simultaneous decrease in the proportion of γ-tocopherol suggested that a nuclear methylation of the latter had taken place, but it is possible that α-tocopherol synthesis and γ-tocopherol degradation may have occurred independently. It would appear to be difficult to distinguish between the two mechanisms, but kinetic studies[1] favor the methylation process being predominant during the early stages of germination.

In the fully photosynthetic organism, α-tocopherol is located, together with α-tocopherylquinone and the plastoquinones, in the chloroplasts. This has been shown to be true both for higher green plants[6] and for *Euglena gracilis*.[7] Booth[6] has studied the ratio of α-, γ-, and δ-tocopherol to chlorophyll in the whole leaf and in the chloroplast fraction of *H. helix* and *T. baccata* and found that most of the γ- and δ-tocopherol is outside the chloroplasts. This finding may be significant in considerations of the possible functional role of these substances in plants. It could mean, for example, that in the mature green plant the α-tocopherol of the chloroplasts is synthesized without the mediation of non-α-tocopherols, a view that could account for the paucity of the latter. Alternatively, differences in membrane permeability to the different tocopherols may exist. Whether the actual site of α-tocopherol synthesis is inside the chloroplast is uncertain at present, although this seems possible, for its formation has been observed[7] to parallel that of plastoquinone and chlorophyll, both of which are of chloroplastal origin. It has recently been shown that the aromatic ring present in the tocopherols and their corresponding quinones is formed by the shikimic acid pathway.[8] Threlfall and Goodwin[9] studied the intracellular distribution and formation of terpinoid quinones in *Euglena gracilis*, strains Z, and found that α-tocopherolquinone and α-tocopherol were mainly located in the chloroplast when the cells were grown in light. They could not demonstrate the incorporation of mevalonic acid into tocopherol (or, in their experiments, into other terpinoid components) but attributed this to the impermeability of the cell wall to the mevalonate, rather than to a novel pathway of terpinoid biosynthesis for tocopherols. However, the incorporation of mevalonic acid into α-tocopherol has not yet been unequivocally demonstrated. Griffiths et al.[10] showed that

[5] T. Baszynski, *Acta. Soc. Bot. Pol.* **30**, 307 (1961).

[6] V. H. Booth, *Phytochemistry* **2**, 421 (1963).

[7] D. R. Threlfall and T. W. Goodwin, *Proc. Biochem. Soc.* **90**, 40P (1964).

[8] G. R. Whistance, D. R. Threlfall, and T. W. Goodwin, *Biochem. Biophys. Res. Commun.* **23**, 849 (1966).

[9] D. R. Threlfall and T. W. Goodwin. *Biochem. J.* **103**, 573 (1967).

[10] W. T. Griffiths, D. R. Threlfall, and T. W. Goodwin, *Biochem. J.* **103**, 589 (1967).

in light-grown maize shoots, α-tocopherolquinone was localized in the chloroplast, but in dark-grown shoots they were unable to detect this quinone. On subsequent illumination of the etiolated shoots all the chloroplastidic quinones, including α-tocopherolquinone, were synthesized in step with chloroplast development. They considered that the quinone was not formed at the immediate expense of α-tocopherol. Pennock et al.[11] have suggested that the four known tocotrienols are intermediates in the biosynthesis of α-tocopherol. They suggest that 8-methyltocotrienol (δ-tocotrienol) is formed first and then methylated to give dimethyltocotrienols (β- and γ-tocotrienols) and trimethyltocotrienol (α-tocotrienol). The final stage of the synthesis is the hydrogenation of the side chain to give a α-tocopherol. According to this hypothesis, β-, γ-, and δ-tocopherol are formed by hydrogenation of the tocotrienol intermediates. It has recently been shown[12] that methionine-^{14}C is incorporated into the α-, β-, and γ-tocotrienol of *Hevea brasiliensis* latex, without incorporation into δ-tocotrienol. This supports the earlier work of Baszynski[5] and suggests that the 5- and 7-methyl groups of α-tocopherol are derived from methionine. It is possible that the 8-methyl group is not derived from methionine, but that the intermediate δ-tocotrienol is formed by cyclization of 3-geranylgeranyl-2,5-toluquinone, formed by prenylation of an aromatic nucleus containing a methyl group. Olsen et al.[13] identified 2-geranylgeranylphenol in *Rhodospirillum rubrum* and suggested that it might be a tocopherol precursor. However, this organism does not contain tocopherols, and the phenol is labeled by p-hydroxy-^{14}C-benzoate,[13] a precursor which apparently is not incorporated into tocopherols.[8]

The work of Booth and his colleagues provides most of the remainder of information relevant to the biogenesis of tocopherols in plants. They have shown that evergreen and slow-growing leaves contain up to 450 ppm of tocopherol, whereas fast-growing leaves contain as little as 7 ppm.[14] Tocopherol concentrations were always found to be higher in parts of plants where growth was less, and dying and fallen leaves contained more tocopherol than fresh green leaves. Winter concentrations were, in general, higher than summer concentrations. In isolated leaves or chloroplasts, tocopherol was destroyed in the presence of light and increased in its absence[15] (but this may depend on the method of isolation[16]). The observations of Sironval and Tannir-Lomba[17] appear to contradict those of Booth, in that they found more

[11] J. F. Pennock, F. W. Hemming, and J. D. Kerr, *Biochem. Biophys. Res. Commun.* **17**, 542 (1964).

[12] K. J. Whittle, B. G. Audley, and J. F. Pennock, *Biochem. J.* **103**, 21C (1967).

[13] R. K. Olsen, G. D. Daves, H. W. Moore, K. Folkers, W. W. Parson, and H. Rudney. *J. Amer. Chem. Soc.* **88**, 5919 (1966).

[14] V. H. Booth and A. Hobson-Frohock, *J. Sci. Food. Ag.* **12**, 253 (1960).

[15] V. H. Booth, *Phytochemistry* **3**, 273 (1964).

[16] R. A. Dilley and F. L. Crane, *Biochem. Biophys. Acta* **75**, 142 (1963).

[17] C. Sironval and J. El Tannir-Lomba, *Nature (London)* **185**, 855 (1960).

"vitamin E" in young leaves than in old ones and more near the apex than near the base of the leaf. However, Sironval and Tannir-Lomba did not use chromatographic methods of separation, and the identity of their reducing compound is not certain. The biosynthesis of tocopherol during flowering has been studied, but the results are likewise contradictory.[14, 17]

Recent studies by several groups of workers[7, 18, 19] have indicated that α-tocopherolquinone occurs in chloroplasts in considerable quantities. The β- and γ-tocopherolquinones have also been found and a metabolic role for them suggested.[19] Whether these substances are formed from the corresponding tocopherols is not known. The reverse is, of course, possible.

VIII. Vitamin E Active Compounds, Synergists, and Antagonists

G. BRUBACHER AND O. WISS

In contrast to other vitamins, the vitamin E activity is not closely related to one single substance. Several of the naturally occurring tocopherols differing from the α-tocopherol by substitutions in the chroman ring system show a considerable vitamin E activity (Table XX).

The artificially produced 3,4-dehydro-α-tocopherol has, in the hemolysis test, 65 % of the activity of the α-tocopherol.[1]

Variations of the structure of the side chain are also possible without losing the whole biological activity of the tocopherol. The naturally occurring ζ_1-tocopherol and ε-tocopherol having unsaturated side chains were found to be partially active in various tests (Table XXI).

Among synthetic isoprenologs of α-tocopherol, the one with one more isoprene unit in the side chain has a marked biological activity. Others with longer and shorter chains, such as, e.g., compounds with one or nine isoprene units, turned out to be completely inactive.[1]

It is generally assumed that esters of α-tocopherol, such as α-tocopheryl acetate and succinate, have, on a molar basis, the same biological activity as the free α-tocopherol.

Of other compounds derived from α-tocopherol, the methyl ether,[2]

[18] C. Bucke, M. Halloway, and R. A. Morton, *Proc. Biochem. Soc.* **90**, 41P (1964).
[19] M. D. Henninger, R. A. Dilley, and F. L. Crane, *Biochem. Biophys. Res. Commun.* **10**, 237 (1963).
[1] H. Weiser, personal communication (1962).
[2] H. S. Olcott, *J. Biol. Chem.* **110**, 695 (1935).

TABLE XX

VITAMIN E ACTIVITY OF HOMOLOGS OF α-TOCOPHEROL IN RATS[a,b]

-Tocopherol	-Tocol	Gestation resorption	Hemolysis
α-	5,7,8-Trimethyl-	100	100
β-	5,8-Dimethyl-	25—40	15—25
γ-	7,8-Dimethyl-	8—19	3—18
ζ_2-	5,7-Dimethyl-	47	60
δ-	8-Methyl-	0.7	0.3
η-	7-Methyl-	3	1
	5-Methyl-	9	3—13
	Tocol		1—5

[a] For references, see J. Bunyan, J. Green, E. E. Edwin, and A. T. Diplock, *Biochem. J.* **75**, 460 (1960).

[b] The values are all related to α-tocopherol on a molar basis. Where the comparison was made between a *dl*-form and a *d*-form or between free tocopherol and the acetate, we have recalculated the values with the assumption that between *d*- and *dl* there exists for all tocopherols a ratio in activity of 1.36 and that the vitamin E activity of the acetate and the free tocopherol are equal on a molar basis.

TABLE XXI

VITAMIN E-ACTIVITY IN RATS OF TOCOPHEROLS WITH UNSATURATED SIDE CHAIN[a,b]

Compounds		Gestation resorption	Hemolysis
ζ_1-Tocopherol	5,7,8-Trimethyl-to-cotrien-3',7',11'-ol	21	17
ε-Tocopherol	5,8-Dimethyltoco-trien-3',7',11'-ol	4	1–4

[a] J. Bunyan, D. McHale, J. Green, and S. Marcinkiewicz, *Brit. J. Nutr.* **15**, 253 (1961).

[b] The values were recalculated as described in footnote b, Table XX.

α-tocopheryl-hydroquinone[3–5] and the potassium iron(III)-cyanide oxidation product of α-tocopherol[6] have to be mentioned. Only α-tocopheryl-hydroquinone has a certain vitamin E-activity, however, it is not yet clear

[3] J. B. Mackenzie, H. Rosenkrantz, S. Ulick, and A. T. Milhorat, *J. Biol. Chem.* **183**, 655 (1950).

[4] J. B. Mackenzie and C. G. Mackenzie, *J. Nutr.* **67**, 223 (1959).

[5] J. B. Mackenzie and C. G. Mackenzie, *J. Nutr.* **72**, 322 (1960).

[6] D. R. Nelan and C. D. Robeson, *J. Amer. Chem. Soc.* **84**, 2963 (1962).

whether this activity is caused by an interconversion of α-tocopherylhydroquinone into α-tocopherol *in vivo*.[5]

Several derivatives of ubiquinone (coenzyme Q) were claimed to have vitamin E activity.[7, 8] Of special interest is the coenzyme Q_4-chromanol which is able to cure the macrocytic anemia caused by vitamin E-deficiency in monkeys and children.[9]

Because of its three asymmetric C-atoms (see formula below) several isomeric forms of α-tocopherol are possible.

The naturally occurring *d*-α-tocopherol is optically active in all three centres [(2*R*, 4′*R*, 8′*R*)α-tocopherol]. Whereas racemization of the carbon 4′ and 8′ has no influence on the biological activity,[10, 11] the *dl*-α-tocopherol with racemic carbon in position 2 has about 75% of the activity of the *d*-form. As described in more detail on page 87, the relative activity of *d*-α-tocopherol versus *dl* has been established in a great number of various trials. When comparing the single compound of the racemic mixture, however, some discrepancies were noticed with regard to the established factor of 1:1.36 of *dl*-α- versus *d*-α-tocopherol, inasmuch as the *l*-compound was found to be less active than was to be expected.[10, 11] This fact can be explained by assuming a synergistic effect of *d*- and *l*-α-tocopherol when given in a mixture. Indeed, a synergism could be demonstrated for the absorption between *d*- and *l*-α-tocopherol from the intestinal tract in rats.[12, 13]

Vitamin E deficiency is characterized by a great variety of symptoms depending on nutritional conditions and animal species. It is generally assumed that vitamin E-active substances structurally related to α-tocopherol despite quantitative differences in the activity are qualitatively equally active for counteracting the various deficiency symptoms. For other categories

[7] B. C. Johnson, Q. Crider, C. H. Shunk, B. O. Linn, E. L. Wong, and K. Folkers, *Biochem. Biophys. Res. Commun.* **5**, 309 (1961).

[8] E. Snødergaard, M. L. Scott, and H. Dam, *J. Nutr.* **78**, 15 (1962).

[9] J. S. Dinning, A. S. Majaj, S. A. Azzam, W. J. Darby, C. H. Shunk, and K. Folkers, *Amer. J. Clin, Nutr.* **13**, 169 (1963).

[10] H. Weiser, G. Brubacher, and O. Wiss, *Science* **140**, 80 (1963).

[11] S. R. Ames, M. I. Ludwig, D. R. Nelan, and C. D. Robeson, *Biochemistry* **2**, 188 (1963).

[12] F. Weber, U. Gloor, J. Würsch, and O. Wiss, *Biochem. Biophys. Res. Commun.* **14**, 186 (1964).

[13] F. Weber, U. Gloor, J. Würsch, and O. Wiss. *Biochem. Biophys. Res. Commun.* **14**, 189 (1964).

—e.g., certain antioxidants such as methylene blue, N,N'-diphenyl-p-phenylenediamine, 2,6-di-*tert*-butyl-p-cresol (BHT), and 1,2-dihydro-6-ethoxy-2,2,4-trimethylquinoline—this is not true. None of these substances can replace vitamin E under all conditions.[14–18] Moreover, it is not established whether these antioxidants have real vitamin E active properties or whether their activity is due merely to a vitamin E sparing effect.[14]

Under certain conditions (white muscle disease, alimentary liver necrosis), vitamin E can be replaced partly by selenium compounds.[19] According to K. Schwarz,[20] selenium and vitamin E act independently in alternate pathways of metabolism, and both of these pathways must be impaired before a fatal deficiency disease develops.

There are no true antagonists of vitamin E. Polyunsaturated fatty acids decrease the absorption rate of vitamin E from the intestine and enhance the consumption of vitamin E in the body.[21] It seems that arachidonic and linoleic, but not linolenic acid, is responsible for this effect.[22, 23] From the data of M. K. Horwitt,[24] it can be concluded that man should ingest for every gram of linoleic acid at least 0.6 mg of α-tocopherol to maintain his α-tocopherol balance.[25] This is in agreement with values found in laboratory trials with rats.[21]

Another compound which was claimed to have an antagonistic effect on vitamin E, o-tricresyl phosphate[26, 27] has, rather, a general toxic effect on the animal metabolism which can be beneficially influenced by administration of α-tocopherol similar to the therapeutic effects of α-tocopherol in carbon tetrachloride pyridine or benzene intoxication in rats.[28–30]

[14] U. Gloor and O. Wiss, *Annu. Rev. Biochem.* **33**, 313 (1964).

[15] M. L. Scott, *Nutr. Abstr. Revs.* **32**, 1 (1962).

[16] S. Krishnamurthy and J. G. Bieri, *J. Nutr.* **77**, 245 (1962).

[17] *Nutr. Rev.* **17**, 174 (1959).

[18] *Nutr. Rev.* **19**, 217 (1961).

[19] K. Schwarz, *Vitam. Horm.* (*New York*) **20**, 463 (1962).

[20] K. Schwarz, *Amer. J. Clin. Nutr.* **9**, Pt. II, 94 (1961).

[21] F. Weber. H. Weiser, and O. Wiss, *Z. Ernaehrungswiss.* **4**, 245 (1964)

[22] H. Dam, G. K. Nielsen, I. Prange, and E. Søndergaard, *Nature* (*London*) **182**, 802 (1958).

[23] H. Dam and E. Søndergaard, *Z. Ernaehrungswiss.* **2**, 217 (1962).

[24] M. K. Horwitt, *Amer. J. Clin. Nutr.* **8**, 451 (1960).

[25] P. L. Harris and N. D. Embree, *Amer. J. Clin. Nutr.* **13**, 385 (1963).

[26] H. Bloch and A. Hottinger, *Z. Vitaminforsch.* **13**, 9 (1942).

[27] P. Meunier, A. Vinet, and J. Jouanneteau, *Bull. Soc. Chim. Biol.* **29**, 507 (1947).

[28] E. L. Hove, *J. Nutr.* **51**, 609 (1953).

[29] O. Selisko, H. Gebauer, and H. Ackermann, *Int. Z. Vitaminforsch.* **28**, 457 (1958).

[30] O. Selisko, H. Gebauer, and H. Ackermann, *Int. Z. Vitaminforsch.* **28**, 234 (1958).

IX. Biochemical Systems

J. GREEN

A. Absorption and Metabolism

Vitamin E is readily absorbed from oil solutions, whether present in free or esterified form. The necessity for bile salts for absorption is uncertain,[1, 2] but dietry phosphatides aid absorption,[3, 4] which appears to take place via the intestinal lacteals into the chyle.[5] A cyclic process of resecretion through the stomach mucosa has been suggested.[2] Tissues such as liver and blood absorb more of the administered dose than other organs, but are depleted more rapidly; on the other hand, heart, lung, and adrenals show a much slower turnover rate and still contain tocopherol after many weeks of depletion.[6-8] Uptake into liver shows a logarithmic relation to the dose and can be used for bioassay purposes.[9-11] Lower homologs of α-tocopherol are absorbed less readily.[12] L-α-Tocopherol is absorbed and excreted more rapidly than D-α-tocopherol,[13] and there is synergism between the two forms in absorption.[14] The plasma plays an important part in tocopherol transport, the vitamin apparently being partly in the neutral fat fraction but mainly attached to the globulin fraction.[2] Intracellular vitamin E is found predominantly in the mitochondrial and microsomal fractions.[7] Heart sarcosomal preparations contain large amounts of α-tocopherol and α-tocopherolquinone, apparently of metabolic origin.[15] The metabolic fate of α-tocopherol has been studied by

[1] J. D. Greaves and C. L. A. Schmidt, *Proc. Soc. Exp. Biol. Med.* **37**, 40 (1937).
[2] J. Sternberg and E. Pascoe-Dawson, *Can. Med. Asso. J.* **80**, 266 (1959).
[3] H. Patrick and C. L. Morgan, *Science* **98**, 434 (1943).
[4] A. Scharf and C. A. Slanetz, *Proc. Soc. Exp. Biol. Med.* **57**, 159 (1944).
[5] P. Johnson and W. F. R. Pover, *Lifr Sci.* **4**, 115 (1962).
[6] E. E. Edwin, A. T. Diplock, J. Bunyan, and J. Green, *Biochem. J.* **79**, 91 (1960).
[7] S. Krishnamuthy and J. G. Bieri, *J. Lipid Res.* **4**, 330 (1963).
[8] U. Gloor, F. Weber, J. Würsch, and O. Wiss, *Helv. Chim. Acta* **46**, 2457 (1963).
[9] H. R. Bolliger and M. L. Bolliger-Quaife, *Vitam. E, Atti. 3rd. Congr. Int.* (*Venice,* 1955) pp. 30–45. Valdonegar, Veronar, 1956.
[10] W. J. Pudelkiewicz, L. D. Matterson, L. M. Potter, L. Webster, and E. P. Singsen, *J Nutr.* **71**, 115 (1960).
[11] M. W. Dicks and L. D. Matterson, *J. Nutr.* **75**, 165 (1961).
[12] M. L. Quaife, W. J. Swanson, M. Y. Dju, and P. L. Harris, *Ann. N.Y. Acad. Sci.* **52**, 300 (1948).
[13] F. Weber, U. Gloor, J. Würsch, and O. Wiss, *Biochem. Biophys. Res. Commun.* **14**, 189 (1964).
[14] F. Weber, U. Gloor, J. Würsch, and O. Wiss, *Biochem. Biophys. Res. Commun.* **14**, 186 (1964).
[15] A. T. Diplock, J. Green, E. E. Edwin, and J. Bunyan, *Biochem. J.* **76**, 563 (1960).

several groups of workers, and, although their conclusions differ, such studies are important when the biochemical role of vitamin E is to be considered. In the rabbit, 70–80 % of an oral dose of D-α-tocopheryl succinate was recovered, mostly unchanged, in the feces within 3 days. Parenteral doses, however, were eliminated more slowly and, apart from substantial amounts of free α-tocopherol in the feces, 20–30 % of the dose appeared as a water-soluble glucuronide metabolite.[16] By giving large doses of α-tocopherol to human subjects, Simon et al.[17] isolated this metabolite in two forms; an acid, 2-(3-hydroxy-3-methyl-5-carboxypentyl)-3,5,6-trimethylbenzoquinone (tocopheronic acid[18]) and its γ-lactone. Although this metabolite has also been found in rat urine,[19] its importance as a normal route of elimination remains uncertain. When D-α-tocopherol-5-Me-^{14}C was given intraperitoneally[20] to rats, mice, or pigs, a substantial quantity (in the rat over half) of the recovered radioactivity in the liver was present as a metabolite, believed to be a dimeric product of a radical oxidation of the tocopherols,[21] but which is possibly a trimeric product.[22] Another metabolic product by this route is α-tocopherol-quinone.[23] However, it is not possible to assess the biochemical significance of these substances at present, since it is clear that the metabolic fate of α-tocopherol is markedly influenced by the dose, the administrative route, the animal species used, and, probably, the dietary regimen; thus, physiological doses of free α-tocopherol given orally to the chick and the rat yield barely significant amounts of tocopheronolactone, tocopherolquinone, or other oxidative products.[9, 19] Indeed the oxidation of tocopherol under normal physiological conditions seems difficult to demonstrate.[24]

B. Antioxidant Effects

Tocopherols are effective in vitro antioxidants for fats, oils, and vitamin A preparations and have been extensively used for their stabilization against autoxidation.[25, 26] Synergistic action occurs in conjunction with small

[16] E. J. Simon, C. S. Gross, and A. T. Milhorat, J. Biol. Chem. 221, 797 (1956).
[17] E. J. Simon, A. Eisengart. L. Sundheim, and A. T. Milhorat, J. Biol. Chem. 221, 807 (1956).
[18] J. Green, A. T. Diplock, J. Bunyan, E. E. Edwin, and D. McHale, Nature (London) 190, 318 (1961).
[19] F. Weber and O. Wiss, Helv. Physiol. Pharmacol. Acta 21, 131 (1963).
[20] H. H. Draper, A. S. Csallany, and S. N. Shah, Biochim. Biophys. Acta 59, 527 (1962).
[21] A. S. Csallany and H. H. Draper, J. Biol. Chem. 238, 2912 (1963).
[22] W. A. Skinner and P. Alaupovic, Science 140, 803 (1963).
[23] A. S. Csallany, H. H. Draper, and S. N. Shah, Arch. Biochem. Biophys. 98, 142 (1962)
[24] C. R. Seward and L. M. Corwin, Arch. Biochem. Biophys. 101, 71 (1963).
[25] W. Heimann and H. V. Pezold, Z. Lebensm.-Untersuch. Forsch. 108, 317 (1958).
[26] W. Heimann and H. V. Pezold, Z. Lebensm.-Untersuch. Forsch. 111, 1 (1959).

amounts of citric acid[27] and amino acids.[28] The optimum concentration range for effective antioxidant action would appear to be about 0.01–0.1 %, and high concentrations may exert pro-oxidant action.[29] Crude natural tocopherol-containing lipids often have enhanced antioxidant activity due to the presence of natural synergists.[30] Studies *in vitro* by many workers have indicated that antioxidant activity increases with diminished nuclear methyl substitution of the tocopherol, a fact apparently at variance with the high biological activity of α-tocopherol as an *in vivo* autoxidant. Lea[31, 32] has summarized much of this work and, in the most extensive studies yet, shown that the order of activity in seven tocopherols was a function of substrate, temperature, and level of oxidation, and, under conditions approaching physiological, α-tocopherol was in fact the most active substance.

C. Interrelationships with Vitamin A and Carotenoids

There are many observations of interrelationships between vitamin A and vitamin E in the rat, the chick, and other animals. Moore[33] has summarized the situation in the rat, which is complex. Thus vitamin E decreases the rate at which hepatic levels of vitamin A are released,[33] but only when the original levels are high (approximately 30,000 IU per liver), not when the starting levels are only one-tenth of this.[34, 35] This may mean that α-tocopherol has a specific effect on the protein binding sites for vitamin A in the liver. In nutritional experiments, many workers have observed marked effects of vitamin E in increasing both the utilization[35a] and storage[35b] of vitamin A in the rat and chick and the effect has long been regarded as due to an antioxidant effect of vitamin E in the gut and in the tissues. However, Green et al.[34] and Cawthorne et al.[35] have demonstrated that vitamin E does not act as an antioxidant for vitamin A *in vivo*. The effect on vitamin A storage is probably due to an antioxidant action in the gut in the presence, especially, of dietary fats sensitive to peroxidation, but there may, in addition, be an effect on the absorption

[27] E. N. Frankel, C. D. Evans, and P. M. Cooney, *J. Agr. Food. Chem.* **7**, 438 (1959).

[28] J. Janicki and M. Gogolewski, *Oleagineux* **13**, 758 (1958).

[29] H. S. Olcott and E. Einest, *J. Amer. Oil Chem. Soc.* **35**, 159 (1958).

[30] R. E. Henze and F. W. Quackenbush, *J. Amer. Oil Chem. Soc.* **34**, 1 (1957).

[31] C. H. Lea and R. J. Ward, *J. Sci. Food. Agr.* **10**, 537 (1959).

[32] C. H. Lea, *J. Sci. Food. Agr.* **11**, 212 (1960).

[33] T. Moore, "Vitamin A" Elsevier, Amsterdam, 1957.

[34] J. Green, I. R. Muthy, A. T. Diplock, J. Bunyan, M. A. Cawthorne, and E. A. Murrell *Brit. J. Nutr.* **21**, 845 (1967).

[35] M. A. Cawthorne, J. Bunyan, A. T. Diplock, E. A. Murrell, and J. Green, *Brit. J. Nutr.* **22**, 133 (1968).

[35a] K. C. D. Hickman, M. W. Kaley, and P. L. Harris, *J. Biol. Chem.* **152**, 303 (1944).

[35b] H. Dam, I. Prange, and E. Sondergaard, *Acta. Pharmacol. Toxicol.* **8**, 1 (1952).

[36] C. G. Mackenzie and E. V. McCollum, *J. Nutr.* **19**, 345 (1940).

or physiological utilization of vitamin A.[34, 45] Moore [33] has summarized the nutritional relationships between vitamin E and carotenoids. While anti-oxidant effects may be exerted in the gut, tocopherols at an optimum level appear to protect β-carotene during its enzymatic oxidation to vitamin A in the region of the intestinal wall; at higher levels, tocopherols may induce an increased destruction of carotene.

D. Biochemical Effects of Deficiency

The great variety of vitamin E deficiency states in different species, im-pinging as they do on so many areas of metabolism, and the lack of agreement as to a unifying mechanistic concept has led to a vast and, over recent years, increasing literature on the biochemical implications of the nutritional dis-orders. In few other fields can there have been so many contradictory findings as in this, and it still remains difficult to delineate what may be the clearest biochemical findings up to the present. The reasons for this are manifold, but probably the most important are (1) the extensive interrelationships among vitamin E metabolism and other nutritional factors and environmental, especially "stress," conditions, (2) the difficulty of deciding whether observed biochemical effects are primary or are secondary to the pathological state, and (3) the difficulty of interpreting results with *in vitro* systems because of the implications of the antioxidant theory itself.

1. MUSCLE AND NITROGEN METABOLISM

Muscle is the most universally affected tissue in vitamin E deficiency. The nutritional myopathies in the rabbit,[36] rat,[37] and several other species are characterized by an increased excretion of creatine in the urine,[38] usually the most readily recognizable sign of early deficiency. Creatinuria is frequently associated with loss of creatine from the muscle of affected animals,[39] and it has been suggested that in vitamin E deficiency there is a diminished capacity to phosphorylate creatine,[40] which eventually leads to muscle degeneration. Homogenates of dystrophic hamster or guinea pig muscle synthesize less phosphocreatine and lactic acid in the presence of glycerophosphate than controls.[41] The histological changes in dystrophic muscle are accompanied in all species by a progressive loss of potassium and iron, accumulation of calcium and sodium, and a fall in total nitrogen but an increase in nucleic acid content.[42] Myosin is greatly reduced in dystrophic rabbit muscle.[43]

[37] F. Verzar, *Schweiz. Med. Wochenschr.* **69**, 738 (1939).
[38] S. Morgulis and H. C. Spencer, *J. Nutr.* **11**, 573 (1936).
[39] A. G. Mulder, A. J. Gatz, and B. Tigerman, *Amer. J. Physiol.* **179**, 246 (1954).
[40] M. R. Heinrich and H. A. Matthill, *J. Biol. Chem.* **178**, 911 (1949).
[41] J. P. Hummel, *J. Biol. Chem.* **172**, 421 (1948).
[42] K. L. Blaxter and F. Brown, *Nutr. Abstr. Rev.* **22**, 1 (1952).
[43] E. Bonetti, M. Aloisi, and P. Merucci, *Experientia* **8**, 69 (1952).

Dinning and his collaborators have studied in some detail the effect of vitamin E on nucleic acid synthesis, recently reviewed.[44] These workers have found that there is an increased turnover of nucleic acids in vitamin E-deficient rabbit muscle. Thus, more formate and less glycine were incorporated,[45] and the effect on DNA was considerably more marked than on RNA. Although nucleotide turnover is also affected by vitamin E deficiency, there is a real effect at the nucleic acid level, since a similar marked elevation of incorporation of guanylic acid[46] and thymidine[44] into the DNA of deficient muscle is found. The results are remarkably specific to muscle and bone marrow, both of which organs are severely affected in the deficiency state, and changes in nucleic acid turnover were not found to be significant in other tissues. Vitamin E may regulate an exchange reaction involving C-2 on the purine ring. Similar effects have been found in the muscle and bone marrow of hamsters, and here the abnormality in DNA turnover disappears 3 days after administration of α-tocopherol in parallel with healing and regeneration of the affected muscle.[47] Increased incorporation of ^{32}P into the nucleic acids of several tissues of the vitamin E-deficient rabbit has also been reported.[48] Prior to the onset of dystrophic symptoms, increased excretion of amino acids takes place into the urine of rabbits,[49] the increase in *l*-methylhistidine being marked.[50] Levels of carnosine and anserine have been observed to decrease in dystrophic muscle, and methionine incorporation is depressed.[50]

In the vitamin E-deficient monkey there seems to be a defect in the ability of skeletal muscle to retain creatine.[50a] Diehl[50b,c] has shown that there is a specific effect of vitamin E deficiency on amino acid transport in the isolated rabbit diaphragm; the effect is probably on the permeability of cell membranes. Protein metabolism in the vitamin A-deficient rat diaphragm is affected by α-tocopherol, also probably through changes in membrane properties.[50d] Brown et al.[50e] have found a defect in the formation of collagen in the skin of the vitamin E-deficient rat. Olson[50f] has suggested that vitamin

[44] J. S. Dinning, *Vitam. Hor.* (*New York*) **20**, 511 (1962).

[45] J. S. Dinning, J. T. Sime, and P. L. Day, *J. Biol. Chem.* **217**, 205 (1955).

[46] J. S. Dinning, J. T. Sime, and P. L. Day, *Biochim. Biophys. Acta* **21**, 383 (1956).

[47] G. B. Gerber, W. G. Aldridge, T. R. Koszalka, and G. Gerber, *J. Nutr.* **78**, 307 (1962).

[48] J. S. Dinning, J. T. Sime, and P. L. Day, *J. Biol. Chem.* **222**, 215 (1965).

[49] J. S. Dinning, K. W. Cosgrove, C. D. Fitch, and P. L. Day, *Proc. Soc. Exp. Biol. Med.* **91**, 632 (1956).

[50] I. R. McManus, *Fed. Proc. Fed. Amer. Soc. Exp. Biol.* **17**, 273 (1958).

[50a] C. D. Fitch and J. S. Denning, *Proc. Soc. Exp. Biol. Med.* **115**, 986 (1964).

[50b] J. F. Diehl, *Biochem. Biophys. Acta* **115**, 239 (1966).

[50c] J. F. Diehl, *Nature* (*London*) **209**, 75 (1966).

[50d] O. A. Roels, A. Guha, M. Trout, U. Vakil, and K. Joseph. *J. Nutr.* **84**, 161 (1964).

[50e] R. G. Brown, G. M. Button, and J. T. Smith, *J. Nutr.* **91**, 99 (1967).

[50f] R. E. Olson, *Amer. J. Clin. Nutr.* **20**, 604 (1967).

E may exert its function by acting at the genetic level as a repressor of certain enzyme syntheses. Such a role may well account for the complex way in which the vitamin affects certain aspects of protein and lipid metabolism.

2. CARBOHYDRATE METABOLISM AND RESPIRATION

Numerous effects of vitamin E on different aspects of carbohydrate metabolism have been described, and, in the opinon of several workers, this area is a primary site of the vitamin's action.[51] Over many years, a great many observations have been made, showing that there is an increase in the oxygen consumption of muscle strips and homogenates (especially in the former and not always in the latter[52]) from vitamin E-deficient animals, such as the rat,[53] chick,[54] or hamster.[55] As shown by Vasington et al.,[56] who have summarized the extensive data, the results are somewhat inconsistent and their interpretation often doubtful as they have sometimes been obtained from animals in extreme deficiency and near death. Moreover, it is often necessary to use special conditions (such as the addition of Ca^{2+} ions[57]) to demonstrate the effect and, unfortunately, in vitro addition of tocopherol usually does not decrease respiration rates. The effect on oxygen uptake is not shared by other tissues: rat liver[54] shows no increase. However, rabbit adrenal cortex and liver slices show an increased respiration, although heart and kidney respiration is unchanged.[57]

Schwarz and his collaborators have carried out the most extensive studies on the effect of tocopherols on the intermediary metabolism of carbohydrate. They consider that dietary necrotic liver degeneration in the rat, which is a combined tocopherol and selenium deficiency state, arises from a primary defect in or near the tricarboxylic acid cycle. Thus, they have demonstrated a serious glucose imbalance in the terminal stage of the disease.[58] In the vitamin E-deficient rabbit, glucose absorption seems to take place at an increased rate and cannot be accounted for as glycogen.[59] Several workers have, in fact, observed decreased levels and, after the administration of glucose, decreased storage of glycogen in the rabbit: diaphragm, gastrocnemius, and sacrospinalis are chiefly affected.[60] Glycogen synthesis in vitro is also affected in

[51] K. Schwarz, Vitam. Horm. (New York) 20, 463 (1962).
[52] D. H. Basinski and J. P. Hummel, J. Biol. Chem. 167, 339 (1947).
[53] I. Friedman and H. A. Mattill, Amer. J. Physiol. 131, 595 (1941).
[54] H. Kaunitz and A. M. Pappenheimer, Amer. J. Physiol. 138, 328 (1943).
[55] O. B. Houchin and H. A. Mattill, J. Biol. Chem. 146, 301 (1942).
[56] F. D. Vasington, S. M. Reichard, and A. Nason Vitam. Horm. (New York) 18, 43 (1960).
[57] H. Rosenkrantz, J. Biol. Chem. 214, 789 (1955).
[58] W. Mertz and K. Scharwz, Fed. Proc. Fed. Amer. Soc. Exp. Biol. 14, 444 (1955).
[59] A. E. Milman, A. M. Treacy, and A. T. Milhorat, Fed. Proc. Fed. Amer. Soc. Exp. Biol. 13, 100 (1954).
[60] A. E. Milman, Amer. J. Phys. Med. 34, 291 (1955).

deficiency,[61, 62] and it has been suggested that there is inhibition at the phosphoglucomutase level.[62] *In vitro* addition of vitamin E to rabbit muscle strips was found to depress glycogen synthesis, but this occurred with tissues from both control and deficient animals: however, α-tocopherol was found to inhibit phosphoglucomutase in an isolated enzyme system.[63]

Rats reared on a diet deficient in both vitamin E and selenium show a metabolic defect. Liver slices from such animals fail to maintain respiration when compared to slices from the livers of rats whose diet has been supplemented with either factor.[51] This respiratory decline can be prevented by intraportal injection of tocopherols shortly before death[64] or by tocopherono-lactone *in vitro*.[65] Although permeability and ion transport mechanisms may be factors influencing the phenomenon (see also McLean[66]), a similar effect exists also in homogenates and mitochondrial preparations. Thus, vitamin E-deficient rat mitochondria show a decline in succinate oxidation in the presence of added diphosphopyridine nucleotide[67] and deficient liver homogenates fail to utilize α-ketoglutarate or succinate as efficiently as control homogenates,[68] and this can also be prevented by tocopherols or tocopherono-lactone. A primary effect of vitamin E on the removal of oxaloacetate has been suggested to account for these findings,[67] but more recently Schwarz[5] has related respiratory decline to a functional role of α-tocopherol (possibly in the form of a quinonoid metabolite) in the protection of the sensitive sulfhydryl sites of specific enzymes: lipoyl dehydrogenase may be a primary site. Several reports suggest that the glycolytic cycle is enhanced in vitamin E-deficient rabbit muscle,[69] rat cornea,[70] and bone marrow.[71]

There is a considerable conflict of opinion as to the effect of vitamin E on oxidative enzymes. Although early studies[72] described increases in succin-oxidase activity in hamster dystrophic muscle, the opposite has been reported.[73] No effect of vitamin E has been observed on the activity of succinic

[61] A. E. Milman and A. T. Milhorat, *Fed. Proc. Fed. Amer. Soc. Exp. Biol.* **14**, 445 (1955).

[62] K. L. Zierler, R. I. Levy, and J. L. Lilienthal, *Bull. Johns Hopkins Hosp.* **92**, 41 (1953).

[63] H. Rosenkrantz and R. O. Laferté, *Proc. Soc. Exp. Biol. Med.* **106**, 391 (1961).

[64] S. S. Chernick, J. G. Moe, G. P. Rodnan, and K. Schwarz, *J. Biol. Chem.* **217**, 829 (1955).

[65] K. Schwarz, W. Mertz, and E. J. Simon, *Biochim. Biophys. Acta* **32**, 484 (1959).

[66] A. E. McLean, *Biochem. J.* **87**, 164 (1963).

[67] L. M. Corwin and K. Schwarz, *J. Biol. Chem.* **234**, 191 (1959).

[68] L. M. Corwin and K. Schwarz, *J. Biol. Chem.* **235**, 3387 (1960).

[69] M. P. Carpenter, P. B. McCay, and R. Caputto, *Fed. Proc. Fed. Amer. Soc. Exp. Biol.* **16**, 162 (1957).

[70] M. D'Esposito, *Ann. ottalmol. Clin. Ocul.* **83**, 283 (1957).

[71] S. Di Bella, *Boll. Soc. Ital. Biol. Sper.* **30**, 1035 (1954).

[72] O. B. Houchin, *J. Biol. Chem.* **146**, 313 (1942).

[73] R. L. Shirley, J. F. Easley, and G. K. Davis, *Abstr. 129th Meet. Amer. Chem. Soc., Dallas* p. 29C (1956).

dehydrogenase in hamster muscle homogenates,[74] or on malic dehydrogenase, cytochrome oxidase, succinic dehydrogenase, lactic dehydrogenase, or fumarase activities in rabbit muscle homogenates.[75] An interesting finding is that citric acid levels are elevated[76] and isocitric dehydrogenase activities decreased[77] in dystrophic rabbit musculature. These reports continue to suggest an effect of vitamin E in the tricarboxylic acid cycle, and this is supported by the observation[78] that exogenous glutamic acid relieves the symptoms of vitamin E deficiency in the rabbit: variation in the glutamic-oxaloacetic transaminase levels suggests that a modified metabolic degradation of glutamic acid to yield more α-ketoglutarate may occur. CoA levels are decreased in dietary hepatic necrosis in the rat.[79]

3. ELECTRON TRANSPORT AND OXIDATIVE PHOSPHORYLATION

α-Tocopherol is to be found, to some considerable extent, in active respiratory coenzyme systems. Horse heart-muscle sarcosomal preparations have been shown to contain 0.1–0.4 μM of α-tocopherol/gm protein[80, 81] and about 0.05 μM of α-tocopherolquinone/gm protein.[81] Most of the former and all of the latter was found in the sarcosomal fragments. The presence of tocopherol has also been confirmed by suitable analytical procedures (which must include partition chromatography) in highly purified NAD–cytochrome c reductase preparations.[56] The question of the role of α-tocopherol in these preparations and whether it is an essential one in electron transport has been extensively discussed since it was originally observed by Nason and Lehman[82] that tocopherols could reactivate particulate NAD–cytochrome c reductase and succinic–cytochrome c reductase preparations that had been extracted with isooctane. These authors have suggested that α-tocopherol might be the antimycin-sensitive factor and a true catalytic factor in electron transport. However, other workers have demonstrated that this effect of tocopherol is, in many respects, nonspecific and is shared by certain other lipids, especially isoprenoid substances, and these views have been summarized by Slater.[80] The phenomenon of enzyme reactivation is generally regarded by most

[74] D. H. Basinski and J. P. Hummel, *J. Biol. Chem.* **167**, 339 (1947).
[75] H. P. Jacobi, S. Rosenblatt, V. M. Wilder, and S. Morgulis, *Arch. Biochem.* **27**, 19 (1950).
[76] H. H. Taussky, A. Washington, E. Zubillager, and A. T. Milhorat, *Nature (London)* **196**, 1100 (1962).
[77] T. A. Barry and H. Rosenkrantz, *J. Nutr.* **76**, 447 (1962).
[78] R. O. Laferté, H. Rosenkrantz, and L. Berlingner, *Can. J. Biochem. Physiol.* **41**, 1423 (1963).
[79] C. S. Yang and R. E. Olson, *Fed. Proc. Fed. Amer. Soc. Exp. Biol.* **13**, 483 (1954).
[80] E. C. Slater, *Proc. 4th Int. Congr. Biochem., Vienna, 1958* **11**, 316 (1960).
[81] A. T. Diplock, J. Green, E. E. Edwin, and J. Bunyan, *Biochem. J.* **76**, 563 (1960).
[82] A. Nason and I. R. Lehman, *J. Biol. Chem.* **222**, 511 (1956).

workers at present as a purely physical effect of tocopherols in removing solvent molecules from sensitive enzyme sites. However, it remains of great interest, and the presence of tocopherol in mitochondria and purified enzyme preparations may imply an important structural, if not a catalytic role, in respiration. The recent report by Nason *et al.* that digitonin inhibition of bovine heart NAD–cytochrome *c* reductase is specifically relieved by tocopherol must revive speculation in this field.[83] Vitamin E deficiency has not been found to affect the NAD–cytochrome *c* reductase level of chick heart muscle[84] or rat liver,[85] and it appears increasingly difficult to postulate a direct role for tocopherol in electron transport. Several workers have found that vitamin E deficiency leads to disturbances of phosphorylation in some tissues. Thus, there is a decrease in the formation of phosphocreatine by dystrophic muscle minces[86] and guinea pig muscle homogenates.[87] Changes in ATPase activity have rarely been reported.[88] Decreased transfer of phosphate from creatine phosphate to hexose monophosphate occurs in vitamin E-deficient rabbit muscle.[89] Increased oxidation of tricarboxylic acid substrates by washed vitamin E-deficient liver homogenates in the presence of ATP has been found.[88] Cell-free preparations from deficient tissues may show a decrease in oxidative phosphorylation [88] or no difference.[90] The problem seems complex, but there is now little support for a direct effect of vitamin E in this area. Many of the findings of earlier workers who used α-tocopheryl phosphate to study *in vitro* phenomena, on the assumption that a hypothetical phosphorylated intermediate of vitamin E might be active biochemically, would appear to be explicable solely in terms of the ionic detergent properties of this substance.[90] There is no evidence for the existence of esterified forms of tocopherol in tissues.

4. FAT METABOLISM AND LIPID PEROXIDATION

Vitamin E appears to play no direct role in either lipogenesis or the breakdown of fat by normal pathways, and the effects of tocopherol on synthesis of fatty acids *in vitro*[91, 92] are probably secondary to other disturbances or to

[83] A. Nason, R. H. Garrett, P. P. Nair, F. D. Vasington, and T. C. Detweiler, *Biochem. Biophys. Res. Commun.* **14**, 220 (1964).

[84] C. J. Pollard and J. G. Bieri, *Biochim. Biophys. Acta* **34**, 420 (1959).

[85] F. Stirpe and K. Schwarz, *Arch. Biochem. Biophys.* **96**, 672 (1962).

[86] P. D. Boyer, Ph.D. Thesis Univ. of Wisconsin, Madison, Wisconsin, 1943.

[87] J. P. Hummel, *J. Biol. Chem.* **172**, 421 (1948).

[88] I. M. Weinstock, I. Shoichet, and A. T. Milhorat, *Fed. Proc. Fed. Amer. Soc. Exp. Biol.* **13**, 482 (1954).

[89] M. P. Carpenter, P. B. McCay, and R. Caputto, *Proc. Soc. Exp. Biol. Med.* **97**, 205 (1958).

[90] M. Rabinovitz and P. D. Boyer, *J. Biol. Chem.* **183**, 111 (1950).

[91] C. Artom, *J. Biol. Chem.* **223**, 389 (1956).

[92] M. Rosecan, G. P. Rodnan, S. S. Chernick, and K. Schwarz, *J. Biol. Chem.* **217**, 967 (1955).

antioxidant effects. The function of α-tocopherol as a cofactor for castor bean lipase[93] does not appear to be specific.[94] There is little evidence that vitamin E affects the overall composition of tissue fatty acids[95] or their metabolism,[96] although an increased synthesis of arachidonic acid from linoleic acid has been observed in vitamin E-deficient rats.[97]

Other effects on specific fatty acids in special tissues have been reported; thus several changes occur in the fatty acid profile of the vitamin E-deficient rat testis, and the deficiency may inhibit the conversion of arachidonate to docosapentaenoate.[97a]

Increased arachidonate synthesis has been found in vitamin E-deficient chick liver,[97b] and Witting and Horwitt[97c] found lower total PUFA in the muscle phospholipids of E-deficient rats given dietary fats varying in their unsaturation. However, in a wide study of the problem, Bunyan et al.[97d] could find no general decrease of PUFA in the tissues of vitamin E-deficient rats and chicks, indicating that lipid peroxidation could not be widespread in such animals.

In spite of the absence of direct involvement, there is a vast and complex relationship between vitamin E and the nutritional stress imposed by the presence of fat, and especially unsaturated fat, in the diet. The most general hypothesis of vitamin E function, that the vitamin acts essentially as a physiological antioxidant, springs essentially from this relationship and although, as already indicated, there are opposing views, it seems to correlate many of the known facts. Thus, it is clear that unsaturated fats exacerbate the onset of vitamin E deficiency in many species (Dam[98] has reviewed the subject); and, not only tocopherols, but certain synthetic antioxidants will prevent or allay the deficiency signs. There has, however, been controversy about whether or how much of the effect of the substances is a protective one on traces of vitamin E. Tappel[99] regards all manifestations of vitamin E deficiency as secondary to in vivo damage of sensitive cell structures, produced by lipid peroxidation: in the absence of tocopherols, free radicals would appear to arise by such reactions as the hematin-catalyzed peroxidation of lipids, and

[93] R. L. Ory and A. M. Altschul, Biochem. Biophys. Res. Commun. 7, 370 (1962).

[94] R. L. Ory, private communication (1969).

[95] R. H. Bunnell, L. D. Matterson, E. P. Singsen, and H. D. Eaton, Poultry Sci. 35, 436 (1955).

[96] K. Bernhard, F. Lindlar, P. Schwed, J.-P. Vuilleumier, and A. Wagner, Z. Ernaehrungswiss. 4, 42 (1963).

[97] K. Bernhard, S. Lersinger, and W. Pedersen, Helv. Chim. Acta 46, 1767 (1963).

[97a] J. G. Bieri and E. L. Andrews, Biochem. Biophys. Res. Commun. 17, 115 (1964).

[97b] J. M. Gilliam and P. B. McCay, Fed. Proc. Fed. Amer. Soc. Exp. Biol. 25, 241 (1966).

[97c] L. A. Witting and M. K. Horwitt, J. Nutr. 82, 19 (1964).

[97d] J. Bunyan, A. T. Diplock, and J. Green, Brit. J. Nutr. 21, 217 (1967).

[98] H. Dam, Pharmacol. Rev. 9, 1 (1957).

[99] A. L. Tappel, Vitam. Horm. (New York) 20, 493 (1962).

these may interact at enzyme sites and structural membranes. Many demonstrations of increased *in vitro* peroxidation in the absence of tocopherol have been made; in many cases, the formation of malondialdehyde on incubation has been used as a criterion. Suitable tissues and systems are rat liver and rabbit heart mitochondria and microsomes,[100, 101] but others have been used. *In vitro* peroxidation is associated with other manifestations of vitamin E deficiency, such as erythrocyte hemolysis[102] and respiratory decline of mitochondria.[99] In a more recent development of the antioxidant hypothesis,[103] the mechanism of muscular dystrophy in deficient animals has been analyzed in terms of release of hydrolytic enzymes from lysosomes after initial lipid peroxidation and invasion of phagocytic cells: large increases of cathepsin, ribonuclease, β-galactosidase, and aryl sulfatase were recorded.

Witting and his co-workers, in a series of papers,[97c, 103a–c] have demonstrated extensive relationships between dietary lipids, selenium, and sulfur amino acid on the one hand and the development of creatinuria and other signs of vitamin E deficiency disease in the rat on the other. They regard vitamin E deficiency diseases as being essentially due to a deficiency of biological antioxidants and closely dependent on the "peroxidizability" of the dietary, and hence the tissue, lipids. Witting[103d,e] has attempted to deal with the role of vitamin E *in vivo* as mechanistically and kinetically identical with its action *in vitro* as a fat antioxidant. However, Green and his colleagues, in another series of papers,[103f–h] have studied the metabolism of D-α-tocopherol-^{14}C in a wide variety of stress conditions in vitamin E-deficient rats and chicks, and their findings cast strong doubts on the primary premises of the biological antioxidant theory. They, and Bunyan et al.[103i,j] question current concepts of "lipid peroxidation" *in vivo* and indicate that such lipid peroxides as are

[100] A. L. Tappel and H. Zalkin, *Arch. Biochem. Biophys.* **80**, 326 (1959).
[101] A. L. Tappel and H. Zalkin, *Nature (London)* **185**, 35 (1960).
[102] J. Bunyan, J. Green, E. E. Edwin. and A. T. Diplock, *Biochem. J.* **77**, 47 (1960).
[103] H. Zalkin, A. L. Tappel, K. A. Caldwell, S. Shilsko, I. D. Desai, and T. A. Holliday, *J. Biol. Chem.* **237**, 267 (1962).
[103a] L. A. Witting and M. K. Horwitt, *J. Nutr.* **84**, 351 (1964).
[103b] L. A. Witting, E. M. Harmon, and M. K. Horwitt, *Proc. Soc. Exp. Biol. Med.* **120**, 718 (1965).
[103c] L. A. Witting and M. K. Horwitt, *Lipids* **2**, 89 (1967).
[103d] L. A. Witting, *Fed. Proc. Fed. Amer. Soc. Exp. Biol.* **24**, 912 (1965).
[103e] L. A. Witting, *J. Amer. Oil Chem. Soc.* **42**, 908 (1965).
[103f] J. Green, A. T. Diplock, J. Bunyan, D. McHale, and I. R. Muthy, *Brit. J. Nutr.* **21**, 69 (1967).
[103g] A. T. Diplock, J. Bunyan, D. McHale, and J. Green, *Brit. J. Nutr.* **21**, 103 (1967).
[103h] J. Green, A. T. Diplock, J. Bunyan, I. R. Muthy, and D. McHale, *Brit. J. Nutr.* **21**, 497 (1967).
[103i] J. Bunyan, E. A. Murrell, J. Green, and A. T. Diplock, *Brit. J. Nutr.* **21**, 475 (1967).
[103j] J. Bunyan, J. Green, E. A. Murrell, A. T. Diplock, and M. A. Cawthorne, *Brit. J. Nutr.* **22**, 97 (1968).

found in most tissues are unaffected by vitamin E, but that those found in adipose tissue, although affected by vitamin E, are of dietary origin.

5. ENZYMES, HORMONES, AND RELATED FACTORS

Vitamin E deficiency has been reported to cause changes in the activities of several enzymes, some of them undoubtedly through secondary effects. One of the most striking changes is the increase in serum transaminases found in dystrophic lambs and calves,[104] rabbits,[78] and other species. These increases are often associated with decreases in transaminase activity of tissues such as muscle[105] and appear to arise through leakage of damaged intracellular membranes. Decreases have been reported in the activity of acid and alkaline phosphatases,[106] cholinesterase,[107] transmethylase,[108] pseudocholinesterase,[109] and kidney transamidinase.[110] Increases have been found in the activity of aldolase,[111] xanthine oxidase,[112] and glutaminase.[113]

Enzyme preparations from the livers of vitamin E-deficient rats and rabbits synthesize 70% to 90% less ascorbic acid than controls.[114] Tocopherol reactivates the synthesis, but the effect is not specific and is given by certain trace metals (Co^{2+}, Mn^{2+}, and Ce^{3+}) and EDTA. The impairment of synthesis is apparently due to the inhibition of a microsomal enzyme, gulonolactone oxidase, which mediates the oxidation of gulonolactone to ascorbic acid, and is associated with an increase of malonaldehyde production after *in vitro* incubation[115]. The effect seems to exist *in vitro* only, tocopherol acting by preventing the formation of an enzyme inhibitor[116] that may be associated with lipid peroxidation, for there is no decrease in the levels of ascorbic acid in vitamin E-deficient animals, nor, apparently, are lipid peroxides to be detected *in vivo*. Vitamin E deficiency has been shown to lead to a decrease in

[104] C. Blincoe and W. B. Dye, *J. Anim. Sci.* **17**, 224 (1958).
[105] M. A. Barber, D. H. Basinski, and H. A. Mattill, *Fed. Proc. Fed. Amer. Soc. Exp. Biol.* **8**, 181 (1949).
[106] L. C. Smith and S. Nehorayan, *Proc. Soc. Exp. Biol. Med.* **98**, 40 (1958).
[107] H. C. Stoerk and E. Morpeth, *Proc. Soc. Exp. Biol. Med.* **57**, 154 (1944).
[108] A. Rabbi, O. Giacalone, M. Marchetti, and R. Viviani, *Int. Z. Vitaminforsch.* **27**, 199 (1956).
[109] J. R. McLean and J. M. R. Beveridge, *Rev. Can. Biol.* **12**, 2 (1953).
[110] J. F. Van Pilsum and R. E. Wahman, *J. Biol. Chem.* **235**, 2092 (1960).
[111] R. Beckmann and E. Buddecke, *Klin. Wochenschr.* **34**, 818 (1956).
[112] R. E. Olson and J. S. Dinning, *Ann. N Y. Acad. Sci.* **57**, 889 (1954).
[113] A. I. Silakova, *Ukr. Biokhim. Zh.* **31**, 338 (1959).
[114] M. P. Carpenter, A. E. Kitabchi, P. B. McCay, and R. Caputto, *J. Biol. Chem.* **234**, 2814 (1959).
[115] I. B. Chatterjee, N. C. Kar, N. C. Ghosh, and B. C. Ghua, *Arch. Biochem. Biophys.* **86**, 154 (1960).
[116] A. E. Kitabchi, P. B. McCay, M. P. Carpenter, R. E. Trucco, and R. Caputto, *J. Biol. Chem.* **235**, 1591 (1960).

ubiquinone levels in certain tissues of the rat,[117] rabbit,[118] and avian species,[119] and it has been suggested that tocopheronolactone may either be or lead to an active metabolite.[120] A pyridine nucleotide–tocopheronolactone reductase has been described.[121] Possible effects of vitamin E on cholesterol metabolism have been summarized.[122] Several reports have suggested that vitamin E activity is associated with hormonal production,[123] and the metabolism of the adrenal appears to be affected in vitamin E-deficient animals. Corticosteroid production may be affected.[124] Vitamin E-deficiency effects are also associated with disturbances in mineral balance,[125] especially molybdenum,[126] and there are several relationships with the metabolism of glutathione and sulfhydryl groups.[51, 99]

6. MEMBRANE DAMAGE AND OTHER FACTORS

There are several indications that the function of vitamin E at the cellular level may be concerned, either solely or mainly, with the preservation of the physical integrity of specialized membranes. Thus, it has been suggested that respiratory defects of tissue slices in the absence of vitamin E may be due to trauma: such defects are commonly associated with disturbances in ion transport mechanisms.[66] Related phenomena may be involved in the protection that vitamin E affords against nutritional hepatic necrosis and the hepatic necrosis produced by the administration of certain damaging agents such as carbon tetrachloride[127] (and perhaps other substances known to produce symptoms resembling those found in vitamin E deficiency, such as o-cresyl phosphate[128] and heated or peroxidized fats). Disturbances in mitochondrial function that have been observed in vitro may also be related to a specialized role for α-tocopherol in the stabilization of the mitochondrial lipid. This could be a simple chemical, and perhaps an antioxygenic, action; it could be a more complex redox function; or a purely physical basis may be involved.

No discussion of the biochemical role of vitamin E would be complete

[117] E. E. Edwin, A. T. Diplock, J. Bunyan, and J. Green, *Biochem. J.* **79**, 91 (1961).
[118] J. Green, A. T. Diplock, J. Bunyan, and E. E. Edwin, *Biochem. J.* **79**, 108 (1961).
[119] A. T. Diplock, J. Bunyan, E. E. Edwin, and J. Green, *Brit. J. Nutr.* **16**, 109 (1962).
[120] J. Green, A. T. Diplock, J. Bunyan, E. E. Edwin, and D. McHale, *Nature (London)* **190**, 318 (1961).
[121] J. Bunyan, J. Green, A. T. Diplock, and E. E. Edwin, *Biochim. Biophys. Acta* **49**, 420 (1961).
[122] R. B. Alfin-Slater, *Amer. J. Clin. Nutr.* **8**, 445 (1960).
[123] H. A. Heinsen, *Vitam. E. Atti 3rd Congr. Int. Venice, 1955* p. 137 Valdonega, Verona, 1956.
[124] H. Rosenkrantz, *J. Biol. Chem.* **123**, 47 (1956).
[125] J. T. King, Y. C. P. Lee, and M. B. Visscher, *Proc. Soc. Exp. Biol. Med.* **88**, 406 (1955).
[126] P. P. Nair and N. G. Magar, *Curr. Sci.* **27**, 208 (1958).
[127] E. L. Hove and J. O. Hardin, *Proc. Soc. Exp. Biol. Med.* **77**, 502 (1951).
[128] H. H. Draper, M. F. James, and B. C. Johnson, *J. Nutr.* **47**, 583 (1952).

without at least a mention of the role of selenium in the complex set of inter-relationships that characterize the vitamin E-deficient state. The discovery by Schwarz and Foltz[129] that factor 3, a hitherto unidentified substance capable of preventing nutritional hepatic necrosis in the rat, was an organic compound of selenium, and the many subsequent demonstrations that inorganic selenium was extraordinarily active in preventing several other conditions of vitamin E deficiency, constitutes a most interesting chapter in the history of this vitamin. Although space is insufficient to discuss the findings in detail, it is clear that the biochemical implications, with their resultant effect on our understanding of the role of α-tocopherol, must be of paramount importance. In another field, the discovery of large amounts of α-tocopherolquinone and probably other tocopherolquinones[130] in chloroplasts must create new fields of study.

X. Effects of Deficiency in Animals

KARL E. MASON AND M. K. HORWITT

A. Introduction

1. GENERAL CONSIDERATIONS

Almost fifty years have passed since the existence of vitamin E (α-tocopherol) was definitely established. Its first recognized function as an antisterility factor for the laboratory rat has been overshadowed by its demonstrated need for maintenance of structural and functional integrity of skeletal muscle, cardiac muscle, smooth muscle, and, in some animals, the peripheral vascular system. Tocopherols play an important role as intra-cellular antioxidants, related especially to the stabilization of ingested fats and possibly of products arising in the metabolic synthesis and degradation of lipids.

Recently, more attention has been paid to the need for tocopherol in protecting subcellular components, such as those involved in maintenance of mitochondrial function and transport mechanisms. Thus, the concept that vitamin E functions as a general protector of structural lipoproteins or of the oxidizable lipid components of enzymes has become more acceptable and serves to explain the great diversity of histopathological lesions which can develop during vitamin E deficiency. Most lesions are dependent upon

[129] K. Schwarz and C. M. Foltz, *J. Amer. Chem. Soc.* **79**, 3292 (1957).
[130] H. D. Henninger, R. A. Dilley, and F. L. Crane, *Biochem. Biophys. Res. Commun.* **10**, 237 (1963).

fat in the diet, and their onset and intensity are accentuated in proportion to the amount and degree of unsaturation of the fat used. There exist the possibilities that unsaturated fats destroy dietary traces of the vitamin in the diet or the gut, and that they or their oxidation products produce a direct cell injury which is superimposed upon any other possible role of vitamin E, other than its antioxidative action.

2. HISTOPATHOLOGIC LESIONS IN DIFFERENT SPECIES

Lesions of skeletal muscles constitute the most universal finding. In the discussion that follows, the absence of recorded lesions in other tissues or organs of certain species does not necessarily mean that a need for vitamin E on the part of these structures does not exist; for the most part, it indicates either that the muscular lesions are so pronounced that the duration and degree of depletion necessary to bring about other tissue dysfunctions have not been attained, or that only a deficiency state during early life of the species has been studied and that little or nothing is known of the effects of prolonged, chronic deficiency during adult phases of life.

3. PIGMENT

Martin and Moore[1] first called attention to the occurrence of this pigment in uterine smooth muscle, skeletal muscle, sex glands, and other organs and tissues of rats maintained for prolonged periods on low E diets, and commented on its insolubility, inert and iron-free nature, and the brownish discoloration of the affected tissues. Its brownish-yellow fluorescence was also recognized.[2] Although its major site of formation appears to be in the musculature, it eventually comes to be acquired by macrophages of the adjacent connective tissues and distributed rather widely throughout the reticuloendothelial system.[3, 4] Chemical analysis of the pigment in rat uteri suggests the presence of oxidation products of protein.[2] Histochemical studies[5] suggest a lipofuchsin type of pigment derived through peroxidation and polymerization of unsaturated fats; except for certain differences in its oxidation potential, it is undistinguishable from a yellowish-brown, waxy pigment commonly observed in association with nutritional cirrhosis of rats on low protein diets and first characterized by Lillie et al.,[6] who proposed for it the term "ceroid." In paraffin sections of tissues exposed to various fixatives and fat solvents, both pigments have similar acid-fast, sudanophilic, and other

---

[1] A. J. P. Martin and T. Moore, *J. Hyg.* **39**, 643 (1939).
[2] T. Moore and Y. L. Wang, *Biochem. J.* **37**, Proc. 1 (1943); *Brit. J. Nutr.* **1**, 53 (1947).
[3] K. E. Mason and A. F. Emmel, *Yale J. Biol. Med.* **17**, 189 (1944).
[4] K. E. Mason and A. F. Emmel, *Anat. Rec.* **92**, 33 (1945).
[5] H. Elftman, H. Kaunitz, and C. A. Slanetz, *Ann. N.Y. Acad. Sci.* **52**, 72 (1949).
[6] R. D. Lillie, L. L. Ashburn, W. H. Sebrell, F. S. Daft, and J. V. Lowry, *Pub. Health Rep.* **57**, 502 (1942).

staining reactions. Furthermore, histochemical studies[7, 8] support the theory that ceroid arises through the autoxidation of unsaturated lipids pathologically accumulated in cells having an insufficiency of biological antioxidants.[8a] Victor and Pappenheimer[9] have pointed out that failure to provide sources of vitamin E, combined with the presence of cod liver oil, in cirrhosis-producing diets, is the primary cause of ceroid production, and that tocopherol supplements suppress or prevent its formation. Pigment accumulation in adipose tissue in low-E rats,[10] which provides the closest morphological counterpart to ceroid formation in the fatty infiltrated liver, is dependent upon the presence in the diet of fatty acids having chain lengths of at least 18 carbon atoms and at least two unsaturated bonds and is accentuated as chain length and unsaturation are increased.[11] The presence of peroxides in the adipose tissue[12] undoubtedly plays a role in pigment formation. The evidence thus indicates that the pigment of vitamin E deficiency and ceroid of nutritional cirrhosis are very similar,[12a] if not identical.

B. Male Reproductive System

1. RATS

In male rats depleted of vitamin E from early life, the seminiferous epithelium shows no injury until active spermatogenesis begins, during the third month of life, when a progressive and relatively rapid degeneration of the epithelium occurs.[13–17] There has been no satisfactory elucidation of the underlying metabolic disturbances, which are irreparable. The latter are so profound that vitamin E therapy must be given 10–15 days prior to first appearance of histological injury in order to give full protection; therapy begun at intermediate periods results in protection of certain seminiferous tubules but progressive degeneration in others, or degeneration in all tubules, depending upon the interval.[18] Degeneration is delayed 30–40 days by a single

[7] W. G. B. Casselman, *J. Exp. Med.* **94**, 549 (1951).

[8] R. D. Lillie, *Stain Technol.* **27**, 37 (1952).

[8a] N. M. Sulkin and P. Srivanij, *J. Gerontol.* **15**, 2 (1960).

[9] J. Victor and A. M. Pappenheimer, *J. Exp. Med.* **82**, 375 (1945).

[10] K. E. Mason, H. Dam, and H. Granados, *Anat. Rec.* **94**, 265 (1946).

[11] L. J. Filer, Jr., R. E. Rumery, and K. E. Mason, *Conf. Biol. Antioxidants, Trans.* **1**, 67 (1946).

[12] H. Dam and H. Granados, *Acta Physiol. Scand.* **10**, 162 (1945).

[12a] W. S. Hartroft and E. A. Porta, *Am. J. Med. Sci.* **250**, 324 (1965).

[13] K. E. Mason, *J. Exp. Zool.* **45**, 159 (1926); *Amer. J. Anat.* **52**, 153 (1933).

[14] H. M. Evans and G. O. Burr, *Mem. Univ. Calif.* **8**, 1 (1927).

[15] A. Juhász-Shäffer, *Virchows Arch. Pathol. Anat. Physiol.* **281**, 3 (1931); *Virchows Arch. Pathol. Anat. Physiol.* **286**, 834 (1932).

[16] A. Ringsted, "Undersögelser over testis' histopathologi ved E-avitaminose; en eksperimentel-morfologisk studie," Dissertation. Nyt. Nord. Forlag, Copenhagen, 1936.

[17] C. Engel and L. H. Britschneider, *Int. Z. Vitaminforsch.* **13**, 58 (1943).

[18] K. E. Mason, *Amer. J. Physiol.* **131**, 268 (1940).

dose of 0.5–1.0 mg of tocopherol fed on day 15 of life;[19] yet daily doses of between 0.5 and 0.75 mg are necessary to protect the testis in rats reared 16–17 months on E-low diets.[20] Prolonged deficiency has no effect on the weight of accessory sex glands.[20]

2. OTHER SPECIES

In the hamster there occurs a much more gradual degeneration of the germinal epithelium, accompanied by accumulation of much acid-fast pigment in the germ cells and macrophages of the interstitial tissue, but, unless injury reaches an advanced stage, vitamin E therapy results in relatively successful restoration of the germinal epithelium.[21] Testicular degeneration, associated with some pigment, occurs also in the guinea pig if a chronic deficiency is maintained such that symptoms of muscular dystrophy are kept minimal until after sexual maturity,[22] but therapeutic response has not been studied. Testis damage resembling early phases of injury in the rat has been observed in the rabbit,[23] the dog,[24] and the monkey.[21a] The testis of the mouse, on the other hand, is remarkably resistant; most investigators have observed no injury after deficiency periods up to 14 months;[25–28] however, Menschik et al.[29] report marked atrophy of the germinal epithelium after about 18 months. In avian forms, testis degeneration has been reported only in cockerels.[30, 31]

C. Female Reproductive System

1. FETAL RESORPTION

Intrauterine death and resorption of the fetus in well-nourished rats represents the phenomenon primarily responsible for the discovery of vitamin E and the basis for its subsequent bioassay and identification. The histopathology is presented in the classic monograph of Evans and Burr[14] and

[19] H. Kaunitz, A. M. Pappenheimer, and C. Schogoleff, *Amer. J. Pathol.* **20**, 247 (1944).

[20] H. M. Evans and G. A. Emerson, *J. Nutr.* **26**, 555 (1943).

[21] K. E. Mason and S. I. Maurer, *Anat. Rec.* **127**, 329 (1957).

[21a] K. E. Mason and I. R. Telford, *Arch. Pathol.* **43**, 363 (1947).

[22] A. M. Pappenheimer and C. Schogoleff, *Amer. J. Pathol.* **20**, 239 (1944).

[23] M. L. Chevrel and M. Cormier, *C. R. Acad. Sci.* **226**, 1854 (1948); *Ann. Endocrinol.* **10**, 19 (1949).

[24] K. M. Brinkhous and E. D. Warner, *Amer. J. Pathol.* **17**, 81 (1941).

[25] W. L. Bryan and K. E. Mason, *Amer. J. Physiol.* **131**, 263 (1940).

[26] M. Goettsch, *J. Nutr.* **23**, 513 (1942).

[27] A. M. Pappenheimer, *Amer. J. Pathol.* **18**, 169 (1942).

[28] C. E. Tobin, *Arch. Pathol.* **50**, 385 (1950).

[29] Z. Menschik, M. K. Munk, T. Rogalski, O. Rymaszewski, and T. J. Szczesniak, *An N.Y. Acad. Sci.* **52**, 94 (1949).

[30] F. B. Adamstone and L. E. Card, *J. Morphol.* **56**, 325, 339 (1934); *Anat. Rec.* **84**, 499 (1942).

[31] E. H. Herrick, I. M. Eide, and M. R. Snow, *Proc. Soc. Exp. Biol. Med.* **79**, 441 (1952).

the later studies of Urner.[32] All reproductive events are normal up to the time of implantation, which occurs at about day 7 after insemination in the rat. Several days later there is retardation of fetal development, diminished hemopoietic activity in yolk sac and liver, and rarefaction of the allantois and mesenchymal tissues of the embryo proper. Either the allantoic placenta fails to properly differentiate and invade the maternal decidua, or else the latter offers unusual resistance to this invasion. In either case, impaired vascular relationships between fetal and maternal components of the placenta appear to be responsible for asphyxia, starvation, and death of the fetus. This is followed by rapid necrosis and resorption of the fetus, more or less persistent but not severe uterine bleeding, and gradual regression of the placenta until little more than a blood clot remains at term.

Fetal resorption can be prevented by administration of adequate vitamin E at any time during the first week of pregnancy. If the dosage is critical there may be delivery of dead as well as viable fetuses, the latter rarely surviving more than a few days Less adequate dosage delays fetal death and resorption for varying periods. Under the latter conditions, fetuses at about day 16 of pregnancy frequently show pronounced changes in the vascular system (stasis, distention, thrombosis, local hemorrhages) and generalized ischemia prior to death, but no obvious lack of hemopoiesis.[33] There are also unconfirmed reports [33a,b] of a high incidence of teratogenic effects in fetuses of vitamin E deficient rats given, on the 10th day of gestation, low levels of tocopherol which would have been fully protective at earlier stages.

With prolonged depletion of vitamin E beyond the first few months of reproductive life, there is a progressive increase in vitamin E requirements for the completion of established pregnancies, and also a progessive interference with implantation of the ovum (i.e., decreased fecundity rate) as age progresses.[34, 35] Evidence points to a uterine, not an ovarian, dysfunction.[36] An eclamptic syndrome which appears to require a specific degree of vitamin E depletion at a specific stage of fetal development has been described.[36a,b]

Fetal death and resorption quite comparable to that in the rat, although not studied in great detail, occur in the mouse[25, 26] and in the hamster.[36c]

[32] J. A. Urner, *Anat. Rec.* **50**, 175 (1931).

[33] K. E. Mason, *Yale J. Biol. Med.* **14**, 605 (1942); and *in* "Essays in Biology (in honor of H. M. Evans)" p. 401, Univ. of California Press, Berkeley, California, 1943.

[33a] D. W. Cheng, L. F. Chang, and T. A. Bairnson, *Anat. Rec.* **129**, 167 (1957).

[33b] D. W. Cheng, T. A. Bairnson, A. N. Rao and S. Subbammal, *J. Nutr.* **71**, 54 (1960).

[34] G. A. Emerson and H. M. Evans, *J. Nutr.* **18**, 501 (1939).

[35] H. Kaunitz and C. A. Slanetz, *Proc. Soc. Exp. Biol. Med.* **66**, 334 (1947); *J. Nutr.* **36**, 331 (1948).

[36] R. J. Blandau, H. Kaunitz, and C. A. Slanetz, *J. Nutr.* **38**, 97 (1949).

[36a] F. W. Stamler, *Amer. J. Pathol.* **35**, 1207 (1959).

[36b] M. A. Kenney and C. E. Roderuck, *Proc. Soc. Exp. Biol. Med.* **114**, 257 (1963).

[36c] K. E. Mason, unpublished studies.

That in the mouse has been attributed to impaired production of histiotrophe.[37] In the guinea pig there may occur necrosis of the placenta and fetal death,[38] or abortion due to premature separation of the placenta.[39]

2. OVARY

In rats reared for a year or more on E-low diets, there are no alterations in behavioral estrus, ovulation, fertilization of the ovum, or its early development and tubal transport.[36] In resorbing rats there is premature regression of corpora lutea, but this is secondary to early termination of pregnancy.[40] Well-controlled observations on mice[41] indicate that lack of vitamin E results in fewer primordial ova, less interfollicular tissue, smaller but more numerous corpora lutea, and absence of neutral fat but marked increase in insoluble lipid complexes.

3. OTHER ENDOCRINES

There is no convincing evidence that vitamin E deficiency exerts any direct effect upon the function or structure of the anterior pituitary. There exists a rather extensive and controversial literature, much of which has been reviewed elsewhere.[42, 43] Alterations observed in the basophiles of the anterior pituitary of male rats, resembling those following castration, are regarded as secondary to the testicular degeneration;[44–46] they are absent in deficient female rats.[47] The pituitary of male chicks with testicular injury of vitamin E deficiency shows changes similar to those of the male rat.[31] Thyroid hypoplasia reported in low-E rats, and attributed to disturbed anterior pituitary functions,[48] seems explicable on the basis of relative inadequacy of dietary iodine.[45]

The adrenal cortex undergoes no significant change as a result of vitamin E deficiency other than an accumulation of acid-fast pigment which closely

[37] P. Soumalainen, *Nature* (*London*) **165**, 364 (1950).

[38] A. M. Pappenheimer and M. Goettsch, *Proc. Soc. Exp. Biol. Med.* **47**, 268 (1941).

[39] A. Ingelman-Sundberg, *Acta Endocrinol.* (*Copenhagen*) **2**, 335 (1949).

[40] B. H. Ershoff, *Anat. Rec.* **87**, 297 (1943).

[41] Z. Menschik, *Quart. J. Exp. Physiol. Cog. Med. Sci.* **34**, 97 (1948).

[42] K. E. Mason, *in* "Sex and Internal Secretions" (E. Allen, C. H. Danforth, and E. A. Doisy, ed.) Ch. 22. Williams & Wilkins, Baltimore, Maryland, 1939.

[43] K. E. Mason, *Vitam. Horm.* (*New York*) **2**, 107 (1944).

[44] A. A. Koneff, *Anat. Rec.* **74**, 383 (1939).

[45] C. Biddulph and R. K. Meyer, *Amer. J. Physiol.* **132**, 259 (1941); *Endocrinology* **30**, 551 (1942).

[46] P. A. T. Tibirica, J. Dutra de Olivera, and A. Aguiar, *Hospital* (*Rio de Janeiro*) **26**, 585 (1944).

[47] S. I. Stein, *J. Nutr.* **9**, 611 (1935).

[48] M. M. O. Barrie, *Lancet* **233**, 251 (1937).

resembles the "wear and tear" pigment normally present to a limited extent in the zona reticularis and may reflect diminished ability of the low-E animal to effectively stabilize cortical lipids of certain types. The accumulation of acid-fast pigment is especially marked in the mouse.[29, 49]

D. Muscular System

1. SKELETAL MUSCLE

Nutritional muscular dystrophy constitutes the most universal manifestation of vitamin E deficiency. Although the histopathological changes vary with the degree of polyunsaturation of the fatty acids in the diet from species to species, and even at different age periods in the same species, there is a fundamental pattern of change which is expressed as an acute type of reaction in young animals and as a chronic type in adult animals. The former type, of which the "late lactation" paralysis of rats is typical, has received most attention because of ease of production experimentally and occasional spontaneous occurrence in domestic animals. Since combined placental and mammary transfer of tocopherol is often barely sufficient to meet the daily needs of the young offspring of mammals, inadequacy of dietary tocopherol during the lactation and early postlactation periods, when there is unusually rapid growth and maturation of muscle fibers, can be expected to have a particularly devastating effect.

a. Late-Lactation Paralysis

When vitamin E reserves of lactating rats are critically low, the suckling young frequently exhibit a generalized paralysis, usually between day 18 and day 25 of life.[50] This often appears rather suddenly. There is clenching of the forepaws, weakness and dragging of the extremities, inability to recover posture when placed on their backs, diminution of respiration and body temperature, listlessness, and death. Spontaneous recovery may occur when symptoms are mild. Vitamin E therapy prevents the symptoms if given as late as day 15 of lactation, but it has little or no beneficial effect once symptoms have appeared. Spontaneous recovery with retention of residual paralysis has been observed,[50, 51] but it is of rare occurrence. Lesions of the brain and spinal cord have been described[52, 52a] but not confirmed. Most investigators favor a purely myogenic origin of the dystrophic process. Immobilization of a muscle by section of its nerve or its tendon prior to day 18 markedly

[49] C. E. Tobin and J. P. Birnbaum, *Arch. Pathol.* **44**, 269 (1947).
[50] H. M. Evans and G. O. Burr, *J. Biol. Chem.* **76**, 273 (1928).
[51] H. M. Evans, *J. Mt. Sinai Hosp. N.Y.* **6**, 233 (1940).
[52] M. D. Lipshutz, *Rev. Neurol.* **65**, 221 (1936).
[52a] W. de Gutierrez-Mahoney, *Southern Med. J.* **34**, 389 (1941).

protects against dystrophy.[53] Death is usually ascribed to serious impairment of the respiratory musculature, but other metabolic dysfunctions may be involved. The pathological changes have been described by Olcott,[54] Telford et al.,[55] Pappenheimer, [53, 56, 57] and Mason.[57a]

Weanling rats low in E but exhibiting no symptoms of paralysis, and rats showing spontaneous recovery from paralysis, usually show considerable muscle damage histologically.[53, 55] Similar muscle changes, unassociated with external symptoms, have been observed in newborn rabbits,[57] in prepubertal mice,[27] and in young pigs.[57b] The muscular dystrophy observed in "stiff-lamb" disease[58–59a] in "white muscle disease" of young calves,[60] and in a similar syndrome in the foal,[61] all of which occur under farm conditions and seem undoubtedly due to inadequacy of vitamin E in early life, closely resembles the early paralysis of laboratory mammals; the same is true of muscle changes observed in puppies,[61a] mink,[62] ducks,[63] goats,[63a] and chicks.[64] Of particular interest are the classic studies of Blaxter and coworkers,[64a–f] who describe in detail the symptomatology, gross pathology,

[53] A. M. Pappenheimer, J. Mt. Sinai Hosp., New York 7, 65 (1940); Physiol. Rev. 23, 37 (1943).

[54] H. S. Olcott, J. Nutr. 15, 221 (1938).

[55] I. R. Telford, G. A. Emerson, and H. M. Evans, Proc. Soc. Exp. Biol. Med. 41, 291 (1939); Proc. Soc. Exp. Biol. Med. 45, 135 (1940).

[56] A. M. Pappenheimer, Amer. J. Pathol. 15, 179 (1939).

[57] A. M. Pappenheimer, "On Certain Aspects of Vitamin E Deficiency," Amer. Lect. Ser. No. 17. Thomas, Springfield, Illinois, 1948.

[57a] K. E. Mason, Proc. 1st & 2nd Med. Conf. Muscular Dystrophy Ass. Amer., New York 1953 p. 25 (1952).

[57b] F. B. Adamstone, J. L. Krider and M. F. James, Ann. N.Y. Acad. Sci. 52, 260 (1949).

[58] J. P. Willman, S. A. Asdell, and P. Olafson, Cornell. Bull. 603, 3 (1934).

[59] J. P. Willman, J. K. Loosli, S. A. Asdell, F. B. Morrison, and P. Olafson, J. Anim. Sci. 4, 128 (1945); Cornell Vet. 36, 200 (1946).

[59a] H. H. Draper, M. F. James, and B. C. Johnson, J. Nutr. 47, 583 (1952).

[60] L. R. Vawter and E. Records, J. Amer. Vet. Med. Ass. 110, 152 (1947).

[61] T. C. Jones and W. O. Reed, J. Amer. Vet. Med. Ass. 113, 170 (1948).

[61a] H. D. Anderson, C. A. Elvejhem, and J. E. Gonce, Jr., Proc. Soc. Exp. Biol. Med. 42, 750 (1939).

[62] K. E. Mason and G. R. Hartsough, J. Amer. Vet. Med. Ass. 119, 72 (1951).

[63] A. M. Pappenheimer and M. Goettsch, J. Exp. Med. 59, 35 (1934).

[63a] L. L. Madsen, C. M. McCay, and L. A. Maynard, Proc. Soc. Exp. Biol. Med. 30, 1434 (1933); Cornell Univ., Agr. Exp. Sta., Mem. 178, 3 (1935).

[64] H. Dam, I. Prange, and E. Sondergaard, Acta Pathol. Microbiol. Scand. 31, 172 (1952).

[64a] K. L. Blaxter, P. S. Watts, and W. A. Wood, Brit. J. Nutr. 7, 125 (1952).

[64b] K. L. Blaxter and W. A. Wood, Brit. J. Nutr. 6, 144 (152).

[64c] A. M. MacDonald, K. L. Blaxter, P. S. Watts, and W. A. Wood, Brit. J. Nutr. 6, 164 (1952).

[64d] K. L. Blaxter, W. A. Wood, and A. M. McDonald, Brit. J. Nutr. 7, 34 (1953).

[64e] K. L. Blaxter, F. Brown, and A. M. MacDonald, Brit. J. Nutr. 7, 105 (1953).

[64f] K. L. Blaxter and F. Brown, Nutr. Abstr. Rev. 22, 1 (1952).

biochemical alterations, and histopathology of a muscular dystrophy produced in Ayrshire calves reared on a low-E diet. Dinning and Day[64g] have extended their studies of dystrophy to young rhesus monkeys to show that the histological picture appeared identical to that found in vitamin E deficient rabbit muscle.

Herbivorous animals as a whole appear to be particularly susceptible to withdrawal of vitamin E, and also to the presence of unsaturated fats in the diet.[63a, 65] It was in the guinea pig and rabbit that nutritional muscular dystrophy was first experimentally produced by Goettsch and Pappen-heimer,[66] although its relationship to lack of vitamin E was not clearly established until a later date.[67-69]

b. Adult, or Chronic, Dystrophy

In young rats which spontaneously recover from late-lactation paralysis there is, within a week or so, a dramatic diminution in the intensity and extent of the muscle lesions. At one month of life only occasional fibers are dystrophic; the remaining musculature is normal and shows little or no connective tissue replacement of degenerated fibers. In rats whose vitamin E reserves prevent the occurrence of early lesions, degenerative changes may not be evident microscopically until the fourth or fifth month, and gross evidence of dystrophy not apparent until the eighth to tenth month of life.

Gross and microscopic details of adult dystrophy in rats have been given by Ringsted,[70] Einarson and Ringsted,[71] Evans et al.,[72] Knowlton et al.,[73] Mackenzie et al.,[73a] Pappenheimer,[56] Martin and Moore,[1] Monnier,[74] and Mason and Emmel.[4]

[64g] J. S. Dinning and P. L. Day, J. Exp. Med. 105, 395 (1957).

[65] L. L. Madsen, J. Nutr. 11, 471 (1936).

[66] M. Goettsch and A. M. Pappenheimer, J. Exp. Med. 54, 145 (1931).

[67] C. G. Mackenzie and E. V. McCollum, Science 89, 370 (1939); J. Nutr. 19, 345 (1940).

[68] C. G. Mackenzie, J. B. Mackenzie, and E. V. McCollum, Science 94, 216 (1941); J. Nutr. 21, 225 (1941).

[69] C. G. Mackenzie, Proc. Soc. Exp. Biol. Med. 49, 313 (1942).

[70] A Ringsted, Biochem. J. 29, 788 (1935).

[71] L. Einarson and A. Ringsted, "Effect of Chronic Vitamin E Deficiency on the Nervous System and Skeletal Musculature in Adult Rats." Levin & Munksgaard, Copenhagen, 1938.

[72] H. M. Evans, G. A. Emerson, and I. R. Telford, Proc. Soc. Exp. Biol. Med. 38, 625 (1938).

[73] G. C. Knowlton, H. M. Hines, and K. M. Brinkhous, Proc. Soc. Exp. Biol. Med. 41, 453 (1939); Proc. Soc. Exp. Biol. Med. 42, 804 (1939).

[73a] C. G. Mackenzie, J. B. Mackenzie, and E. V. McCollum, Proc. Soc. Exp. Biol. Med. 44, 95 (1940).

[74] M. Monnier, C. R. Soc. Phys. Hist. Nat., Geneva 57, 252 (1940); Int. Z. Vitaminforsch. 11, 235 (1941).

The reader is referred to a recent publication by Telford[75] for a well documented review and splendidly illustrated analysis of skeletal muscle lesions observed after vitamin E deficiency in twelve different species of laboratory and farm animals. Consideration is given to electron microscopical and histochemical observations, as well as to those based upon light microscopy. The effects of deficiency of vitamin E, and of other dietary factors, upon skeletal, cardiac and smooth muscle have been recently reviewed by Mason.[76]

It is of some interest that ultrastructural studies of skeletal muscle from vitamin E deficient rats[77] and rabbits[78] present convincing evidence that vitamin E is necessary for maintenance of the biochemical and structural integrity of mitochondria, which are the first cell constituents to manifest alterations. This stands in contrast to smooth muscle cells whose mitochondria appear to be little affected by the deficiency state.

Somewhat apart from these observations are those of Kakulus pertaining to the Rottnest quokka (*Setonix brachyurus*), a small nocturnal wallaby of Western Australia. When subjected to captivity and fed for a month or two a high protein diet designed for sheep, there develops a progressive myopathy which responds very effectively to vitamin E therapy.[79] The muscle lesions are quite comparable to those seen in laboratory animals deficient in vitamin E.[80] However, the finding that decreasing the size of the enclosure markedly accentuates onset and severity of the myopathy[80a] stands in contrast to other observations[53] that in young vitamin E deficient rats section of the nerve supply to a muscle, or immobilization of a limb, significantly reduces the severity of muscle lesions.

Peripheral nerves and motor end plates are reported as normal in nutritional myodegeneration of ducklings,[81] guinea pigs,[82, 82a] and young[56] and old[82b] rats; but Telford[83] finds that loss of end plates, secondary to degeneration of muscle fibers, occurs in young rats. Einarson and Ringsted[71] observed

[75] I. R. Telford, " Experimental Muscular Dystrophies in Animals. A comparative Study." Thomas, Springfield, Illinois, 1971.

[76] K. E. Mason, *in* " The Structure and Function of Muscle" (G. H. Bourne, ed.) III, Academic Press, New York, 1972 (in press).

[77] E. L. Howes, Jr., H. M. Price, and J. M. Blumberg, *Amer. J. Pathol.* **45**, 599 (1964).

[78] J. F. Van Vleet, B. V. Hall, and J. Simon, *Amer. J. Pathol.* **51**, 815 (1967); *Amer. J. Pathol.* **52**, 1067 (1968).

[79] B. A. Kakulus, *Nature* **191**, 402 (1961).

[80] B. A. Kakulus and R. D. Adams, *Ann. N. Y. Acad. Sci.* **138**, 90 (1966).

[80a] B. A. Kakulus, *Nature* **198**, 673 (1963).

[81] A. M. Pappenheimer, M. Goettsch, and E. Jungherr, *Conn., Storrs Agr. Exp. Sta., Bull.* **229** (1939).

[82] W. M. Rogers, A. M. Pappenheimer, and M. Goettsch, *J. Exp. Med.* **54**, 167 (1931).

[82a] H. Chor and R. E. Dolkart, *Arch. Pathol.* **27**, 497 (1939).

[82b] N. Malamud, M. M. Nelson, and H. M. Evans, *Ann. N. Y. Acad. Sci.* **52**, 135 (1949).

[83] I. R. Telford, *Anat. Rec.* **81**, 171 (1941).

some atrophic muscle spindles in dystrophic muscle of adult rats which they imply may be related to alterations noted by them in ventral root fibers.

2. CARDIAC MUSCLE

Hyaline necrosis and replacement fibrosis of cardiac muscle, closely resembling the changes occurring in skeletal muscle, have been observed in the vitamin E-deficient rabbit,[63a, 84, 85] guinea pig,[63a, 86] young calf,[60, 64a-c] cow,[87, 88] sheep,[59, 89] goat,[63a] rat,[4, 90-92] and mouse.[28] The myocardial lesions are usually rapid in onset in herbivorous animals (rabbit, guinea pig, sheep, and cattle), not associated with acid-fast pigment, and frequently the cause of sudden death through myocardial failure. This is in striking contrast to other laboratory animals (rat, hamster, and cotton rat) in which extensive focal necrosis and scarring of the myocardium, with accumulation of pigment in muscle fibers and macrophages, may exist for many months without serious effects. Electrocardiographic changes of varying degrees, indicative of myocardial damage without involvement of the conducting system (Purkinje fibers), have been found in the rat, guinea pig, rabbit, cattle, and monkey. The most dramatic picture is seen in sudden collapse of cattle in cardiac failure, usually with little or no symptomatology prior to exitus.[88]

3. SMOOTH MUSCLE

Rats deprived of vitamin E for several months exhibit a yellowish discoloration of the uteri which gradually increases to a chestnut brown color as deficiency progresses, due to the accumulation of brownish, fluorescent, acid-fast pigment granules in the smooth muscle cells and macrophages of the myometrium.[1, 2, 4, 92-95] A similar but somewhat less pronounced change occurs in the smooth musculature of the fallopian tube, cervix, vagina, seminal vesicle, prostate, vas deferens, ureter, trabeculae and capsule of the

[84] A. J. Gatz and O. B. Houchin, *Anat. Rec.* **110**, 249 (1951).

[85] J. H. Bragdon and H. D. Levine, *Amer. J. Pathol.* **25**, 265 (1949).

[86] S. Americano Freire and B. Figueiredo Magalhaes, *Rev. Brasil. Biol.* **2**, 91 (1943).

[87] T. W. Gullickson and C. E. Calverley, *Science* **104**, 312 (1946).

[88] T. W. Gullickson, *Ann. N.Y. Acad. Sci.* **52**, 256 (1949).

[89] R. Culick, F. A. Bacigalupo, F. Thorp, Jr., R. W. Luecke, and R. H. Nelson, *J. Anim. Sci.* **10**, 1006 (1951).

[90] S. Americano Freire, *Brasil-Med.* **55**, 308 (1941).

[91] G. J. Martin and F. B. Faust, *Exp. Med. Surg.* **5**, 405 (1947).

[92] W. Ruppel, *Naunyn-Schmiedebergs Arch. Exp. Pathol. Pharmakol.* **206**, 584 (1949).

[93] W. Hessler, *Int. Z. Vitaminforsch.* **11**, 9 (1941).

[94] V. Demole, *Int. Z. Vitaminforsch.* **8**, 338 (1939); *Schweiz. Med. Wochenschr.* **71**, 1251 (1941).

[95] J. C. Radice and M. L. Herraiz, *Ann. N.Y. Acad. Sci.* **52**, 126 (1949).

spleen, small intestine, bronchi, and uterine and pulmonary veins.[1, 4, 92-94]

The uterine changes constitute a prototype for those observed in smooth muscle elsewhere. Pigment granules appearing first at each pole of the nucleus gradually push the myofibrillae peripherally, eventually distending and even distorting the muscle cells so that they are difficult to distinguish from intervening pigment-laden macrophages. Electronmicroscopical studies[77, 95a,b] indicate that in the affected smooth muscle cells unsaturated lipids accumulate in the region of the Golgi apparatus, where metabolic activities are particularly high, and are oxidized and polymerized in increasing amounts; they are subsequently bound to proteins to variable degrees.

4. EFFECT OF PEROXIDATION AND SELENIUM ON THE DEVELOPMENT OF MUSCULAR DYSTROPHY

Recent studies of the effects of varying the level of unsaturation of fats and of selenium in the diet have focused attention on how the needs for tocopherol may be modified by altering the lipid composition of the tissues. Using the onset of creatinuria in rats as an assay technique, Century and Horwitt[96] and Horwitt et al.,[96a] related the degree of unsaturation of different fats to the rate of development of experimental myopathy. To quantitize such effects, Witting and Horwitt[96b] fed synthetic fats to certify the close relationships between the estimated peroxidizability of fats fed, the type of fats that accumulate in the tissues, and the rate of production of creatinuria.

The ability of trace amounts of selenium to inhibit the development of classic signs of vitamin E deficiency[97] is not completely explainable in biochemical terms. Possibly the most logical explanation, especially to those who consider that tocopherol is primarily or solely a tissue antioxidant, is related to recent observations that seleno-organic compounds are strong antioxidants. Data to support the antioxidant function of seleno-amino acids have been reported by Olcott et al.,[98] Bieri and Andrews,[98a] and Zalkin et al.[98b] Most convincing is the report by Hamilton and Tappel[98c] which included

[95a] P. Gedigk and R. Fischer, Virchow's Arch. Pathol. Anat. 332, 431 (1959).
[95b] P. Gedigk and W. Wessel, Virchow's Arch. Pathol. Anat. 337, 367 (1964).
[96] B. Century and M. K. Horwitt, J. Nutr. 72, 357 (1960).
[96a] M. K. Horwitt, C. C. Harvey, B. Century, and L. A. Witting, J. Amer. Diet. Ass. 38, 231 (1961).
[96b] L. A. Witting and M. K. Horwitt, J. Nutr. 82, 19 (1964).
[97] K. Schwarz and C. M. Foltz, J. Amer. Chem. Soc. 79, 3292 (1957).
[98] H. S. Olcott, W. D. Brown, and J. Van der Veen, Nature (London) 191, 1201 (1961).
[98a] J. G. Bieri and E. L. Andrews, J. Amer. Oil Chem. Soc. 40, 365 (1963).
[98b] H. Zalkin, A. L. Tappel, and J. P. Jordon, Arch. Biochem. Biophys. 91, 117 (1960).
[98c] J. W. Hamilton and A. L. Tappel, J. Nutr. 79, 493 (1963).

observations that the protein tissue fractions from selenium-fed animals strongly inhibited the hematin catalyzed oxidations of linoleates *in vitro*. Additions of selenium below toxic levels can stimulate the growth of rats fed casein diets deficient in tocopherol.[99] Some selenium may be required as an essential nutrient, but increased levels of either tocopherol or selenium decrease the requirement for the other. Zalkin *et al.*[99a] have shown that large increases in lysosomal hydrolytic enzymes appear in the leg muscles of rabbits during nutritional muscular dystrophy. Whether this is a symptom, like creatinuria and aminoaciduria, or a cause of the syndrome, is not yet clear. It remains logical that the primary pathology is associated with damage to the cells due to lipid peroxidation, and that this is followed by the invasion of phagocytic cells which in turn bring the lysosomal enzymes to the site of tissue damage. There is also an extensive literature, recently reviewed,[76] relative to interrelationships between vitamin E and selenium in previously recognized manifestations of vitamin E deficiency, especially in farm animals and poultry. Most recent evidence points toward the essentiality of selenium for the absorption of lipids and of vitamin E from the digestive tract.[99b]

E. Nervous System

Skeletal muscle lesions of vitamin E deficiency in various species studied have generally been regarded as purely myogenic. However, Einarson and Ringsted[71] and Monnier[74] first reported that after prolonged deficiency in the rat there occurs demyelinization of axons and gliosis in posterior spinal fasciculi (gracilis and cuneatus) and dorsal nerve roots; also noted was an accumulation of acid-fast pigment, decrease in Nissl substance, and atrophy of anterior horn cells suggestive of late spinal atrophy superimposed upon the myopathic lesions. Einarson[100] later concluded that the myopathic and neuropathic lesions represented separate and unrelated manifestations of vitamin E deprivation. The same can be said of the widespread "lipodystrophy" and atrophy of neurons in the spinal cord motor nuclei, reticular formation of the brain stem, and cerebral cortex observed by Einarson and Telford[100a] in the deficient monkey.

Alterations in the fasciculi gracilis and cuneatus, sometime referred to as "systemic axonal dystrophy," have since been reported in the rat by various investigators.[100b–d] Recent evidence of similar lesions in vitamin E deficient

[99] L. A. Witting and M. K. Horwitt, *Lipids* 2, 89 (1967).

[99a] H. Zalkin, A. L. Tappel, K. A. Caldwell, S. Shibko, I. D. Desai, and T. A. Holliday, *J. Biol. Chem.* 237, 2678 (1962).

[99b] M. L. Scott, G. Olson, L. Krook, and W. R. Brown, *J. Nutr.* 91, 573 (1967).

[100] L. Einarson, *Acta Psychiat. Neurol. Scand. Suppl.* 78, 9 (1952).

[100a] L. Einarson and I. R. Telford, *Anat. Skrifter*, III, 1 (1960).

[100b] C. N. Luttrell and K. E. Mason, *Ann. N.Y. Acad. Sci.* 52, 113 (1949).

[100c] A. Pentschew and K. Schwarz, *Acta Neuropathol.* 1, 313 (1962).

[100d] P. Lampert and A. Pentschew, *Acta Neuropathol.* 4, 158 (1964).

dogs,[101, 101a] in association with rather minimal changes in skeletal muscles, supports the concept of the unrelated nature of neural and muscle alterations in vitamin E deficiency. Neural changes have not been observed in the guinea pig, rabbit, hamster, lambs or calves, where lesions of skeletal muscle have received much attention.

F. Vascular System

1. CHICKS

a. Embryonic Mortality

According to Adamstone,[102] inadequate vitamin E in the chick egg results in embryonic death at about the fourth day of incubation, due to disintegration of blood vessels of the blastoderm, hemorrhage into the coelom and exocoelom, and cellular proliferations in the blastoderm which interrupt the vitelline circulation. If this critical period is passed, there may be spontaneous rupture of vascular channels at various sites within the embryo, usually associated with clusters of pycnotic histiocyte-like cells at the points of extravasation. Whether these cells are responsible for the vascular rupture or represent a protective reaction at the site of injury has not been satisfactorily established.

b. Exudative Diathesis

Chicks reared from hatching on low-E diets usually exhibit a state of exudative diathesis or of nutritional encephalomalacia, or sometimes both, during the first two months of life. The two manifestations appear to be secondary to dysfunctions of the capillary bed, sometimes regress spontaneously, and are influenced considerably by variations in fats and other dietary components.

Exudative diathesis, as described by Dam and Glavind,[103] is characterized grossly by the appearance of large patches of subcutaneous edema on the breast and abdomen, and less frequently on the neck, legs, or wings. These represent local subcutaneous and interfascial accumulations of a plasm-like fluid frequently tinged greenish by decomposed hemoglobin. The affected tissues show edema, hyperemia, and increased permeability of the capillaries as indicated by increased absorption of intravenously injected Trypan blue.

[101] K. C. Hayes, S. W. Nielsen, and J. E. Rousseau, J. Nutr. 99, 196 (1969).
[101a] K. C. Hayes, J. E. Rousseau, and D. M. Hegsted, J. Amer. Vet. Med. Ass. 157, 64 (1969).
[102] F. B. Adamstone, J. Morphol. 52, 47 (1931); Arch. Pathol. 31, 622 (1941).
[103] H. Dam and J. Glavind, Nature (London) 143, 810 (1939); Skand. Arch. Physiol. 82, 299 (1939).

The subcutaneous tissue at the site of old lesions retains a buff color for some time.[104] Bird and Culton[105] describe more severe manifestations of a similar disorder in which edema of brain and lungs, marked distention of heart and pericardium, generalized ascites, and coronary and intestinal hyperemia usually terminate in stupor and death of the chicks.

c. Nutritional Encephalomalacia

This disorder of the nervous system, as described by Pappenheimer et al.,[57, 81, 106, 107] and by Adamstone,[108] is characterized by motor incoordination, ataxia, head retraction, coarse tremors, opisthotonos, prostration with legs spastic and claws strongly flexed, somnolence, stupor, and death. At necropsy there is gross swelling, flattening, irregular distortion, and greenish-brown discoloration of the cerebral convolutions. Similar lesions frequently occur in the cerebrum, midbrain, and medulla. They vary from small focal areas to large confluent patches of ischemic necrosis. The cerebellar lesions, microscopically, show edema and disruption of cellular and fibrillar elements of the gray matter, degenerative necrosis of Purkinje cells[108a] and the small cells of the granular layer, capillary thrombi which are especially abundant where the blood vessels make a pronounced right-angle turn at the Purkinje cell level, and small hemorrhages in the cortical white matter. Although capillary thrombosis seems to be the primary cause of the ischemic necrosis, it is possible that some of the symptomatology may be secondary to prolonged vasoconstriction or vasomotor paralysis of larger blood vessels.[107] During spontaneous or induced recovery there is active ingrowth of new blood vessels, gliosis and reparative reorganization in the softened tissues, and appearance of phagocytes with brownish pigment. The symptoms and lesions described are identical to those of "crazy chick disease." long recognized by poultrymen in brooder-stage chicks.[81]
diet it is possible to produce these two manifestations separately or

d. Influence of Variations in Diet

According to Dam,[104] exudative diathesis is rare and encephalomalacia never occurs in chicks fed purified E-deficient diets containing no added fats; furthermore, dietary unsaturated fats accentuate both manifestations, and by varying the type and proportion of fats and other components of the

[104] H. Dam, J. Nutr. 27, 193 (1944).
[105] H. R. Bird and T. G. Culton, Proc. Soc. Exp. Biol. Med. 44, 543 (1940).
[106] A. M. Pappenheimer and M. Goettsch, J. Exp. Med. 53, 11 (1931).
[107] A. Wolf and A. M. Pappenheimer, J. Exp. Med. 54, 399 (1931).
[108] F. B. Adamstone, Arch. Pathol. 31, 602 (1941); Arch. Pathol. 43, 301 (1947).
[108a] B. Century, M. K. Horwitt, and P. Bailey, AMA Arch. Gen. Psychiat. 1, 420 (1959).

concomitantly. Essentially the same diet may give a very different incidence of the two symptoms in the hands of different investigators.[109] The presence of substances such as ascorbic acid,[109] xanthophyll,[110] or redox substances of various types,[111] by virtue of their capacity to replace tocopherol as an antioxidant, may confer considerable protection against the symptoms. Thus it appears that in addition to lack of vitamin E there is a delicate balance of dietary factors which operate to determine the onset and severity of the vascular dysfunctions and the anatomic site at which they occur. In this connection reference may be made to the lymphoblastoma-like growths observed by Adamstone[112] in the liver, the intestine, and other visceral organs of the chick, sometimes leading to hemorrhage by invasion of blood vessels, when cod liver oil or sardine oil, but not halibut oil, was added to diets previously treated with ferric chloride to destroy traces of vitamin E. Century and Horwitt[113] have shown that fresh cod liver oil fed at 8% level inhibited the production of encephalomalacia unless 1% arachidonic acid was added to the diet. This was explained on the basis that cod liver oil inhibits the conversion of linoleate to arachidonate and higher essential polyunsaturated fatty acids. Scott[113a] has reviewed the interaction of vitamin E and selenium in preventing exudative diathesis and muscular dystrophy in the chick, and the ineffectiveness of selenium in preventing encephalomalacia. Century and Horwitt[113b] showed that while selenium addition did not completely prevent encephalomalacia, it did prolong the time of its development in those chicks which succumed. In interpreting results of earlier studies there is need to consider recent evidence[113c] that in the chick dietary deficiency of selenium can result in degeneration of the exocrine component of the pancreas and impaired absorption of lipids, including vitamin E.

2. MAMMALS

a. Hemorrhage

The vascular stasis and hemorrhage occurring in the rat fetus, as described in an earlier section, bears a certain resemblance to the vascular dysfunction in chicks. So also do the interfascial, subcutaneous, and thymic hemorrhages observed during the second month of life in rats reared from birth on low-E

[109] L. Zacharias, P. Goldhaber, and V. E. Kinsey, *J. Nutr.* **42**, 359 (1950).
[110] P. Goldhaber, L. Zacharias, and V. E. Kinsey, *J. Nutr.* **42**, 453 (1950).
[111] H. Dam, I. Kruse, I. Prange, and E. Søndergaard, *Acta Physiol. Scand.* **22**, 299 (1951).
[112] F. B. Adamstone, *Amer. J. Cancer* **28**, 540 (1936); *Arch. Pathol.* **31**, 717 (1941).
[113] B. Century and M. K. Horwitt, *Arch. Biochem. Biophys.* **104**, 416 (1964).
[113a] M. L. Scott, *Vitam. Horm. (New York)* **20**, 621 (1962).
[113b] B. Century and M. K. Horwitt, personal communication.
[113c] J. N. Thompson and M. L. Scott, *J. Nutr.* **100**, 797 (1970).

diets high in total unsaturated fatty acids of cod liver oil,[114] and also the hemorrhages into cranial and visceral cavities, lungs, and intestine observed by Elvehjem et al.[115] in puppies born of mothers fed mineralized milk diets low in vitamin E. As in the chick studies just discussed, there are again the three factors to be considered—inadequate vitamin E, early age of animal, and some type of metabolic stress or local insult to tissues. The latter may be related to the levels of polyunsaturated lipids deposited in the tissues. Nishida et al.[115a] have suggested that vitamin E protects chicks against encephalomalacia by preventing the breakdown of linoleic acid to 12-oxy-cis-9-octodecanoic(keto)acid.

Holman[116] has demonstrated that a necrotizing arteritis in dogs, produced by induction of renal insufficiency after prior feeding of a high fat diet, can be retarded or prevented by tocopherol. Here vitamin E seems to protect against chemical injury resulting from the presence of abnormal lipids deposited in the vascular wall. Difference of opinion exists as to whether α-tocopherol does[117] or does not[118] protect dogs against stilbestrol-induced thrombocytopenic purpura. In rats, tocopherols prevent increased capillary fragility due to α-irradiation.[119]

b. Hemolysis

György and Rose have shown that hemoglobinuria, intravascular hemolysis, and death occurring in alloxan-treated rats are readily prevented by dietary tocopherols, although the diabetic phenomena are not affected,[120] and that dialuric acid, a decomposition product of alloxan, and several related compounds produce hemolysis of erythrocytes.[121, 122] α-Tocopherol, through its function as an antioxidant, protects the red cell against this chemical injury, perhaps by counteracting a free radical or peroxide formed as an intermediate of the oxidation–reduction system of dialuric acid and alloxan. On the basis of these reactions they have developed an hemolysis test which can be applied either in vivo or in vitro as a measure of the biological activity of tocopherols and of vitamin E depletion in the rat.[122, 122a] Modifications of this test have demonstrated increased tendency to hemolysis in

[114] R. E. Rumery, Ph.D. Thesis. Univ. of Rochester, Rochester, New York, 1952.

[115] C. A. Elvejhem, J. E. Gonce, Jr., and G. W. Newell, J. Pediat. 24, 436 (1944).

[115a] T. Nishida, H. Tsuchiyama, M. Inoue, and F. A. Kummerow, Proc. Soc. Exp. Biol. Med. 105, 308 (1960).

[116] R. L. Holman, Proc. Soc. Exp. Biol. Med. 66, 307 (1947); S. Med. J. 42, 108 (1949).

[117] F. Skelton, E. Shute, H. G. Skinner, and R. A. Waud, Science 103, 762 (1946).

[118] A. J. Richtsmeier, M. Spooner, and O. O. Meyer, Proc. Soc. Exp. Biol. Med. 65, 2 (1947).

[119] S. R. Ames, J. G. Baxter, and J. Q. Griffith, Jr., Int. Z. Vitaminforsch. 22, 401 (1951).

[120] P. György and C. S. Rose, Science 108, 716 (1948).

[121] C. S. Rose and P. György, J. Nutr. 39, 529 (1949); Blood 5 1962 (1950).

[122] P. György and C. S. Rose, Ann. N.Y. Acad. Sci. 52, 231 (1949).

[122a] C. S. Rose and P. György, Amer. J. Physiol. 168, 414 (1952).

red cells of premature infants,[123] full-term infants, and newborn rats.[124] Although hemolysis can be produced by many other compounds and can be prevented by other antioxidants, α-tocopherol is unquestionably a most effective natural intracellular antioxidant. Dinning[125] has reported a pronounced leukocytosis in low-E rabbits, responding to tocopherol therapy, which he concedes may reflect leukocytic infiltration of dystropic muscle. In later studies, Dinning and associates[125a,b] noted a pronounced anemia in monkeys due to inadequate erythropoiesis. Many multinucleated erythroid precursors were reported. These disappeared after tocopherol administration, and there was a marked reticulocyte response with subsequent improvement in the peripheral blood picture.

G. Other Manifestations

1. ADIPOSE TISSUE

Prolonged vitamin E deficiency in rats results in considerable diminution in body fat, accounting in part for the plateau in body weight occurring during early adulthood and for the rather emaciated appearance of rats showing advanced stages of paresis. Menschik et al.[29, 126] have studied this phenomenon in mice, reporting that adipose tissue develops normally during early life but that after about 9 months of deficiency little or no body fat is evident—except for the brown glandular fat of the interscapular region which is often increased in amount and of deeper brown color than in control mice.

A strikingly different reaction occurs in the adipose tissues of the rat when low-E diets contain high levels (about 20%) of cod liver oil[10] or highly unsaturated fractions of this oil,[127] or methyl esters of linseed, corn, or soybean oils.[11] Under such circumstances there is a brownish discoloration of the subcutaneous and intraperitoneal adipose tissue. Peroxides are usually demonstrable either by chemical[12] or histochemical[128–130] methods. Microscopically,[10, 127] the adipose tissue first appears studded with yellowish-brown islets. The latter represent clusters of fat cells in various stages of development in which small fat globules and the peripheral portions of

[123] H. H. Gordon, and J. P. de Metry, Proc. Soc. Exp. Biol. Med. **79**, 446 (1952).

[124] P. György, G. N. Cogan, and C. S. Rose, Amer. J. Dis. Child. **82**, 237 (1951).

[125] J. S. Dinning, Proc. Soc. Exp. Biol. Med. **79**, 231 (1952).

[125a] J. S. Dinning, Rev. Can. Biol. **21**, 501 (1962).

[125b] F. S. Porter, C. D. Fitch, and J. S. Dinning, Blood **20**, 471 (1962).

[126] Z. Menschik, Edinburgh Med. J. **51**, 486 (1944).

[127] H. Granados, K. E. Mason, and H. Dam, Acta Pathol. Microbiol. Scand. **24**, 86 (1947).

[128] H. Granados and H. Dam, Acta Pathol. Microbiol. Scand. **27**, 591 (1950).

[129] J. Glavind, H. Granados, S. Hartmann, and H. Dam, Experientia **5**, 84 (1949).

[130] H. Dam, Ann. N.Y. Acad. Sci. **52**, 195 (1949).

larger fat vacuoles are composed of acid-fast pigment; pigment-laden macrophages are also present in increased numbers. At later stages these cells, and possibly other connective elements, participate in complex foreign-body type of reactions leading to the formation of large, pigment-laden giant cells which eventually dominate the picture. Tocopherol therapy arrests the process but in most locations brings about no more than a limited reduction in pigment and very little change in other cellular reactions.

Similar alterations of adipose tissue have been observed in the mouse,[28] hamster,[36c] pig[131, 132] and mink;[62, 133] it is of interest that the naturally occurring "yellow fat disease" or "steatitis" of mink, frequently causing serious losses of kits prior to the pelting season, fits into this picture. In all instances a dietary intake of highly unsaturated fats and inadequacy of vitamin E have been involved. The most satisfactory explanation for the histopathological reactions described above is that unsaturated dietary fats incorporated into adipose tissue cells which lack sufficient tocopherol as an antioxidant to stabilize them, or to counteract peroxides which accumulate in the tissues, undergo polymerization or combine with cell proteins, or both, to form acid-fast pigment which provokes giant cell reactions and perhaps a certain amount of cell necrosis.

2. LIVER

Certain histopathological changes in the liver have been observed in a few species, but in most instances lack of vitamin E is merely one of several factors involved. In chicks there has been reported a phenomenon of "erythropagocytosis," in which the liver shows brownish discoloration and, microscopically, enlargement of hepatic cells, widening of sinusoids, and much hemosiderin in hepatic and Kupffer cells; there is also hyperplasia of myeloid tissue.[112] Its occurrence only when ferric chloride-treated diets are supplemented with halibut liver oil raises questions as to its specificity.

After prolonged vitamin E depletion in mice (14 months or more) Menschik et al.[29, 134] have noted progressive accumulation of coarse "lipoproteic" globules, swelling, and nuclear pycnosis in hepatic cells; they also describe sinusoidal dilation, extravasation of erythrocytes or obvious hemorrhage, hemosiderin in Kupffer cells, and disorganization of the parenchyma. Histochemically, the lipoproteic globules are composed of a mixture of unsaturated fatty acids, phospholipids, and cholesterol, probably combined with protein, resembling the "ceroid" of nutritional cirrhosis referred to before and suggesting abnormal metabolic changes in liver fat.

[131] K. L. Robinson and W. E. Coey, Nature (London) 168, 997 (1951).
[132] J. R. Gorham, N. Boe, and G. A. Baker, Cornell Vet. 41, 332 (1951).
[133] J. R. Gorham, G. A. Baker, and N. Boe, Vet. Med. 46, 100 (1951).
[134] Z. Menschik and T. J. Szczesniak, Anat. Rec. 103, 349 (1949).

In nutritional cirrhosis (diffuse hepatic fibrosis) of rats fed diets low in lipotropic factors (methionine, choline) there is an extensive fatty infiltration of the liver followed by a progressive deposition of fibrous tissue in the form of irregular trabeculae with extensive disorganization of the parenchyma. If such diets are low in vitamin E, as was usually the case in the early studies, the livers become grossly brownish-yellow and on histological examination show accumulations of ceroid pigment in cells of the parenchyma and fibrotic areas, especially in the latter.[6, 135, 136] As mentioned previously this ceroid is generally indistinguishable from the acid-fast pigment of vitamin E deficiency. Tocopherols have no influence on the fatty or fibrotic changes but retard or prevent ceroid formation.[9] The cellular reactions which occur in areas of fatty infiltration of hepatic cells are essentially the same as those described above for adipose tissue and indicate the need for tocopherols to prevent undesired oxidative changes in the infiltrating lipids. Dietary unsaturated fats such as cod liver oil accentuate ceroid formation.[137]

A different type of liver injury, known as acute or massive hemorrhagic necrosis, occurs in rats reared on diets low in vitamin E and deficient in sulfur-containing amino acids (alkali-treated casein or low casein diets)[138-141] or containing as their protein component certain yeasts (high yeast diets)[142-144] which lack an unidentified protective substance (factor 3 of Schwarz)[144] present in most American yeasts. Factor 3 has since been identified as a selenium containing compound.[97] It apparently functions in some association with the sulfur-amino acids and although vitamin E can replace it, and the possibility that seleno-organic compounds serve as antioxidants has been suggested,[98, 98c] it is not yet clear how these substances act in protecting the rat against the rather sudden onset of massive necrosis and hemorrhage in the liver[138, 141-144] or massive lung hemorrhages,[140] which cause death. In addition to widespread centrolobular necrosis of the liver, there have been noted dystrophic changes in skeletal muscles,[139, 141] ulcers of the forestomach,[143, 144] kidney lesions, and hemorrhage in lymph nodes and intestine.[144] The story of how selenium came to be recognized as an essential nutrient has been reviewed by Schwarz.[144]

[135] P. György, *Amer. J. Clin. Pathol.* **14**, 67 (1944).

[136] H. Popper, P. György, and H. Goldblatt, *Arch. Pathol.* **37**, 161 (1944).

[137] M. Wachstein, *Proc. Soc. Exp. Biol. Med.* **59**, 73 (1945).

[138] P. György and H. Goldblatt, *J. Exp. Med.* **89**, 245 (1949).

[139] K. Schwarz, *Hoppe-Seyler's Z. Physiol. Chem.* **281**, 106 (1944); *Hoppe-Seyler's Z. Physiol. Chem.* **283**, 106 (1948); *Ann. N.Y. Acad. Sci.* **52**, 225 (1949).

[140] E. L. Hove, D. H. Copeland, and W. D. Salmon, *J. Nutr.* **39**, 397 (1949).

[141] M. Goettsch, *J. Nutr.* **44**, 443 (1951).

[142] L. Lindan and H. P. Himsworth, *Brit. J. Exp. Pathol.* **31**, 651 (1950).

[143] P. György, C. S. Rose, R. M. Tomarelli, and H. Goldblatt, *J. Nutr.* **41**, 265 (1950).

[144] K. Schwarz, *Nutr. Rev.* **18**, 193 (1960).

3. KIDNEY

Martin and Moore[1] were first to describe in the kidney of rats reared on diets deficient in vitamin E and containing 20% lard, a progressive necrosis of the proximal convoluted tubules. These changes were apparent after 3 to 4 months, and be came quite widespread after 10 months or more of deficiency. According to later studies of Emmel,[144a,b] these changes reflect a tendency for the kidney to manifest an unusually rapid rate of postmortem autolysis, recognizable as early as 6 weeks post-weaning in rats fed deficient diets containing 15.5% (30 caloric percent) of free fatty acids of linseed oil. This renal abnormality is most conspicuous in the proximal convoluted tubules, is characterized by a rapid rise in tissue non-protein nitrogen, and is not readily reversed by α-tocopherol therapy. These indications of interrelationships between vitamin E and unsaturated lipids in maintaining morphological integrity and function of the kidney have received rather limited consideration.

4. TOOTH DEPIGMENTATION

Depigmentation of the maxillary incisors of the rat is recognized as a common manifestation of vitamin E deficiency; mandibular incisors are also involved if dietary protein is low.[145] This iron-containing, nonfluorescent pigment is continuously formed and deposited by the enamel organ as the incisor is worn away by attrition. The depigmentation is secondary to atrophic changes in the enamel organ.[146, 147] According to Pindborg,[148] there is edema and disorganization of the papillary layer, probably caused by capillary damage in this region, followed by epithelial derangement and cyst formation in the ameloblast layer. There is also a progressive deposition of acid-fast pigment in macrophages of the highly vascular periodontal connective tissue.[147] After vitamin E therapy, function of the enamel organ is restored and newly deposited enamel acquires its normal color. Depigmentation of maxillary incisors occurs also in the hamster,[147] but no histopathological studies have been reported.

[144a] V. M. Emmel, *J. Nutr.* **61**, 51 (1957).
[144b] V. M. Emmel and P. L. LaCelle, *J. Nutr.* **75**, 335 (1961).
[145] T. Moore, *Biochem. J.* **37**, 112 (1943); *Ann. N.Y. Acad. Sci.* **52**, 206 (1949).
[146] J. T. Irving, *Nature (London)* **150**, 122 (1942).
[147] H. Granados, K. E. Mason, and H. Dam, *J. Dent. Res.* **24**, 197 (1945); *J. Dent. Res.* **25** 179 (1946).
[148] J. J. Pindborg, *J. Dent. Res.* **29**, 212 (1950); *J. Dent. Res.* **31**, 805 (1952).

XI. Effects of Deficiency in Man

KARL E. MASON AND M. K. HORWITT

A. General Considerations

There are similarities between certain manifestations of vitamin E deficiency in experimental animals (such as fetal resorption, dystrophic changes in skeletal muscle) and certain clinical disorders in man (habitual abortion, progressive muscular dystrophy); yet, it has not been established that the latter are either due to lack of vitamin E or benefited by therapeutic use of the vitamin. If tocopherol actually does exert a beneficial effect in such disorders, the high dosage levels reported as necessary suggest a true pharmacological action on particular tissues or local regions of the body, perhaps through some influence upon deranged metabolic processes at the affected site.

Deficiency states are of two general types: natural deficiency, due to inadequate intake of a nutrient over prolonged periods of time which, in the case of fat-soluble vitamins, are measured in terms of years, if previous intake and body storage have been reasonably normal; and "conditioned" deficiency, arising through factors which chronically diminish the absorption or storage or increase the rate of metabolic utilization of the vitamin. To establish whether suboptimal or marked deficiency of vitamin E occurs in man there must be acquisition of many data on the vitamin E status of normal individuals and of others whose status might be considered suboptimal on the basis of dietary habits or organic disease. Such data must relate primarily to four major aspects of vitamin E nutriture: (1) the dietary intake over a period of years, (2) the extent of intestinal absorption and excretion (3) capacity for tissue storage, and (4) rate of metabolic utilization. In such considerations, it is customary to express vitamin E in terms of d-α-tocopherol which constitutes about 90% of the total tocopherol in human tissues and seems to be absorbed and retained more efficiently than, or preferentially to, the non-α forms, which represent about one-half the usual dietary supply.[149]

1. DIETARY INTAKE

Chemical and biological analyses indicate that tocopherols are present in essentially every article of diet; the richest sources are vegetable oils and unmilled cereals. It has been estimated that the average American dietary

[149] M. L. Quaife, W. J. Swanson, M. Y. Dju, and P. L. Harris, *Ann. N.Y. Acad. Sci.* **52**, 300 (1949).

provides approximately 14–19 mg of d-α-tocopherol daily,[150] and that the better diets probably do not provide more than 25 mg.[149] More important than the actual level of tocopherol in the diet is the ratio of tocopherol to polyunsaturated fats. The tocopherol linoleic acid ratio of experimental diets have been calculated by Harris and Embree.[150a] The losses of tocopherol which may occur during storage, commercial handling, and cooking, may be quite large.[151]

2. INTESTINAL ABSORPTION AND EXCRETION

It has been recognized that little or no tocopherol is excreted in the urine[152] and that appreciable amounts are lost in the feces.[152–154] The tocopherol content of bile is of about the same magnitude as that of the blood, and undoubtedly some absorbed tocopherol is re-excreted into the intestinal tract via the biliary tract.[152, 153] Klatskin and Molander,[153] have shown that normal individuals excrete approximately two-thirds of ingested tocopherol in the feces; they are also of the opinion that there is little or no destruction in the gastrointestinal tract, and concur with others that intestinal synthesis of tocopherol is quite unlikely. On the assumption that approximately 50% of ingested tocopherol is absorbed, it appears that a normal adult on an average American diet would have a net absorption of about 7–10 mg of d-α-tocopherol, daily.

3. TISSUE STORAGE

Most tissues and organs of man contain tocopherol, chiefly in the form of α-tocopherol, as first reported by Abderhalden who carried out a series of analyses on organs from human fetuses, newborn infants, and adults.[155] These findings have been generally verified and extended by other studies[156–159a] which begin to give a fairly satisfactory picture of tocopherol distribution and concentration in man. Unlike vitamin A, which is stored largely in the liver, tocopherol is stored chiefly in the adipose tissue. On the

[150] P. L. Harris, M. L. Quaife, and W. J. Swanson, J. Nutr. 40, 367 (1950).
[150a] P. L. Harris and N. D. Embree, Amer. J. Clin. Nutr. 13, 385 (1963).
[151] R. S. Harris, Vitam. Horm. (New York) 20, 603 (1962).
[152] G. Klatskin and D. W. Molander, J. Clin. Invest. 31, 159 (1952).
[153] G. Klatskin and D. W. Molander, J. Lab. Clin. Med. 39, 802 (1952).
[154] K. C. D. Hickman, M. W. Kaley, and P. L. Harris, J. Biol. Chem. 152, 321 (1944).
[155] R. Aberhalben, Int. Z. Vitaminforsch. 16, 309, 319 (1945).
[156] M. L. Quaife and M. Y. Dju, J. Biol. Chem. 180, 263 (1949).
[157] K. E. Mason, M. Y. Dju, and L. J. Filer, Jr., Fed. Proc. Fed. Amer. Soc. Exp. Biol. 11, 449 (1952).
[158] M. Y. Dju, K. E. Mason, and L. J. Filer, Jr., Etud. Neo-Natales 1, 49 (1952).
[159] K. E. Mason and M. Y. Dju, Nutr. Symp. Ser., Nat. Vitam. Found., New York 7, 1 (1953).
[159a] M. Y. Dju, K. E. Mason, and L. J. Filer, Jr. Am. J. Clin. Nutr. 4, 50 (1958).

basis of tocopherol content of a wide variety of tissues from two healthy adults, both cases of accidental death, total body storage has been estimated to be 3.4 gm for a 20-year-old male and 8 gm for a 40-year-old female.[156] Accepting 5 gm as the average body storage in well-nourished adults, an individual of 70 kg body weight would possess approximately 70 mg of tocopherol per kilogram of body mass. For comparison there are reported levels of 5.6 mg per kilogram in a newborn infant analyzed *in toto*, and of 3.1 mg per kilogram in fetuses of 2–6 months gestation age (average of 20 fetuses).[157, 158] Analyses of separate tissues and organs of man, as discussed later, suggest that the tocopherol content of adipose tissue provides a much more reliable index of vitamin E nutriture than that of other tissues.

B. Vitamin E in Early Life

For some 25 years considerable attention has been given to the vitamin E status of man during prenatal and early postnatal life. Tocopherol concentration is low in tissues of the fetus and newborn infant[155, 157–159a] but somewhat higher in the placenta,[157, 158, 160, 161] which, as in lower mammals, appears to have but a limited capacity to transfer tocopherol to the fetus. Tocopherol levels are also low in cord blood[160–166] and in blood of the newborn,[167, 168] generally ranging from one-third to one-fifth those of the mother; yet maternal blood levels show a natural increment during the latter part of gestation.[164, 165, 169–171] Human breast milk has a considerably higher content of tocopherol than does cow's milk;[165, 171–174] furthermore, in both species colostrum is much richer in tocopherol than is later milk.

There is thus unquestionable evidence that the newborn infant has a rather small endowment of tocopherol at birth. Analysis of one full-term infant *in toto*[157, 158] has indicated a total content of about 25 mg, or approximately

[160] R. Abderhalben, *Schweiz. Med. Wochenschr.* **75**, 281 (1945).

[161] G. Athanassiu, *Klin. Wochenschr.* **24**, 170 (1946); *Klin. Wochenschr.* **25**, 362 (1947).

[162] J. Varangot, H. Chailley, and N. Rieux, *C. R. Soc. Biol.* **137**, 210 (1943); *C. R. Soc. Biol.* **138**, 24 (1944).

[163] W. Neuweiler, *Int. Z. Vitaminforsch.* **21**, 83 (1949).

[164] J. V. Straumfjord and M. L. Quaife, *Proc. Soc. Exp. Biol. Med.* **61**, 369 (1946).

[165] P. Cattaneo and A. Mariani, *Rend. Ist. Super. Sanita (Ital. Ed.)* **13**, 424 (1950).

[166] F. Gerloczy, B. Bencze, J. Szenasy, and D. Kuncz, *Experientia* **7**, 427 (1951).

[167] W. T. Moyer, *Pediatrics* **6**, 893 (1950).

[168] S. W. Wright, L. J. Filer, Jr., and K. E. Mason, *Pediatrics* **7**, 386 (1951).

[169] N. S. Scrimshaw, R. B. Greer, and R. I. Goodland, *Ann. N.Y. Acad. Sci.* **52**, 312 (1949).

[170] W. J. Darby, M. E. Ferguson, R. H. Furman, J. M. Lemley, C. T. Ball, and G. R. Meneely, *Ann. N.Y. Acad. Sci.* **52**, 328 (1949).

[171] L. Rauramo, *Acta Obstet. Gynecol. Scand.* **24**, 193 (1944); *Acta Obstet. Gynecol. Scand. Suppl.* **27**, 1 (1947).

[172] W. Neuweiler, *Int. Z. Vitaminforsch.* **20**, 108 (1948).

[173] M. L. Quaife, *J. Biol. Chem.* **169**, 513 (1947).

[174] P. L. Harris, M. L. Quaife, and P. O'Grady, *J. Nutr.* **46**, 459 (1952).

the daily intake of an adult on a high-quality diet. It also appears that tocopherol concentration in tissues shows no significant increase during the first three years of postnatal life.[159a] It is pertinent at this point to call attention to the fact that certain manifestations of vitamin E deficiency have been produced only during relatively early phases of life of the species, and that in producing states of experimental vitamin E deficiency it has always been a practice to initiate the deficient diet early in life, before any appreciable tissue storage has occurred, because of the recognized difficulty in depleting tissue reserves of the vitamin.

1. SUSCEPTIBILITY OF ERYTHROCYTES TO HEMOLYSIS

György and his associates[175, 176] have demonstrated that erythrocytes of low-E adult rats, and of newborn rats from mothers on stock diets, are readily hemolyzed *in vivo* or *in vitro* by small amounts of dialuric acid, alloxantin (both reduction products of alloxan), or hydrogen peroxide, and that small amounts of α-tocopherol protect the cells against these effects.

Furthermore, György *et al.*[176] reported that the red blood cells of full-term infants at birth show mild hemolysis when exposed to small amounts of hydrogen peroxide, that incubation of washed erythrocytes with α-tocopherol makes them resistant to this effect, and that tocopherol fed to the infant (but not when given to the pregnant mother) accelerates the disappearance of this fragility, which normally occurs during the first week or so of postnatal life. They speculate that "the physiologic vitamin E deficiency of the fetus and the newborn may have practical clinical implications in Rh-incompatibility as well as in the development of erythroblastosis in newborn infants of diabetic and prediabetic mothers." Of additional significance are the reports by Gordon and deMetry[177] and Mackenzie[178] describing hemolysis of red cells, by the hydrogen peroxide test, in premature infants bottle-fed for periods up to 30 days after birth, and disappearance of this fragility within 2–5 days after tocopherol administration to the infant. They emphasize the low tocopherol content of most artificial formulas for infants, compared to that of breast milk, as have Wright *et al.*,[168] who showed that in bottle-fed full-term infants the postnatal increase in serum tocopherol is much more gradual than in breast-fed infants, and that in bottle-fed prematures during the first month or so of postnatal life there is a gradual decline in serum

[175] C. S. Rose and P. György, *J. Nutr.* **39**, 529 (1949); *Blood* **5**, 1062 (1950); *Amer. J. Physiol.* **168**, 414 (1952).

[176] P. György, G. M. Cogan, and C. S. Rose, *Amer. J. Dis. Child.* **82**, 237 (1951); *Proc. Soc. Exp. Biol. Med.* **81**, 536 (1952).

[177] H. H. Gordon and J. P. de Metry, *Proc. Soc. Exp. Biol. Med.* **79**, 446 (1952).

[178] J. B. Mackenzie, *Pediatrics* **13**, 346 (1954).

tocopherols until they reach levels comparable to those which in the experimental animal are associated with manifestations of vitamin E deficiency. It seems, therefore, that the bottle-fed premature infant, denied the benefit of placental transfer of vitamin E during the latter phases of gestation, physiologically handicapped from the standpoint of suckling and other postnatal adaptations, and usually reared on a low-fat formula (because of poor tolerance for fats) rarely providing more than one-fourth to one-fifth the tocopherol present in breast milk, represents a close approach to a natural avitaminosis E in man.

2. RETROLENTAL FIBROPLASIA

In view of what has been said regarding the tocopherol status of the fetus and the newborn infant, it is natural that considerable attention has been given to the possible implication of an inadequacy of vitamin E in the etiology of retrolental fibroplasia.[179-181] This disorder is characterized by unusual proliferative activity in retinal capillaries, followed by edema and small hemorrhages which rupture into the vitreous, separation of the retina, and, with further proliferation, the formation of a disorganized membrane-like mass in the vitreous. Its etiology is unknown, but it is generally regarded as related to some metabolic disorder of prenatal or early postnatal life.

There are many observed facts which provide quite logical reasons for suspecting that inadequacy of vitamin E might be involved, as outlined by Owens and Owens.[179] Although the latter investigators found no significant difference in serum tocopherol levels between infants with normal eyes and those who developed retrolental fibroplasia, prophylactic tocopherol therapy given to alternate premature infants with birth weights of 3 pounds or less gave results which were at least encouraging; so also did the use of α-tocopherol in infants showing early stages of the disease. Unfortunately, however, their subsequent experience, and that of other investigators,[180, 181] has raised doubt as to whether tocopherol has therapeutic value in preventing or ameliorating the lesions. Capillary changes due to physiological immaturity and electrolyte imbalance[182] and failure to maintain proper oxygenation[183] during early postnatal life are currently considered to be causal.

3. OTHER IMPLICATIONS

Impressed by the frequency with which fetal death in prematures, especially in those with birth weights under 1.5 kg, can be related to cerebromeningeal

[179] W. C. Owens and E. U. Owens, *Amer. J. Opthalmol.* **32**, 1631 (1949).
[180] W. E. Kinsey and J. F. Chisholm, Jr., *Amer. J. Ophthalmol.* **34**, 1259 (1951).
[181] W. O. La Motte, Jr., G. S. Tyner, and H. G. Scheie, *Arch. Ophthalmol.* **47**, 556 (1952).
[182] A. C. Krause, *Amer. J. Ophthalmol.* **34**, 1003 (1951).
[183] T. S. Szewczyk, *Amer. J. Ophthalmol.* **34**, 1649 (1951); *Amer. J. Ophthalmol.* **35**, 301 (1952).

hemorrhages due to multiple rupture of capillary vessels, Minkowski[184, 185] has attempted to measure the vascular resistance of such infants (on the basis of petechiae produced by vacuum cup applied to skin of the back) and its response to vitamin P-like substances and to α-tocopherol. When mothers were given large doses (600–900 mg) of α-tocopherol several hours prior to premature delivery, there was a definite increase in vascular resistance of the premature infant as compared to that observed in infants of comparable weight from untreated mothers; tocopherol also lessened the visibility of the capillary network of the skin, as visualized by the capillaroscope.[185] There were 4 instances of intracranial hemorrhages in the treated group and 12 in the untreated group, each represented by 105 infants; Minkowski considers these results suggestive of beneficial effects but recognizes the need for additional data before more conclusive statements can be made.

Children with steat-orrhea resulting from cystic fibrosis of the pancreas or biliary atresia have shown not only pronounced "peroxide hemolysis" but also a marked creatinuria.[186, 187] Children with similar signs brought about by inadequate diets, showed a marked reticulocyte response after tocopherol administration.[187a] The creatinuria in these children was repaired by giving tocopherol.

One case of nutritional encephalomalacia quite similar to chick encephalo-malacia has been reported[187b] in an infant. This child had been given, daily for 20 days, a lipid preparation, intravenously, which provided a high concentration of linoleic acid without compensatory high levels of tocopherol. Necropsy did not reveal abnormalities in the cerebral hemispheres, but the cerebellum was the site of widespread hemorrhages, proliferation of capillaries and absence of Purkinje cells.

Ceroid pigment, a product of autoxidation of unsaturated lipids, has been found in the smooth muscle of the intestine, bronchial wall, and bladder of children dying of cystic fibrosis of the pancreas.[187c,d] It is presumed that these children were tocopherol deficient, not only because of generalities associated with the malabsorption syndrome, but because these observations were similar to those found in experimental animals.

[184] A. Minkowski, *Arch. Fr. Pediat.* **6**, 276 (1949); *Ann. Paediat.* **174**, 80 (1950).

[185] A. Minkowski, *Sang* **22**, 701 (1951).

[186] H. H. Gordon, H. M. Nitowsky, and J. T. Tildon, *Trans. Amer. Clin. Climatol. Ass.* **68**, 155 (1956).

[187] H. M. Nitowsky, K. S. Hsu, and H. H. Gordon, *Vitam. Horm.* (*New York*) **20**, 559 (1956).

[187a] A. S. Majaj, J. S. Dinning, S. A. Assam, and W. J. Darby, *Amer. J. Clin. Nutr.* **12**, 374 (1963).

[187b] M. K. Horwitt and P. Bailey, *AMA Arch. Neurol.* **1**, 312 (1959).

[187c] W. A. Blanc, J. D. Reid, and D. H. Anderson, *Pediatrics* **22**, 494 (1958).

[187d] I. Kerner and R. B. Goldbloom, *AMA J. Dis. Child.* **99**, 597 (1960).

C. Vitamin E in Later Life

It had seemed unlikely that a natural deficiency of tocopherol occurrs in man. To test this, the Food and Nutrition Board of the National Research Council sponsored a long-term study of the tocopherol requirements of adult men[188-191] at the Elgin State Hospital (hereafter referred to as the " Elgin Project ") the results of which more clearly demonstrate the relationships between the levels of polyunsaturated fatty acids in the tissues and the need for tocopherol to protect these compounds. Such relationships might become unbalanced as a result of a prolonged and severe impairment of fat absorption or as a consequence of dietary choices which increase the consumption of polyunsaturated fats without compensatory increases of α-tocopherol.

To evaluate the state of tocopherol nutriture in man, one depends largely upon information pertaining to (1) dietary history, (2) plasma tocopherol levels, (3) susceptibility of erythrocytes to peroxide hemolysis and other factors affecting the life of the erythrocyte, and (4) histopathological changes which are comparable to those found in experimental animals, particularly those associated with creatinuria. Blood levels represent the interplay of many factors and while not necessarily indicative of the tocopherol status of the individual, since a single recent ingestion may give a false indication of adequacy, they constitute the most widely used criterion for evaluating vitamin E nutriture in man.

1. PLASMA (OR SERUM) TOCOPHEROLS

a. Normal Levels

Most of our information on plasma tocopherols is based upon blood samples analyzed by the method of Quaife and Harris,[192, 193] utilizing the Emmerie and Engel color reaction. A micromethod later developed by Quaife *et al.*,[194] and requiring minute samples of blood, has been of particular value in studies with infants.[168, 195]

[188] M. K. Horwitt, C. C. Harvey, G. D. Duncan, and W. C. Wilson, *Amer. J. Clin. Nutr.* **4**, 408 (1956).

[189] M. K. Horwitt, *Amer. J. Clin. Nutr.* **8**, 451 (1960).

[190] M. K. Horwitt, C. C. Harvey, B. Century, and L. A. Witting, *J. Amer. Diet. Ass.* **38**, 231 (1961).

[190a] M. K. Horwitt, *Borden's Rev. Nutr. Res.* **22**, 1 (1961).

[190b] M. K. Horwitt, *Amer. J. Clin. Nutr.* **12**, 99 (1963).

[191] M. K. Horwitt, *Vitam. Horm.* (*New York*) **20**, 541 (1962).

[192] M. L. Quaife and P. L. Harris, *J. Biol. Chem.* **156**, 499 (1944).

[193] M. L. Quaife and R. Biehler, *J. Biol. Chem.* **159**, 663 (1945).

[194] M. L. Quiafe, N. S. Scrimshaw, and O. H. Lowry, *J. Biol. Chem.* **179**, 1229 (1949).

[195] L. J. Filer, Jr., S. W. Wright, M. P. Manning, and K. E. Mason, *Pediatrics* **8**, 328 (1951).

Plasma tocopherol levels in newborn infants are approximately one-third to one-fourth those found in healthy adults. Average values of 0.23 mg/100 ml (SD ± 0.13),[167] 0.37 mg/100 ml (SD ± 0.15),[168] and 0.43 mg/100 ml (SD ± 0.12)[164] have been reported. For young and adolescent children, values of about 1 mg/100 ml are considered normal.[196] Plasma tocopherol levels for healthy adults usually fall within the range of 1.0–1.2 mg/100 ml. During pregnancy there is a rather pronounced increment in plasma tocopherols,[164, 165, 169–171] which declines only gradually during lactation.[168, 171] A tendency for values to increase with age has been reported.[170, 197]

b. Effect of Disease

Compared to normal healthy adults, clinic patients[198] and convalescent hospital patients randomly selected[197, 199, 200] have somewhat lower levels of plasma tocopherol. Patients with liver disease also tend to show low values,[200, 201] but they are not significantly different from those of convalescent patients with no evidence of liver disease;[152, 200] the same is true of cardiac patients.[199] Lower-than-usual values are also commonly observed in diseases where intestinal absorption is defective, as in sprue,[202, 203] celiac disease, fibrocystic disease of the pancreas, biliary obstruction, and diarrhea associated with achlorhydria.[170, 195] This is in accord with experimental evidence that surgical production of a biliary fistula leads to a state of vitamin E deficiency in the rat and dog. On the other hand, higher-than-usual values are frequently observed in diseases associated with hypercholesteremia and in cardiovascular disease and pregnancy, both of which are often associated with increased blood lipids (Fig. 30). These deviations from normal might be explained on the basis of differences in intestinal absorption[170] or differences in lipid-carrying power of the blood.[204]

The effectiveness of intestinal absorption of vitamin E has been measured by the tocopherol "absorption curve" (also termed "tolerance curve," "tolerance test," "blood persistence curve"). Subjects are given a single, large, oral dose of tocopherol (usually 5–20 mg of α-tocopherol/kg of body weight) and blood samples are taken at 0, 3, 6, 9, 12, and 24 hours. The curve

[196] A. S. Minot, J. Lab. Clin. Med. 29, 772 (1944).
[197] M. Chieffi and J. E. Kirk, J. Gerontol. 6, 17 (1951).
[198] P. L. Harris, K. C. D. Hickman, J. L. Jensen, and T. D. Spies, Amer. J. Pub. Health Nat. Health 36, 155 (1946).
[199] J. M. Lemley, R. G. Gale, R. H. Furman, M. E. Cherrington, W. J. Darby, and G. R. Meneely, Amer. Heart J. 37, 1029 (1949).
[200] G. Klatskin and W. A. Krehl, J. Clin. Invest. 39, 1528 (1950).
[201] H. Popper, A. Dubin, F. Steigmann, and F. P. Hesser, J. Lab. Clin. Med. 34, 648 (1949).
[202] W. J. Darby, M. E. Cherrington, and J. M. Ruffin, Proc. Soc. Exp. Biol. Med. 63, 310 (1946).
[203] W. J. Darby, E. Jones, H. F. Warden, and M. M. Kaser, J. Nutr. 34, 645 (1947).
[204] K. C. D. Hickman and P. L. Harris, Advan. Enzymol. 6, 469 (1946).

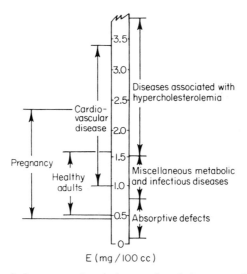

E (mg / 100 cc)

FIG. 30. Range of plasma tocopherols in man in relation to good health, pregnancy and certain broadly classified diseases. From Darby *et al.*[170]

obtained by plotting the tocopherol values, or the planimeter measurement of the area under the curve, provides a basis for comparing individual responses. Low response curves have been reported in some, but not all, cases of liver disease,[200, 201] in primary fibrositis,[205] and in sprue;[196, 202, 203] low responses have been observed in cases of fibrocystic disease of the pancreas, diarrhea and cirrhosis in infants, and in children with celiac syndrome and lupus erythematosus, and rather high responses in metabolic disorders with associated hypercholesteremia.[195]

The relationship between plasma tocopherol and the peroxide hemolysis test was determined in the " Elgin Project " during 6 years of restriction of a representative group of male adults to a diet which provided approximately 3 mg of α-tocopherol/day. Figure 31 (from reference 191) gives the results obtained on a single representative patient who provided data that were similar to the average of the depleted group.[189] Note that although the peroxide hemolysis reached a maximum after two years on the original basal diet in which stripped lard was the basic fat used, the plasma tocopherol level continued to decrease when stripped corn oil (which, although low in vitamin E, provided slightly more total tocopherol than the lard) was substituted. The corn oil contained about five times as much linoleic acid as an equivalent amount of lard.[190, 190a]

Paradoxically, the simplicity with which many signs of vitamin E deficiency can be produced in experimental animals has served to belittle the

[205] C. L. Steinberg, *Med. Clin. N. Amer.* **30**, 221 (1946).

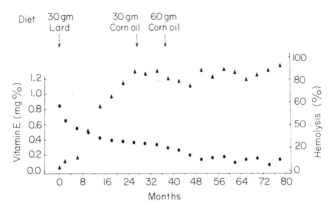

FIG. 31. Changes in plasma tocopherol (●) and peroxide hemolysis (▲) on a single representative subject from the group on a low-E basal diet. From Horwitt.[191]

less dramatic needs of man for α-tocopherol. Although there were suggestions of creatinuria in some of the depleted subjects, which could not be proved statistically because several of the control subjects also had increased ex- cretions of creatine, the only definite signs of pathology were decreases in the erythrocyte survival time and the finding of a reticulocyte response after the administration of tocopherol to the depleted subjects.[190b] The first report of a reticulocyte response from tocopherol in man was recorded in the Proceed- ings of the Food and Nutrition Board in 1958 which cites "the case of one tocopherol-depleted patient whose reticulocyte count increased from 1.3 to 4.7 per cent when supplemented with 100 mg. of α-tocopherol after a blood loss episode which had reduced his hemoglobin level from 14 to 9 gm. per cent." Subsequent attempts[190, 190b] to establish the validity of this reticulo- cyte response to tocopherol using rigid controls during the counting pro- cedures did produce statistically significant differences but the increases obtained were in so-called normal ranges because the patients used were not anemic. However, quite large reticulocyte responses recently obtained by Dinning[205a] and his collaborators when tocopherol was given to anemic children have served to validate the observations made on the adult subjects. The data obtained from these children who were subsisting in a refugee camp[187a] are important and should stimulate additional research on other groups of children on inadequate diets.

2. TISSUE TOCOPHEROLS

The usual method for analysis of tocopherols in foods and tissues[206] is laborious and time-consuming. Tissues obtainable are limited to postmortem material, except where generous biopsy samples can be secured. Although

[205a] J. S. Dinning, Nutr. Rev. 21, 289 (1963).
[206] M. L. Quaife and P. L. Harris, Anal. Chem. 29, 1221 (1948).

d-α-tocopherol is the predominant type found in tissues, variable but usually not very large amounts of γ- and δ-tocopherols are also present;[156-159] however, results are generally expressed in terms of total tocopherols.

Information concerning tocopherols in human tissues is limited to analyses carried out by Abderhalden[155] on a variety of tissues from fetuses, newborn, and adults, those of Quaife and Dju[156] on two cases of accidental death, and a more extensive series of analyses covering the period from early fetal life to old age.[157-159a] The results of these studies indicate that tocopherols are widely distributed in human tissues from early fetal life to advanced old age. Tocopherol levels, expressed as milligrams per 100 grams of fresh tissue, are low in fetuses of 2 to 6 months' gestation age, and only slightly higher in premature and full-term infants at birth. The data obtained are in accord with other evidence that during the early postnatal period of life states of suboptimal vitamin E nutriture may occur. During early postnatal life, tissue levels tend to increase slowly unless suppressed by disease of various types. During childhood and adolescence they reach levels comparable to those of adults which, for muscle, heart, liver, and certain other visceral organs, are approximately twice those at birth, and for adipose tissue are considerably higher than in other tissues, with the exception of the adrenals. Both pituitary and testis contain about four times as much tocopherol per unit of fresh tissue as do other visceral organs, but only about one-third as much as the adrenals. During the latter few decades of life there appears to be a tendency for tocopherols to diminish somewhat in liver and in adipose tissue It is also of interest that total tocopherols (expressed as milligrams per 100 grams of fresh tissue) in skeletal muscle, heart, liver, and other visceral organs, except the endocrine glands mentioned, are of about the same order as observed in the circulating blood.

On the other hand, when tocopherols are expressed as milligrams per gram of extractable fat, the values for adipose tissue are considerably lower than for most of the tissues just mentioned, whereas the values for pituitary, testis, and adrenal appear to be considerably higher. Although tocopherols in adipose tissue appear to increase during early life on the basis of tocopherols per unit of fresh tissue, and to diminish in terms of tocopherols per unit of extractable fat, from a quantitative standpoint the adipose tissue of the body appears to represent the major site of tocopherol deposition and may therefore best reflect the tocopherol status of the body as a whole.

3. HISTOPATHOLOGY

Histopathological approaches to the question of vitamin E deficiency in man have been generally twofold. One is based upon the occurrence of an acid-fast pigment commonly associated with the lesions of experimental vitamin E deficiency; the other relates to striking similarities between the muscle lesions of progressive muscular dystrophy in man and those common to the various species of animal in which vitamin E deficiency has been produced.

a. Acid-Fast Pigment (Ceroid)

An acid-fast pigment, referred to as ceroid (see p. 109), occurs in the smooth and striated musculature and becomes disseminated throughout the reticuloendothelial system after prolonged vitamin E deficiency in certain animals; in organs such as the sex glands and the adrenal, where small amounts of this pigment occur normally, there may be a conspicuous increase. Excess of intracellular, unsaturated lipids or fat peroxides and inadequacy of tocopherols as antioxidants are considered primary factors in the genesis of this pigment. A comparable pigment has been described by Wolf and Pappenheimer[207] in various parts of the central nervous system, and by Pappenheimer and Victor[208] in a variety of other tissues and organs from routine autopsies. They report that, in general, the occurrence of acid-fast pigment in human tissues tends to be associated with hepatic cirrhosis and hemochromatosis, celiac disease, pancreatic fibrosis, and nontropical sprue, except for its occasional location about focal degenerative lesions such as atheromatous placques and areas of follicular atresia. It is of interest that acid-fast pigment, some of which may be derived from red blood cells,[209] is commonly associated with atheromatous lesions of the aorta and other vessels,[209, 210] and that atheromatous aortas are said to contain peroxides[211] such as are associated with sites of ceroid formation in vitamin E-deficient animals. A ceroidlike pigment in the human ovary has also been described by Brenner[212] and by Reagan,[213] usually in association with follicular atresia, and regarded as an oxidation product of vitamin A (or carotene) and unsaturated fats, catalyzed perhaps by lipoxidase of the ovarian tissues.

It should be made clear that in the studies describing ceroid in human tissues no claim is made that an avitaminosis E is involved. Ceroid may arise in tissues where, in association with unsaturated fats, there are local oxidative disturbances similar to those occurring in vitamin E deficiency but due to other causes; there is also the possibility of a localized destruction of intracellular tocopherol due to metabolic stress or chemical insult even though the tocopherol status of the body in general is normal.

There are several reports which present more definite suggestions that human beings may approach a state of conditioned avitaminosis E. Pappenheimer and Victor[208] have presented in considerable detail the postmortem

[207] A. Wolf and A. M. Pappenheimer, *J. Neuropathol. Exp. Neurol.* **4**, 402 (1945).
[208] A. M. Pappenheimer and J. Victor, *Amer. J. Pathol.* **22**, 395 (1946).
[209] W. S. Hartroft, *Amer. J. Pathol.* **28**, 526 (1952).
[210] R. C. Burt, *Amer. J. Clin. Pathol.* **22**, 135 (1952).
[211] J. Glavind, S. Hartmann, J. Clemmesen, K. E. Jessen, and H. Dam, *Acta Pathol.* **30**, 1 (1952).
[212] S. Brenner, *S. Afr. J. Med. Sci.* **11**, 173 (1946).
[213] J. W. Reagan, *Amer. J. Obstet. Gynecol.* **59**, 433 (1950).

findings on four individuals exhibiting chronic nutritional disorders (idiopathic hypoproteinemia, gastrocolic fistula subsequent to gastroenterostomy, nontropical sprue, and chronic jejunitis with cirrhosis) in which there was found an abundance of acid-fast pigment having much the same localization as that seen in vitamin E-deficient animals. In all cases, there was pronounced pigmentation of the muscular coats of the esophagus, stomach, and small intestine, such as are seen in the E-deficient monkey and in dogs with biliary fistulas. Acid-fast pigment was also noted in liver cells, Kupffer cells, uterine muscle, phagocytes of ovarian stroma, cardiac and skeletal muscle, media of small arteries, and the Sertoli tissue and interstitial cells of the degenerate testes of the one male of the series. Tverdy et al.,[214] present a detailed clinical history and postmortem findings in a case of nontropical sprue, in which they noted acid-fast pigment with essentially the same distribution in intestinal smooth muscle, liver, degenerate testes, and macrophages of various organs and tissues. Histopathological changes were also noted[214a] in the central nervous system, including the presence of much acid-fast pigment, especially in relation to blood vessels and the choroid plexus epithelium. They consider these changes to be strongly indicative of an avitaminosis E associated with sprue. Possible association of vitamin E deficiency with the so-called "brown bowel" syndrome has also been suggested.[215a,b]

Surveys of human autopsy material have revealed ceroid pigment in varying amounts in a wide variety of lesions affecting many organs.[214b] The amount may be significant in sites in which hemorrhage has occurred in or around accumulations of abnormal stainable fat. Fatty cirrhosis and ischemic infarcts affecting brain, spleen, kidney, heart, and lung provide excellent examples of this type of ceroid deposition. The pigment is a constant component of atheromatous plaques in which both abnormal lipid accumulation and hemorrhage have developed.[214c] Necrosis of tissues that do not contain excess abnormal fat also leads to deposits of small amounts of ceroid, probably secondary to hemorrhage into minimal quantities of fat liberated from death of cells containing only normal amounts of lipid.

Reference has been made (p. 109) to the low serum tocopherol levels and flat type of absorption curve observed in sprue, celiac disease, and similar disorders. Also of interest is the comment of Frazer[215] that "Dietary

[214] G. Tverdy, A. L. Froehlick, and B. Fierens, Acta Gastro-Enterol. Belg. **12**, 221 (1949).

[214a] L. van Bogaert and G. Tverdy, Monatsschr. Psychiat. Neurol. **120**, 301 (1950).

[214b] W. S. Hartroft, personal communication.

[214c] W. S. Hartroft, R. M. O'Neal, and W. A. Thomas, Fed. Proc. Fed. Amer. Soc. Exp. Biol. **18**, Pt. II, 36 (1959).

[215] A. C. Frazer, Brit. Med. J. **ii**, 731 (1949).

[215a] A. H. Toffler, P. B. Hulkill, and H. M. Spiro, Ann. Int. Med. **58**, 872 (1963).

[215b] M. B. Bauman, J. D. DiMase, F. Oski, and J. R. Senior, Gastroenterology **54**, 93 (1968).

inadequacy is certainly not a common cause of vitamin deficiency in the sprue syndrome. It may account for the occasional case of vitamin E deficiency, especially since oxidative rancidity of fats may be one of the precipitating causes in tropical sprue."

b. Progressive Muscular Dystrophy

Many investigators have been impressed by the striking similarity between the skeletal muscle lesions of progressive muscular dystrophy and dermatomyositis in man and those of nutritional myodegeneration which represent the most characteristic manifestation of vitamin E deficiency in experimental animals. This applies also to myocardial lesions, which constitute a rather characteristic finding in progressive muscular dystrophy[216, 217] as they do in many animal species deficient in vitamin E. Nevertheless, it is necessary to make a clear distinction between progressive muscular dystrophy and nutritional myopathy while recognizing that there may be some pathological and biochemical similarities.

There is evidence of a common biochemical defect, in the form of urinary excretion of ribose-phosphorus-containing complexes which appear to be rather specific for human muscular dystrophy[218, 218a] and which occur also in dystrophic vitamin E-deficient rabbits.[219] The suggestion that these complexes may reflect disturbances in nucleotide metabolism is in keeping with other evidence of disturbed nucleic acid metabolism in the vitamin E-deficient rabbit[220] and monkey.[221] Of interest is the observation of Minot et al.[218] that "pentose-containing complexes were detected in the urine of an apparently normal 3 year old brother of one of our patients with muscular dystrophy." A generalized aminoaciduria observed in muscular dystrophy[222] may, like creatinuria, reflect muscle breakdown, not a primary metabolic disturbance.

Despite many hopes that vitamin E might prove beneficial in at least retarding or arresting the course of human progressive muscular dystrophy, therapeutic efforts have provided no valid evidence that this is so. This is

[216] W. G. Nothacker and M. G. Netsky, *Arch. Pathol.* **50**, 578 (1950).

[217] J. Zatachni, E. E. Aegerter, L. Molthan, and C. R. Shuman, *Circulation* **3**, 846 (1950).

[218] A. S. Minot, H. Frank, and D. Dziewiatkowski, *Arch. Biochem.* **20**, 394 (1949).

[218a] W. F. Orr and A. S. Minot, *Arch. Neurol. Psychiat.* **67**, 483 (1952).

[219] A. S. Minot and M. Grimes, *J. Nutr.* **39**, 159 (1949).

[220] J. M. Young and J. S. Dinning, *J. Biol. Chem.* **193**, 743 (1951).

[221] J. S. Dinning, L. D. Seager, and P. L. Day, *Fed. Proc. Fed. Amer. Soc. Exp. Biol.* **10**, 380 (1951).

[222] S. R. Ames and H. A. Risley, *Proc. Soc. Exp. Biol. Med.* **68**, 131 (1948).

not surprising in view of the normal levels of tocopherol found in the blood[196] and in various tissues and organs[159, 223] of dystrophic subjects. The oxidation-reduction product of α-tocopherol, α-tocohydroquinone, has been shown to have antidystrophic properties in the rabbit[223a] and the Syrian hamster[223b] deficient in vitamin E. On the premise that in progressive muscular dystrophy there might be a defect in the conversion of a-tocopherol to its hydroquinone, Harris and Mason[223c] carried out a series of studies comparing the effects of placebo and of α-tocohydroquinone therapy of 12 to 18 months duration upon 12 dystrophic children. The results of treatment, based upon a variety of motor activities recorded by split-frame photography at six-month intervals[223d] were indisputably negative.

Of special interest is a recent report by Vester and Williams[223e] about a 46-year-old male with progressive muscular weakness and a pronounced creatinuria who demonstrated marked improvement after receiving 100 mg of α-tocopherol three times per day. When tocopherol administration was halted, the symptoms returned and could again be reversed by giving this vitamin. Muscle biopsy showed focal regeneration and sarcolemmal proliferation not consistent with muscular dystrophy. Later studies on the same patient showed that he could not absorb fats effectively because of a pancreatic insufficiency. Administering lipases[223f] apparently made it possible for him to absorb the carrier lipids and tocopherol more efficiently.

4. DISORDERS OF REPRODUCTION

The discovery of vitamin E and the long-established method for its bio-assay are based upon the phenomenon of fetal resorption in the rat. It is not surprising that over the past 40 years there have appeared numerous clinical reports on the therapeutic use of vitamin E in habitual abortion, threatened abortion, threatened miscarriage, premature labor, and eclamptic states. The results are conflicting and are confused by differences in definition, vitamin E dosage, and extent to which other therapeutic measures are employed and often not recorded. As is so often the case with unestablished therapeutic agents, favorable reports considerably exceed those which relay negative findings.

[223] K. E. Mason, M. Y. Dju, and S. J. Chapin, *Fed. Proc. Fed. Amer. Soc. Exp. Biol.* **12**, 422 (1953); *Proc. 1st & 2nd Med. Conf. Muscular Dystrophy Ass. Amer., New York, 1951–1952* p. 94 (1952).

[223a] J. B. Mackenzie and C. G. Mackenzie, *J. Nutr.* **67**, 223 (1959).

[223b] W. T. West and K. E. Mason, *Am. J. Phys. Med.* **34**, 223 (1955).

[223c] P. L. Harris and K. E. Mason, *Am. J. Clin. Nutr.* **4**, 402 (1956).

[223d] R. P. Schwartz, K. E. Mason, and T. Tyler, *Am. J. Phys. Med.* **34**, 183 (1955).

[223e] J. W. Vester and L. R. Williams, *Clin. Res.* **11**, 180 (1963).

[223f] J. W. Vester and E. Moody, personal communication.

a. Habitual Abortion

A habitual aborter is usually defined as one who has spontaneously aborted before the 16th week during three successive pregnancies. It is estimated that 4% of all spontaneous abortions are habitual, and that about 10% of all pregnancies terminate in abortion, amounting to 240,000 yearly in the United States.[224] Bacharach,[225] in a statistical analysis of reported cases of habitual abortion treated with vitamin E up to 1940, felt that the chance of a successful pregnancy was definitely increased by this therapeutic measure. Hertig and Livingstone[226] later stated: "Vitamin E, judging from the literature, has an important effect on the favorable outcome of pregnancy in cases of habitual abortion—this in spite of the fact that the average human dietary cannot be shown to be deficient in vitamin E." Only about 16% of habitual aborters show plasma tocopherol levels below the average normal range, and these are effectively raised to normal by as little as 25 mg of α-tocopherol, daily.[227] An 80% salvage in 211 patients with from 3 to 11 previous abortions, by correction of contributory conditions of varied type, has been reported by Javert et al.[228] The present status of the problem is well summarized in their statement: "There is such a maze of literature that proper cognizance cannot be taken of all the pertinent articles. As the reader reviews them in order to develop his own philosophy, let him be reminded of three important matters: the high percentage of success irrespective of which vitamin, hormone or method is employed; the lack of specific information as to the pathogenesis of human spontaneous abortion. . . ."

b. Threatened Abortion and Miscarriage

Evan Shute, although dubious about the merits of vitamin E in habitual abortion, has reported its therapeutic usefulness in threatened abortion and threatened miscarriage,[229, 230] premature labor,[231] abruptio placentae,[232] and noneclamptic late toxemias of pregnancy,[233] and is of the opinion that tocopherol may in some way counteract the effects of high blood estrogen rather than compensate for a true avitaminosis E. Other clinicians have

[224] C. Mazer and S. L. Israel, "Diagnosis and Treatment of Menstrual Disorders and Sterility," 3rd Ed. Harper & Row (Hoeber), New York, 1951.
[225] A. L. Bacharach, *Brit. Med. J.* i, 890 (1940); *Brit. Med. J.* i, 567 (1948).
[226] A. Hertig and R. A. Livingstone, *New Engl. J. Med.* 230, 797 (1944).
[227] E. Delfs and G. E. S. Jones, *Obstet. Gynecol. Surv.* 3, 680 (1948).
[228] C. T. Javert, W. F. Finn, and H. J. Stander, *Amer. J. Obstet. Gyncecol.* 57, 878 (1949).
[229] E. Shute, *Urol. Cutaneous Rev.* 47, 239 (1943).
[230] E. Shute and W. E. Shute, *J. Obstet. Gynaecol. Brit. Emp.* 49, 534 (1942).
[231] E. Shute, *Amer. J. Obstet. Gynecol.* 44, 271 (1942); *J. Obstet. Gynaecol. Brit. Emp.* 52, 571 (1945).
[232] E. Shute, *Surg. Gynecol. Obstet.* 75, 515 (1942).
[233] E. Shute, *Amer. J. Surg.* 71, 470 (1946).

reported similar success with tocopherol, frequently combined with pro-
gesterone therapy; the reason that so much doubt still exists concerning these
claims is due not so much to other reports in the negative as it is to failure to,
or inability to, satisfactorily validate these clinical experiences by control
data or by basic information regarding the tocopherol status of the patients.

c. Sterility in the Male

The other classic manifestations of experimental vitamin E deficiency,
namely, testicular degeneration in the rat, has no known counterpart in
man. Although Shute [234] holds the opinion that vitamin E therapy causes an
increase in sperm count and enhances the possibilities that infertility in
males can frequently be overcome by vitamin E therapy, largely through
improvement in the number and quality of the sperm, Farris[235] reported
that vitamin E concentrates have no significant effect on sperm concentration,
motility, or cytological aberrations in infertile men. Three other studies,
yielding somewhat contradictory results, are summarized by Swyer.[236]

XII. Pharmacology and Toxicology

M. K. HORWITT AND KARL E. MASON

Largely through the pioneer researches of Mattill[1] and his associates, the
tocopherols have come to be recognized as widely distributed and important
biological antioxidants, both *in vivo* and *in vitro*. Compared to other toco-
pherols (β, γ, δ), α-tocopherol possesses the greatest biological activity *in vivo*
and is regarded as the prototype of vitamin E. It represents 90% or more of
the tocopherols in animal tissues.

Both the *d* and *dl* forms of α-tocopherol, like ascorbic acid, are among the
few antioxidants capable of passing the intestinal barrier, reaching intracellular sites, and exerting regulatory control over cell oxidations. Despite hopes
and a certain amount of evidence that tocopherol might prove to function in
some oxidation–reduction system, or participate in some specific manner in
certain enzyme systems, no indisputable evidence has been produced that α-
tocopherol exerts biological effects unrelated to its important functions as an
intracellular antioxidant.

[234] E. Shute, *Urol. Cutaneous Rev.* **48**, 423 (1944).
[235] E. J. Farris, *Ann. N.Y. Acad. Sci.* **52**, 409 (1949).
[236] G. I. M. Swyer, *Brit. J. Nutr.* **3**, 100 (1949).
[1] H. A. Mattill, *Nutr. Rev.* **10**, 225 (1952).

A. Hypervitaminosis E

No state or syndrome of hypervitaminosis E has been described, nor is there evidence that tocopherols per se exert any deleterious effect in animals or man. Demole[2] has shown that mice will tolerate oral doses of 50 gm/kg, and rats doses of 4 gm/kg daily for 2 months. Adult humans have tolerated oral doses of 1 gm/day for months, or larger doses for shorter periods, with no undesirable effects.

B. Mode of Administration

The natural and synthetic forms of α-tocopherol and their acetate esters are viscous oils. Intramuscular injections, frequently used in clinical practice, have sometimes led to painful reactions locally and to oleogranulomas at a later date;[3] "solubilized" preparations may be less reactive in these respects. Tocopherol ointments have been used to only a limited extent. In animals, implanted pellets of the crystalline esters (palmitate, succinate, and phosphate) produce marked local tissue reactions;[4] so also does injection of the slightly water-soluble phosphate ester. Neither in animals nor in man are there reliable data concerning the relative effectiveness of absorption and utilization of tocopherols administered in these various ways, as compared to oral dosage, which appears to be the most effective mode of administration.

C. Metabolic Stress in Animals

There is a considerable body of evidence that α-tocopherol has a remarkable capacity to protect experimental animals against a variety of metabolic stresses, including those induced by anoxia, high intake of unsaturated fats, low protein intake, restricted intake of other vitamins (A, B_6, and essential fatty acids), irradiation,[5] and the toxic or otherwise detrimental effects of such substances as alloxan, lead,[6] selenium,[7] silver nitrate, o-cresyl phosphate, and carbon tetrachloride.[8] In many instances, additional tocopherol means the difference between death of the animal or continued survival in good health. Presumably these beneficial effects relate to the antioxidant functions of tocopherol, operating sometimes in the intestinal tract and at other times at sites where local tissue injury would otherwise occur. Furthermore, tocopherol can enhance the curative action of critical amounts of vitamin A and

---

[2] V. Demole, *Int. Z. Vitaminforsch.* **8**, 338 (1939).
[3] C. L. Steinberg, *Ann. N.Y. Acad. Sci.* **52**, 380 (1949).
[4] C. E. Tobin, *Proc. Soc. Exp. Biol. Med.* **73**, 475 (1950).
[5] Z. M. Bacq, *Experientia* **7**, 11 (1951).
[6] H. Chiodi and A. F. Chardeza, *Arch. Pathol.* **48**, 395 (1949).
[7] E. A. Sellers, R. W. You, and C. C. Lucas, *Proc. Soc. Exp. Biol. Med.* **75**, 118 (1950).
[8] E. L. Hove, *Amer. J. Clin. Nutr.* **3**, 328 (1955).

essential fatty acids, possibly by protecting them up to the point of intestinal absorption.

D. Therapeutic Use

There exists an extensive but rather controversial literature dealing with the therapeutic efficacy of tocopherol in a wide variety of disease states, many of which have little or nothing in common with experimentally induced manifestations of vitamin E deficiency and are not associated with any evidence of a significant inadequacy of tocopherol in the patient. Furthermore, the effects reported are usually obtained only with relatively high doses over a period of many weeks or months. As expressed by Hickman[9] in an interesting review of this subject, "The discrepancy between the few milligrams a day that suffice to maintain the majority of people in health and the hundreds of milligrams being used clinically gives cause for serious thought.... Only time and continued study can resolve the dosage paradox with this vitamin...."

Those who report benefit in certain clinical disorders usually stress the importance of sustained, high daily dosage, generally amounting to between 200 and 600 mg of α-tocopherol; this represents about 12 to 36 times the average daily intake from diet. There is also the common observation that only in a certain proportion of patients suffering from a specified disorder is there a significant remission of symptoms, the remainder showing no benefit other than perhaps an improved sense of well-being and physical vigor. Observations such as these suggest that in certain instances high tocopherol dosage may, through its capacity to prevent undesirable oxidation and regulate the oxidation–reduction milieu, greatly improve states of lowered or otherwise altered metabolism at various localized sites in tissues and organs of the body. The location of the latter, and their relation to the etiology and sequelae of the disease entity under consideration, would of course, vary widely from patient to patient. In other words, as in its protective effect in enabling the experimental animal to resist and overcome the effects of a variety of metabolic stresses, the clinical value of tocopherol may lie in large part in its ability to counteract localized metabolic and toxic stresses which may be either primary or secondary to, or quite independent of, a primary disease process.

Marks[10] has made a critical appraisal of the therapeutic value of α-tocopherol in which he attempted to distinguish between claims based upon well-founded evidence and those that are not too well supported. Included under the classification of "claims supported by good evidence" are the sprue syndrome and other nutritional deficiency disorders conditioned by either the poor absorption of fats or the abnormally large ingestion of

[9] K. C. D. Hickman, Rec. Chem. Progr. 9, 104 (1948).
[10] J. Marks, Vitam. Horm. (New York) 20, 573 (1962).

polyunsaturated fats without compensatory increases in tocopherol. In intermittent claudication of moderate severity there have been many reports on the benefits of large doses of tocopherol which are difficult to discount completely. To eliminate problems involved in evaluating subjective interpretations, Marks[10] has compared survival in intermittent claudication, in 1476 patients who were treated with about 400–600 mg of synthetic α-tocopherol/day, with recent reports of survival rates in an equivalent number of patients to show that survival in the tocopherol series was significantly better. It was noted that these large amounts of α-tocopherol could not be administered easily by feeding wheat germ oil since newer methods of analysis have shown a much lower content of α-tocopherol in wheat germ oil than previously thought.

There have been over 2000 papers on the clinical use of tocopherol for almost every disorder in the medical dictionary. Unfortunately, so many of these are so difficult to substantiate that anything useful may be buried in the backwash of contrary opinions. If it were not for the fact that, in experimental animals, stressful situations, unrelated to nutritional variables, are often remarkably ameliorated by tocopherol administration, one would be tempted to take the easy way out and discount all of them. Perhaps the answers will come when we know more about the effects of disease processes on oxidation–reduction potentials in the body.

XIII. Requirements of Microbes and Animals

STANLEY R. AMES

A. Microbes and Invertebrates

Vitamin E is apparently not specifically required for the growth of microorganisms. Microorganisms have been isolated which grow on d-α-tocopheryl acetate and are isomer specific.[1] Higher phyla of invertebrates have a requirement for vitamin E. In the rotifer *Asplanchna*, vitamin E induces sexual reproduction and body wall out growths in the offspring.[1a] The latter response was developed into an isomer-specific quantitative bioassay for d-α-tocopherol.[1b] The crustacean *Daphnia magna* needs vitamin E for normal

[1] C. T. Goodhue, *Biochemistry* 4, 1822 (1965).
[1a] J. J. Gilbert and G. A. Thompson, Jr., *Science* 159, 734 (1968).
[1b] J. J. Gilbert and C. W. Birky, Jr., *J. Nutr.* 101, 113 (1971).

reproduction.[2] The larval forms of some insects such as the European corn borer[3] the beet worm, the cotton bollworm, and the mallow moth[4] apparently need α-tocopherol when raised on purified diets.

B. Birds and Mammals

The determination of the vitamin E requirements of various species of animals has been handicapped by lack of convenient and specific analytical procedures to establish the dietary intake of d-α-tocopherol. A need for vitamin E has been established for many species of birds and mammals, but it has been difficult to ascertain a quantitative requirement. The requirement varies markedly with a given species, depending on the particular deficiency symptom studied. Furthermore, a quantitative requirement will apply only to a specific set of environmental, physiological, genetic, and dietary conditions.

Several dietary factors can have major effects on the vitamin E requirement, including fat, polyunsaturated fatty acids, selenium, amino acids, and antioxidants. A diet high in fat appears to increase the need for vitamin E,[5, 6] whereas poultry on a fat-free diet appear to have a relatively low requirement.[7] Certain vitamin E deficiency symptoms are accentuated by high dietary levels of unsaturated fatty acids,[8] especially the polyunsaturated fatty acids (PUFA). The feeding of cod liver oil has traditionally been used to induce more rapid appearance of vitamin E deficiency. There is a high positive correlation of PUFA level with vitamin E requirement in many species of animals.[9] Under certain conditions, selenium supplementation has been shown to affect the vitamin E requirement. Selenium supplementation decreased the amount of vitamin E needed for the prevention of exudative diathesis in chicks,[10-12] and enzootic muscular dystrophy in sheep,[13, 14] but was ineffective in most experimentally produced dystrophies[14] and in

[2] A. Viehoever and I. Cohen, *Amer. J. Pharm.* **110**, 297 (1938).

[3] S. D. Beck, J. H. Lilly, and J. F. Stauffer, *Ann. Entomol. Soc. Amer.* **42**, 483 (1949).

[4] E. M. Sumakov, N. M. Edel'man, and A. E. Borisova, *Dokl. Akad. Nauk. SSSR* **130**, 237 (1960).

[5] H. Gottlieb, F. W. Quackenbush, and H. Steenbock, *J. Nutr.* **25**, 433 (1943).

[6] G. A. Emerson and H. M. Evans, *J. Nutr.* **27**, 469 (1944).

[7] J. G. Bieri, G. M. Briggs, C. J. Pollard, and M. R. S. Fox, *J. Nutr.* **70**, 47 (1960).

[8] H. Dam, *Vitam. Horm.* (*New York*) **20**, 527 (1962).

[9] P. L. Harris and N. D. Embree, *Amer. J. Clin. Nutr.* **13**, 385 (1963).

[10] E. L. R. Stokstad, E. L. Patterson, and R. Milstrey, *Poultry Sci.* **36**, 1160 (1957).

[11] M. L. Scott, J. G. Bieri, G. M. Briggs, and K. Schwarz, *Poultry Sci.* **36**, 1155 (1957).

[12] K. Schwarz, J. G. Bieri, G. M. Briggs, and M. L. Scott, *Proc. Soc. Exp. Biol. Med.* **95**, 621 (1957).

[13] O. H. Muth, J. E. Oldfield, L. F. Remmert, and J. R. Schubert, *Science* **128**, 1090 (1958).

[14] K. L. Blaxter, *Vitam. Horm.* (*New York*) **20**, 633 (1962).

rat reproduction.[15] Dietary levels of cystine and arginine affect vitamin E requirements. Under specific dietary conditions, cystine supplementation reduced the amount of vitamin E needed to prevent muscular dystrophy in the chick,[16] and the appearance of dystrophy was in part dependent on adequate arginine levels.[17] Some vitamin E deficiencies, such as encephalomalacia in chicks, can be accentuated by unsaturated fatty acids, and these can be moderated by the addition of synthetic antioxidants.[18, 19] Dietary sources of antioxidants appear to delay but do not prevent the onset of such deficiency conditions as muscular dystrophy in guinea pigs[20] and fetal resorption in rats.[21, 22] Synthetic antioxidants appear to have a sparing action on the vitamin E requirement, but do not appear to substitute for vitamin E in function.[8, 22, 26]

Environmental and physiological factors can also effect the vitamin E requirement. For the rat, the daily needs for males and females are about equal for reproduction,[23] but the female requires less vitamin E than the male to prevent erythrocyte hemolysis.[24] Growing animals appear to need somewhat less vitamin E than breeding or lactating animals. Particularly with lactating animals, higher levels of vitamin E are needed to produce normal viable young. As in many other physiological functions, the vitamin E requirement appears to be quantitatively related to the 0.7 power of body weight.[25] The age of the animal is important in determining vitamin E requirements. The vitamin E requirement to prevent fetal resorption in rats increased logarithmically with the age of the animals.[26]

In spite of the limitations in the determination of the quantitative requirements for vitamin E, various estimates have been made. Examples of such estimates are summarized in Table XXII.

[15] P. L. Harris, M. I. Ludwig, and K. Schwartz, *Proc. Soc. Exp. Biol. Med.* **97**, 686 (1958).

[16] M. L. Scott, *Nutr. Abstr. Rev.* **32**, 1 (1962).

[17] M. C. Nesheim, C. C. Calvert, and M. L. Scott, *Proc. Soc. Exp. Biol. Med.* **104**, 783 (1960).

[18] H. Dam, I. Kruse, I. Prange, and E. Søndergaard, *Biochim. Biophys. Acta* **2**, 501 (1948).

[19] E. P. Singsen, R. H. Bunnell, L. D. Matterson, H. Kozeff, and E. L. Jungherr, *Poultry Sci.* **34**, 262 (1955).

[20] R. Shull, R. B. Alfin-Slater, H. J. Deuel, Jr., and B. H. Ershoff, *Proc. Soc. Exp. Biol. Med.* **95**, 263 (1957).

[21] F. Christensen, H. Dam, and R. A. Gortner, *Acta. Physiol. Scand.* **36**, 87 (1956).

[22] S. R. Ames, M. I. Ludwig, W. J. Swanson, and P. L. Harris, *Proc. Soc. Exp. Biol. Med.* **93**, 39 (1956).

[23] K. E. Mason, *Amer. J. Physiol.* **131**, 268 (1940).

[24] R. J. Ward, *Brit. J. Nutr.* **17**, 135 (1963).

[25] P. L. Harris, *Ann. N.Y. Acad. Sci.* **52**, 240 (1949).

[26] S. R. Ames and M. I. Ludwig, *Fed. Proc. Fed. Amer. Soc. Exp. Biol.* **23**, 291 (1964).

TABLE XXII

ESTIMATES OF VITAMIN E REQUIREMENTS

Species	Level (α-tocopherol)	References
Man, infant	5 IU/day	27
adult	20–30 IU/day	27
Monkey	0.7–3 mg/kg body wt/day	28
Dog	44 mg/kg feed	29
Cat	34–136 IU/kg/feed	30
Mink	6–10 mg/day	31, 32
Cattle, beef	44–176 IU/100 kg body wt/day	33
dairy	165 mg/100 kg body wt/day	34
Swine	40 mg/kg feed	35, 36
Rat, growth	60 mg/kg feed	30
gestation	30 mg/kg feed	30
Chickens, grower diets	15–31 IU/kg feed	19, 37, 38
breeding diets	41 IU/kg feed	39
Turkeys, grower diets	15–20 IU/kg feed	40, 41
breeding diets	31–44 IU/kg feed	42, 43

[27] "Recommended Dietary Allowances," 7th Ed., *Nat. Acad. Sci.—Nat. Res. Counc., Publ.* **1964**, (1968).

[28] C. D. Fitch and J. S. Dinning, *J. Nutr.* **79**, 69 (1963).

[29] "Nutrient Requirements of Dogs," Rev. Ed., *Nat. Acad. Sci.—Nat. Res. Counc., Publ.* **989**, (1962).

[30] "Nutrient Requirements of Laboratory Animals," *Nat. Acad. Sci.—Nat. Res. Counc., Publ.* **990**, (1962).

[31] J. R. Gorham, G. A. Baker, and N. Boe, *Vet. Med.* **46**, 100 (1951).

[32] H. C. Momberg-Jørgensen, *Dan. Pelsdyravl* **16**, 44 (1953).

[33] "Nutrient Requirements of Beef Cattle," Rev. Ed., *Nat. Acad. Sci.—Nat. Res. Counc., Publ.* **1137**, (1963).

[34] J. W. Thomas and M. Okamoto, *J. Dairy Sci.* **39**, 928 (1956).

[35] A. G. Hogan and G. C. Anderson, *J. Nutr.* **36**, 437 (1948).

[36] R. G. Eggert, E. Patterson, W. T. Akers, and E. L. R. Stokstad, *J. Anim. Sci.* **16**, 1037 (1957).

[37] M. L. Scott, L. C. Norris, G. F. Heuser, and T. S. Nelson, *Poultry Sci.* **34**, 1220 (1955).

[38] T. W. Griffiths, *Brit. J. Nutr.* **15**, 271 (1961).

[39] E. P. Singsen, L. D. Matterson, A. Kozeff, R. H. Bunnell, and E. L. Jungherr, *Poultry Sci.* **33**, 192 (1954).

[40] M. L. Scott, *Poultry Sci.* **32**, 670 (1953).

[41] S. J. Slinger, W. F. Pepper, and I. Motzok, *J. Nutr.* **52**, 395 (1954).

[42] R. L. Atkinson, T. M. Ferguson, J. H. Quisenberry, and J. R. Couch, *J. Nutr.* **55**, 387 (1955).

[43] L. S. Jensen, M. L. Scott, G. F. Heuser, L. C. Norris, and T. S. Nelson, *Poultry Sci.* **35**, 810 (1956).

XIV. Requirements of Man

M. K. HORWITT

Any previous doubt that man may need α-tocopherol, or an equivalent fat-soluble antioxidant, has been dispelled recently by both depletion studies in adult men and by studies of creatinuria in patients who have difficulty absorbing fats. The problem that remains is determining more exactly how much α-tocopherol is required under the different circumstances of varying diets and stresses.

Harris and Embree[1] have compared the published data on the tocopherol requirement of animals with data on average diets in the United States and with the results found in depletion studies on man[2] and have suggested that a ratio of α-tocopherol to polyunsaturated fatty acids of approximately 0.6 will protect against vitamin E deficiency.

As a part of the National Research Council sponsored Elgin Project[2] on human requirements, animal studies were designed to quantitize the recognized[3] relationships between unsaturated fat and tocopherol. With chick encephalomalacia[4] used as an end point, and varying the amounts of the same stripped corn oil that was fed to the human subjects, it was noted that the requirement for tocopherol increased as the corn oil was increased up to a level of the consumption of 4% linoleic acid in the diet of the chicks. Using creatinuria in rats as an end point but employing a variety of fats, Century and Horwitt[5] obtained confirmation that it was not the amount of fat fed, but the degree of unsaturation, that was primary. The oxidative process both *in vivo* and *in vitro* behaves as though it were a free-radical initiated reaction (Tappel[6]) occurring in an isolated lipid phase. In an extension of this work which attempted to establish this relationship in the tissues more quantitatively, Witting and Horwitt[7] showed that the rate of development of creatinuria could be mathematically related to the *in vitro* oxidation rates[8] of different unsaturated fats. The data obtained in the tocopherol-deficient rats were consistent with relative *in vivo* rates of fatty acid peroxidation of monoenoic, dienoic, trienoic, tetraenoic, pentaenoic, and hexaenoic fatty

[1] P. L. Harris and N. D. Embree, *Amer. J. Clin. Nutr.* **13**, 385 (1963).

[2] M. K. Horwitt, *Amer. J. Clin. Nutr.* **8**, 451 (1960).

[3] L. J. Filer, R. E. Rumery, and K. E. Mason, *J. Amer. Oil Chem. Soc.* **24**, 240 (1947).

[4] B. Century, M. K. Horwitt, and P. Bailey, *AMA Arch. Gen. Psychiat.* **1**, 420 (1959).

[5] B. Century and M. K. Horwitt, *J. Nutr.* **72**, 357 (1960).

[6] A. L. Tappel, *Vitam. Horm.* (*New York*) **20**, 493 (1962).

[7] L. A. Witting and M. K. Horwitt, *J. Nutr.* **82**, 19 (1964).

[8] R. T. Holman, *Prog. Chem. Fats Other Lipids* **2**, 73 (1961).

acids in the ratios 0.025, 1, 2, 4, 6, and 8, respectively. The relative amounts of tocopherol required for a constant diminution of the rate of *in vivo* peroxidation were approximately in the ratios of 0.3, 2, 3, 4, 5, and 6, respectively. Accordingly, if such data are translated to human requirements one would have to discuss the needs for tocopherol in terms of relative peroxidizability of the fatty acids in the diet and in the tissues instead of in terms of the total amount of polyunsaturated fatty acids.

Present approximations of tocopherol requirements of adult man are stated as varying between 10 mg and 30 mg/day depending upon the lipids in the diet.[9] The lower level is related to the amount usually found in diets low in vegetable fats and high in animal protein.[10] The higher level is taken from the observations that patients who have been depleted of tocopherol and who were consuming the equivalent of 30 gm of linoleic acid/day (60 gm of stripped corn oil) required a supplement of 30 mg of α-tocopherol/day for many months to keep their plasma tocopherol levels and peroxide hemolysis tests within normal ranges.[2] In such patients, a supplement of 15 mg of α-tocopherol, even after 4 months of continuous supplementation, was not sufficient to protect the erythrocytes from peroxide hemolysis; the plasma levels had returned to a normal range but that this was more a reflection of the residuals from the daily ingestion of the supplement than of any true balance was shown by withdrawing the supplement for a few days to produce a rapid drop in the plasma tocopherol levels.

How much other factors, such as protein deficiency,[11] and the level of other potential antioxidants in the diet, such as selenium,[12] affect the human tocopherol requirement is at present an open question.

[9] "Recommended Dietary Allowances," *Nat. Acad. Sci.—Nat. Res. Counc., Publ.* **1146,** (1963).
[10] P. L. Harris, M. L. Quaife, and W. J. Swanson, *J. Nutr.* **40,** 367 (1950).
[11] J. S. Dinning, *Nutr. Rev.* **21,** 289 (1963).
[12] J. W. Hamilton and A. L. Tappel, *J. Nutr.* **79,** 493 (1963).

CHAPTER 17

NEW AND UNIDENTIFIED GROWTH FACTORS

I. Lipoic Acid (Thioctic Acid)

VERNON H. CHELDELIN AND ANNETTE BAICH

The body of information that has formed the basis for the preceding chapters has enabled us to obtain a clear outline of the chemistry and function of several of the vitamins that have been discussed. Although the pioneer work on vitamins was done only half a century ago, the intensity of research, particularly during the past two decades, has so overcome the time disadvantage that several vitamin systems are now as well or better understood than many of the more classic compounds of biochemical importance.

Research on new growth factors must, like the discovery of gold, come some time to an end; and it is proposed herewith to end their formal discussion with the present discourse, reserving the right, of course, to reopen the subject if future events should warrant it. The "new factors" have not increased in number since the last previous edition of this volume,[1] and although the last word has probably not been written on this subject, it is proposed that germane new material can be covered most easily in the future under a title that refers more directly to it. Meanwhile, the emphasis is shifting from research on new factors to a search for (new) mechanisms of biological action, as the new information may appropriately be added.

Lipoic acid is selected for initial consideration because it typifies well what has already been said. As most of the previous investigators have turned to other, more fruitful kinds of investigation, only Reed and his co-workers remain actively studying new forms of lipoic acid; two reviews by Reed[2,3] and another by Wagner and Folkers[4] contain most of the pertinent informa-

[1] V. H. Cheldelin, in "The Vitamins" (W. H. Sebrell, Jr. and R. S. Harris, eds.), Vol. 3, pp. 575–600. Academic Press, New York, 1954.
[2] L. J. Reed, *Vitam. Horm.* (*New York*) 20, 1 (1962).
[3] L. J. Reed, in "The Enzymes" (P. D. Boyer, H. Lardy, and K. Myrbäck, eds.), 2nd Ed., Vol. 3, pp. 195–223. Academic Press, New York, 1960.
[4] A. F. Wagner and K. Folkers, "Vitamins and Coenzymes," pp. 244–63. Wiley (Interscience), New York, 1964.

tion that has been amassed regarding this factor. Together with the work of Reed may now be added that of Sanadi and co-workers,[5] as attempts were made to describe a meaningful enzymatic role for this compound. The work of Calvin[6] should be mentioned, not because it has yet been proved to be experimentally meaningful, but because the interesting possibility that he has raised previously still has not been disproved. Finally, the work of Breslow[7] deserves mention here because it indicates some possibilities for continued research on the closely related problem of thiamine activity.

Studies on the probable role of lipoic acid in metabolism have clustered about two closely related, although different, conditions: those that involve the free vitamin added to systems in substrate amounts,[8, 9] and others involving (partially) purified enzyme systems in which the lipoic acid came largely from natural sources.[10–13] The results are largely in agreement, and are condensed in Fig. 1, although it should be remembered that the contribution of Gunsalus and co-workers to this scheme was made with the aid of free, added lipoic acid, whereas Reed and co-workers employed the vitamin largely as obtained in bound form from the extracts studied.

Interest in lipoic acid metabolism was heightened by the possibility, alluded to previously,[5] that lipoic acid might play a part in the primary quantum conversion act of photosynthesis. This suggestion was made by Calvin and seemed especially noteworthy. Unfortunately, subsequent experimental attempts at verification of this idea have not been rewarding, despite the authors' continued interest in the problem. In spite of the attractiveness of the idea and the seeming logic behind some suppositions that were made, including possible structures of intermediates, results have not borne them out. The negative reaction expressed by Wagner and Folkers[4] seemingly must still prevail, in assessment of a possible role for this vitamin: that there is no clear evidence for a deficiency of lipoic acid. While Folkers' statement applied to mammalian nutrition, it would seem logical now to extend it to other systems—remembering meanwhile that only one bona fide positive result is needed to revive interest in any compound and dispel many doubts of its role in other systems.

[5] D. R. Sanadi, M. Langley, and F. White, *J. Biol. Chem.* **234**, 183 (1959).
[6] M. Calvin, *in* "The Vitamins" (W. H. Sebrell, Jr. and R. S. Harris, eds.), Vol. 3, pp. 575–600. Academic Press, New York, 1954.
[7] R. Breslow, The Mechanism of Thiamine Action: Evidence from Studies on Model Systems. *CBA Found. Study Group (Pap.)* **11**, pp. 65–79.
[8] I. C. Gunsalus, *in* "The Mechanism of Enzyme Action" (W. D. McElroy and B. Glass, eds.), p. 553. Johns Hopkins Press, Baltimore, Maryland.
[9] I. C. Gunsalus, L. S. Barton, and W. Gruber, *J. Amer. Chem. Soc.* **78**, 1763 (1956).
[10] L. J. Reed, M. Koike, M. E. Levitch, and F. R. Leach, *J. Biol. Chem.* **232**, 143 (1958).
[11] M. Koike, L. J. Reed, and W. R. Carroll, *J. Biol. Chem.* **235**, 1924 (1960).
[12] M. Koike and L. J. Reed, *J. Biol. Chem.* **235**, 1931 (1960).
[13] M. Koike, P. C. Shah, and L. J. Reed, *J. Biol. Chem.* **235**, 1939 (1960).

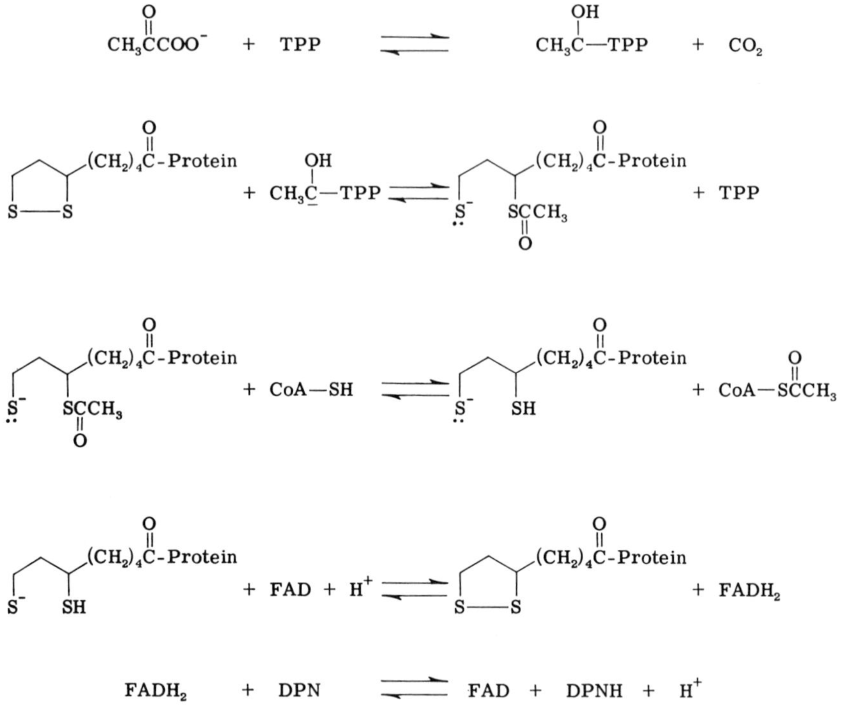

$$CH_3\overset{O}{\overset{\|}{C}}COO^- + TPP \rightleftharpoons CH_3\overset{OH}{\overset{|}{C}}-TPP + CO_2$$

$$\text{(structure)} + CH_3\overset{OH}{\overset{|}{C}}-TPP \rightleftharpoons \text{(structure)} + TPP$$

$$\text{(structure)} + CoA-SH \rightleftharpoons \text{(structure)} + CoA-S\overset{O}{\overset{\|}{C}}CH_3$$

$$\text{(structure)} + FAD + H^+ \rightleftharpoons \text{(structure)} + FADH_2$$

$$FADH_2 + DPN \rightleftharpoons FAD + DPNH + H^+$$

FIG. 1. Role of lipoic acid in oxidative decarboxylation.[8-13] TPP, thiamine pyrophosphate; COA-Sh, coenzyme A; FAD, flovin adenine dinucleotide; DPN (= NAD), diphosphopyridine nucleotide.

II. Peptides in Metabolism and Nutrition

VERNON H. CHELDELIN AND ANNETTE BAICH

The advantage gained by using peptides as opposed to free amino acids in microbial nutrition may be explained by a consideration of at least four factors. First, the administration of a single amino acid may antagonize the absorption, use, or synthesis of another amino acid; second, the administration of a single amino acid may be inefficient, because it is rapidly degraded; and third, a peptide may be a more effective nutrient if the concentration mechanism for the amino acid, but not the peptide, is impaired. In addition, it has been suggested by some workers that peptides per se are required for the growth of certain organisms.

A direct involvement of a dipeptide in metabolism was demonstrated by Neuhaus,[14] who described the purificaton of the enzyme which forms the dipeptide D-Ala·D-Ala, in the synthesis of cell walls. The reaction is

$$ATP + 2\ \text{D-Ala} = \text{D-Ala} \cdot \text{D-Ala} + ADP + P_i$$

Comb[15] has described the enzyme which adds D-Ala·D-Ala to the nucleotide UDP-N-acetylglucosamine-3-O-lactyl-Ala·Glu·DAP, also in cell wall synthesis. Ito and Strominger[16,17] have studied the stepwise addition of L-Ala, L-Glu, and L-Lys and D-Ala·D-Ala to UDP-N-acetylglucosamine by *Staphylococcus aureus* extracts. These authors consider the synthesis of this nucleotide peptide to be analogous to the synthesis of glutamine or glutathione, since free amino acids do not catalyze an exchange reaction with ATP.

Recently, Gilvarg and Katchalski[18] tested the effect of size of a peptide on its nutritional usefulness. Using a strain of *Escherichia coli* which requires lysine, they found that the organism can use di-, tri-, and tetrapeptides. Peptides larger than this are discriminated against, apparently at the entry site. An unsubstituted α-amino group was also critical to peptide utilization.

Strepogenin.[19–24] Considerable interest was created by the discovery by Woolley and Sprince[25,26] of a peptide-like fraction of natural materials that was necessary for growth of a strain of hemolytic streptococci. The material, which was called strepogenin, was also shown to be needed for early growth of *Lactobacillus casei* and to promote growth in mice.[27] However, its structure is still unknown, and to the writer's knowledge no pure samples of strepogenin have been prepared. It is probably a mixture, perhaps of structurally closely related peptides. The best information has been derived indirectly from degradation studies of insulin,[28,29] which was thought to have a strepogenin-like pattern in a portion of its structure, together with inhibition studies on lycomarasmin, the tomato-wilting agent of *Fusarium lycopersici* SACC.

[14] F. C. Neuhaus, *J. Biol. Chem.* **237**, 778 (1962).
[15] D. G. Comb, *J. Biol. Chem.* **237**, 1601 (1962) [*Chem. Abstr.* **58**, 707C].
[16] E. Ito and J. L. Strominger, *J. Biol. Chem.* **235**, PC5 (1960).
[17] E. Ito and J. L. Strominger, *J. Biol. Chem.* **235**, PC7 (1960).
[18] C. Gilvarg and E. Katchalski, *J. Biol. Chem.* **240**, 3093 (1965).
[19] *Nutr. Rev.* **4**, 273 (1946).
[20] *Nutr. Rev.* **5**, 218 (1947).
[21] *Nutr. Rev.* **6**, 223, 277 (1948).
[22] D. W. Woolley, *Annu. Rev. Biochem.* **16**, 376 (1947).
[23] E. L. R. Stokstad and T. H. Jukes, *Annu. Rev. Biochem.* **17**, 474 (1949).
[24] E. E. Snell and L. D. Wright, *Annu. Rev. Biochem.* **19**, 305 (1950).
[25] D. W. Woolley, *J. Exp. Med.* **73**, 487 (1941).
[26] H. Sprince and D. W. Woolley, *J. Exp. Med.* **80**, 213 (1944).
[27] D. W. Woolley, *J. Biol. Chem.* **162**, 383 (1946).
[28] D. W. Woolley, *J. Biol. Chem.* **171**, 443 (1947).
[29] D. W. Woolley, *J. Biol. Chem.* **179**, 593 (1949).

Lycomarasmin activity in tomatoes could be duplicated by tripeptides containing serine, glycine, and aspartic acid.[30] These peptides were also antagonistic to strepogenin for *L. casei*. Serylglycylglutamic acid was then synthesized and found to possess strepogenin activity, about one-fortieth that of strepogenin concentrates. It was concluded that the latter peptide may be a fragment or a relative of strepogenin.

Support for the concept of an intrinsic growth-promoting property associated with the serine–glycine–glutamic acid structure is provided by the experiments of Chattaway and co-workers.[31, 32] They found that extracts of liver and yeast contained growth-promoting agents for *Corynebacterium diphtheriae gravis*, *Streptococcus faecalis R.*, and *L. casei*, which upon concentration proved to be of a peptide nature. Two peptides, labeled P_1 and P_2, contained the bulk of the activity; P_2 upon hydrolysis was found to yield serine, glycine, and glutamic acid. Finally, the experiments of Krehl and Fruton[33] have confirmed the activity of L-serylglycyl-L-glutamic acid for *L. casei* and have shown that the closely related L-seryl-L-alanyl-L-glutamic acid was inactive.[33a] Also inactive were several related peptides of glutamic acid, glycine, and tyrosine.

Peptides of other amino acids have also been shown to be more active than their constituent moieties in supporting microbiol growth. Malin *et al.*[36] reported that certain peptides of glycine were utilized more readily by several lactobaccilli than was glycine itself. Simmonds and Fruton observed[37, 38] that a prolineless mutant of *E. coli* was more responsive to any of several proline peptides tested than it was to proline, and that an isolated species of *Alcaligenes*, termed " SF,"[39] required leucyl peptides for growth; with these in the medium, no other nitrogen or carbon source was needed. Other peptide

[30] D. W. Woolley, *J. Biol. Chem.* **166**, 783 (1946).

[31] F. W. Chattaway, F. C. Happold, and M. Sanford, *Biochem. J.* **38**, 111 (1944).

[32] F. W. Chattaway, D. E. Dolby, D. A. Hall, and F. C. Happold, *Biochem. J.* **45**, 592 (1949).

[33] W. A. Krehl and J. S. Fruton, *J. Biol. Chem.* **173**, 479 (1948).

[33a] Although reports on the structure of insulin [34, 35] fail to reveal a serine-glycine-glutamic acid sequence, the closest relatives are a cysteine-glycine-glutamic acid, and a cystein-glycine-serine series. Both of these are found in the " phenylalanine" fraction of insulin rather than in the " glycine" fraction where strepogenin activity was first reported.[28] However, the similarity of the first sequence listed here to the strepogenin-active compound (serine replaced by cysteine) may warrant the testing of additional peptides.

[34] F. Sanger and H. Tuppy, *Biochem. J.* **49**, 481 (1951).

[35] F. Sanger and E. O. P. Thompson, *Biochem. J.* **53**, 366 (1953).

[36] R. B. Malin, M. N. Camien, and M. S. Dunn, *Arch. Biochem. Biophys.* **32**, 106 (1951).

[37] S. Simmonds and J. S. Fruton, *J. Biol. Chem.* **174**, 705 (1948).

[38] S. Simmonds and J. S. Fruton, *J. Biol. Chem.* **180**, 635 (1949).

[39] S. Simmonds and J. S. Fruton, *Science* **109**, 561 (1949).

requirements have been demonstrated by Kihara *et al.*[40-42] in a medium in which D-alanine satisfied the vitamin B_6 requirement; *L. casei* could be shown also to depend upon a peptide factor for its nutrition. Fractionation of the factor from partly hydrolyzed casein produced a mixture of dipeptides, thought to be the alanyl and tyrosyl peptides of valine, leucine, and isoleucine. Also, Sloane and McKee[43] have shown that the *Staphylococcus albus* factor of Hughes[44] is replaceable by an intact plasma protein fraction, the activity of which may be due to special peptide structures, especially those of cysteine.

Apart from this, it has been shown that in *L. casei,*[41] when D-alanine was present in the medium it inhibited the utilization of the L-isomer; however, D-alanine had no effect on L-alanine peptides. A similar effect was then suggested for other systems, i.e., an antagonism among certain related amino acids that may not be experienced when peptides are employed instead. The destructive action of tyrosine decarboxylase[42] upon free tyrosine, but not on its peptides, was also noted and offered as an explanation of the greater response of *S. faecalis* to tyrosine peptides. Finally, it should be pointed out that many peptides have been shown to be *less* active than their constituents.[45,46] These may simply become digested, assimilated, and re-synthesized into protein patterns in which the peptide sequences in question may not appear at all. Some peptides (in addition to the antibiotic polypeptides) actually delay or inhibit bacterial growth,[47] perhaps by interference with the synthesis of peptides and proteins within the cells.

The role of strepogenin and other peptides in animal nutrition is doubtful. Although Womack and Rose[48] were able to produce more rapid weight gains in rats fed intact protein (casein) than in those maintained on nineteen amino acids, these differences have been eliminated by employing acid-hydrolyzed casein supplemented with tryptophan and cystine (Ramasarma *et al.*[49]). The casein hydrolyzate was devoid of strepogenin activity. Other workers[50,51] have also shown that properly balanced amino acid mixtures supported good growth of mice and that these mixtures were not improved by the addition of strepogenin-rich proteins. It is possible that lower taste acceptability may have been chiefly responsible for the poorer performance

[40] H. Kihara, W. G. McCullough, and E. E. Snell, *J. Biol. Chem.* **197**, 783 (1952).
[41] H. Kihara and E. E. Snell, *J. Biol. Chem.* **197**, 791 (1952).
[42] H. Kihara, O. A. Klatt, and E. E. Snell, *J. Biol. Chem.* **197**, 801 (1952).
[43] N. H. Sloane and R. W. McKee, *J. Amer. Chem. Soc.* **74**, 987 (1952).
[44] T. P. Hughes, *J. Bacteriol.* **23**, 437 (1932).
[45] J. S. Fruton and S. Simmonds, *Cold Spring Harbor Symp. Quant. Biol.* **14**, 55 (1949).
[46] V. Nurmikko and A. I. Virtanen, *Acta Chem. Scand.* **5**, 97 (1951).
[47] S. Simmonds, J. I. Harris, and J. S. Fruton, *J. Biol. Chem.* **188**, 251 (1951).
[48] M. Womack and W. C. Rose, *J. Biol. Chem.* **162**, 735 (1946).
[49] G. B. Ramasarma, L. M. Henderson, and C. A. Elvehjem, *J. Nutr.* **38**, 177 (1949).
[50] E. Brand and D. K. Bosshardt, *Abstr. Amer. Chem. Soc., 114th Meet.* p. 38C (1948).
[51] K. H. Maddy and C. A. Elvehjem, *J. Biol. Chem.* **177**, 577 (1949).

Organism	Peptide–source	References
Lactobacillus	Alanine, glycine	41, 59
	Casein hydrolyzates	60, 62–65
	Human serum	66
	Chymotrypsinogen	67
	Pronulan	68
	Oxytocin, insulin	61, 69, 70
	Cow spleen	71
	L. casei	72
L. delbrueckii	Serine peptides	58
	Histidine, protein	73, 74
Leuconostoc mesenteroides	Peptides, glycyl peptides	75–77
Streptococcus faecalis	Soybeans, D-Ala-Gly	40
	Tyrosine peptides	42
	p-Aminobenzoyl peptides	81
Escherichia coli, K12	Serine dipeptides	82
E. coli	Glucosylglycine	83
	Proline peptides	84
	Peptides	79
Bacillus subtilis	Glycine peptides	85
P. cerevisiae	Casein	86
Pasteurella pestis	Methionine and phenyl alanine peptides	87
Lactobacillus bulgaricus	Protein digests	88
Streptococcus	Peptides	89
Tomato root tips	5-OHTrp-Glu-Arg-Ala-Val-Leu	90
Salmonella pullorum	Glycine peptides	91
Pediococcus soyae	Casein	92
Gram-negative bacillus	Glycine dipeptide	93
Lactobacillus sake	Casein	94
Paramecium aurelia	Yeast	95
Homo sapiens	Bovine blood	96
Milk starter culture	Peptides	97
Mouse cells	Tripeptide	98
Erysipelothrix rhusiopathiae	Peptides	99
L. arabinosus	*p*-Aminobenzylpeptides	81
Lactic acid bacteria	Pancreas	100
Saccharomyces carlsbergensis	Alanine dipeptides	101
Mammalian cells	Dipeptide	102
Chick heart cells	Peptide	103
Staphylococci	Peptide	104
Hiochi-kin	Rice	105
Bacillus alkaliphilus	Peptide	106
Bacteroides ruminicola	Peptides	107
Mycoplasma laidlawii	Thr-Thr-Glu · NH_2-Ala-Asp · NH_2-Lys	108

on amino acid mixtures.[49, 52] The need for special peptides such as strepogenin thus seems to be best established for microbial species. Even with these, the proportion of peptides that is utilized per se is probably very small; in *L. casei*, strepogenin activity has been claimed for glutamine[53] (although this is not in agreement with the findings of others[54–56]). Below are listed some additional reports of peptides which have been found to be effective in nutritional studies.

The study of peptides was begun, as so much of biochemistry, in the study of nutrition, with the idea that peptides had a possibly unique role in the nourishment of an organism, apart from the constituent amino acids. The study of peptides as growth factors has led, however, to an intense examination of the general subject of amino acid competition and amino acid transport. Only now, with the work of Umbarger, Changeux, Stadtman, and many others is there an adequate explanation for the amino acid antagonisms which were discovered during the earlier nutritional studies.

[52] L. P. Snipper, Ph.D. Thesis, Oregon State College, Corvallis, Oregon, 1951.
[53] H. T. Peeler, L. J. Daniel, L. C. Norris, and G. F. Heuser, *J. Biol. Chem.* **177**, 905 (1949).
[54] L. D. Wright and H. R. Skeggs, *J. Bacteriol.* **48**, 117 (1944).
[55] E. Kodicek and S. P. Mistry, *Biochem. J.* **51**, 108 (1951).
[56] E. Kodicek and S. P. Mistry, *Arch. Biochem. Biophys.* **44**, 30 (1953).
[57] M. Harris, *Growth* **16**, 215 (1952) [*Chem. Abstr.* **47**, 82222d].
[58] J. M. Prescott, V. J. Peters, and E. E. Snell, *J. Biol. Chem.* **202**, 533 (1953) [*Chem. Abstr.* **47**, 8832b].
[59] F. R. Leach and E. E. Snell, *Biochim. Biophys. Acta* **34**, 292 (1959) [*Chem. Abstr.* **53**, 20270c].
[60] J. Gonin, P. Baudet, and E. Cherbuliez, *Pharm. Acta Helv.* **37**, 425 (1962) [*Chem. Abstr.* **57**, 12842a].
[61] G. L. Tritsch and D. W. Woolley, *J. Amer. Chem. Soc.* **80**, 1490 (1958).
[62] P. Baudet and E. Cherbuliez, *Helv. Chim. Acta* **43**, 904 (1960) [*Chem. Abstr.* **55**, 5602a].
[63] O. Mikeš and F. Šorm, *Collect. Czech. Chem. Commun.* **24**, 1897 (1959) [*Chem. Abstr.* **54**, 606f].
[64] B. N. Mashelkar and K. Sohonie, *Ann. Biochem. Exp. Med.* **18**, 183 (1958) [*Chem. Abstr.* **53**, 13442d].
[65] O. Mikeš, V. Schuh, and F. Šorm, *Chem. Listy* **52**, 1801 (1958) [*Chem. Abstr.* **53**, 3339c].
[66] V. V. Mosolov, I. V. Skarlat, and P. V. Afanasiev, *Biokhimiya* **27**, 219 (1962).
[67] O. Mikeš and F. Šorm, *Chem. Listy* **52**, 1975 (1958) [*Chem. Abstr.* **53**, 3339e].
[68] O. Mikeš and F. Šorm, *Chem. Listy* **52**, 2160 (1958) [*Chem. Abstr.* **53**. 3339i].
[69] D. W. Woolley, R. B. Merrifield, C. Ressler, and V. du Vigneaud, *Proc. Soc. Exp. Biol. Med.* **89**, 669 (1955).
[70] R. B. Merrifield and D. W. Woolley, *J. Amer. Chem. Soc.* **78**, 358 (1956).
[71] G. Ågren, *Acta Pathol. Microbiol. Scand.* **35**, 97, 136 (1954).
[72] P. Baudet and E. Cherbuliez, *Helv. Chim. Acta* **44**, 1142 (1961).
[73] V. J. Peters, J. M. Prescott, and E. E. Snell, *J. Biol. Chem.* **202**, 521 (1953).
[74] V. J. Peters and E. E. Snell, *J. Bacteriol.* **67**, 69 (1954).
[75] T. P. O'Barr, H. Levin, and H. Reynolds, *J. Bacteriol.* **75**, 429 (1958).

[76] Ko Aida, Tadayuki Kajiwara, and Toshinobu Asai, *Nippon Nogei Kagaku Kaishi* **35**, 292 (1961) [*Chem. Abstr.* **61**, 3440a].

[77] D. C. Shelton and W. E. Nutter, *J. Bacteriol* **88**, 1175 (1964).

[78] P. N. Davis, L. C. Norris, and F. H. Kratzer, *J. Nutr.* **76**, 223 (1962).

[79] H. Kihara and E. E. Snell, *J. Biol. Chem.* **212**, 83 (1955) [*Chem. Abstr.* **49**, 4790f].

[80] T. A. Nevin, *J. Bacteriol.* **67**, 217 (1954).

[81] P. R. Pal, B. N. Banerjee, and B. C. Guha, *Ann. Biochem. Exp. Med.* **17**, 151 (1957) [*Chem. Abstr.* **52**, 11171e].

[82] J. O. Meinhardt and S. Simmonds, *J. Biol. Chem.* **216**, 51 (1955).

[83] D. Rogers, *J. Bacteriol.* **80**, 794 (1960).

[84] David Stone and H. D. Hoberman, *J. Biol. Chem.* **202**, 203 (1953) [*Chem. Abstr.* **47**, 8831a].

[85] A. L. Demain and D. Hendlin, *J. Bacteriol.* **75**, 46 (1958) [*Chem. Abstr.* **52**, 5539h].

[86] H. A. Florsheim, S. Makineni, and S. Shankman, *Arch. Biochem. Biophys.* **97**, 243 (1962) [*Chem. Abstr.* **57**, 7719a].

[87] J. L. Smith and K. Higuchi, *J. Bacteriol.* **77**, 604 (1959).

[88] K. M. Jones and D. W. Woolley, *J. Bacteriol.* **83**, 797 (1962).

[89] E. N. Fox, *J. Biol. Chem.* **236**, 166 (1961).

[90] A. Winter and H. E. Street, *Nature (London)* **198**, 1283 (1963) [*Chem. Abstr.* **59**, 5386g].

[91] H. Shoji, *Nisshin Igaku* **49**, 819 (1962) [*Chem. Abstr.* **59**, 11926c].

[92] Kenji Sakaguchi, *Bull. Agr. Chem. Soc. Jap.* **23**, 438 (1959) [*Chem. Abstr.* **54**, 2653a].

[93] S. Simmonds and J. S. Fruton, *Yale J. Biol. Med.* **23**, 407 (1951),

[94] K. Kitahara and A. Ohayashi, *Nippon Nogei Kagaku Kaishi* **33**, 524 (1959) [*Chem. Abstr.* **57**, 3773h].

[95] V. A. Tarantola and W. J. Van Wagtendonk, *J. Protozool.* **6**, 189 (1959) [*Chem. Abstr.* **54**, 25335a].

[96] K. Raczńska-Bojanowska and I. Chmielewska, *Bull Acad. Pol. Sci., Ser. Sci. Biol.* **6**, 1 (1958) [*Chem. Abstr.* **53**, 22453h].

[97] W. E. Sandine and J. K. McAnelly, *Milk Plant Mon.* **46**, 23 (1957).

[98] K. K. Sanford, W. T. McQuilkin, M. C. Fioramonti, V. J. Evans, and W. R. Earle, *J. Nat. Cancer Inst.* **20**, 775 (1958).

[99] G. Zimmermann and K. H. Kludas, *Arch. Exp. Veterinäermed* **10**, 237 (1956) [*Chem. Abstr.* 2116b].

[100] W. E. Sandine, M. L. Speck, and L. W. Aurand, *J. Dairy Sci.* **39**, 1532 (1956) [*Chem. Abstr.* **51**, 3734e].

[101] A. Betz, *Arch. Mikrobiol.* **44**, 253 (1962) [*Chem. Abstr.* **58**, 9433g].

[102] H. Eagle, *Proc. Soc. Exp. Biol. Med.* **89**, 96 (1955) [*Chem. Abstr.* **49**, 1180f].

[103] R. E. Winnick and T. Winnick, *J. Nat. Cancer Inst.* **14**, 519 (1953) [*Chem. Abstr.* **48**, 2801c].

[104] S. Goto, C. Niwa, Y. Onuma, S. Kuwahara, and H. Shoji, *Nisshin Igaku* **49**, 274 (1962) [*Chem. Abstr.* **57**, 10343a].

[105] S. Teramoto, W. Hashida, and Y. Endo, *Hakko Kogaku Zasshi* **35**, 32 (1957) [*Chem. Abstr.* **51**, 18101a].

[106] Y. Takasaki, Y. Takasaki, and O. Tanabe, *Kogyo Gijutsuin, Hakko Kenkyusho Kenkyu Hokoku* **22**, 85 (1962) [*Chem. Abstr.* **60**, 14858h].

[107] K. A. Pittman and M. P. Bryant, *J. Bacteriol* **88**, 401 (1964).

[108] M. E. Tourtellotte, H. J. Morowitz, and P. Kasimir, *J. Bacteriol.* **88**, 11 (1964).

III. Carnitine

STANLEY FRIEDMAN[1] AND G. S. FRAENKEL[2]

A. Introduction

The history of carnitine, β-hydroxy-γ-butyrobetaine $(CH_3)_3N^+CH_2$-$CHOHCH_2COO^-$ is different from that of almost all other vitamins in that its discovery and identification preceded recognition of its vitamin function by almost fifty years. The reasons for this are two: (1) it is found in large amounts in a natural product of commercial value, i.e., meat extract; and (2) until very recently, investigations concerned with its activity as a vitamin were confined to work on a small group of insects.

The record of carnitine research can be divided into four relatively independent periods, each governed by some observation that renewed speculation concerning its function. An initial flurry of interest leading to its isolation from meat extract and approximate characterization (1905–1910)[3–5] was followed by an interval of intermittent activity which lasted until 1927,[6] when its structure was finally established. It then disappeared from the literature to be disinterred when the physiological roles of acetylcholine and choline were recognized in the early 1930's. At that time, a number of quaternary ammonium compounds, including carnitine, became objects of intensive study, especially by a group associated with E. Strack at the University of Leipzig. This phase was at an end by 1939, and twelve years passed before a third round of inquiry began, this time as a result of the discovery of its function as an insect growth factor.

In 1948,[7] Fraenkel's research on the dietary requirements of the mealworm, *Tenebrio molitor*, led to the recognition of a new B vitamin, B_T, which, in 1952, was identified as carnitine (Carter *et al.*[8]). With the aid of a sensitive assay procedure and new isolation methods (Friedman *et al.*[9]), a large number

[1] Part of the preparation of this contribution was assisted by NIH grant AI-06345.
[2] Supported by a Public Health Service research career award from the Division of General Medical Sciences.
[3] V. S. Gulewitsch and R. Krimberg, *Hoppe-Seyler's Z. Physiol. Chem.* **45**, 326 (1905).
[4] F. Kutscher, *Z. Unters. Nahr. Genussm. Gebrauchsgegenstaende* **10**, 528 (1905).
[5] R. Krimberg, *Hoppe-Seyler's Z. Physiol. Chem.* **53**, 514 (1907).
[6] M. Tomita and Y. Sendju, *Hoppe-Seyler's Z. Physiol. Chem.* **169**, 263 (1927).
[7] G. Fraenkel, *Nature (London)* **161**, 981 (1948).
[8] H. E. Carter, P. K. Bhattacharyya, K. R. Weidman, and G. Fraenkel, *Arch. Biochem. Biophys.* **38**, 405 (1952).
[9] S. Friedman, J. E. McFarlane, P. K. Bhattacharyya, and G. Fraenkel, *Arch. Biochem. Biophys.* **59**, 484 (1955).

of organisms and tissues were studied and the ubiquity of this compound in living material was uncovered (Fraenkel[10–12]). These studies led logically to investigations of the specificity of structure (Bhattacharyya et al.[13]).

The current (fourth) phase, which is involved with the physiological role of carnitine, stems from the fact that it is of universal occurrence in biological systems and is required as a vitamin in a small number of cases. "Since the vital function of carnitine is obvious in those animals in which it plays the role of a vitamin, there is a strong possibility that its function in the majority of animals which synthesize it is also vital."[14] The first clue to this role arose from the finding that γ-butyrobetaine inhibited the action of carnitine, which resulted in recognition of the physiological importance of the hydroxy group in the β-position (Bhattacharyya et al.[13]). This was followed by the discovery of an enzyme in animal tissue capable of reversibly acetylating carnitine by transfer from acetylcoenzyme A (Friedman and Fraenkel[15]), and a concurrent observation by Fritz[16] that carnitine increased the rate of fatty acid oxidation by rat liver homogenates. The present main stream of research into the function of carnitine in fatty acid metabolism is a direct outcome of these bits of evidence. Other areas now under investigation are concerned with its presence as a constituent of phosphatides and its importance in nervous activity.

An exhaustive review of various aspects of carnitine synthesis, function, etc., has been published in the recent past (Fraenkel and Friedman,[14]) and much of the detail of its content will not be repeated here. Reviews on more specific subjects that have been released since that time include descriptions of the isolation and purification procedures of carnitine (Carter and Bhattacharyya[17]) and procedures for the preparation of natural carnitine (Friedman et al.[18]). Many aspects of the carnitine problem were discussed at a conference held in 1959[19] and general reviews of carnitine, with special emphasis on clinical aspects, have been published since by Deltour,[20] and Reynier.[21] A comprehensive discussion of the work dealing with the physiological role of

[10] G. Fraenkel, Arch. Biochem. Biophys. 34, 457 (1951).

[11] G. Fraenkel, Biol. Bull. 104, 359 (1953).

[12] G. Fraenkel, Arch. Biochem. Biophys. 50, 486 (1954).

[13] P. K. Bhattacharyya, S. Friedman, and G. Fraenkel, Arch. Biochem. Biophys. 54, 424 (1955).

[14] G. Fraenkel and S. Friedman, Vitam. Horm. (New York) 15, 73 (1957).

[15] S. Friedman and G. Fraenkel, Arch. Biochem. Biophys. 59, 491 (1955).

[16] I. B. Fritz, Acta Physiol. Scand. 34, 367 (1955).

[17] H. E. Carter and P. K. Bhattacharyya, Methods Enzymol. 3, 660 (1957).

[18] S. Friedman, J. E. McFarlane, P. K. Bhattacharyya, and G. Fraenkel, Biochem. Prep. 7, 26 (1960).

[19] H. Peeters, ed., Protides Biol. Fluids, Proc. 1959 Colloq. 7, 235 (1960).

[20] G. Deltour, Ind. Chim. Belge 25, 1329 (1960).

[21] M. Reynier, Rev. Agressol. 4, 361 (1963).

carnitine has recently appeared (Fritz[22]), as has a compilation of papers presented at a symposium concerned with carnitine occurrence and function (Wolf[23]).

B. Structure, Chemical Synthesis, Isolation Methods, and Properties

Since a detailed historical and systematic account of the chemical identification and various methods of synthesis of carnitine has been previously given,[14] a very abbreviated description follows here. The discovery of carnitine in meat extracts and the assignment of the correct empirical formula $C_7H_{15}NO_3$ was made independently by Gulewitsch and Krimberg,[3] and Kutscher,[4] in 1905. Krimberg,[5] as early as 1907, after establishing a number of facts regarding its structure, proposed the correct formula, but in spite of the efforts of some of the best organic chemists of the time, including Engeland, Fischer, and Willstaetter, it was 1927 before Tomita and Sendju[6] separated the two isomers of β-hydroxy-γ-butyrobetaine and demonstrated that the levorotatory isomer was identical with natural carnitine. It was later shown by Friedman *et al.* that the levorotatory form alone is active as a vitamin for *Tenebrio*.[24]

Methods of synthesis of carnitine, including those of Tomita[25] and Tomita and Sendju,[6] Carter and Bhattacharyya,[26] Strack *et al.*,[27] and Dechamps *et al.*,[28] have been set forth elsewhere in some detail.[14] Jellinek and Strength[29] have reported what is described as a "simplified procedure," and recently Binon *et al.*[30] have reviewed the steps in these methods and added the results of a scan of the patent literature. Since all chemical methods of synthesis end up with the racemic mixture which has been difficult to resolve into its components (although, see below), and since only the levorotatory form is biologically active in certain contexts, a number of laborious procedures for isolation of *l*-carnitine from natural materials have been developed. The methods of Gulewitsch and Krimberg (1905),[3] Strack *et al.*,[31] Fraenkel,[32]

[22] I. B. Fritz, *Advan. Lipid Res.* 1, 285 (1963).
[23] G. Wolf, ed., "Recent Research on Carnitine." MIT Press, Cambridge, Massachusetts, 1965.
[24] S. Friedman, A. B. Galun, and G. Fraenkel, *Arch. Biochem. Biophys.* 66, 10 (1957).
[25] M. Tomita, *Hoppe-Seyler's Z. Physiol. Chem.* 124, 253 (1923).
[26] H. E. Carter and P. K. Bhattacharyya, *J. Amer. Chem. Soc.* 75, 2503 (1953).
[27] E. Strack, H. Röhnert, and I. Lorenz, *Chem. Ber.* 86, 525 (1953).
[28] G. Dechamps, N. P. Buu-Hoi, H. Le Bihan, and F. Binon, *C. R. Acad. Sci.* 283, 826 (1954).
[29] M. Jellinek and D. R. Strength, *Fed. Proc. Fed. Amer. Soc. Exp. Biol.* 19, 255 (1960).
[30] F. Binon, P. Bruckner, and G. Deltour, *in* "Recent Research on Carnitine" (G. Wolf, ed.), pp. 7–10 MIT Press, Cambridge, Massachusetts, 1965.
[31] E. Strack, P. Wördehoff, and H. Schwaneberg, *Hoppe-Seyler's Z. Physiol. Chem.* 238, 183 (1936).
[32] G. Fraenkel, *Arch. Biochem. Biophys.* 34, 468 (1951).

Carter et al.,[8] and Friedman et al.[18] are presented elsewhere.[14] A "simplified" method has lately been reported by Jellinek and Strength,[29] as has a method for obtaining small amounts from single animals (Wolf and Berger.[33]).

Isolation of d-carnitine from DL-carnitine has been achieved by growing a bacterium isolated from a polluted stream bed on a synthetic medium containing DL-carnitine chloride as the sole carbon source. The organism (tentatively identified as a pseudomonad), utilized only the l form of the racemic mixture, and d-carnitine was isolated from the medium (Friedman et al.[24]). This work has been repeated, using another pseudomonad, by Aurich and Lorenz.[34]

The chemical method originally used to resolve the two isomers of synthetic carnitine, i.e., the brucine method of Tomita and Sendju,[6] has been found to be very difficult to handle (see Bhattacharyya, in Fraenkel and Friedman),[14] but Strack and Lorenz[35] have recently been able to separate both d- and l-carnitine nitrile from a racemic mixture using D-camphor sulfonic acid to precipitate the d form and then dibenzoyl-D-tartaric acid to remove the l form. Brendel and Bressler[36] have slightly modified Strack's procedure to obtain higher yields and have also improved the yields of resolved acyl-carnitines. A patent has recently been taken out on a process for resolving DL-carnitine using N-acetyl-d-glutamic acid to sequentially precipitate the nitrile isomers.[37]

PROPERTIES OF CARNITINE DERIVATIVES

DL-Carnitine (free base)—$C_7H_{15}O_3N$ (161.20)—very hygroscopic, easily soluble in H_2O, ethanol; m.p. 195–197°C (Carter and Bhattacharyya[26]).

DL-Carnitine hydrochloride—$C_7H_{15}O_3N \cdot HCl$ (197.67)—very soluble in H_2O, slightly soluble in cold ethanol, easily soluble in hot ethanol, poorly soluble in acetone, insoluble in ether. Crystallizes from ethanol in stellately ordered, compact, short needles; m.p. 196°C (decomp.) (Strack et al.[27]).

DL-Carnitine chloroaurate—$C_7H_{15}O_3N \cdot HAuCl_4$ (501.04)—slightly soluble in cold H_2O, freely soluble in hot H_2O, soluble in acetone. Needles or prisms crystallize slowly from HCl solution; m.p. 145°C (decomp.) (Strack et al.[27]), m.p. 153–155° (Carter and Bhattacharyya[26]).

DL-Carnitine reineckate—$C_7H_{15}O_3N \cdot C_4H_7N_6S_4Cr \cdot H_2O$ (498.64)—poorly soluble in cold H_2O, somewhat soluble in warm H_2O, soluble in dilute alkali (pH 8–9), somewhat soluble in ethanol, freely soluble in acetone. Red leaves appear upon cooling a water solution heated to 50°C; m.p. 155–156°C (Strack et al.[27]).

[33] G. Wolf and C. R. A. Berger, Arch. Biochem. Biophys. **92**, 360 (1961).
[34] H. Aurich and I. Lorenz, Acta Biol. Med. Ger. **3**, 272 (1959).
[35] E. Strack and I. Lorenz, Hoppe-Seyler's Z. Physiol. Chem. **318**, 129 (1960).
[36] K. Brendel and R. Bressler, Biochim. Biophys. Acta **137**, 98 (1967).
[37] Otsuka Pharmaceutical Co., Chem. Abstr. **67**, 64702W (1967).

l-Carnitine—$C_7H_{15}O_3N$—crystalline, hygroscopic solid. $[\alpha]_D^{22} = -23.5°$ (0.5% solution in H_2O) (Carter *et al.*[8]).

l-Carnitine hydrochloride—$C_7H_{15}O_3N \cdot HCl$—$[\alpha]_D^{22} = -20.4°$ (Carter *et al.*[8]), $[\alpha]_D^{22} = -20.9°$ (Krimberg[38]); $[\alpha]_D^{22} = -23.7°$ (Strack and Lorenz[35]); m.p. 137–139°C. (Carter *et al.*[8]), m.p. 142° (Strack *et al.*[31]). On standing in a desiccator, the hydrochloride gradually forms an intermolecular ester which gives an oily gold salt. The changed hydrochloride also gives a reineckate which is less soluble in alcohol and acetone than the normal derivative (Strack *et al.*[31]).

l-Carnitine chloroaurate—$C_7H_{15}O_3N \cdot HAuCl_4$—soluble to 2.5% in dilute HCl. Solubility decreases in the presence of excess $HAuCl_4$ and NaCl. In air, carnitine chloroaurate gradually changes to crotonobetaine (Strack *et al.*[31]). On recrystallization from warm H_2O with slow cooling, an oil appears, changing slowly to short, thick, dark orange plates on the bottom of the tube. Farther up in the solution crystallization takes place in the form of citron-yellow needles up to 1 cm long; m.p. 151–153°C. (Krimberg[39]); m.p. 142°C (Strack and Lorenz[35]).

d-Carnitine hydrochloride—$C_7H_{15}O_3N \cdot HCl$—very soluble in H_2O, slightly soluble in cold ethanol, somewhat more soluble in hot ethanol, insoluble in ether. Large stellate crystals from alcohol-ether; m.p. 137–138°C (uncorrected), $[\alpha]_D^{22} = +22.3°$ (5% solution in H_2O) (Friedman *et al.*[24]); m.p. 142°C, $[\alpha]_D^{22} = +23.7°$ (Strack and Lorenz[35]).

C. The Vitamin Function of Carnitine

1. Carnitine as a Vitamin in the Nutrition of the Yellow Mealworm *Tenebrio molitor* (Coleoptera, Tenebrionidae)

The first indication of nutritional deficiency ultimately attributed to a lack of carnitine arose in work by Fraenkel and Blewett on the nutrition of the mealworm *Tenebrio molitor*.[40] The larvae failed to grow or survive on a diet previously found adequate for a number of other insects, (casein, glucose, cholesterol, a salt mixture and nine B vitamins), while optimal growth ensued upon addition of certain yeast or liver preparations. For full growth and survival two fractions from yeast or liver extract, separable by charcoal adsorption, were required. In the presence of the active factor in the charcoal eluate, eventually identified as folic acid, growth was enhanced, but death occurred even more rapidly than in the absence of both materials. In the presence of the unadsorbed fraction alone, survival was good, but the larvae failed to grow (Fig. 2). This filtrate factor was named "vitamin B_T"

[38] R. Krimberg, *Hoppe-Seyler's Z. Physiol. Chem.* **55**, 466 (1908).
[39] R. Krimberg, *Hoppe Seyler's Z. Physiol. Chem.* **48**, 412 (1906).
[40] G. Fraenkel and M. Blewett, *Biochem. J.* **41**, 469 (1947).

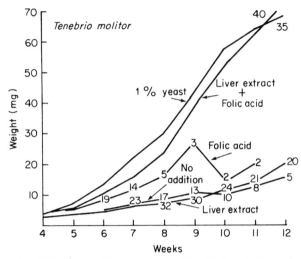

FIG. 2. Growth of *Tenebrio molitor* on a basic diet with the addition of brewer's yeast, a charcoal filtrate from liver extract, and/or folic acid. The numbers on the lines indicate the numbers of beetle larvae alive, out of 40 larvae (from Fraenkel and Blewett[40]).

to indicate its place in the group of B vitamins ("T" for *Tenebrio*), and further isolation finally led to recognition of its identity with carnitine.[8]

2. OTHER SPECIES OF TENEBRIONIDAE

A requirement for carnitine, with very similar deficiency symptoms, has been demonstrated in every representative of the family Tenebrionidae studied up to the present time. Included are the following species: *Tenebrio obscurus*,[14] *Palorus ratzeburgi* (Cooper and Fraenkel[41]), *Tribolium confusum* (Fröbrich,[42] French and Fraenkel[43]), *Tribolium castaneum* (Magis[44]), *Gnathocerus cornutus* (Leclercq[45]), and *Tribolium obstructor* (Naton[46]).

3. OTHER INSECTS

With regard to insects other than Tenebrionidae, there have been claims of dietary carnitine requirements in only two instances. In the larva of the yellow fever mosquito, *Aedes aegypti*, the duration of the first larval instar was increased from 3.9 to 6.5 days in the absence of carnitine, and a high mortality became manifest from the 4th instar onward (Singh and Brown[47]).

[41] M. I. Cooper and G. Fraenkel, *Physiol. Zool.* **25**, 20 (1952).
[42] G. Fröbrich, *Naturwissenschaften* **40**, 344 (1953).
[43] E. W. French and G. Fraenkel, *Nature (London)* **173**, 173 (1954).
[44] N. Magis, *Arch. Int. Physiol.* **62**, 505 (1954).
[45] J. Leclercq, *Arch. Int. Physiol. Biochim.* **65**, 337 (1957).
[46] E. Naton, *Zool. Beitr.* **8**, 95, 173 (1963).
[47] K. R. P. Singh and A. W. A. Brown, *J. Insect Physiol.* **1**, 199 (1957).

This result was not confirmed by Akov,[48] who obtained optimal growth on purified diets in the absence of carnitine. Further, carnitine did not replace choline in choline-free diets, nor were *Aedes* larvae affected by the addition of the "anticarnitine" γ-butyrobetaine, in quantities highly lethal to *Tenebrio* larvae. In a beetle, *Oryzaephilus surinamensis*, the absence of carnitine led to a decrease in the number of larvae pupating (from 77% to 62%) and an increase of the larval + pupal period (from 22 to 26 days) (Davis[49]).

There is no evidence that any other insect has a requirement for carnitine. Addition of carnitine to carnitine-free diets did not affect the growth rate of the larvae of two species of flies, *Phormia regina*[50] and *Musca domestica*,[51] or a beetle, *Dermestes vulpinus*, and in the latter case the carnitine content of the insect grown in the presence or absence of the compound was about the same.[11] Little *ad hoc* work has been performed with insects, other than tenebrionids, with a carnitine requirement in mind. In many studies the absence of an indication of a carnitine deficiency may not be too significant since it is present in relatively large amounts in some purified casein preparations. Microbial synthesis in the intestine must also be considered a possibility in certain instances. However, a number of insects, including the fruit fly *Drosophila*, the blow fly *Phormia regina*, the house fly *Musca domestica*, and the onion maggot *Hylemya antiqua*, have been successfully grown in axenic culture on diets lacking protein.[52] The absence of serious deficiency symptoms in these cases points, by implication, to the fact that carnitine is not required in the diet.

The apparent restriction of a carnitine requirement to a group of taxonomically closely related species (family Tenebrionidae) represents a striking example of biochemical evolution. Since four genera belonging to two different subfamilies are affected, it is probable that the ability to synthesize· carnitine was lost very early in the evolution of this family.

4. MICROORGANISMS

Up to a short time ago no evidence existed of a nutritional requirement for carnitine by a microorganism. The fact that *E. coli* could be grown in the absence of carnitine and did not contain measurable quantities of the compound (by the *Tenebrio* assay), discouraged attempts to isolate a carnitine-less mutant of this organism. Recently, however, Sakaguchi[53] has demonstrated that *Pediococcus soyae*, the soy sauce lactic acid bacterium, requires two

[48] S. Akov, *J. Insect Physiol.* **8**, 337 (1962).
[49] G. R. F. Davis, *Arch. Int. Physiol. Biochim.* **72**, 70 (1964).
[50] M. Brust and G. Fraenkel, *Physiol. Zool.* **28**, 186 (1955).
[51] V. J. Brookes and G. Fraenkel, *Physiol. Zool.* **31**, 208 (1958).
[52] Conference on Axenic Culture of Invertebrate Metazoa: A Goal, New York, 1958, *Ann. N.Y. Acad. Sci.* **77**, 25 (1959).
[53] K. Sakaguchi, *Agr. Biol. Chem.* **26**, 72 (1962).

factors for growth and salt tolerance, an unidentified one, and carnitine, for which glycine–betaine can be substituted. The optimal concentration for carnitine is 10 μg/ml. A far higher activity of carnitine has been shown in the case of a carnitine-less mutant of a yeast, *Candida bovina*, which requires it for growth in quantities ranging from 1 to 2 μg/100 ml (Travassos *et al.*[54]). None of the following possible carnitine precursors can substitute for it, γ-aminobutyric acid, γ-amino-β-hydroxybutyric acid, β-hydroxybutyric acid, choline, γ-butyrobetaine, proline, or hydroxyproline. O-Acetylcarnitine is as effective as carnitine, but γ-butyrobetaine does not seem to be a competitive antagonist. The specificity of the requirement is, therefore, astonishingly similar in this bacterium and the beetle *Tenebrio* (see below). The possibility of using *Pediococcus soyae* or *Candida bovina* in the biological assay of carnitine has been suggested by the respective authors.

D. Specificity of Action

In order to obtain information about the structural specificity of carnitine in a first attempt to throw light on its physiological function, studies were made by Bhattacharyya *et al.*[13] of the effects of a number of carnitine derivatives, analogs, etc., on the development of *Tenebrio molitor*. Modifications of chain length were produced and substitutions made on or for the carboxyl, hydroxyl, and quaternary ammonium groups. Of all compounds tested only four showed any activity, and of these, only two, a carboxy and a hydroxy ester were active at the same level as the parent. The results of testing led to the conclusions that (1) the γ-amino group must be present and substituted, (2) three carbon atoms must separate the nitrogen atom from the carboxyl carbon, (3) a hydroxyl group must be present in the β position, and (4) the carboxyl group must be present.

Of all the compounds assayed, only one, γ-butyrobetaine, showed a decisive toxicity, the inhibition being competitive in nature; carnitine completely reversed the toxicity, even at high levels of γ-butyrobetaine. At the lower concentrations of γ-butyrobetaine (33 and 100 μg/gm diet) the inhibition index was of the order of 100; and with 1500 μg of γ-butyrobetaine, it was of the order of 1000. The specific inhibitory effect of γ-butyrobetaine has since been used to study the effect of carnitine in systems in which carnitine is normally synthesized, e.g., the developing chick embryo.[154] The inhibitor, γ-butyrobetaine, does not appear to affect the growth of *P. regina* larvae, and, in fact, will substitute completely for carnitine or choline through a single generation in both *P. regina*[55] and *D. melanogaster*.[56]

[54] L. R. Travassos, E. N. Suassuna, A. Cury, R. L. Hausman, and M. Miranda, *An. Microbiol.* **9**, 465 (1961).
[55] E. Hodgson, V. H. Cheldelin, and R. W. Newburgh, *Arch. Biochem. Biophys.* **87**, 48 (1960).
[56] B. W. Geer and G. F. Vovis, *J. Exp. Zool.* **158**, 223 (1965).

Fritz et al.,[57] working with a partially purified enzyme, carnitine acetyl-transferase, which catalyzes the reaction

$$\text{Acetyl CoA} + \text{carnitine} \rightleftharpoons \text{acetyl carnitine} + \text{CoA}$$

have noted that removal of a methyl group from the nitrogen of carnitine to produce the dimethylamino compound (norcarnitine) decreases the velocity of the reaction, while any substitution for the carboxyl group abolishes the reaction completely. Tables of K_m and K_i values for various substrates and inhibitors of this reaction have recently appeared (Fritz and Schultz[58, 59]).

E. Occurrence and Distribution

1. METHODS OF ASSAY

Methods developed for the assay of carnitine are of three general types, biological, chemical, and enzymatic, and can be taken up in that order.

a. Biological

The biological test for carnitine by the Tenebrio assay method (Fraenkel[10–12, 60, 61]) is based on the fact that Tenebrio on a basic diet in the absence of carnitine survive and grow to a weight of 2–3 mg during the first 3–4 weeks after hatching from the egg, whereupon mortality starts rising and most of the larvae die within the following 2–3 weeks. The addition of 0.35 to 0.7 μg carnitine/gm diet ensures optimal survival up to a weight of about 60 mg at an age of 10 weeks, while for successful growth to maturity (150 mg after about 20 weeks) 1.5 μg/gm is required. In the routine assays, a diet on which the larvae exhibit maximum survival up to 10 weeks (60 mg) with a somewhat suboptimal growth rate, is assumed to contain 0.35 μg carnitine/gm.

With this method the carnitine content of a great many natural materials was determined (see Table III), but after 1954 the procedure failed to give meaningful results for a variety of reasons which were ultimately recognized as (a) deficiencies of zinc and potassium in the basic diet, (b) impurities of carnitine in casein, (c) the possible presence of carnitine in a commercially obtained salt mixture, and (d) differences in the requirements of different strains of insects. The basic diet was then redesigned to contain 20 parts of casein, 80 parts glucose, 1 part cholesterol, 4 parts Wesson salt mixture, 0.02% $ZnCl_2$, and nine vitamins of the B complex.[52] A carnitine deficiency developed again on this diet.

[57] I. B. Fritz, S. K. Schultz, and P. A. Srere, J. Biol. Chem. 238, 2509 (1963).
[58] I. B. Fritz and S. K. Schultz, in "Recent Research on Carnitine" (G. Wolf, ed.), pp. 113–115 MIT Press, Cambridge, Massachusetts, 1965.
[59] I. B. Fritz and S. K. Schultz, J. Biol. Chem. 240, 2188 (1965).
[60] G. Fraenkel, Methods Enzymol. 3, 662 (1957).
[61] G. Fraenkel, J. Nutr. 65, 361 (1958).

In addition to the *Tenebrio* test there are some potential microbiological methods based on the carnitine requirements of a mutant of *Candida bovina*[54] and a bacterium, *Pediococcus soyae*.[53]

A chemical–biological method developed by Strack and Lorenz[62] depends upon converting carnitine to crotonobetaine methyl ester by dehydration and subsequent esterification and then assaying this compound by measuring the contraction of a frog rectus abdominus in a physiological saline to which it has been added.

b. Chemical

Chemical methods of historical interest are those of Lintzel and Fomin,[63] Lintzel,[64] and Dyer,[65] which depended upon the liberation of trimethylamine from carnitine and analysis as the picrate; of Strack and Lorenz,[62] which measured crotonobetaine formed from carnitine by permanganate titration; and of Binon and Deltour[66] and Binon,[67] which gravimetrically determined carnitine after reineckate precipitation. Aside from being long, drawn-out procedures, these methods were all relatively insensitive and required fairly pure samples.

In the method most recently developed by the Strack group[68] carnitine is converted to crotonobetaine and measured as such photometrically or polarographically. According to the authors, as little as 1.5 μg of carnitine can be measured with an error of $\pm 5\%$, but the sample to be analyzed requires elaborate purification.

The assay most extensively used until 1964 (Broekhuysen and Deltour,[69] Wolf and Berger,[33] Mehlman and Wolf[70, 71]) was that of Friedman,[72] which involved esterification of carnitine and its colorimetric determination as a bromophenol blue complex. It had the advantages of rapidity and sensitivity (down to 6 μg/sample), but was not specific (Deltour *et al.*[73]). Modifications were made to improve its reproducibility, and the preassay purification used by the author was extended to remove interfering compounds (Mehlman and Wolf,[70] Deltour *et al.*,[73] Broekhuysen and Deltour[69]).

[62] E. Strack and I. Lorenz, *Hoppe-Seyler's Z. Physiol. Chem.* **298**, 27 (1954).

[63] W. Lintzel and S. Fomin, *Biochem. Z.* **238**, 438 (1931).

[64] W. Lintzel, *Biochem. Z.* **273**, 243 (1934).

[65] W. J. Dyer, *J. Fish. Res. Bd. Can.* **6**, 359 (1945).

[66] F. Binon and G. Deltour, *C. R. Soc. Biol.* **149**, 932 (1955).

[67] F. Binon, *Voeding* **16**, 781 (1955).

[68] E. Strack and W. Kunz, *Hoppe-Seyler's Z. Physiol. Chem.* **333**, 46 (1963).

[69] J. Broekhuysen and G. Deltour, *Ann. Biol. Clin.* (*Paris*). **19**, 549 (1961).

[70] M. A. Mehlman and G. Wolf, *Arch. Biochem. Biophys.* **98**, 146 (1962).

[71] M. A. Mehlman and G. Wolf, *Arch. Biochem. Biophys.* **102**, 346 (1963).

[72] S. Friedman, *Arch. Biochem. Biophys.* **75**, 24 (1958).

[73] G. Deltour, J. Broekhuysen, and L. Dierickx, *Clin. Chim. Acta* **5**, 181 (1960).

c. Enzymatic

An enzymatic method based on the release of CoA from acetyl-CoA in the presence of limiting amounts of carnitine and the enzyme carnitine acetyltransferase has been described by Fritz et al.,[57] Fritz,[22] and Marquis and Fritz,[74] and appears to provide the ultimate solution for the determination of this compound. The assay is simple, sensitive, quite specific at the level of enzyme purification achieved by the authors, and, most important, does not seem to require extensive preassay purification. Some data on the carnitine content of various mammalian tissues obtained by this method are presented in the following section.

2. DISTRIBUTION

It is no accident that carnitine was originally discovered in and isolated from meat extract since this material constitutes one of the richest known sources of the compound. Strack et al.[31] have reported a yield of 1.8%, Carter et al.[8] a yield of 1.5%, and Friedman[72] a yield of 1.5%.

With the discovery of the Tenebrio assay the field was opened for more accurate measurements of materials in which the carnitine content was too low for isolation procedures. By this method, carnitine was found to be almost universally distributed in biological substances (Fraenkel[10–12]), and Table I contains representative examples of the main groups of organisms upon which assays have so far been conducted. (In using this table, however, it must be understood that all the figures determined by the Tenebrio method express vitamin B_T activity. This assumes that carnitine, or one of its esters, is the only compound with vitamin B_T activity present in natural materials, an assumption which up to the present time has not been disputed.) The figures in the table are based on the supposition that a diet on which Tenebrio larvae show a maximum survival up to a weight of about 60 mg contains 0.35 μg carnitine/gm of the dry diet. It is self-evident that the accuracy of such a method cannot be very high.

Two general conclusions can be drawn from the table: (a) Animal tissues contain very much higher levels of carnitine than do microorganisms or plants. (b) The richest source of carnitine is muscle, both vertebrate and invertebrate. The only biological materials in which carnitine could not be demonstrated were two microorganisms, Escherichia coli and Tetrahymena geleii (both grown on synthetic diets in the absence of carnitine), corn (seed), the hen's egg before embryonic development, and, as one would expect, Tenebrio larvae grown on an artificial diet in the virtual absence of carnitine. Whether carnitine was, in fact, completely absent, or present only in minute quantities could not be decided, since the lower limit of the testing method lies at about 1–3 μg/gm. For clinical investigations involving routine analysis

[74] N. R. Marquis and I. B. Fritz, J. Lipid Res. 5, 184 (1964).

TABLE I

THE CARNITINE CONTENT OF A NUMBER OF MATERIALS OF BIOLOGICAL ORIGIN,
DETERMINED BY THE *Tenebrio* ASSAY[a]

Organism	Carnitine (μg/gm dry matter)	Description of material	Reference (Fraenkel)
Microorganisms			
Escherichia coli	None?	Grown on synthetic medium	11
Streptococcus hemolyticus	28	Medium not entirely synthetic	11
Torula yeast	17.5–35		11
Brewers' yeast	17.5–35		11
Neurospora crassa	28	Grown on synthetic medium	11
Tetrahymena geleii	None?	Grown on synthetic medium	11
Plants			
Wheat	7–14	Seeds	11
Corn	None?	Seeds	11
Alfalfa concentrate	20	Spray-dried	11
Invertebrates (excluding insects)			
Aurelia aurita (medusa)	700	Muscular rim	12
Nereis pelagica (Annelida)	175	Whole	12
Venus mercenaria (Pelecypoda)	85–175	Foot	12
	1120–2240	Striated and smooth adductor muscles	12
Libinia emarginata (Decapoda)	112–224	Hepatopancreas	12
	560–1120	Muscle	12
Limulus polyphemus (horseshoe crab)	8800–35,000	Muscle	12
	2100	Hepatopancreas	12
Asterias forbesi (sea urchin)	35	Whole	12
Insects			
Tenebrio molitor	17.5	Grown in presence of carnitine	11
	None?	Grown in absence of carnitine	11
Dermestes vulpinus	140	Grown in presence of carnitine	11
	70–140	Grown in absence of carnitine	11
Phormia regina: larvae	560	Grown on liver	11
Pupae and adults	17.5	Grown in absence of carnitine	11
Vertebrates			
Fishes			
Mustelus canis (dogfish)	700	Muscle	12
	420	Liver	12

TABLE I—*continued*

Organism	Carnitine (μg/gm dry matter)	Description of material	Reference (Fraenkel)
Tautoga onitis	224	Muscle	12
	70	Liver	12
Birds			
Chick	175–350	Muscle	12
	22.4	Liver	12
	None?	Egg	11
Mammals			
Dog	1120	Muscle of leg	11
	140–280	Liver	11
Rat	560–1120	Muscle of leg, laboratory diet	11
	350–700	Muscle of leg, carnitine-free diet	11
	100–200	Liver, laboratory diet	11
	112–224	Liver, carnitine-free diet	11
Rabbit	700	Leg muscle	11
	370	Liver	11
Beef muscle extract	4860–29,200	Several commercial preparations	11
Homo sapiens, urine	14–56	Diet high in vegetables and fruit	11
	56	High protein diet	11
	132–264	After 3 days of starvation	11
Homo sapiens, blood	7–14	Pooled sample	11

[a] All figures are based on the dry weights of the materials in question, except for urine and blood. Figures are taken from[11] G. Fraenkel, *Biol. Bull.* **104**, 359 (1953) and[12] G. Fraenkel, *Arch. Biochem. Biophys.* **50**, 486 (1954).

of muscle, urine, and blood, the *Tenebrio* method is out of the question because of the size of the samples required (with muscle) and the time and labor involved.

Renewed interest in carnitine has led in recent years to assays based on different principles (see preceding sections). Measurements made on rat tissues by a modification of Friedman's[72] chemical method, resulted in values very close to those found earlier by the *Tenebrio* method (muscle 120–180 μg/gm wet weight, brain 20 μg, liver 60–90 μg) (Mehlman and Wolf[70]). Good agreement between the two methods was also obtained in assays of carnitine during embryonic development of the chick. [Results obtained on "horse meat" by the chemical method developed by

Friedman[72] gave indications of quantities of carnitine 3–8 times higher than those previously (Fraenkel[11]) found in rat, rabbit, or dog muscle. The horse meat used in this study, a commercial preparation containing bone, various organs, and glandular material as well as muscle, has since been equated with horse muscle,[22, 69] an erroneous synonymy that should be corrected.]

With a still different method, that of Fritz,[74] virtually the same results were obtained for the following rat tissues: muscle 250 μg/gm dry weight, liver 142 μg, brain 66 μg. In this investigation by far the highest carnitine content of any vertebrate tissue was demonstrated in adrenal, about 6604 μg/gm dry tissue. The significance of this finding is unknown (Abdel-Kader and Wolf[75]).

Broekhuysen et al.,[76] have summarized the results of a number of investigators and indicated how closely these methods agree.

3. TURNOVER OF CARNITINE

The turnover time of 97 days reported for a single rat by Wolf and Berger[33] has been critically reexamined in Wolf's laboratory with quite different answers. It is apparent that some of the assumptions made in the original calculation were invalidated by the large quantity of carnitine injected, since the latest figures (Khairallah and Mehlman[77]) obtained from a number of rats injected with physiological doses of carnitine are of the order of 6–12 days. These values may be high, the work having been done with DL-carnitine (see Fritz[22] for additional comment).

Results of others using doses within the physiological range have inclined toward a slow rate of turnover, but no quantitative evaluations have been made (Yue and Fritz,[78] Lindstedt and Lindstedt[79]).

4. BOUND CARNITINE

Attempts to ascertain the presence of bound carnitine in a wide array of tissues have met with the usual uncertainties associated with methods of isolation and determination.

Binon and Deltour,[80–82] using indirect assay methods, stated that carnitine

[75] M. M. Abdel-Kader and G. Wolf, in " Recent Research on Carnitine " (G. Wolf, ed.), pp. 147–156 MIT Press, Cambridge, Massachusetts, 1965.

[76] J. Broekhuysen, C. Rozenblum, M. Ghislain, and G. Deltour, in " Recent Research on Carnitine " (G. Wolf, ed.), pp. 23–25 MIT Press, Cambridge, Massachusetts, 1965.

[77] E. A. Khairallah and M. A. Mehlman, in " Recent Research on Carnitine " (G. Wolf, ed.), pp. 57–62 MIT Press, Cambridge, Massachusetts, 1965.

[78] K. T. N. Yue and I. B. Fritz, Amer. J. Physiol. 202, 122 (1962).

[79] G. Lindstedt and S. Lindstedt, Biochem. Biophys. Res. Commun. 6, 319 (1961).

[80] F. Binon and G. Deltour, C. R. Soc. Biol. 149, 932 (1955).

[81] F. Binon and G. Deltour, Experientia 12, 357 (1956).

[82] F. Binon and G. Deltour, Rev. Ferment. Ind. Aliment. 11, 14 (1956).

was present in high concentrations in serum phospholipid and lipocaic (a crude pancreatic extract), but these claims were not confirmed by Deltour et al.,[73] Adams et al.,[83] or Bender and Adams,[84] who were also unable to find any carnitine bound in ox liver or muscle phospholipid by chemical analysis.

In 1960, Hosein and Proulx[85, 86] chemically identified carnitine as a compound bound in rat brain as a CoA ester and released by chloroform treatment. Strack et al.,[87] using a bioassay, claimed that 10–40 % of carnitine present in muscle and liver was " bound," and released upon treatment with methanolic HCl. Broekhuysen and Deltour[69] treated various dog tissues with chloroform and petroleum ether and were able to demonstrate that much higher quantities of carnitine were bound in brain, pancreas, and thymus lipid and released by hydrolysis than were present in the residue hydrolyzed after lipid extraction. The method used for analysis consisted of a preliminary purification on an ion-exchange resin, followed by paper electrophoretic separation of carnitine from other nitrogenous bases, and finally estimation by the bromophenol blue method of Friedman.[72] Mehlman and Wolf,[70] using an assay method which involved an ion exchange purification followed by a modified bromophenol blue estimation, examined a number of rat tissues for free and bound carnitine. Their methods of release of bound carnitine were based mainly on treatment of TCA extracts with HCl for various times and at various temperatures, although attempts were made to repeat the results of Hosein and Proulx[85] using their procedure. They were unable to find any carnitine bound in muscle, liver, testis, or brain, but an investigation of chick egg yolk sac proved more profitable, in that 42 % of the compound was shown to be in the form of phospholipid carnitine. Upon reinvestigation of various tissues they found carnitine in phospholipid fractions at a level of 8 % of total in rat liver and 79 % of total in chick liver.[71] These authors isolated and identified the phospholipid as phosphatidyl-carnitine containing palmitic, stearic, and, in pregnant rat liver, arachidonic acid, and also stated that β-methylcholine (a decarboxylation product of carnitine) could be found in rat embryo phospholipid. Proulx[88] also showed carnitine in a phospholipid fraction of cow brain. Recently, Soderberg, Therriault, and Wolf,[89] in an attempt to obtain large amounts of the egg yolk material for characterization, have shown that the compound in the

[83] E. P. Adams, P. E. Ballance, and A. E. Bender, Nature (London) 185, 612 (1960).
[84] A. E. Bender and E. P. Adams, Biochem. J. 82, 232 (1962).
[85] E. A. Hosein and P. Proulx, Nature (London) 187, 321 (1960).
[86] E. A. Hosein and P. Proulx, J. Agr. Food Chem. 8, 428 (1960).
[87] E. Strack, W. Rotzsch, and I. Lorenz, Protides Biol. Fluids, Proc. 1959 Colloq. 7, 235 (1960).
[88] P. Proulx, Nature (London) 200, 1210 (1963).
[89] J. Soderberg, D. G. Therriault, and G. Wolf, in "Recent Research on Carnitine" (G. Wolf, ed.), pp. 165–171 MIT Press, Cambridge, Massachusetts, 1965.

lipid bound fraction identified by Mehlman and Wolf as phosphatidyl-carnitine is, in reality, O-acylcarnitine, probably palmityl carnitine. Fritz[90] has confirmed this using a slightly different isolation method.

Bieber et al.[91] have identified β-methylcholine in phospholipid derived from Phormia regina larvae grown on a diet in which carnitine replaced choline. Their results indicate carnitine decarboxylation and incorporation into phospholipid as β-methylcholine (although not necessarily in that order). Mehendale et al.[92] have been able to isolate carnitine (not as O-acylcarnitine), as well as β-methylcholine in the phospholipid fraction when trimethyl (3-hydroxypropyl) ammonium acetate is added to P. regina larval diets containing carnitine. Larval growth is inhibited when this compound is used. They have postulated that the decarboxylation of carnitine to yield β-methylcholine takes place on the phosphatide since the ratio of carnitine: β-methylcholine in the H_2O fraction of the isolation procedure is 95:5 in both inhibited and noninhibited larvae. Recently, Khairallah and Wolf[93] have isolated carnitine decarboxylase from a number of rat organs. The enzyme which splits free carnitine to β-methylcholine is present in mitochondrial extracts and requires ATP and Mg^{2+} for maximum activity.

F. Biosynthesis of Carnitine

1. Evidence of Biosynthesis of Carnitine in Various Organisms

The presence of carnitine, often in large quantities, in all forms of life, together with the failure to demonstrate its nutritional importance in any but a minute sector of the living world, strongly points to its general origin. It has been shown in a number of cases that the level of carnitine in tissues is not greatly affected by dietary supply. Thus, the beetle Dermestes vulpinus when grown on a synthetic diet lacking carnitine has approximately the same content as when raised on a mixture of a fishmeal and yeast which is rich in carnitine.[11] (On the other hand, the beetle Tenebrio, one of the few animals known to have a nutritional requirement for carnitine, contains less in the body than can be demonstrated by the biological assay when grown on a minimal quantity of carnitine. Controls fed large amounts of the compound assay high[11].) Rat muscle and liver contain about the same level of carnitine whether the rats are grown on an ordinary laboratory diet or on a synthetic diet without added carnitine.[11] Muscle and livers from chicks grown in the absence of bacteria, but on a practical diet which probably

[90] I. B. Fritz, in "Recent Research on Carnitine" (G. Wolf, ed.), pp. 173–174 MIT Press, Cambridge, Massachusetts, 1965.

[91] L. L. Bieber, V. H. Cheldelin, and R. W. Newburgh, J. Biol. Chem. 239, 1262 (1963).

[92] H. M. Mehendale, W. C. Dauterman, and E. Hodgson, Nature (London) 211, 759 (1966).

[93] E. A. Khairallah and G. Wolf, J. Biol. Chem. 242, 32 (1967).

contained some carnitine, have the same carnitine levels as those from conventionally grown chicks.[11]

The avian embryo is an example of proof of carnitine synthesis, in that it is a self-contained developing sterile system with a carnitine content at day 1 of less than 52.5 μg and a level in the fully developed embryo of ca. 420 μg.[11] Mehlman and Wolf[70] have also investigated the chick embryo using a different assay system and report results of a similar magnitude.

2. Pathways of Carnitine Biosynthesis

A number of routes have been proposed for the synthesis of carnitine (Guggenheim,[94] Strack et al.,[95]) but evidence has been forthcoming for only a single one up to now. In 1929 Linneweh[96] found that γ-butyrobetaine injected into dogs led to an increase in carnitine in the urine and proposed a β-oxidation mechanism of formation. The basic work was repeated in rats by Lindstedt and Lindstedt[79] using ^{14}C-carboxy-labeled γ-butyrobetaine, and it was shown that within 30 hours over 70% of the labeled compound had been converted into carnitine. (Bremer, in 1962, demonstrated the same in vivo oxidation of γ-butyrobetaine[97].) Lindstedt and Lindstedt,[98] and Lindstedt[99] have since been able to obtain a 50-fold purification of an enzyme from rat liver which is capable of hydroxylating γ-butyrobetaine in the presence of O_2 when supplied with the cofactors NADPH (or NADP), ascorbate, and Fe^{2+}.

The question of formation of γ-butyrobetaine is one which remains completely unanswered. Hosein et al.[100] investigated this in in vitro experiments and obtained a very small amount of γ-butyrobetaine from incubation of γ-aminobutyric acid and S-adenosylmethionine with rat muscle homogenates. The significance of these findings has been severely criticized by Fritz,[22] and it is obvious that further work must be done before this pathway of synthesis is accepted as worthy of consideration. In vivo labeling experiments have shown practically no incorporation into carnitine after injection into rats of carboxy-labeled γ-N,N-dimethyl aminobutyrate and none on injection of carboxy-labeled γ-aminobutyric acid, γ-amino-β-hydroxybutyrate, 2-^{14}C-homocarnosine (Lindstedt and Lindstedt,[101]) or glutamic acid

[94] M. Guggenheim, "Die Biogenen Amine," 3rd Ed. 564 pp. and 4th Ed. 619 pp. Karger, Basel, 1940 and 1951.

[95] E. Strack, P. Wördehoff, E. Neubauer, and H. Geissendörfer, Hoppe-Seyler's Z. Physiol. Chem. 233, 189 (1935).

[96] W. Linneweh, Hoppe-Seyler's Z. Physiol. Chem. 181, 42 (1929).

[97] J. Bremer, Biochim. Biophys. Acta 57, 327 (1962).

[98] G. Lindstedt and S. Lindstedt, Biochem. Biophys. Res. Commun. 7, 394 (1962).

[99] G. Lindstedt, Biochemistry 6, 1271 (1967).

[100] E. A. Hosein, M. Smart, K. Hawkins, S. Rochon, and Z. Strasberg, Arch. Biochem. Biophys. 96, 246 (1962).

[101] G. Lindstedt and S. Lindstedt, Biochem. J. 84, 84 (1962).

3,4-[14]C (Bremer[97]). Others have shown that radioactivity from carboxy-labeled betaine (Fraenkel and Friedman[14]) and carboxy-labeled glycine (Wolf and Berger[33]) are very slowly transferred to carnitine. The incorporation of label from methyl-labeled methionine proceeds very slowly according to Cantoni (see Wolf and Berger,[33] Bremer[102]). However, Strength and Yu[103] and Strength, Yu, and Davis,[104] using choline- and methionine-deficient rats in which liver carnitine is only 30% of normal, have found that injection of methyl-labeled methionine increases the activity of carnitine in deficient animals to more than 15 times that of carnitine from control rats injected with the same compound. Incorporation was maximal at 3 hours, and all the activity was recovered in the methyl groups.

G. Biochemical Activity of Carnitine

The paucity of evidence[14] for the involvement of carnitine as a methyl donor in transmethylation reactions does not invite our serious consideration of this as a possible function for the compound. Within the past ten years, however, a great body of information has been built up concerning an entirely different and perhaps very important role in the metabolism of fatty acids.

In 1955, Fritz[16] observed that addition of carnitine to a reaction mixture containing palmitic acid and a rat liver homogenate caused an increase in the rate of oxidation of the fatty acid. Isolation of mitochondria from rat heart for further study of the influence of carnitine on fatty acid oxidation revealed a marked stimulation by the compound and a requirement for CoA, Mg^{2+}, ATP, and NAD for maximum oxygen uptake both in its presence and absence (Fritz and Kaplan,[105] Fritz et al.[106]). The effect of carnitine appeared to be limited to fatty acids with chain lengths greater than C_8. There was considerable structural specificity, so that removal of one methyl group resulted in a marked decrease in activity, and activity completely disappeared when the carboxyl was replaced by any of a number of end groups, the β-hydroxyl was reduced, or two of the methyl groups were removed from the quaternary nitrogen.[106] (This paralleled the results of Bhattacharyya et al.[13] on carnitine requirements in the nutrition of Tenebrio molitor.)

The discovery that carnitine increased the rate of palmityl-CoA oxidation by mitochondria (Fritz and Yue[107]) coupled with some thoughts concerning the observation (Friedman and Fraenkel[15]) that an enzyme present in pigeon liver catalyzed a reversible acetylation of carnitine by acetyl-CoA, led two

[102] J. Bremer, Biochim. Biophys. Acta 48, 622 (1961).
[103] D. R. Strength and S. Y. Yu, Fed. Proc. Fed. Amer. Soc. Exp. Biol. 21, 1 (1962).
[104] D. R. Strength, S. Y. Yu, and E. Y. Davis, in "Recent Research in Carnitine" (G. Wolf, ed.), pp. 45–56 MIT Press, Cambridge, Massachusetts, 1965.
[105] I. B. Fritz and E. Kaplan, Protides Biol. Fluids, Proc. 1959 Colloq. 7, 252 (1960).
[106] I. B. Fritz, E. Kaplan, and K. T. N. Yue, Amer. J. Physiol. 202, 117 (1962).
[107] I. B. Fritz, and K. T. N. Yue, The Physiologist 5, 144 (1962).

groups of workers to consider the possibility that carnitine might function to carry both short- and long-chain acyl groups across mitochondrial membranes (Bremer,[108, 109] Fritz and Yue[107, 110]). This was borne out by the finding that there was, indeed, a reversible acylation of carnitine by mitochondria in the presence of palmityl-CoA, and by the fact that synthetic palmitylcarnitine was oxidized much more rapidly by mitochondria than was palmityl-CoA or palmitic acid.

The presence of two chain-length specific enzymes active in acyl transfer to and from carnitine was inferred from work on whole mitochondria and from the substrate limitations of an acyltransferase studied by Fritz et al.[57] Norum,[111] at the same time, succeeded in separating two substrate specific activities from fractionated ox heart mitochondria.

Fritz et al.,[57] have partially purified and studied in some detail the short-chain acyltransferase (probably the same enzyme described by Friedman and Fraenkel[15]) from pig heart. This enzyme catalyzes the reaction

$$\text{Acetylcarnitine} + \text{CoA} \rightleftharpoons \text{acetyl-CoA} + \text{carnitine}$$

The Keq of the reaction has been established as 0.6 in the direction of acetyl-CoA, and the enzyme is equally active from C_2 to C_4, showing a decrease in activity to practically nil at C_{10}. Chase et al.[112] have crystallized the enzyme from pigeon breast muscle, and Chase and Tubbs[113] have examined the kinetics of the reaction. Their results have led them to conclude, in contrast to Fritz et al.,[57] that the enzyme mechanism involves binary and ternary complexes in rapid equilibrium with free substrates rather than ordered substrate addition. Chase[114, 115] has made an analysis of other parameters: substrate specificity and pH optimum, with a view to establishing the nature of the active site.

The long-chain acyltransferase has been purified about 22 times from calf liver mitochondria (Norum[116]), and catalyzes the reaction

$$\text{Palmityl-CoA} + \text{carnitine} \rightleftharpoons \text{palmitylcarnitine} + \text{CoA}$$

The Keq of the reaction is ca. 0.5 in the direction of palmityl carnitine. The enzyme at a 12-fold purification is about 17 times as active with palmitylcarnitine as with butyrylcarnitine. Palmityl-CoA is not only a substrate for the enzyme, but also competitively inhibits carnitine attachment

[108] J. Bremer, J. Biol. Chem. 237, 2228 (1962).
[109] J. Bremer, J. Biol. Chem. 237, 3628 (1962).
[110] I. B. Fritz and K. T. N. Yue, J. Lipid Res. 4, 279 (1963).
[111] K. R. Norum, Acta Chem. Scand. 17, 1487 (1963).
[112] J. F. A. Chase, D. J. Pearson, and P. K. Tubbs, Biochim. Biophys. Acta 96, 162 (1965).
[113] J. F. A. Chase and P. K. Tubbs, Biochem. J. 99, 32 (1966).
[114] J. F. A. Chase, Biochem. J. 104, 503 (1967).
[115] J. F. A. Chase, Biochem. J. 104, 510 (1967).
[116] K. R. Norum, Biochim. Biophys. Acta 89, 95 (1964).

to the enzyme at very low concentrations, making for a delicately balanced system that might be easily subject to regulation (Bremer and Norum[117]).

Experiments concerned with enzymatic localization within tissues initially showed a skewed distribution of short- and long-chain acyltransferases between the cytoplasm and mitochondria, with a higher concentration of both enzymes in the mitochondria (Norum,[118] Bremer[119]). This general distribution was, of course, in line with the idea concerning transport function across mitochondrial membranes, in that an activated long-chain fatty acid such as palmityl-CoA could be transferred to carnitine extramitochondrially, moved across the mitochondrial membrane as the carnitine ester, and be reconstructed as the CoA derivative within the mitochondrion at the site of fatty acid oxidation.[107, 109, 110, 119] The same series of reactions could take place with acetyl-CoA, which is formed within the mitochondrion as a result of pyruvate or fatty acid oxidation and transported outward for various cytoplasmic functions such as fatty acid and sterol synthesis. In view of the fact that long-chain fatty acids, long- and short-chain acyl-CoA compounds, and free CoA move across the mitochondrial membrane with difficulty, if at all, this appeared to be a clear-cut biochemical function for carnitine, an idea which was supported by *in vitro* and *in vivo* data gathered by Bressler and his colleagues.[120–122]

Recent work has caused questions to be raised concerning this mechanism, since it appears that all of the enzymatic activity concerned with transacylation involving carnitine takes place intramitochondrially.[123–125] This finding coupled with the observation that washed fresh mitochondria from rat liver show an activation of palmitate oxidation by carnitine in the absence of CoA have led Klingenberg and Bode[126, 127] to propose an alternative scheme for the movement of fatty acids across the mitochondrial membrane. Their scheme which requires both long- and short-chain acyltransferases and the presence of an unknown acylcarnitine transferase to move long-chain fatty acids into the mitochondrion has been taken to task by Fritz and Marquis,[128]

[117] J. Bremer and K. R. Norum, *J. Biol. Chem.* **242**, 1744 (1967).
[118] K. R. Norum, *Acta Chem. Scand.* **17**, 896 (1963).
[119] J. Bremer, *Acta Chem. Scand.* **17**, 902 (1963).
[120] R. Bressler and S. J. Friedberg, *J. Biol. Chem.* **239**, 1364 (1964).
[121] R. Bressler and R. I. Katz, *in* "Recent Research on Carnitine" (G. Wolf, ed.), pp. 65–81 MIT Press, Cambridge, Massachusetts, 1965.
[122] R. Bressler, R. Katz, and B. Wittels, *Ann. N.Y. Acad. Sci.* **131**, 207 (1965).
[123] A. M. T. Beenakkers and M. Klingenberg, *Biochim. Biophys. Acta* **84**, 205 (1964).
[124] J. M. Lowenstein, *in* "Recent Research on Carnitine" (G. Wolf, ed.), pp. 97–112 MIT Press, Cambridge, Massachusetts, 1965.
[125] K. R. Norum and J. Bremer, *J. Biol. Chem.* **242**, 407 (1967).
[126] M. Klingenberg and C. Bode, *in* "Recent Research on Carnitine" (G. Wolf, ed.), pp. 87–95 MIT Press, Cambridge, Massachusetts, 1965.
[127] C. Bode and M. Klingenberg, *Biochem. Z.* **341**, 271 (1965).
[128] I. B. Fritz and N. R. Marquis, *Proc. Nat. Acad. Sci. U.S.* **54**, 1226 (1965).

who have shown that long-chain fatty acids can be oxidized at a carnitine activated rate when the short-chain acyltransferase is inhibited. It is probable that, as both Fritz and Marquis,[128] and Norum and Bremer[125] have suggested, recent information regarding the permeability of intramitochondrial membranes and the contents of various mitochondrial compartments should be taken into account in attempting to evaluate the meaning of Klingenberg's experiments. If there are membranes separating compartments involved in fatty acid activation and fatty acid oxidation, it would be on these membranes that the acyltransferases might be expected to be situated, acting as permeases or translocases. Norum et al.[129] have, in fact, demonstrated that the long-chain acyltransferase is localized on an inner membrane of rat liver mitochondria.

Other arguments have been made against the importance of the short-chain acyltransferase in moving acetate out of mitochondria for use in fatty acid synthesis, etc., based on the absence of this transferase from high speed rat liver supernatant, and the generally low activity of the enzyme in rat liver mitochondria compared to that of the citrate cleavage enzyme in the supernatant (Lowenstein[124]). Norum and Bremer[125] have shown, however, that the transferase assay method used by Lowenstein is somewhat low in crude systems. It also appears that the concentration of the enzyme in ox, sheep, and guinea pig liver is 10–20 times its concentration in rat liver (Sauer and Erfle[130]). Conversely, citrate cleavage activity has been shown to be lower in guinea pig liver than rat liver (Hardwick and Lowenstein[131]).

Fritz and Hsu[132, 133] have recently made an observation from which a new function for carnitine in fat metabolism may be derived. Having noted that palmitylcarnitine stimulates fat synthesis in rat liver homogenates, they have been able to demonstrate a direct activation of acetyl-CoA carboxylase by this compound. They have proposed that palmitylcarnitine in tandem with palmityl-CoA (which inhibits acetyl-CoA carboxylase), may be involved in the regulation of lipogenesis.

Childress et al.,[134] working with blow fly flight muscle mitochondria, have shown that carnitine increases the rate of oxidative decarboxylation of pyruvate (see also Bremer[135]). This animal does not have the capacity to oxidize fatty acid for flight energy but does maintain high concentrations of carnitine and short-chain acyltransferase in its mitochondria, and it may be

[129] K. R. Norum, M. Farstad, and J. Bremer, *Biochem. Biophys. Res. Commun.* **24**, 797 (1966).

[130] F. Sauer and J. D. Erfle, *Fed. Proc. Fed. Amer. Soc. Exp. Biol.* **25**, 769 (1966).

[131] D. C. Hardwick and J. M. Lowenstein, *Fed. Proc. Fed. Amer. Soc. Exp. Biol.* **25**, 340 (1966).

[132] I. B. Fritz and M. P. Hsu, *Biochem. Biophys. Res. Commun.* **22**, 737 (1966).

[133] I. B. Fritz and M. P. Hsu, *J. Biol. Chem.* **242**, 866 (1967).

[134] C. C. Childress, B. Sacktor, and D. R. Traynor, *J. Biol. Chem.* **242**, 754 (1966).

[135] J. Bremer, *Biochim. Biophys. Acta* **104**, 581 (1965).

that here carnitine takes on the role of a device for conserving CoA. The authors suggest that at the inception of flight this insect stores acetyl groups produced from pyruvate plus CoA as acetylcarnitine. Glycolysis may then proceed without inhibition due to excess pyruvate formation (as a result of low levels of free CoA) until the level of oxaloacetate reaches the value necessary for maximal rates of citrate synthesis.

H. Physiological Activity of Carnitine

1. NERVE FUNCTION

The proposal that betaine-CoA esters are involved in pathological nervous activity was originally made by Hosein and his co-workers[136-140] on the basis of analyses of brains taken from rats convulsed with central nervous system poisons and electroshock. These investigators found carnitine, γ-butyrobetaine, crotonobetaine, and their CoA derivatives in water extracts of brain from treated rats, but neither free nor esterified bases in water extracts from normal rats. Chloroform extraction of brain of normal rats released CoA esters of these bases from what was called a " bound " form.[137] Since the methyl, ethyl, choline, and CoA esters of these betaines had been shown to be pharmacologically active both *in vivo* and *in vitro*[137-139, 141] and damage to brain mitochondria during convulsons could be demonstrated, the thesis was put forth that esters are released from mitochondria damaged by administration of central nervous system stimulants or electroshock and are then responsible for the electrical activity associated with convulsions.[137] Convulsive perturbations would be expected to cease when the CoA esters were hydrolyzed by enzymes found in the cytoplasm of the afflicted cells.[140]

An objection to Hosein's argument was raised by the results of assays made by Mehlman and Wolf,[70] Fritz,[22] and Abdel-Kader and Wolf,[75] all of whom identified and quantitatively measured carnitine in water extracts of normal rat brain by colorimetric or enzymatic methods. An explanation for this might be found in the fact that the methods used by Hosein for the isolation and identification of the betaines were the usual chemical ones, so that small amounts of these compounds could easily have been missed. However, a more serious question came up as a result of the inability of Mehlman and Wolf[70] to show any " bound " carnitine in normal rat brain using extraction methods much like Hosein's, coupled with more sensitive techniques of

[136] E. A. Hosein, *Protides Biol. Fluids*, *Proc. 1959 Colloq.* **7**, 275 (1960).
[137] E. A. Hosein and P. Proulx, *Nature (London)* **187**, 321 (1960).
[138] E. A. Hosein, M. Smart, and K. Hawkins, *Can. J. Biochem. Physiol.* **38**, 837 (1960).
[139] E. A. Hosein, P. Proulx, and R. Ara, *Biochem. J.* **83**, 341 (1962).
[140] E. A. Hosein, *Arch. Biochem. Biophys.* **100**, 32 (1963).
[141] E. Strack and K. Försterling, *Hoppe-Seyler's Z. Physiol. Chem.* **286**, 207 (1950).

analysis. McLennan *et al.*,[142] and Crossland and Redfern[143] were also unable to confirm Hosein's findings, and both groups of·investigators suggested that his results were due to isolation artifacts. More recently, Mehlman and Therriault[144] have isolated lipid-bound carnitine from rat brain, and Hosein, continuing work along lines similar to those he had been doing, claims to have found acetyl-L-carnityl-CoA in particles of narcotized rat and rabbit brain (Hosein and Koh,[145] Hosein *et al.*[146]).

McCamen *et al.*[147] have shown that carnitine acetyltransferase is found uniformly distributed within the brain while choline acetyltransferase is localized within the nerve ending particle fraction. They believe that this argues against the hypothesis that acetylcarnitine is a neurohumoral agent.

Fritz[22] and his colleagues have made a number of observations which, if confirmed and extended, will open a somewhat different route of carnitine utilization in mammals. They have found that small quantities of acetyl-carnitine injected directly into the brains of rats and cats cause hyperexcitability and increased motor activity, results that cannot be duplicated with either free carnitine or systemic injections of the acetyl derivative. They have also shown that application of acetylcarnitine directly to the lateral geniculate body of cats under anesthesia produces an increase in the amplitude of evoked cortical potentials in both the association and visual cortical area, an effect not reproduced by injection of acetylcholine, carnitine, or NaCl. In view of the known presence of carnitine and carnitine acyl transferase in the brain, these findings assume an even greater significance and demand further inquiry.

2. OTHER FUNCTIONS

a. On the Isolated Muscle

Hayashi in 1956[148] made the observation that if freshly excised skeletal muscle (which normally undergoes prolonged spontaneous "salt contractions" in Ringer's solution) were placed into a bath in which a previously excised muscle had contracted until becoming inactive, it would never begin contracting. The compounds released from an isolated muscle and responsible for the series of contractions and finally twitch inhibition were identified as

[142] H. McLennan, L. Curry, and R. Walker, *Biochem. J.* **89**, 163 (1963).
[143] J. Crossland and P. H. Redfern, *Life Sci.* **2**, 711 (1963).
[144] M. A. Mehlman and D. G. Therriault, *in* "Recent Research on Carnitine" (G. Wolf, ed.), pp. 35–43 MIT Press, Cambridge, Massachusetts, 1965.
[145] E. A. Hosein and T. Y. Koh, *Arch. Biochem. Biophys.* **114**, 94 (1966).
[146] E. A. Hosein, A. Orzeck, and S. Jacobson, *Biochem. Pharmacol.* **15**, 1429 (1966).
[147] R. McCamen, M. W. McCamen, and M. L. Stafford, *J. Biol. Chem.* **241**, 930 (1966).
[148] T. Hayashi, "Chemical Physiology of Excitation in Muscle and Nerve," 1st Ed. Nakayama Shoten, Tokyo, 1956.

carnosine (Excitine) and carnitine (Inhibitine), respectively. In 1960,[149] he claimed, on the basis of further experiments, that mixtures of the two compounds in different proportions were the real factors, and in 1961[150] he revised this once again to reveal that carnitine corresponded to Excitine and carnosine to Inhibitine. Hayashi has recently extended and clarified his ideas in a 1965 symposium on carnitine,[151] although no additional data have been offered.

It may be noted here that Friebel[152] corroborated the fact that DL-carnitine was not inhibitory, but showed that addition of small quantities of KCl to fresh Ringer's would inhibit contraction of fresh muscle. Analysis of Ringer's solution which had accommodated contracting muscle until it became inactive revealed that enough K^+ ion had been released by the contracting muscle to produce the same effects on fresh muscle as Hayashi's Inhibitine.

b. Effect of Carnitine on Growth and Metabolism of Vertebrates

Strack and Rotzsch[153] have reported various effects of carnitine on total metabolism and growth of vertebrates. Tadpoles grew faster when kept in water in which carnitine had been dissolved whereas there were no such effects in the presence of betaine or γ-butyrobetaine, and choline or crotonobetaine caused toxic symptoms to appear. Carnitine also acted as a partial antagonist to thyroxine; thyroxine reduced growth and induced early metamorphosis in tadpoles, and carnitine addition partly relieved these symptoms. The precocious metamorphosis remained unaffected but growth approached normal levels. In rats, the N balance, which becomes strongly negative with thyroxine, was restored with carnitine and excretion of urea reduced. Carnitine also increased weight in young rats, presumably owing to increased food uptake.

The effect of carnitine on development of the chick embryo has been demonstrated by the indirect method of inhibiting growth through the administration of γ-butyrobetaine. This effect could be reversed upon addition of carnitine (Ito and Fraenkel[154]).

Liébecq-Hutter, in 1956,[155] claimed an effect of carnitine on the development of embryonic chick bone in organ explants, but on reinvestigation in 1960[156] this effect was shown to have been due to crotonobetaine, while carnitine did not significantly affect bone growth.

Partially starving rabbits, fed intravenously with an insufficient supply of

[149] T. Hayashi, *Protides Biol. Fluids, Proc. 1959 Colloq.* 7, 239 (1960).

[150] T. Hayashi, *in* "Nervous Inhibition," Proc. 2nd Friday Harbor Symp. (E. Florey, ed.), p. 378. Pergamon, Oxford, 1961.

[151] T. Hayashi, *in* "Recent Research on Carnitine" (G. Wolf, ed.), pp. 183–191 MIT Press, Cambridge, Massachusetts, 1965.

[152] H. Friebel *Protides Biol. Fluids, Proc. 1959 Colloq.* 7, 263 (1960).

[153] E. Strack and W. Rotzsch, *Protides Biol. Fluids, Proc. 1959 Colloq.* 7, 263 (1960).

[154] T. Ito and G. Fraenkel, *J. Gen. Physiol.* 41, 279 (1957).

[155] S. Liébecq-Hutter, *J. Embryol. Exp. Morphol.* 4, 279 (1956).

[156] S. Liébecq-Hutter, *Protides Biol. Fluids, Proc. 1959 Colloq.* 7, 245 (1960).

glucose and β-hydroxybutyrate have been shown to survive for a longer time with a lower rate of nitrogen catabolism if carnitine was added to the diet (Reynier[21]).

I. Clinical Effects of Carnitine

Extensive work on the effect of carnitine in human disease has been reported from France, Belgium, and Germany. Statements (see above) that carnitine increased digestive secretion, was a growth factor for certain insects, stimulated the growth of bones *in vitro* (later disclaimed by its authors), and enhanced, in general, metabolic processes led to the suggestion that investigations be made of its value in cases of loss of appetite and delayed growth in premature babies, retarded infants, and small children. Early claims of positive results with appetite and growth (Canlorbe et al.[157]) have been, according to the authors, confirmed and extended. Infants and children, aged 1.5–6 months, suffering from malnutrition due to infections were treated with 20 % carnitine solution, with a consequent recovery of appetite, acceleration of growth, and return of the protein constitution to normalcy.[158] Alexander et al.[159] have reported significant increases in weight of tuberculous children, 3–6 years old upon daily oral administration of 600 mg of carnitine for periods of 2 to 6 months. Strack et al.,[87] similarly have recorded increased growth in infants as a result of carnitine administration. Not only did prematurely born infants lose less weight following birth, but they also regained their initial weight sooner.

Since carnitine has been shown partially to antagonize the effect of thyroxine in animal experiments, its influence on patients with a hyperfunctioning thyroid has been investigated, and favorable results have been reported (Strack et al.,[160] Deltour[20]). Duriez and Beaumond[161] have noted a regression of rickets upon administration of carnitine. Bekaert and Deltour[162] have reported a relief of hyperlipidemy in the diabetic by administration of carnitine for several weeks.

Favorable effects of carnitine have also been claimed in cases of loss of appetite in adults and the aged (Jacquel et al.[163]).

In view of such widespread reports of curative effects of carnitine in various types of diseases, it is not surprising that the compound is available in pharmaceutical preparations in several countries of Europe. However, it should be mentioned here that Bender and Adams[84] in an *ad hoc* investigation,

[157] P. Canlorbe, G. Deltour, P. Borniche, and R. Scholler, *Sem. Hop.* 32, 276 (1956).
[158] P. Borniche and P. Canlorbe, *Clin. Chim. Acta* 5, 171 (1960).
[159] F. Alexander, H. Peeters, and P. Vuylsteke, *Protides Biol. Fluids, Proc. 1958 Colloq.* 6, 306 (1959).
[160] E. Strack, G. Woratz, and W. Rotzsch, *Endokrinologie* 38, 218 (1959).
[161] J. Duriez and A. de Beaumont, *Presse Med.* 68, 1393 (1960).
[162] J. Bekaert and G. Deltour, *Clin. Chim. Acta* 5, 177 (1960).
[163] G. Jacquel, G. Robert, and B. Saade, *Presse Med.* 70, 763 (1962).

have failed to reproduce many of the above observations in rats. Carnitine had no effect on protein synthesis or growth of weanling and young rats, nor did it stimulate acid secretion in the isolated mucosa of the toad. Similarly, Deltour[20] has been unable to confirm favorable effects on growth in rats on a protein-poor regime. Reynier,[21] with reference to these findings, has emphasized that this type of metabolic effect of carnitine applies only to conditions of negative nitrogen balance and need not necessarily become manifest in the normally functioning organism. Lack of space does not allow a presentation of multifarious reports and speculations on curative effects of carnitine (see, e.g., Deltour,[20] Reynier,[21]), mostly claims based on limited material and never independently confirmed. From a general examination of the literature extant, it is our present feeling that the usefulness of carnitine in the treatment of metabolic disorders and disease still remains to be significantly demonstrated.

J. Conclusions

Over ten years ago,[14] in another review, the authors expended a large amount of space on chemistry, methods of determination, requirements for, and distribution of carnitine, and could find almost nothing to say about biosynthesis, intracellular location, and physiological function. While the situation is not completely reversed, enough has been learned within this time to give us new insights into precursors, sites of accumulation, and biochemical activity.

It is generally accepted that carnitine is produced almost universally, and recent evidence indicates that its mode of formation proceeds through γ-butyrobetaine. The biosynthetic pathway of this latter compound is still virtually unknown, however, and remains a fruitful field for investigation.

The implication of carnitine in fat metabolism, about which there were only hints in 1957, appears to be a reality on at least two levels, i.e., as a precursor of a constituent of phospholipids and as a catalytic agent in the transfer of fatty acids across mitochondrial membranes. When it replaces choline in the diet of blow fly larvae, it can be isolated from the phospholipids in the form of β-methylcholine, and it may normally be present in phospholipid in this decarboxylated form as well as in its native form. Its activity as a catalyst is best described in terms of two enzymes which have been isolated from mammalian muscle, long-chain and short-chain carnitine acyltransferase. These enzymes are involved in the transfer of acyl groups from CoA to carnitine and vice versa, and it appears that carnitine activity in this system may rest in the fact that carnityl derivatives of fatty acids pass across mitochondrial membranes at a more rapid rate than do CoA derivatives, leading to an enhancement of utilization of fatty acid moieties. It may also be involved with the regulation of lipogenesis through its effectiveness as palmitylcarnitine in activating acetyl-CoA carboxylase.

Other functions of carnitine even less well understood are those concerning nervous activity, and here it is probable that some derivative is more active that the parent compound when applied directly to nervous tissue. This area of investigation is only now being explored, but, from all indications, there will be results of some importance in the near future.

Whether any of the clinical effects attributed to the administration of carnitine are involved with the activities described above is beyond our present state of knowledge. Certainly, however, the important biochemical and physiological functions of this compound uncovered within the past few years should lead to greater interest among responsible clinicians and with it, we hope, some significant findings at this level.

IV. Ubiquinone (Coenzyme Q)[1]

R. A. MORTON

A. Introduction

This subject has now a considerable literature, and reference is made to some general articles.[1a-12]

[1] In respect to the Liverpool University contribution to the work reviewed in this section, grateful acknowledgement is made to the Nuffield Foundation, The Rockefeller Foundation, The Department of Scientific and Industrial Research, The Medical Research Council, The Agricultural Research Council and the U.S. Public Health Service (Contract No. AM 05282) and the British Egg Marketing Board, for grants at different times to the research work of the Department of Biochemistry. Revision of this account was done during the tenure of a Leverhulme Emeritus Fellowship.

[1a] *Quinones Electron Transp., Ciba Found. Symp.*, **1960** (G. E. W. Wolstenholme and C. M. O'Connor, eds.). Churchill, London, 1961.

[2] "Biochemistry of Quinones" (R. A. Morton, ed.). Academic Press, New York, 1965.

[3] B. Chance, *in* "Biological Structure and Function" (T. W. Goodwin and O. Lindberg, eds.), Vol. II, p. 119. Academic Press, New York, 1961.

[4] F. L. Crane, *Biochemistry* **1**, 510 (1962).

[5] D. E. Green, *Proc. 5th Int. Congr. Biochem., Moscow*, 1961 IX.9 (1963). (IUB Series Vol. 29).

[6] D. E. Green and S. Fleischer, *in* "Horizons in Biochemistry" (M. Kasha and B. Pullman, eds.), p. 381. Academic Press, New York, 1962.

[7] Y. Hatefi, *Advan. Enzymol. Relat. Subj. Biochem.* 275 (1963).

[8] F. W. Hemming and R. A. Morton, *in* "Enzyme Chemistry of Phenolic Compounds" (W. D. Ollis, ed.), pp. 57 Pergamon, Oxford, 1963.

[9] R. A. Morton, *Nature (London)* **182**, 1764 (1958).

[10] R. A. Morton, *Vitam. Horm. (New York)* **19**, 395 (1961).

[11] E. R. Redfearn, *Annu. Rep. Chem. Soc.* **57**, 395 (1961).

[12] E. C. Slater, *Advan. Enzymol. Relat. Subj. Biochem.* **20**, 147 (1958).

The ubiquinones (coenzymes Q) were discovered independently at Liverpool and at Madison by very different routes, in the one case via the study of fat-soluble vitamins and the other via enzymatic processes in mitochondria.

Before World War II, work directed primarily to the distribution of vitamins A_1 and A_2 led to the recognition in halibut spleen of a new substance with λ_{max} 275 mμ in ethanol.[13] Interest had been aroused in a claim[14] that the symptoms of agranulocytosis (usually induced by drugs) could be greatly alleviated by administering orally the unsaponifiable matter from yellow bone marrow. Dr. A. L. Stubbs and the writer fractionated the unsaponifiable matter from about 100 lb of ox bone marrow. In addition to cholesterol and carotene, the material yielded *inter alia* batyl alcohol and a very pale substance with λ_{max} 275 mμ resembling the halibut spleen constituent. Attempts by the late Professor T. B. Davie to produce experimental agranulocytosis in animals failed to give a bioassay method, and projected trials had to be abandoned when war broke out in 1939. (It was subsequently shown that batyl alcohol was the active principle.) Further study of the 275 mμ absorbing substance was deferred because of wartime duties.

Moore and Rajagopal[15] observed that the unsaponifiable lipid from rat liver sometimes had an absorption peak at 275 mμ and that the selective absorption disappeared on further digestion of the unsaponifiable matter with alkali.

The devious ways in which research topics become interlocked have always held particular interest for students of vitamins. At Liverpool it had been found[16] that the oils extracted from the intestines of many fish species were rich in vitamin A. In particular, the oil from halibut intestinal tissue contained up to 8 % of vitamin A. Later, Glover and Morton[17] discovered that the lipid extracted from the *tunica propria* layer of halibut pyloric caecae could contain as much as 40 % by weight of esterified vitamin A. A parallel study of intestinal tissue was carried out on domestic animals, and it soon became clear that mammals do not store vitamin A esters in the intestinal mucosa. It was observed, however, that vitamin A aldehyde (then newly available) was converted to vitamin A in the animal intestinal wall. This led to other work which proved that carotene could be converted to vitamin A in mammalian intestinal mucosa, a conclusion reached also by other groups of workers led by Kon and by Deuel.

These investigations on processes occurring in the lining of the gut influenced thinking on another problem, i.e., the origin of provitamin D. Glover[18] proved that, in guinea pigs, cholesterol undergoes enzymatic

[13] J. A. Lovern, R. A. Morton, and J. H. Ireland, *Biochem. J.* **33**, 327 (1939).
[14] C. M. Marberg and H. C. Wiles, *Arch. Intern. Med.* **61**, 408 (1938).
[15] T. Moore and K. R. Rajagopal, *Biochem. J.* **34**, 335 (1940).
[16] J. A. Lovern, J. R. Edisbury, and R. A. Morton, *Nature (London)* **140**, 276 (1937).
[17] J. Glover and R. A. Morton, *Biochem. J.* **42**, 63P (1948).
[18] M. Glover, J. Glover and R. A. Morton, *Biochem. J.*, **51**, 1 (1952).

dehydrogenation in the gut wall to form 7-dehydrocholesterol. The guinea pig is here peculiar only because of the unexplained fact that a larger proportion than usual of the provitamin remains at the site of origin with the cholesterol. The enzyme must occur in most species.

B. Substance A (SA) and Substance C (SC)

Various other animal species were studied, and Festenstein et al.[19, 20] worked on horse intestine. They scraped the mucosal tissue from lengths of small intestine and fractionated the extracted lipids and unsaponifiable matter derived therefrom. One fraction had the following spectroscopic properties in cyclohexane: λ_{max} 272 mμ, inflexion 330 mμ, flat peak 400 mμ ($E_{1\,cm}^{1\%}$ values 195, 14, 8, respectively). This product was chromatographically homogeneous on alumina, but although nearly pure it did not give crystals stable at room temperature. Further attempts to isolate the new substance were made using liver tissue from ox, sheep, and horse, but the presence of carotenoids, vitamin A, and decomposition products made large-scale adsorption chromatography on alumina difficult.[21]

The mode of action of vitamin A, a problem which even today remains intractable, was also being studied by the Liverpool group. Lowe et al.[22] reported that two unidentified substances with characteristic absorption spectra in the ultraviolet region could be recognized as constituents of the liver unsaponifiable matter from vitamin A-deficient rats. As the vitamin depletion progressed and the symptoms of deficiency became more severe, the concentrations of the two new substances rose significantly.

Fractionation of the liver unsaponifiable by chromatography on alumina (Brockmann, Grade 3) separated the two materials which were provisionally designated substance A (SA) and substance C (SC), respectively.[23, 24] The purest SA from rat liver showed λ_{max} 272, inflexion 330, 400–410 mμ, $E_{1\,cm}^{1\%}$ 182, 14, 8, respectively. It was very like Festenstein's horse intestine constituent. The purest SC showed λ_{max} 232, 275, 283, 332 mμ, $E_{1\,cm}^{1\%}$ 192, 84, 79.4, and 34.3, respectively. The two substances have since become known as ubiquinone (or coenzyme Q) and ubichromenol.[25, 26]

Substance A occurred in livers of both normal and vitamin A-deficient

[19] G. N. Festenstein, Ph.D. Thesis, Univ. of Liverpool, 1950.
[20] G. N. Festenstein, F. W. Heaton, J. S. Lowe, and R. A. Morton, Biochem. J. 59, 558 (1955).
[21] J. C. Cain and R. A. Morton, Biochem. J. 60, 274 (1955).
[22] J. S. Lowe, R. A. Morton, and R. G. Harrison, Nature (London) 172, 716.
[23] F. W. Heaton, J. S. Lowe, and R. A. Morton, Biochem. J. 60, 18P (1955).
[24] F. W. Heaton, J. S. Lowe, and R. A. Morton, Biochem. J. 67, 208 (1957).
[25] R. A. Morton, G. M. Wilson, J. S. Lowe, and W. M. F. Leat, Chem. Ind. (London) p. 1649 (1957).
[26] D. L. Laidman, R. A. Morton, J. Y. F. Paterson, and J. F. Pennock, Chem. Ind. (London) p. 1019 (1959).

rats.[20, 27] Heaton et al.[24] observed that weanling rats given a vitamin-A-free diet became xerophthalmic and began to lose weight after 40–50 days. The deficiency state was accompanied by an increase in SA which (recalculated from published data) corresponded with a rise of 117–278 μg ubiquinone/gm liver tissue. There was a smaller rise in submaxillary glands, but not in kidney tissue. The liver SC also rose (recalculated) from 74.9 to 161.4 μg ubichromenol/gm tissue.

The distribution of SA was studied carefully; it was always present in liver,[28, 29] kidney,[30, 31] spleen and pancreas.[32] Heaton et al.,[33] in testing a claim that yeast contained vitamin A, did not find the vitamin but succeeded in isolating a fraction with the spectroscopic and other properties of SA: λ_{max} 272 mμ, $E_{1\,cm}^{1\%}$ 167 in cyclohexane. [In retrospect this was an impure specimen of a second ubiquinone (Q-6) (see Gloor et al.[56]). Hemming et al.[34] found ubiquinone in mitochondria.]

It is well known that in different species the symptoms of vitamin A deficiency are not all the same and do not occur in the same order. Thus the domestic fowl does not readily show xerophthalmia or loss of appetite and weight although it may be fully depleted and unable to stand and, indeed, may die suddenly. Lowe et al.,[35] found that, as compared with controls, vitamin A-deficient birds showed little change in liver levels of ubiquinone or ubichromenol. Cunningham and Morton,[28] and Phillips[36] studied the tissues of vitamin A-deficient guinea pigs to observe any rise in the ubiquinone concentrations in tissues. In fact, Cunningham found less ubiquinone in guinea pig liver as a result of deprivation, and Phillips found reduced incorporation of isotope from ^{14}C-labeled mevalonate in the livers of vitamin A-depleted guinea pigs.

These results with poultry and with guinea pigs negated the attractive idea that ubiquinone and ubichromenol levels in liver were directly and necessarily related to vitamin A status. The experimental evidence for rats, however, is quite definite. Thus Morton and Phillips[37] analyzed livers from animals killed after varying times on a vitamin A-free diet. The weanling at first con-

[27] R. J. Ward and T. Moore, Biochem. J. 59, xv (1955).

[28] N. F. Cunningham and R. A. Morton, Biochem. J. 72, 92 (1958).

[29] J. S. Lowe, R. A. Morton, N. F. Cunningham, and J. Vernon, Biochem. J. 67, 215 (1957).

[30] J. S. Lowe, R. A. Morton, and J. Vernon, Biochem. J. 67, 228 (1957).

[31] L. Mervyn and R. A. Morton, Biochem. J. 68, 26P (1958); Biochem. J. 72, 106 (1959).

[32] R. A. Morton and N. I. Fahmy, Biochem. J. 72, 99, (1959).

[33] F. W. Heaton, J. S. Lowe, and R. A. Morton, J. Chem. Soc. p. 4094 (1956).

[34] F. W. Hemming, J. F. Pennock, and R. A. Morton, Biochem. J. 68, 29P (1958).

[35] J. S. Lowe, R. A. Morton, N. F. Cunningham, and J. Vernon, Biochem. J. 67, 215 (1957).

[36] W. E. J. Phillips, Can. J. Biochem. Physiol. 39, 855 (1961).

[37] R. A. Morton and W. E. J. Phillips, Biochem. J. 73, 416 (1959).

TABLE II

UBIQUINONE AND UBICHROMENOL IN LIVERS OF RATS ON A VITAMIN A-FREE
DIET FROM WEANING

Stage	Ubiquinone		Ubichromenol, μg/liver
	μG/g liver	μG/liver	
5 days after weaning	82	304	25
11 days after weaning	136	558	—
20 days after weaning	207	972	—
28 days after weaning	245	994	—
At weight plateau	299	1225	123
Post-plateau	409	1390	144

[a] Data were recalculated from data by Morton and Phillips.[37]

tinues to grow, then the weight curve flattens to a plateau and later the rat begins to lose weight and will finally die. Table II shows the effects on ubiquinone and ubichromenol levels. Moore and Sharman[38] noted a distinct fall in liver weight as a late sign of vitamin A deficiency. This effect somewhat exaggerates the large rise in ubiquinone and the results are perhaps best expressed as micrograms per liver. The rise in ubichromenol occurs mainly in the later stages of deficiency. Hemming[34] found that in normal rats the liver ubiquinone was mainly in mitochondria whereas in vitamin A-deficient rats there was a good deal in the microsomes and the supernatant fraction. Aiyar and Sreenivasan[39] found a definite increase in liver mitochondrial ubiquinone in vitamin A deficiency, but most of the increase in liver tissue occurred in other subcellular fractions.

Stoffel and Martius[40] claim that the biosynthesis of ubiquinone is completed in mitochondria.

C. Nature of SA-Ubiquinone

The problem of the structure of SA (ubiquinone) was first tackled by Wilson[41] (see Morton et al.[42]). The substance has an ultraviolet absorption spectrum resembling very closely that of 8,9-ene-7,11-diones in the steroids, but Wilson showed that SA was not a steroid. Molecular weight determinations by different methods failed to agree. The Rast method gave values near 650 but the Barger method of isothermal distillation indicated 870–995 and cryoscopic determinations (cyclohexane as solvent) 890–1000. Wilson had

[38] T. Moore and I. M. Sharman, Brit. J. Nutr. 14, 473, (1960).
[39] A. S. Aiyar and A. Sreenivasan, Nature (London) 190 344 (1961).
[40] W. Stoffel and C. Martius, Biochem. Z. 333, 440 (1960).
[41] G. M. Wilson, Ph.D. Thesis, Univ. of Liverpool, 1956.
[42] R. A. Morton, G. M. Wilson, J. S. Lowe, and W. M. F. Leat, Chem. Ind. (London) p. 1659 (1957); Biochem. J. 68, 16P (1958).

obtained crystalline preparations from pig liver and other sources but the melting points (34°–41°) were variable. The compound was easily reducible with a change in ultraviolet absorption λ_{max} 291 mμ, $E_{1\,cm}^{1\%}$ 52), but it was quickly reoxidized in air (λ_{max} 272 mμ). The reduction product could be acetylated and thereby rendered more stable. The oxidation–reduction potential of the system SA–reduced SA was $E_0 = 0.542$ V.

On the basis of a molecular weight of about 860, perbenzoic acid titration indicated 10 double bonds in the molecule. Catalytic hydrogenation led on the same basis to an uptake of 11 molecules of hydrogen per mole. The fully hydrogenated product was oxidized (e.g., by methanolic ferric chloride) to a product having almost the same ultraviolet absorption spectrum as the original substance. If now it was subjected to catalytic hydrogenation, the uptake of hydrogen was only 1/11 of that first observed. Alkoxy determinations suggested the presence of two alkoxyl groups in a molecular weight of 860 with two other oxygen atoms. These could well belong to a quinone of the p-benzoquinone series because substituents could have reduced E_0 from 0.71 to 0.542 V. Vitamin K analogs were excluded on spectroscopic evidence as well as on the magnitude of the redox potentials.

It seemed likely that SA was a p-benzoquinone derivative with a long polyisoprenoid side chain, and at this stage the writer approached Dr. O. Isler of Hoffmann-La Roche at Basel because of his special experience in the synthesis of vitamins A and K$_2$ and similar products. The polyisoprenoid chain is not itself a source of selective absorption in the ultraviolet region and will not influence the *molecular* extinction coefficient. The Craven test[43] indicated that SA was a fully substituted benzoquinone. From the literature it was found that aurantiogliocladin (2,3-dimethoxy,5,6-dimethyl-p-benzo-quinone I) had been isolated by Vischer[44] and synthesized by Baker, McOmie, and Miles.[45] Professor Baker kindly provided a specimen of aurantioglio-cladin which on examination showed the expected absorption spectrum λ_{max} 272 mμ, $E_{1\,cm}^{1\%}$ 775 or ε_{max} 15,190. If SA had the same ε_{max} and its molecular weight was 860, the $E_{1\,cm}^{1\%}$ value would be 176—very close to that observed. Comparisons with the spectra of other substituted toluquinones confirmed the positions of the alkoxy groups:

[43] R. Craven, *J. Chem. Soc.* p. 1605 (1931).
[44] E. B. Vischer, *J. Chem. Soc.* p. 815 (1953).
[45] W. Baker, J. F. W. McOmie and D. Miles, *J. Chem. Soc.* p. 820 (1953).

D. Coenzyme Q from Mitochondria

By this time an exchange of information had made it practically certain that Crane and Lester's group,[46–48] working at Madison on heart muscle mitochondria, had independently discovered the same substance and had made progress in recognizing it as a quinone with two alkoxy groups. The investigation at the Enzyme Institute at Wisconsin had been hampered in exactly the same way as the Liverpool work by ambiguous results in the determinations of molecular weights. The help of Dr. K. Folkers of Merck, Sharp, and Dohme had been sought over characterization and synthesis of the new quinone.

The important work done at Madison by D. E. Green's School depended in part on facilities for obtaining large amounts of mitochondria, the convenient sources being heart muscle or liver tissue. The new quinone (Q_{275} from its absorption peak at 275 mμ in ethanol) was obtained by fractionating mitochondrial lipids and crystallization (m.p. 48°–49°). It was present in various electron transport particle preparations, and it quickly became recognized as a new member of the mitochondrial electron transport sequence (Hatefi et al.,[47] Lester et al.,[48] Pumphrey et al.[49]). It has been designated Q_{275}, mitoquinone, coenzyme Q, and ubiquinone. It seems likely that the abbreviation Q and the trivial name ubiquinone will be retained.

The Madison workers established the quinone-like properties, prepared a crystalline diacetate of the corresponding quinol, and proved the presence of two methoxyl groups and a long unsaturated side chain.

Lester and Crane[50] found that many microbial species contained substances akin to that found in animals. Four substances were isolated (Lester et al.[51]) which turned out to be isoprenologs of coenzyme Q differing from one another in the length of the polyisoprenoid side chain. The notation Q-10 means a coenzyme Q or ubiquinone with a C_{50} side chain (10 isoprenoid C_5 groups), similarly Q-9 is a ubiquinone with a C_{45} side chain, and so on to Q-6 for the yeast ubiquinone with a C_{30} side chain.

Crane and his colleagues (Crane et al.,[52] Hatefi et al.,[53] Lester and

[46] F. L. Crane, Y. Hatefi, R. L. Lester, and C. Widmer, Biochim. Biophys. Acta 25, 220 (1957).
[47] Y. Hatefi, R. L. Lester, and T. Ramasarma, Fed. Proc. Fed. Amer. Soc. Exp. Biol. 17, 238 (1958).
[48] R. L. Lester, F. L. Crane, and Y. Hatefi, J. Amer. Chem. Soc. 80, 4751 (1958).
[49] A. M. Pumphrey, E. R. Redfearn, and R. A. Morton, Chem. Ind. (London) p. 978 (1958).
[50] R. L. Lester and F. L. Crane, Biochim. Biophys. Acta 32, 492 (1959).
[51] R. L. Lester, Y. Hatefi, C. Widmer, and F. L. Crane, Biochim. Biophys. Acta 33, 169 (1959).
[52] F. L. Crane, C. Widmer, R. L. Crane, and Y. Hatefi, Biochim. Biophys. Acta 31, 476 (1959).
[53] Y. Hatefi, R. L. Lester, F. L. Crane, and C. Widmer, Biochim. Biophys. Acta 31, 490 (1959).

Fleischer[54]) early showed it to be probable that Q (coenzyme Q or ubiquinone) was indispensable for electron transport in many types of mitochondrial preparations, i.e., for the oxidation of succinate or reduced nicotine adenine dinucleotide (NADH) via the cytochrome system.

E. Proof of Structure of Ubiquinone or Coenzyme Q

The structures of the ubiquinones were proved by Isler's group jointly with the Liverpool workers and by Folkers' team jointly with the group from the Enzyme Institute at Madison (Morton et al.,[55] Gloor et al.,[56] Rüegg et al.,[57] Wolf et al.,[58] Shunk et al.[59]).

In isolating ubiquinone it is important to saponify the tissue rather than to extract the lipid beforehand, and it is also necessary to add pyrogallol fairly generously (1–2%) as an antioxidant before heating with ethanol and alkali. On a fairly large scale (200 kg) it is possible to obtain 1 gm of Q-10 per 20 kg of pig heart tissue.

The methoxy group was determined by the standard procedure; the resulting methyl iodide was allowed to react with silver 3,5-dinitrobenzoate, and the methyl ester was rigorously identified. The evidence for the structure is shown in part in Fig. 3. The quinol derived from Q-10 was acetylated, and the dimethyl ester of ubiquinol was degraded and the structure confirmed. Gloor et al.[56] obtained from bakers' yeast a pure ubiquinone (m.p. 19°–20°, $E_{1\,cm}^{1\%}$ 272 mμ 246 –OMe 10.22%) which from its physical properties seemed to be Q-6 (i.e., C_{30} side chain).

This was confirmed by condensing the quinol from 2,3-dimethoxy-5-methyl-1,4-benzoquinone with all-*trans* farnesylnerolidol using zinc chloride. The product, after purification, was identical with the yeast ubiquinone. The polyisoprenoid alcohol $C_{45}H_{73}OH$ obtained from tobacco similarly leads to Q-9, the coenzyme or ubiquinone with a nonaprenyl (C_{45}) side chain.

F. Ubichromenol (SC)

Substance C appears to have a much more restricted distribution than

[54] R. L. Lester and S. Fleischer, *Arch. Biochem. Biophys.* **80**, 470 (1959).

[55] R. A. Morton, U. Gloor, O. Schindler, G. M. Wilson, L. H. Chopard-dit-Jean, F. W. Hemming, O. Isler, W. M. F. Leat, J. F. Pennock, J. Rüegg, U. Schwieter, and O. Wiss, *Helv. Chim. Acta* **41**, 2343 (1958).

[56] U. Gloor, O. Isler, R. A. Morton, R. Rüegg, and O. Wiss, *Helv. Chim. Acta* **41**, 2357 (1958).

[57] R. Rüegg, U. Gloor, R. N. Goel, R. Ryser, O. Wiss, and O. Isler, *Helv. Chim. Acta* **42**, 2616 (1959).

[58] D. E. Wolf, C. H. Hoffman, N. R. Trenner, B. H. Arison, C. H. Shunk, O. B. Linn, J. F. McPherson, and K. Folkers, *J. Amer. Chem. Soc.* **80**, 4752 (1958).

[59] C. H. Shunk, B. O. Linn, E. L. Wong, P. E. Wittreich, F. M. Robinson, and K. Folkers, *J. Amer. Chem. Soc.* **81**, 2026 (1959).

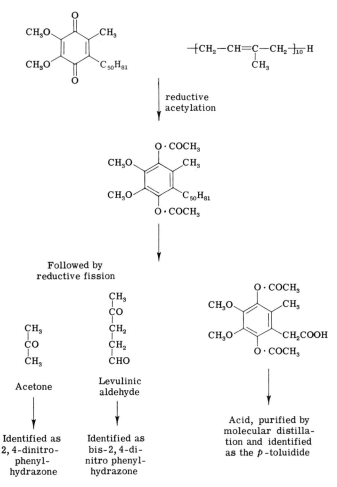

FIG. 3. Evidence for the structure attributed to ubiquinone-coenzyme Q.

ubiquinones (Cunningham and Morton,[28] Festenstein et al.,[20] Lowe et al.,[30] Lowe et al.,[29] Mervyn and Morton,[31] Morton and Fahmy,[32]).

In normal animal organs it is never present in more than very small amounts, and even in the liver of the vitamin A-deficient rat it is still a very minor constituent. After many tissues from various species had been studied, the best source was found to be "normal" human kidney, i.e., tissues obtained at post-mortem examinations from persons who had died from conditions other than disease of the kidneys. With the help of a number of pathologists, 46.5 kg of human kidney tissue was obtained. The unsaponifiable matter was chromatographed on alumina after removal of most of the cholesterol

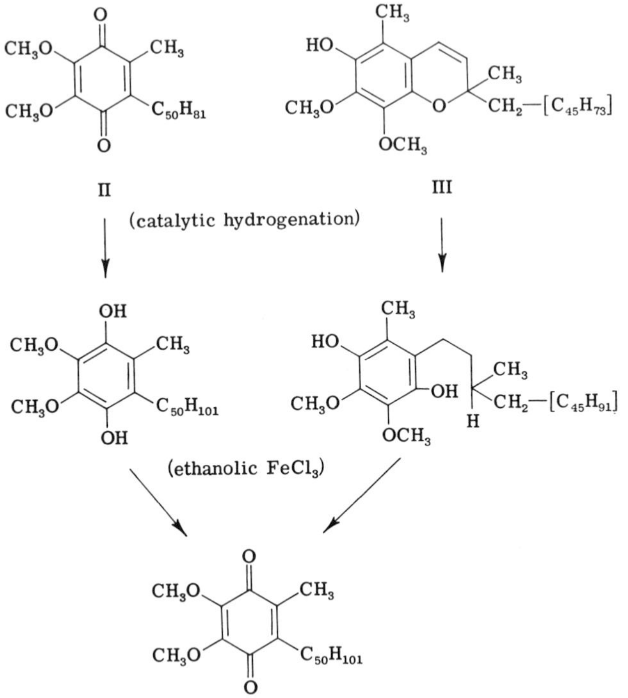

FIG. 4. Evidence for the structure attributed to ubichromenol.

by crystallization. The fractions were examined for ultraviolet absorption, and those exhibiting the SC spectrum were combined and rechromatographed on magnesia. The impurities were less strongly adsorbed than SC which was eluted from the magnesia by means of methylal. It was then crystallized from ethanol (0.153 gm, m.p. 18°). The absorption spectrum (Fig. 4) λ_{max} 233, 275, 283, 332 mμ, $E_{1\ cm}^{1\%}$ 233, 76.1, 91.4, and 38.6, respectively, suggested the presence of a styrene chromophore. Infrared absorption pointed to an aromatic ring, a double bond conjugated to the ring (1575 cm^{-1}), OH (3546 cm^{-1}) —OCH$_3$ (1272, 1098 cm^{-1}) and —CH(CH$_3$)$_2$ (1179, 1359, and 1389 cm^{-1}). SC formed a crystalline acetate. Analysis gave:

SC   C 81.93, H 10.67 —OCH$_3$ 7.34%
SC-acetate C 80.81, H 10.59 —OCH$_3$ 7.05%

The molecular weight was near 850. The above and other considerations led to structure III (Laidman et al.[60]). Fully hydrogenated SC (H$_2$ uptake equal to 11 double bonds) could be oxidized (ferric chloride) to give a product showing λ_{max} 279 and 407 mμ ($E_{1\ cm}^{1\%}$ 160 and 4.3). This in turn could be

[60] D. L. Laidman, R. A. Morton, J. Y. F. Paterson, and J. F. Pennock, Biochem. J. 24, 541 (1960).

reduced (by KBH_4) to yield a product with λ_{max} 290 mμ ($E_1^{1\%}$ $_{cm}$ 50). Perhydro-ubiquinone behaved in exactly the same manner. Ubiquinone can be converted to ubichromenol in various ways (Links,[61] Draper and Csallany[62]). The most convenient method is to reflux ubiquinone with pyridine (McHale and Green[63]) or piperidine.

Some workers have suggested that ubichromenol may be an artifact. Against this is the fact that the product isolated from kidney was optically active.

G. Plastoquinones

Kofler[64] and Kofler et al.[65] obtained a new quinone from lucerne (*Medicago sativa*) and concluded that it was a trisubstituted *p*-benzoquinone (λ_{max} 254, 263 mμ $E_1^{1\%}$ $_{cm}$ approximately 250) with a long side-chain making the molecular weight about 800. Autumnal leaves from horse chestnut and pine needles were good sources. The substance was independently rediscovered by Crane and Lester[66] and more fully described by Crane.[67] Dried lucerne gave ubiquinone (Q-10) and the new quinone. Further investigations led to the formula

H₃C

H₃C

[CH₂—CH=C—CH₂]₉H

CH₃

Plastoquinone

IV

Crane gave to this quinone the name plastoquinone because he found it to be concentrated in chloroplasts. It can be synthesized from 2,3-dimethyl-1,4-quinol and the polyisoprenoid alcohol solanesol ($C_{45}H_{73}OH$), obtainable from tobacco.

Kegel et al.[68] isolated two further quinones (plastoquinones B and C, A being the original compound). Reversed phase paper chromatography showed that A (plastoquinone PQ-9) was predominant (Table III). Henninger

[61] J. Links, *Biochim. Biophys. Acta* **38**, 193 (1960).

[62] H. H. Draper and A. S. Csallany, *Biochem. Biophys. Res. Commun.* **2**, 307 (1960).

[63] D. McHale and J. Green, *Chem. Ind. (London)* p. 1867 (1962).

[64] M. Kofler, *Festschr. Emil Barell* p. 199. Hoffmann-La Roche, Basel, 1946.

[65] M. Kofler, A. Langemann, R. Rüegg, L. H. Chopard-dit-Jean, A. Rayroud, and O. Isler, *Helv. Chim. Acta* **42**, 1283 (1959).

[66] F. L. Crane and R. L. Lester, *Plant Physiol.* **33**, Suppl. VII (1958).

[67] F. L. Crane, *Plant Physiol.* **34**, 546 (1959).

[68] L. P. Kegel, M. D. Henninger, and F. L. Crane, *Biochem. Biophys. Res. Commun.* **8**, 294 (1962).

TABLE III

A. PLASTOQUINONE (PQ-9) ABSORPTION SPECTRA

	Solvent	λ_{max}	$E_{1\ cm}^{1\%}$	ε_{max}
PQ-9	Ethanol	254–255	210	15,720
		263		
	Light petroleum	254	253	18,940
Reduced PQ-9 (plastoquinol)		290	46	3,450

B. QUINONES IN SPINACH CHLOROPLASTS

	M.p. (°C)	λ_{max}	$E_{1\ cm}^{1\%}$	Mole/mole total chlorophyll
PQ A (PQ-9)	44	255	246	0.16
PQ B	35	255	202	0.08
PQ C	Oil	255	66	0.10
Phylloquinone	—	—	—	0.008

et al.[69] found that in spinach chloroplasts plastoquinone B and C were present in about one-fifth the concentration of plastoquinone A.

Bishop,[70, 71] Redfearn and Friend,[72, 73] Arnon *et al.*,[74] Arnon and Horton,[75] Crane *et al.*,[76] and Witt *et al.*[77] have all made contributions showing that plastoquinone functions in electron transport in plants and algae and in particular catalyzes reactions concerned with the photosynthetic processes in which water is the source of reducing power and $NADPH_2$ and ATP are formed in chloroplasts.

Morton[77a] has reviewed the state of knowledge concerning quinones in photosynthesis and photosynthetic phosphorylation. Arnon and Crane[77b]

[69] M. D. Henninger, R. A. Dilley, and F. L. Crane, *Biochem. Biophys. Res. Commun.* **10**, 237 (1963).

[70] N. I. Bishop, *Proc. Nat. Acad. Sci. U.S.* **45**, 1696 (1959).

[71] N. I. Bishop, *Quinones Electron Transp.*, Ciba Found. Symp., 1960 p. 383 (1961).

[72] E. R. Redfearn and J. Friend, *Nature (London)* **191**, 806 (1961).

[73] E. R. Redfearn and J. Friend, *Biochem. J.* **84**, 34P (1962).

[74] D. I. Arnon, F. R. Whatley, and A. A. Horton, *Fed. Proc. Fed. Amer. Soc. Exp. Biol.* **21** 91 (1962).

[75] D. I. Arnon and A. A. Horton, *Acta Chem. Scand.* **17s**, 135 (1963).

[76] F. L. Crane, B. Ehrlich, and P. L. Kegol, *Biochem. Biophys. Res. Commun.* **3**, 37 (1960).

[77] H. T. Witt, A. Müller, and B. Rumberg, *Nature (London)* **197**, 987 (1963).

[77a] R. A. Morton, *Biol. Rev. (Cambridge)* **46**, 47 (1971).

placed plastoquinone between the two light reactions. Henninger and Crane[77c] also found a role for PQ-C since 40% of the PQ-9 (PQ-A) could be removed (by extraction of freeze-dried chloroplasts) before Hill reaction activity fell whereas it decreased in proportion to the extraction of PQ-C. Restoration was optimal only when PQ-9 (0.1 μmole/mg. chlorophyll) and PQ-C (0.01 μmole/mg. chlorophyll) were added. PQ-C perhaps links cytochrome b with the copper protein plastocyanin. Schmidt-Mende and Rumberg[77d] exposed chloroplasts to continuous far-red light of wave-length 718 nm., absorbed by "chlorophyll a_2". Chlorophyll a_1 and substances between it and chlorophyll a_2 were all oxidised. Additional light (hν_2, 620–700 nm.) then excites only chlorophyll a_2 since the continuous light keeps chlorophyll a_1 fully oxidised. Changes in absorption at 254 nm. indicate that plastoquinone forms the quinol (PQH$_2$ or PQ^{--}) and that there is a plastoquinone pool of ten electron capacity. The School of Witt, using the method of flash photolysis, confirms the essential role of plastoquinone in photosynthesis and a quantitative treatment has been advanced, (Stiehl and Witt,[77,e,f]; Schmidt-Mende and Witt[77g]; Vater et al.[77h]; Reinwald et al.[77i,j]). A twin molecule PQ-PQ is postulated and is thought to become a semiquinone PQ$^-$-PQ$^-$ on reduction by chlorophyll a_2 followed by a dismutation to PQ^{--} (quinol) and PQ.

Preparations of PQ-C exhibited a hydroxyl peak in their infrared absorption spectra (Threlfall et al.[77k]. By means of thin layer chromatography Griffiths obtained six PQ-B fractions and resolved PQ-C into six fractions PQ-C$_1$ . . . . . PQ-C$_6$ (Griffiths et al.[77l]). Barr et al. [77m] found spinach PQ-C to be mainly PQ-C$_2$ and PQ-C$_3$ (see also Das et al.[77n,o]; Threlfall and Griffiths[77p]).

[77b] D. I. Arnon and F. L. Crane in *Biochemistry of Quinones* R. A. Morton, Ed. Academic Press, New York & London. pp. 433–438 (1965).

[77c] M. D. Henninger and F. L. Crane, *J. Biol. Chem.* **141**, 5190 (1966).

[77d] P. Schmidt-Mende and B. Rumberg, *Z. Naturforsch.* **23b**, 255 (1968).

[77e] H. H. Stiehl and H. T. Witt, *Z. Naturforsch*, **23b**, 220 (1968).

[77f] H. H. Stiehl and H. T. Witt, *Z. Naturforsch*, **24b**, 1588 (1969).

[77g] P. Schmidt-Mende and H. T. Witt, *Z. Naturforsch.* **23b**, 228 (1968).

[77h] J. Vater, G. Renger, H. H. Stiehl and H. T. Witt, *Naturwissenschaften* **55**, 220 (1968).

[77i] E. Reinwald, U. Siggel and B. Rumberg, *Naturwissenschaften* **55**, 221 (1968).

[77j] E. Reinwald, H. H. Stiehl and B. Rumberg, *Z. Naturforsch* **23b**, 1616 (1968).

[77k] D. R. Threlfall, W. T. Griffiths and T. W. Goodwin, *Biochim. biophys. Acta* **102**, 614 (1965).

[77l] W. T. Griffiths, J. C. Wallwork and J-F. Pennock, *Nature, London* **211**, 1037 (1966).

[77m] R. Barr, M. D. Henninger and F. L. Crane, *Plant Physiol. Wash.*, **42**, 1246 (1967).

[77n] B. C. Das, M. Lounasma, C. Tendille and E. Lederer, *Biochem. Biophys. Res. Commun.* **21**, 318 (1965).

[77o] B. C. Das, M. Lounasma, C. Tendille and E. Lederer, *Biochem. Biophys. Res. Commun.* **26**, 211 (1967).

[77p] D. R. Threlfall and W. T. Griffiths in *Biochemistry of Chloroplasts* Vol. II, p. 255. T. W. Goodwin, Ed. Academic Press, New York and London.

The heterogeneity of plastoquinones is thus much greater than was at first thought. Wallwork and Pennock[77q] now postulate two types of plastoquinone C: (a) eight hydroxylated quinones each having a secondary alcohol grouping at a different point in the side-chain (PQ-C-$_2$ type) and (b) eight hydroxylated quinones each having a tertiary hydroxyl in an isoprene unit other than that adjacent to the ring (PQ-C-$_3$ type). When the secondary alcohols are esterified with a fatty acid they form PQ-B series. There is as yet no evidence that more than one hydroxyl enters the side-chain.

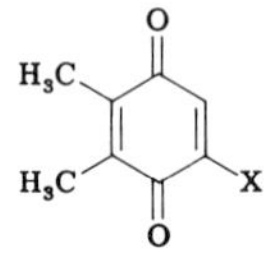

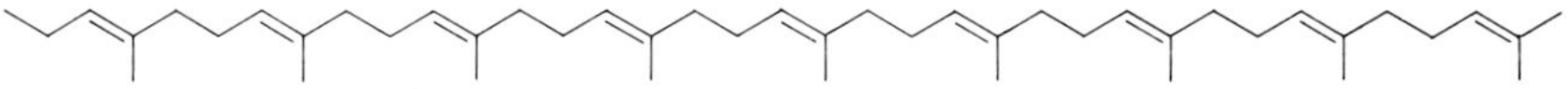

PQ-9

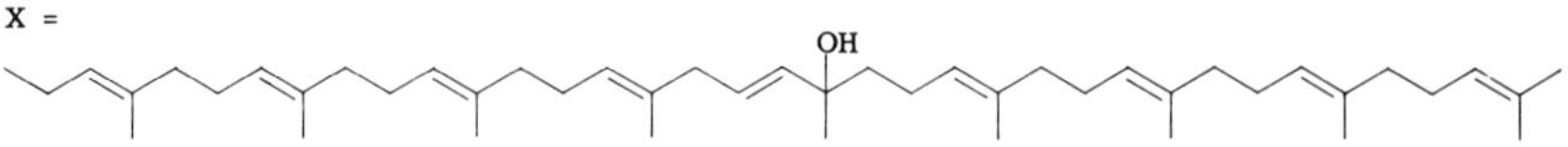

a PQ-C$_3$

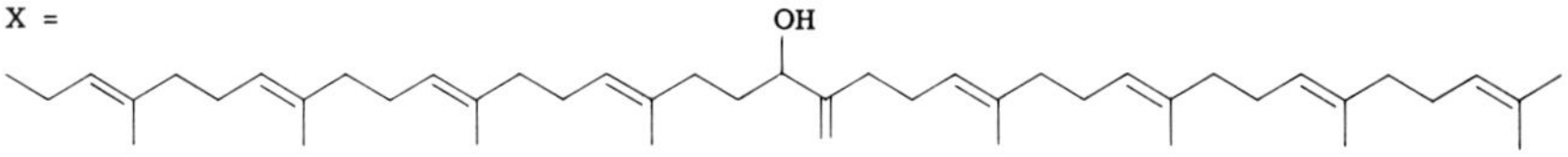

a PQ-C$_2$

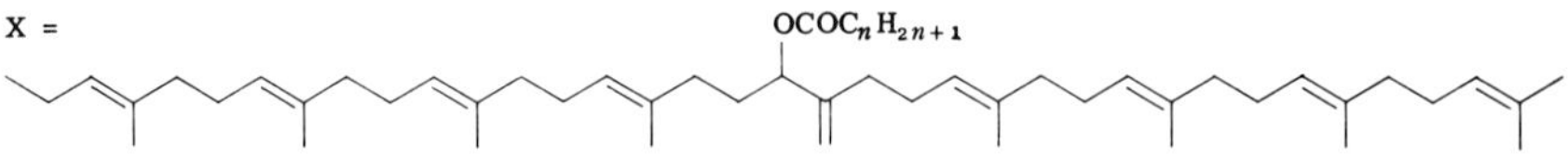

a PQ-B (ester of PQ-C$_2$)

Fuller and Nugent[77r] showed that pteridine is needed for photosynthesis in green bacteria, and that it plays a part in the initial photochemical transfer step. Excited chlorophyll facilitates the transfer of an electron from a reduced cytochrome (type c) to pteridine. Green and Baum[77s], discussing this,

[77q] J. C. Wallwork and J. F. Pennock, *Chem. & Ind.* 1571 (1968).
[77r] R. C. Fuller and N. A. Nugent, *Proc. Nat. Acad. Sci. U.S.* **63**, 1311 (1969).
[77s] D. E. Green and H. Baum, Energy and the Mitochondrion. Academic Press, New York and London, (1970).

suggested that the photosynthetic electron transfer chain could be formulated:

pteridine $\rightarrow$ ferredoxin $\rightarrow$ flavoprotein $\rightarrow$
coenzyme Q $\rightarrow$ cytochrome b, c_1 $\rightarrow$ cytochrome c

Green bacteria present a special case; the evidence is that in the chloroplast the quinone is plastoquinone (PQ-9) and not ubiquinone. They go on to say however that "all the available evidence is compatible with the assumption that the mechanism of photosynthetic phosphorylation is identical with that of oxidative phosphorylation in mitochondria... the photochemical evolution of oxygen will also be accompanied by coupled phosphorylation ... reduced coenzyme Q generated in this process will be oxidized via the electron transfer chain and this oxidation will lead to ATP synthesis".

The photosynthetic bacteria (*Rhodospirillum rubrum, Chlorobium, Chromatium*) do not contain plastoquinone. The organisms do, however, produce ubiquinone freely (Lester and Crane,[78] Fuller *et al.*[79]). It seems that plastoquinones are associated with organisms producing oxygen from water whereas ubiquinones are concerned in processes ending with cytochrome oxidase and molecular oxygen.

An interesting plant tissue is the mature spadix of *Arum maculatum*. It is a site of metabolic activity on a scale sufficient for a time to raise its temperature 15°C above the ambient temperature. This tissue is rich in cytochromes and ubiquinone and very poor in plastoquinone and chlorophyll. Other parts of the plant have the normal preponderance of chloroplast function (Hemming *et al.*[80]).

It is obvious that many species of animals must ingest dietary plastoquinones. Whether the isoprenoid side chain is firmly fixed or can be exchanged has not been determined, and possible nutritional or biosynthetic interlocking with ubiquinones or tocopherol-quinones is a matter on which speculation is legitimate if it stimulates new experiments.

H. Distribution of Ubiquinones

Quinones occur widely in microorganisms.[78, 81, 82] Some contain a number of the vitamin K_2 series, some contain one of the ubiquinones, and others contain a representative of both series. Finally there are organisms that seem to be practically devoid of quinones of either family. The following abbreviations will be used: vitamins K_2 MK-n, ubiquinones Q-n

[78] R. L. Lester and F. L. Crane, *J. Biol. Chem.* **234**, 2169 (1959).
[79] R. C. Fuller, R. M. Smillie, N. Rigolpoulos, and V. Yount, *Arch. Biochem. Biophys.* **95**, 197 (1961).
[80] F. W. Hemming, R. A. Morton, and J. F. Pennock, *Proc. Roy. Soc. Ser. B* 291 (1963).
[81] D. H. L. Bishop, K. P. Pandya, and H. K. King, *Biochem. J.* **83**, 606 (1962).
[82] D. H. L. Bishop and H. K. King, *Biochem. J.* **85**, 550 (1962).

Menaquinones	MK	
$n = 4$	MK-4	(tetraprenol)
$n = 5$	MK-5, etc.	(pentaprenol)

Ubiquinones	(coenzymes Q)	
$n = 10$	Q-10	(decaprenol)
$n = 9$	Q-9, etc.	(nonaprenol)

The following organisms can produce both ubiquinones and menaquinones: *Azotobacter vinelandii* (Q-8, some MK); *Escherichia coli* (Q-8, MK-8 variable with strain); *Proteus vulgaris* (Q-8, MK-8 each approximately 0.65 μmoles/gm dry weight); *Chromatium* strain D (Q-7 2.9 μmoles/gm dry weight, some MK).

The following bacteria produce ubiquinone but not vitamin K_2; *Rhodospirillum rubrum* Q-10 (? Q-9); *Pseudomonas denitrificans* Q-10; *P. fluorescens*, *P. aeruginosa*, *P. fragi*, *P. geniculata*, *P. mildenborgii*, *P. putida*, all Q-9; *Azotobacter chroococcum*, *Chromobacterium prodigiosum*, *Aerobacter* 418, *Pasteurella pseudotuberculosis*, *Serratia marcescens*, *Neisseria catarrhalis*, *Hydrogenomonas* sp., *Thiobacillus thiooxidans*, *Thiobacillus thioparus*, all Q-8.

Two outstandingly good sources are *Rhodospirillum* and *Thiobacillus thiooxidans*, both producing about 4.3 μmoles/gm dry weight (3–4 mg/gm).

Among the organisms which produce vitamin K_2 but not ubiquinone are: *Bacillus subtilis*, *B. megaterium*, *B. mesentericus*, *Staphylococcus albus* (all MK-7); *Sarcina lutea* (MK-8), *Corynebacterium diphtheriae*, *Mycobacterium tuberculosis*, *M. smegmatis* (all MK-9).

A number of anaerobic organisms do not appear to produce Q or MK quinones. Ubiquinones occur in many fungi at 0.2–0.6 μmole/gg dry weight:

Q-10: *Neurospora crassa, Aspergillus fumigatus, Ustilago zea* [dihydro Q-10 in *Gibberrella fujikuroi*]

Q-9: *Mucor corymbifer, Torula* yeast (*Candida utilis*), *Penicillium chrysogenum, P. brevicompactum, Agaricus campestris*

Q-8: *Mycoderma nonosa*

Q-7: *Saccharomyces cerevisiae, Endomyces lindnerii, Endomycopsis fibuliger, Mycoderma nonosa*

Q-6: *Saccharomyces cerevisiae, S. cavalieri, S. fragilis, S. ludwigii, Ashbya gossypii, Zygosaccharomyces barkeri*

A great many plant tissues have been shown to contain quite small amounts of ubiquinones (0.005 to approximately 0.05 μmole/gm dry weight). Plastoquinone is in general much more plentiful, and vitamin K_1 (phylloquinone) is also present albeit often in amounts so small as to be detectable by isolation procedures only with difficulty. In leaves the normal ubiquinone is Q-10, but Q-9 has been claimed as a constituent of corn oil (*Zea mays* seed oil). Crane[83] found both plastoquinone (PQ) and ubiquinone (Q) in plants. Finely comminuted spinach leaves were suspended in sucrose solution and subjected to differential centrifugation; PQ accompanied chlorophyll in the chloroplast fraction while Q went into the mitochondrial fraction. Further work on variegated leaves of *Pandanus* and on the roots and shoots of maize seedlings confirmed the distribution. The mitochondria, which contain most of the Q-10 are concerned in oxidative processes and the chloroplasts mediate photosynthetic phosphorylation. Good preparations of chloroplasts from spinach or lilac leaves did not contain ubiquinone (Dilley and Crane[84]). In the animal kingdom Q-10 is extremely widely distributed. Although only a very incomplete survey has been made a variety of fishes (Pennock et al.[85]), birds and mammals have been studied and Q-10 has been found in liver, kidney, spleen, pancreas, heart, brain, and skeletal muscle. Q-10 has been determined in egg yolk, in embryos, subcellular particles, and in chromatophores. The rat is abnormal in having a mixture of ubiquinones in which Q-9 predominates over Q-10 and Q-8. Among the favored sources of ubiquinones are ox or pig heart (ca. 0.9 μmole/gm wet weight), liver (ca. 0.35 μmole/gm wet weight), mitochondria from heart, liver, or kidney and *R. rubrum* preparations. Investigations on invertebrates indicate that ubiquinones (Q-9 or Q-10) occur in insects (Laidman and Morton[86]), annelids, echinoderms, and protozoans, such as Tetrahymena.

It will be recalled that the original work by Crane and Lester concerned the lipids of mitochondria, and it is not therefore surprising to find high concentrations of ubiquinone in the Keilin–Hartree preparation in purified heart mitochondria and in electron transport particles (see page 379). There is thus a *prima facie* case that the ubiquinones play an essential role in oxidative metabolism in a very wide range of living organisms. Nevertheless there are strong pointers away from an exclusive occurrence in mitochondria. Leonhauser et al.[87] found Q in liver and adrenal microsomes while Rajagopalan et al.[88] found Q associated with liver alcohol oxidase (a soluble flavoprotein).

There are, however, still unsolved problems in connection with the distribution of ubiquinones and ubichromenols. As an example *Candida utilis*

[83] F. L. Crane, *Plant Physiol.* **34**, 128 (1959).
[84] R. A. Dilley and F. L. Crane, *Plant Physiol.* **38**, 452 (1963).
[85] J. F. Pennock, R. A. Morton, D. E. M. Lawson, and D. L. Laidman, *Biochem. J.* **84**, 637 (1962).
[86] D. L. Laidman and R. A. Morton, *Biochem. J.* **84**, 386 (1962).
[87] S. Leonhauser, K. Leybold, K. Krisch, H. Standinger, P. H. Gale, A. C. Page, Jr., and K. Folkers, *Arch. Biochem. Biophys.* **96**, 580 (1962).
[88] K. V. Rajagopalan, I. Fridovich, and P. Handler, *J. Biol. Chem.* **237**, 922 (1962).

grown under controlled conditions produces ubiquinone plentifully but no ubichromenol. The fresh dried yeast contains no ubichromenol but storage (of a material which probably had all its enzymes inactivated by heat) witnesses a slow but steady transformation of ubiquinone to ubichromenol (Diplock et al.,[89] Stevenson et al.,[90] McHale et al. [91]).

Again Packter and Glover[92] worked on *Aspergillus fumigatus* Fres. which produces fumigatin and probably spinulosin and secretes them into the medium. Extraction of the thallus yielded ubiquinone (Q-10, 0.6 μmole per gram dry weight after 7–10 days of growth).

Fumigatin
VI

Spinulosin
VII

Addition to the culture medium of L-leucine suppressed formation of fumigatin and spinulosin but increased the formation of ubiquinone, while ubichromenol also appeared. Thus the control experiment produced about 150 mg fumigatin/liter of medium and 5.85 mg of Q-10 in the thalli; with 0.25–0.50% of leucine in the medium the weight of ether extract fell by about 80% and there was no fumigatin produced, but in the thalli the ubiquinone production rose to about 10 mg and the ubichromenol to 1–2 mg/liter of medium. The ubichromenol was not an artifact as the amount present in the thalli in the control experiment was negligible. *E. coli* is particularly interesting in containing both Q-8 and MK-8. Brodie[93] separated two subcellular fractions, one rich in larger particles contained Q-8 and displayed succinoxidase activity, the other made up of smaller particles contained MK-8 as well. Bishop and King,[82] working on another strain of *E. coli* subjected frozen cells to shock in a Hughes bacterial press and separated the hulls, i.e., insoluble cell residues representing cell walls plus membranes. Both Q and MK were found exclusively in these residues.

Micrococcus lysodeikticus treated with lysozyme undergoes hydrolysis of cell wall material, but the membranes from the ruptured cells can be collected by centrifugation. This organism, which produces a menaquinone and no Q, retained all its quinone in the cell membranes. Both *E. coli* and *M. lysodeik-*

[89] A. T. Diplock, J. Green, E. E. Edwin, and J. Bungar, *Nature (London)* **189**, 740 (1961).
[90] J. Stevenson, P. J. Hayward, F. W. Hemming, and R. A. Morton, *Nature (London)* **196**, 1291 (1962).
[91] D. McHale, J. Green, and A. J. Diplock, *Nature (London)* **196**, 1293 (1962).
[92] N. M. Packter, and J. Glover, *Nature (London)* **187**, 413 (1960).
[93] A. F. Brodie, *Fed. Proc. Fed. Amer. Soc. Exp. Biol.* **20**, 995 (1961).

ticus were subjected to progressive ultrasonic disintegration. The liberation of quinones by this method of differential release indicated that Q-8 and MK-8 were both equally characteristic "hull" components. Bishop *et al.*[81] grew *E. coli* and *Proteus vulgaris*, both under aerobic and anaerobic conditions, and in all cases Q-8 and MK-8 were produced in approximately the same amounts.

If Q and MK are interchangeable catalysts in these microbial systems there is little reason to expect them to be associated with different subcellular fractions. If, however, they both occur because both are necessary a separation might be anticipated. If the distinction between aerobiosis and anaerobiosis sometimes lies in the biosynthesis of cytochrome components the persistence of quinone biosynthesis under anaerobic conditions may not be totally surprising.

I. Biosynthesis of Ubiquinones

In plants and microorganisms there is total biosynthesis of ubiquinones. In animals there is no doubt that the isoprenoid side chain can be synthesized, but present-day ideas run counter to the notion that the aromatic ring system can be formed by higher animals. On this basis ubiquinones would rank not as vitamins, but as essential metabolites. On the other hand, if it is discovered that some specific and relatively scarce constituent containing a benzenoid ring system is a necessary precursor, it might qualify for vitamin status. If, however, a number of aromatic dietary constituents not in short supply will serve equally well, the vitamin issue cannot be very relevant.

It is now agreed that mevalonate can be synthesized from acetate. The 5-pyrophosphate yields Δ^3-isopentenyl pyrophosphate (Lynen *et al.*,[94] Agranoff *et al.*,[95] Popják,[96] Bloch,[97] Witting and Porter[98]). See Fig. 5.

This compound leads to farnesyl pyrophosphate and thence to squalene, lanosterol, and cholesterol, and it seems possible that vitamin A has a role in this biosynthetic sequence.

When the polyisoprenoid side chains present in vitamins K_2 (menaquinones), ubiquinones, and plastoquinones are considered, they are seen to be regularly linked and all-trans. The irregular (tail-to-tail) linkage of two C_{15} units in squalene is a special process without which there would be no sterols. Similarly the irregular linkage of two C_{20} units leads to the C_{40}

[94] F. Lynen, H. Eggerer, U. Henning, and L. Kessel, *Angew. Chem.* **70**, 738 (1958).
[95] B. H. Agranoff, H. Eggerer, U. Henning, and F. Lynen, *J. Amer. Chem. Soc.* **81**, 1254 (1959).
[96] G. Popják, *Annu. Rev. Biochem.* **27**, 533 (1958).
[97] K. Bloch, *Biosyn. Terpenes and Sterols, Ciba Found. Symp.*, 1958 p. 4 (1959).
[98] L. A. Witting and J. W. Porter, *J. Biol. Chem.* **234**, 2841 (1959).

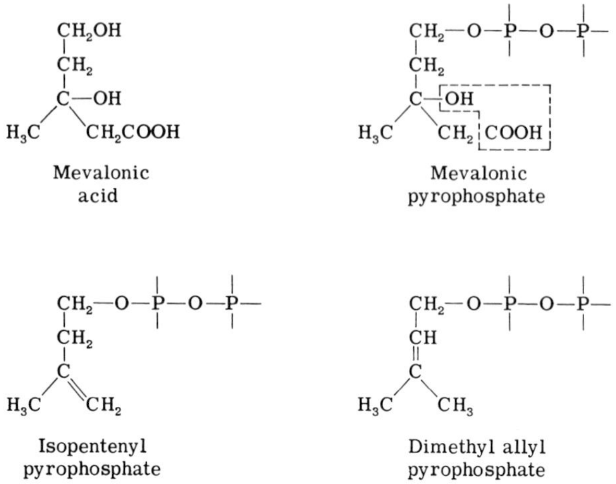

$$
\begin{array}{ccc}
CH_2OH & & CH_2-O-P-O-P- \\
| & & | \\
CH_2 & & CH_2 \\
| & & | \\
C-OH & & C-[OH] \\
H_3C \quad CH_2COOH & & H_3C \quad CH_2 | COOH |
\end{array}
$$

Mevalonic   Mevalonic
acid   pyrophosphate

Isopentenyl   Dimethyl allyl
pyrophosphate   pyrophosphate

FIG. 5. Precursors of polyprenoid side-chain

carotenoids and makes possible symmetrical compounds like lycopene and β-carotene. See Fig. 6.

Gloor, et al.[99–101] and Wiss et al.[102] proved that ^{14}C-labeled mevalonate was used in the biosynthesis of ubiquinones as well as of squalene and cholesterol. In vitamin A-deficient rats, incorporation of ^{14}C into ubiquinone was greater than that shown by control rats given vitamin K. The more developed the deficiency syndrome, the greater was the incorporation of ^{14}C into liver Q. In relation to total incorporation the radioactivity in Q rose from 2% to 20%. Incorporation into squalene rose even faster (2–30%) while the counts for cholesterol fell from 93 to 50% of the total in the unsaponifiable fraction. A dose of vitamin A reversed the effects within a few hours. Gloor and Wiss however failed in experiments with liver tissue in vitro to incorporate radioactive carbon from mevalonate into Q. This is the general experience. It seems that in the rat liver vitamin A deficiency limits the conversion of squalene to cholesterol. An accumulation of substances derived from mevalonate may be diverted to the synthesis of ubiquinone and other isoprenoid compounds. Phillips[103] found, however, that addition of vitamin A alcohol to homogenates of vitamin A-deficient rat liver did not influence incorporation of isotope into sterols. In the vitamin A-deficient guinea pig, however, Phillips found decreased incorporation from mevalonate

[99] U. Gloor and O. Wiss, Experientia 14, 410 (1958).
[100] U. Gloor and O Wiss, Biochem. Biophys. Res. Commun. 1, 182 (1959).
[101] U. Gloor, O. Schindler, and O. Wiss, Helv. Chim. Acta 43, 2089 (1960).
[102] O. Wiss, U. Gloor, and F. Weber, Amer. J. Clin. Nutr. 9, 27 (1961).
[103] W. E. J. Phillips, Can. J. Biochem. Physiol. 39, 855 (1961).

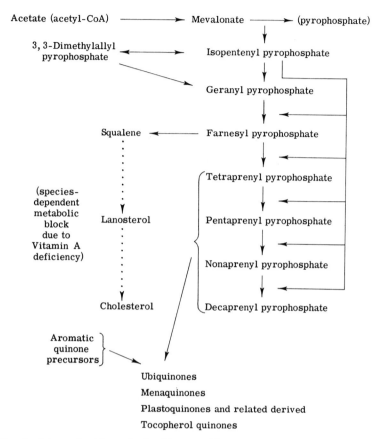

Fig. 6. Scheme for biosynthesis of isoprenoid quinones and related substances.

into Q and squalene and increased incorporation into cholesterol. The Q concentration in liver did not change, so a decreased turnover was probable (see page 358). Sugimura and Rudney[104] prepared Q-6 from yeast grown on a medium containing ^{14}C-labeled formate and found that the isotope was present in the methoxyl groups. When this Q-6 was injected into rats and the animals were later killed, both Q-6 and Q-9 were isolated, but only the former was radioactive. The same authors found that the rat could not introduce ^{14}C from labeled formate into the methoxyl groups of Q-9. Olson and Dialameh[105] established that Q-9 was the main endogenous ubiquinone in the rat and that it incorporated carbon from labeled acetate.

[104] T. Sugimura and H. Rudney, *Biochim. Biophys. Acta* **37**, 560 (1959).
[105] R. E. Olson, and G. H. Dialameh, *Biochem. Biophys. Res. Commun.* **2**, 198 (1960).

The possibility that phenylalanine is the source of the aromatic ring has been explored (Olson et al.[106a]).

Phenylalanine and tyrosine are in fact precursors of the quinone portion of ubiquinone since when ^{14}C-labeled acids are fed to rats the isotope is found only in the ring (Olson et al.[106a]; Bentley et al. [106b]). Dietary protein provides the aromatic amino acids and there is little ubiquinone formation on a protein-free diet (Joshi et al.[106c]). Q-O, i.e. ubiquinone without an isoprenoid side-chain is not used (Gloor and Wiss[106d]) but p-hydroxybenzoic acid or p-hydroxybenzaldehyde are effective precursors in animals (Olson et al.[106e]; Rudney and Parson[106f]) and in plants can be formed via shikimate. In Rhodospirillum rubrum a new intermediate was found to be 2-decaprenyl-phenol (Olson et al.[106g,h]) derived from decaprenyl-p-hydroxybenzoic acid. The methoxyl group enters via S-adenosylmethionine (Lawson and Glover[106i]) and the methyl group via formate. In maize shoots the pathway has been tested using labeled shikimic acid and labeled phenylalanine and tyrosine as well as p-hydroxybenzoic acid (Whistance[106j]). Labeled methionine did not provide all the methyl groups.

Although the precise pathway in animals has not been finally settled the scheme given below is probably substantially correct (cf Friis et al.[106k]).

Gloor and Wiss had found that neither synthetic α-tocopherol nor 2,3-dimethoxy-5-methyl-1,4-benzoquinone (Q-0) were precursors of ubiquinones in the rat. In both cases tritium labeling was used, but the results were negative. This, however, is not absolutely conclusive.

The fact that microorganisms can synthesize ubiquinones and that animals may be coprophagous lends significance to the work of Bieri and McDaniel[107] on germfree rats. The liver content of ubiquinone may fall (expressed as micromoles per gram of tissue) but the total amount present rises to an extent which proves that the synthesis does not depend on microorganisms.

[106a] R. E. Olson, G. H. Dialameh & R. Bentley, Fed. Proc. 19, 220 (1960).
[106b] R. Bentley, V. G. Ramsey, C. M. Springer, G. H. Dialameh, and R. E. Olson, Biochem. Biophys. Res. Commun. 5, 443 (1961).
[106c] V. C. Joshi, J. Jayaraman, and T. Ramasarma, Biochem. J. 85, 25 (1963).
[106d] U. Gloor and O. Wiss, Arch. Biochem. Biophys. 83, 216 (1959).
[106e] R. E. Olson, R. Bentley, A. S. Aiyar, G. H. Dialameh, R. H. Crold, V. G. Ramsey, and C. M. Springer, J. Biol. Chem. 238, PC. 3146 (1963).
[106f] R. Rudney and W. W. Parson, J. Biol. Chem. 238, PC. 3137 (1963).
[106g] R. K. Olsen, G. D. Daves, H. W. Moore, K. Folkers, W. W. Parson, and H. Rudney, J. Amer. Chem. Soc. 88, 5919 (1966a).
[106h] R. K. Olsen, G. D. Daves, H. W. Moore, K. Folkers, and H. Rudney, J. Amer. Chem. Soc. 88, 2346 (1966b).
[106i] D. E. M. Lawson and J. Glover, Biochem. Biophys. Res. Commun. 4, 223 (1961).
[106j] G. R. Whistance, D. R. Threlfall, and T. W. Goodwin, Biochem. J. 105, 145 (1967).
[106k] P. Friis, G. D. Daves and K. Folkers, J. Amer. Chem. Soc. 88, 4754 (1966).
[107] J. G. Bieri and E. G. McDaniel, Biochim. Biophys. Acta 56, 602 (1962).

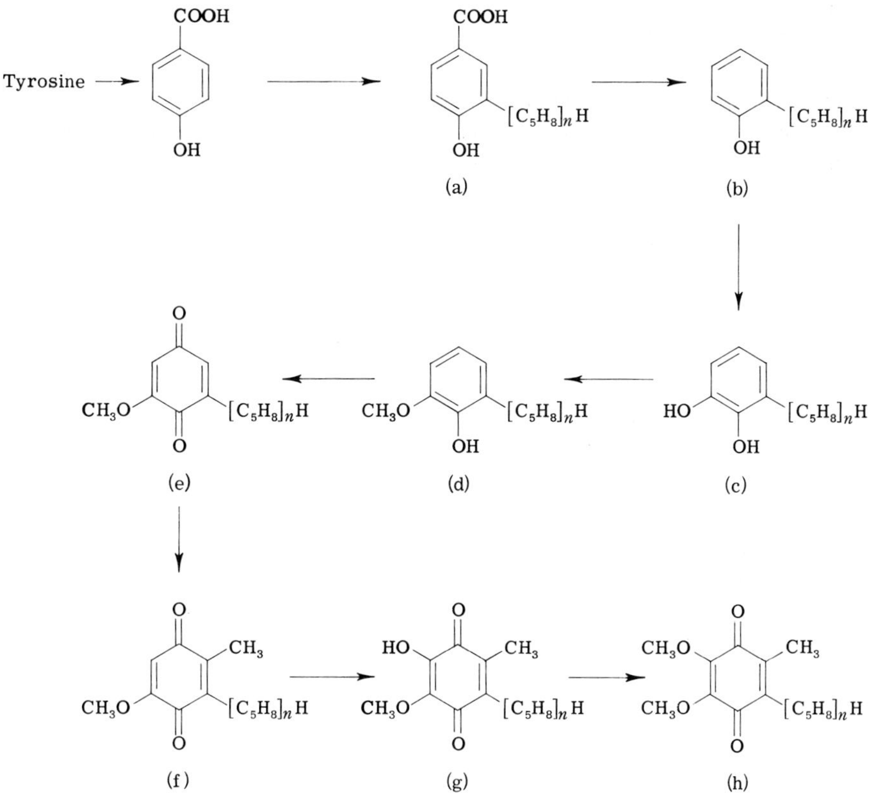

FIG. 7. Probable Biosynthetic pathway for ubiquinones. Intermediates, (a) 4-Carboxy-2-Polyprenylphenol, (b) 2-Polyprenylphenol, (c) 5-Hydroxy-2-Polyprenylphenol, (d) 6-Methoxy-2-Polyprenylphenol, (e) 2-Methoxy-6-Polyprenyl-1,4-Benzoquinone, (f) 2-Methoxy-5-Methyl-6-Polyprenyl-1,4-Benzoquinone, (g) 3-Desmethyl Ubiquinone, (h) Ubiquinone.

Ramasarma et al.[108] have shown that the yolk of hen eggs contains Q-10 which is transferred to the embryo. There is also a de novo synthesis of Q-10 in the developing embryo.

Jayaraman and Ramasarma[109, 110] and Pennock, Neiss, and Mahler[111] studied the developing chick embryo in more detail. Disappearance of Q from the yolk is slow and after 19 days half the original amount (i.e., about 60 μg) remains in the yolk sac. In the embryo, Q content rises only slowly for 15 days, but by the time of hatching the embryo contains more than four times as much as was originally present in the yolk. It is important

[108] T. Ramasarma, J. Jayaraman, and P. S. Sarma, Naturwissenschaften 48, 102 (1961).
[109] J. Jayaraman and T. Ramasarma, J. Sci. Ind. Res., Sect. C, 69 (1961).
[110] J. Jayaraman and T. Ramasarma, Ind. J. Exp. Biol. 1, 1 (1963).
[111] J. F. Pennock, G. Neiss, and H. R. Mahler, Biochem. J. 85, 530 (1962).

that the chick embryo exhibits aerobic metabolism as early as day 4 and that Q can enter the embryo from the yolk. Pennock *et al.* were able to show that tocopherol, vitamin A, cholesterol, and 7-dehydrosterol also entered the embryo in the last 4 or 5 days of incubation.

Jayaraman, Joshi, and Ramasarma[112] administered to rats ^{14}C-labeled Q-10 orally or intracardially and observed that almost all of it reached the liver. The resultant radioactivity in liver fell rapidly, but there was no corresponding rise in the activity of Q in other tissues. Labeled Q was synthesized from mevalonate-2-^{14}C in other tissues including kidney, spleen, heart, and brain (in that order of activity). These authors consider that exogenous ubiquinones may be absorbed and transported to liver and spleen, but not distributed. They favor the view that Q is independently synthesized in each tissue but suggest that in the rat ^{14}C-labeled Q-10 in the diet can reach the fetus via the bloodstream.

Lawson *et al.*[113] had previously observed a net synthesis of Q in rat skin and in everted intestinal sacs if small amounts of ubiquinone were already present. It is conceivable that Q can be degraded to yield an aromatic nucleus to which a newly synthesized isoprenoid moiety can be attached. There is no doubt that microorganisms can effect total synthesis of ubiquinones from acetate as carbon source, and there is special interest in the fact that *Rhodospirillum rubrum*, a photosynthetic organism, suffers inhibition of ubiquinone synthesis and of photosynthetic capacity in the presence of diphenylamine (Rudney[114]). This substance also inhibits carotene biosynthesis in molds, but the mechanism is not fully clear. Bentley *et al.*[115] found in animals that phenylalanine could be used as a source of the aromatic nucleus for mammalian Q, although tyrosine can also be used. It may be doubted, however, whether either is the main natural precursor.

Jayaraman *et al.*[112] found that ^{14}C-labeled Q-10 given to rats orally or intracardially went exclusively to the liver, where it was metabolized but not transferred to other tissues. The radioactivity persisting in the liver for 24–48 hours was due to Q-10, not to ubichromenol. Injected into the bloodstream, ^{14}C-labeled Q-10 was able to pass through the placental barrier to the fetus. It must be remembered, however, that Q-9 is the characteristic ubiquinone of rats (see page 375).

Packter and Glover[116] found that *Aspergillus fumigatus*, which secretes fumigatin into the medium, produces Q in the thalli. If the medium is enriched with L-leucine, L-isoleucine, and L-valine, total lipid and ubiquinone

[112] J. Jayaraman, V. C. Joshi, and T. Ramasarma, *Biochem. J.* **88**, 369 (1963).
[113] D. E. M. Lawson, D. R. Threlfall, J. Glover, and R. A. Morton, *Biochem. J.* **79**, 201 (1961).
[114] H. Rudney, *J. Biol. Chem.* **236**, PC39 (1961).
[115] R. Bentley, V. G. Ramsey, C. M. Springer, G. H. Dialameh, and R. E. Olson, *Biochem. Biophys. Res. Commun.* **5**, 443 (1961).
[116] N. H. Packter and J. Glover, *Biochim. Biophys. Acta* **58**, 531 (1962).

synthesis both increase while the excretion of fumigatin decreases. The corresponding keto acids are also effective presumably because they yield acetyl-CoA and acetoacetyl-CoA leading to mevalonic acid. Only L-phenylalanine among the aromatic amino acids stimulated Q production. Methionine also had a stimulatory effect, but fumigatin is apparently not a Q precursor.

Threlfall and Glover[117] prepared ubiquinone U-^{14}C by growing *Rhodospirillum rubrum* on a medium containing acetate-carboxy-^{14}C and isolated pure crystalline Q-10 (15–20 μC/mmole). The labeled Q-10 contained about one-fifth of the isotope in the quinone ring and four-fifths in the $C_{50}H_{81}$ side chain. The Q-10 was given by mouth to rats which were killed at 3.5 hours and 24 hours later. Analysis of tissues showed that the radioactive Q-10 was found only in intestine and liver. A small portion (6%) of the total liver Q-activity was Q-9, the 94% being still in Q-10. After 24 hours the proportion had risen only to 11%. Fragments from ubiquinone-10-U-^{14}C were used to form newly synthesized Q-9, but as no radioactivity was detected in sterols, the polyisoprenoid chain was probably not used. There was no radioactivity in the Q of heart or kidney. Exogenous Q cannot be very important for the rat, and probably no more than one-third is absorbed.

J. Ubiquinones and Electron Transport

Prolific research activity by many groups and particularly that led by D. E. Green has emphasized the revolutionary effects of Crane and Lester's discovery of coenzyme Q or ubiquinone as a constituent of mitochondria. When Q occurs in bacteria it is present in the cell membrane, which, like the mitochondria of plant and animal cells, contains the enzymes concerned in electron transfer whereby substrates are oxidized. It is important that Q is not water soluble but is a normal lipid congener physically associated with other lipids in the mitochondrion.

Certain enzyme-rich preparations, such as the well-known Keilin–Hartree heart muscle preparation, contain damaged or fragmented mitochondria. Intact mitochondria in the living cell can catalyze oxidative phosphorylation but "uncoupling" occurs in many types of derived particles so that although oxidation occurs, there is no concomitant production of ATP. This fact has not been wholly disadvantageous to research because the elucidation of the electron transfer itself has been difficult enough.

Electron microscopy of mitochondria together with shrewd interpretations of enzymatic processes has led to the view that mitochondria contain membranes comprising or structurally loaded with the enzymes and coenzymes needed for the smooth working of the Krebs citric acid cycle producing ATP from ADP and inorganic phosphate. The energy is provided by the oxidation of substrates through the cytochrome system. The dehydrogenases

[117] D. Threlfall and J. Glover, *Biochem. J.* **82** 14P (1962).

of the tricarboxylic acid cycle are all linked to NAD with the exception of NADP–isocitric dehydrogenase and succinate dehydrogenase which conducts electrons via flavoprotein to the cytochrome system.

The electron transport system can be abbreviated:

$$\begin{array}{c}
NADH \rightarrow flavoprotein_1 \searrow \\
\hspace{3cm} Q \rightarrow Cyt\ c_1 \rightarrow \quad Cyt\ c \rightarrow Cyt\ a \rightarrow O_2 \\
Succinate \rightarrow flavoprotein_2 \nearrow
\end{array}$$

the position of Q and cytochrome b being for our present purposes open to discussion.

The placing of cofactors in order owes much to the use of inhibitors. Thus the reduction of ubiquinones by succinate or NADH is not prevented by cyanide or by antimycin A. Both inhibitors prevent the oxidation of added ubiquinol by oxygen (via cytochrome oxidase and cytochromes c and c_1). On the other hand, amytal and malonate prevent reduction of the quinone by NADH or succinate but do not interfere with oxidation of ubiquinol (Fig. 8) (Redfearn,[11] see also Pumphrey et al.,[119] Pumphrey and Redfearn,[120, 121] Redfearn and Pumphrey[122, 123] Joel, et al.[125]).

If mitochondria are subjected to violent mechanical treatment (e.g., strong ultrasonic vibrations) smaller particles are formed and can be separated by differential centrifugation. Many of the Krebs cycle enzymes catalyzing the oxidation of pyruvate, malate, isocitrate, and α-ketoglutarate pass into the aqueous medium, but the derived particles can still oxidize NADH and succinate. By observing certain special precautions particles can be obtained which retain the capacity to produce ATP. Electron transport particles predominate in the activity of the Keilin–Hartree preparation. They consist very largely of membranes from mitochondria and contain about 40% (calculated on the dry weight) of lipid and of this over 90% is phospholipid and 5–6% cholesterol (Bouman and Slater[124]).

Analysis of mitochondrial components[127] (Table IV) shows that Q is present in relatively large amount. No wholly satisfactory hypothesis for this apparent excess is yet available. Crane[4] thinks that clear evidence for the role of Q in NADH oxidase activity is still lacking, and Redfearn[11] and Chance[126] have advanced the idea that Q has a site of action that is off the main pathway. Extraction studies, however, strongly indicate that

[119] A. M. Pumphrey, E. R. Redfearn, and R. A. Morton, Chem. Ind. (London) p. 978 (1958).
[120] A. M. Pumphrey and E. R. Redfearn, Biochem. J. 72, 2P (1959).
[121] A. M. Pumphrey and E. R. Redfearn, Biochem. J. 76, 61 (1960).
[122] E. R. Redfearn and A. M. Pumphrey, Biochem. J. 73, 3P (1959).
[123] E. R. Redfearn and A. M. Pumphrey, Biochem. J. 76, 64 (1960).
[124] J. Bouman and E. C. Slater, Biochim. Biophys. Acta 26, 624 (1957).
[125] C. D. Joel, M. L. Kornovsky, E. G. Ball, and O. Cooper, J. Biol. Chem. 233, 1565 (1958).
[126] B. Chance, in Quinones Electron Transp., Ciba Found. Symp. 1960 p. 327 (1961).
[127] D. E. Green and D. C. Wharton, Biochem. Z. 338 335, (1963).

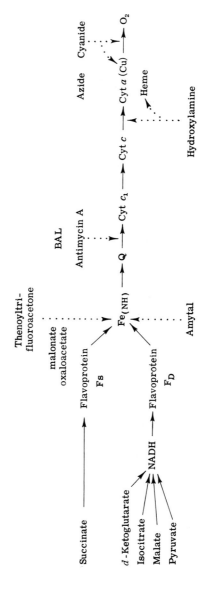

FIG. 8. Electron transport system showing sequences and inhibitors.

TABLE IV

COMPONENTS OF THE ELECTRON TRANSPORT CHAIN IN
MITOCHONDRIA

Component	Amount (mmoles/mg of protein)
Succinic flavoprotein	0.20
Acid-extractable flavin	0.46
Flavin mononucleotide[a]	0.15
Ubiquinone (Q)	3.4–4.0
Cytochrome b	0.68
Cytochrome c_1	0.21
Cytochrome c	0.45
Cytochrome a	1.31
Copper	1.47
Nonheme iron	3.3

[a] May reflect the content of NADH flavoprotein.

Q functions on the main path in succinate oxidation. If nonpolar solvents like isooctane are used to remove Q from electron transport particles at 0°C, with prolonged vigorous shaking about half the ubiquinone is removed and there is a marked fall in succinoxidase activity in the residue. Addition of lipid cytochrome c alone restores about half the activity, addition of Q alone about 25%, while addition of both at once restores the full activity. Aqueous cytochrome c also restores activity completely; presumably the residual Q can be "mobilized." Extraction with isooctane at room temperature not only removes Q almost completely, it also eliminates phospholipid and neutral lipids, all of which appear to be necessary for full activity. Residual solvent acts as an inhibitor and it is essential to remove all the isooctane under reduced pressure before trying to restore activity.

Extraction with acetone is in some ways a better procedure, it removes Q plus neutral lipid and both are needed for fully restored activity. Acetone extraction also induces a requirement for cytochrome c. Redfearn has suggested that the solvent probably leads to considerable displacements of mitochondrial components; in intact mitochondria this leads to loss of phosphorylative activity, but on restoration of Q-10 and cytochrome c, electron transport may even be stimulated considerably above that shown originally. Q-10 certainly seems not to be strongly adsorbed to a specific protein, as is often the case for water-soluble coenzymes and it may indeed function as a "free component of a lipid matrix," which includes phospholipid and neutral lipid (Brierley et al.,[128] Fleischer et al.,[129] Wharton

[128] G. P. Brierley, A. J. Marola, and S. Fleisher, *Biochim. Biophys. Acta* **64**, 205, 218 (1962).
[129] S. Fleischer, G. P. Brierley, H. Klouwen, and D. B. Slautterback, *J. Biol. Chem.* **237**, 3264 (1962).

and Griffiths[130]). Both forms of lipid appear to be essential. There can be no doubt at all that Q functions in electron transport in the succinoxidase system, but many other aspects of the wider problem remain to be clarified.

D. E. Green[5] has discussed the interpretation of electron micrographs of mitochondria (Fernández-Morán,[131] Palade,[132] Sjöstrand,[133] Ziegler et al.[134]). He accepts a three-dimensional scheme due to Anderson-Cedergren[135] and has welded together the enzymology and the physical evidence.

The mitochondrion is shaped like a sausage. The external membrane has three layers, and there are internal membranes called septa or cristae. The space between the cristae may be a large or a small proportion of the volume, depending on the source from which the mitochondria are obtained. Heart mitochondria are more tightly packed with cristae than liver mitochondria. The major components are (a) lipid, about 30% (b) structural protein, about 50%. The cofactors are thought to be arranged in order on the membranes; those concerned in electron transport being less readily detached than those concerned in fat metabolism and Krebs cycle processes. Green and Fleischer[136] regard the electron transfer chain as made up of four segments or complexes:

I—transfer of electrons from NADH to Q (NADH-Q reductase)

II—transfer of electrons from succinate to Q (succinate-Q reductase)

III—transfer of electrons from QH_2 to cytochrome c (QH_2-cytochrome c reductase)

IV—transfer of electrons from reduced cytochrome c to molecular oxygen (cytochrome c oxidase)

In each case the minimum molecular weight of the complex is between 2 and 5×10^5 (Green and Wharton[127]). Each is made up of a number of protein molecules and cofactors ranged in order. Although separable, the four complexes can be reassembled on mixing in the natural proportions. The fact that neutral lipids, phosphatides, cholesterol, d-tocopherol, and carotenoids all occur in addition to Q reminds us, if reminder were necessary, how much remains to be discovered concerning the modes of action of minor unsaponifiable constituents.

The catalysts are part of lipoprotein phospholipid micelles, and Q is thought to be in true solution. It is nevertheless regarded as undergoing oxidation-reduction–reduction by complex I or II and oxidation by complex

[130] D. C. Wharton and D. E. Griffiths, *Arch. Biochem. Biophys.* **96**, 103 (1962).

[131] H. Fernández-Morán, *Rev. Mod. Phys.* **31**, 319 (1959).

[132] G. E. Palade, *in* "Enzymes: Units of Biological Structure and Function" (O. H. Gaebler, ed.), p. 185. Academic Press, New York, 1956.

[133] F. S. Sjöstrand, *Radiat. Res. Suppl.* **2**, 349 (1960).

[134] D. M. Ziegler, A. W. Linnane, D. E. Green, C. M. Dass, and H. Ris, *Biochim. Biophys. Acta* **28**, 524 (1958).

[135] A. Anderson-Cedergren, *J. Ultrastruct. Res. Suppl.* **1**, (1959).

[136] D. E. Green and S. Fleischer, *in* "Horizons in Biochemistry" (M. Kasha and B. Pullman, eds.), p. 381. Academic Press, New York, 1962) 381.

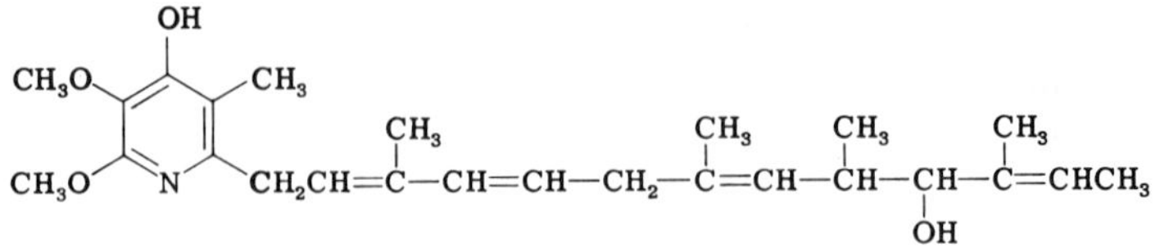

FIG. 9. Structures of piericidins A and B.

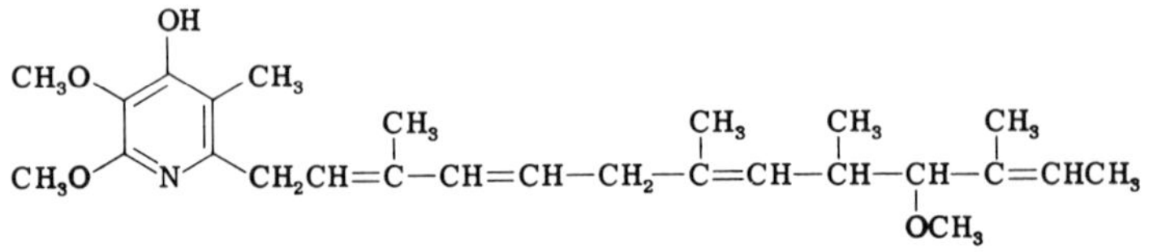

III. Cytochrome c acts as a similar link and a picture emerges of Q and cytochrome c as mobile substances found in the lipid layer between complexes. Hatefi et al.[137] studied the NADH-Q reductase by electron paramagnetic resonance spectroscopy and obtained results which might mean that one-electron transfer $(Q + e^\bullet \rightleftharpoons Q^\bullet)$ was occurring.

NADH–cytochrome c reductase preparations can be split into two: (a) NADH–Q-reductase and (b) QH_2-cytochrome c reductase. The former complex is virtually free from cytochromes but contains an iron flavoprotein (rich in FMN). It catalyzes the oxidation by NADH by Q-1, but Q-10 does not work, possibly because it cannot reach the site of action. The second derived particle obtained by treating the parent enzyme preparation with cholate and salt is richer in cytochromes and works best with QH_2-2 (C_{10} side chain) although QH_2-10 (the quinol from Q-10) is also oxidized. On mixing (a) and (b) the original activity is restored. The endogenous Q-10 is almost certainly functioning in this general way.

The piericidins isolated from Streptomyces mobaraensis (Takahashi et al.[137a]) possess structures with certain resemblances to that of ubiquinone. The similarity prompted investigation of piericidin as a competitive inhibitor of ubiquinone. Jeng et al.[137b] observed that electron transport in ox heart muscle mitochondria displayed clear-cut inhibition by piericidin A at a site near the nicotine adenine dinucleotide (NADH) dehydrogenase and that very low concentrations were effective. Much higher concentrations of piericidin A inhibited the succinic dehydrogenase and the effect tended to be reversed by ubiquinone. The formation of ubiquinol from ubiquinone by the two

[137] Y. Hatefi, A. G. Hasvik, and D. E. Griffiths, J. Biol. Chem. 237, 1676 (1962).
[137a] N. Takahashi, A. Auzuika, S. Tamura, J. Amer. Chem. Soc. 87, 2066 (1965).
[137b] M. Jeng, C. Hall, F. L. Crane, N. Takahashi, S. Tamura and K. Folkers, Biochemistry 7, 1311 (1968).

dehydrogenase systems was inhibited by piericidin A and the block occurred between ubiquinone and the flavoprotein. The inhibitory effect is largely retained when as in piericidin B the side-chain hydroxyl is methylated. On the other hand acetylation of the ring hydroxyl destroys inhibitory activity as does replacement of the side-chain by a carboxyl group. It is said that with NADH as substrate, reduction in the presence of piericidin A results in reduction of cytochrome c, whereas when succinate is the substrate cytochrome b is reduced.

The recent work on the role of ubiquinone has been reviewed (Morton[77a]). A special point of view presenting an "integrated interpretation of the mitochondrion as an operational and transducing unit and as a prototype of membrane sytems" is seen in a new book by Green & Baum[77s].

Succinic-Q-reductase (Ziegler and Doeg[138]) contains when purified one flavin molecule of cytochrome b and 8 atoms of nonheme iron and 18–20% of lipid (on dry weight). Q-2 has a little water solubility and works better than Q-10 which is soluble only in lipid. The role of cytochrome b is very uncertain, but oxidation–reduction of nonheme iron occurs between succinate and Q (see Singer and Kearney,[139] Basford et al.[140]).

The problem (Hatefi[141]) of the mechanism of oxidative phosphorylation is very much in the air and is perhaps near to solution for menaquinone in bacterial systems. In oxidative phosphorylation the initial reaction is the esterification of inorganic phosphate. In the menaquinones the naphthoquinol seems to go to naphthochroman, which can form a high-energy phosphate (Brodie,[93] Russell and Brodie[142]). In animals there is no direct proof that ubiquinone acts as an intermediate. NAD is very likely to be involved (Griffiths and Chaplain[143]) and a role for Q would be very attractive. Theoretical schemes have been advanced (Harrison,[144] Clark et al.[145]). Very promising work has been done concerning the involvement of quinone derivatives in photosynthetic phosphorylation.

If the work on the modes of action of plastoquinone and phylloquinone in the plant and the work on the role of menaquinones (MK-6 to MK-9) in bacteria are elucidated, there will probably be new advances in understanding the roles of ubiquinone. Much very elegant work has been done but more remains to be discovered.

[138] D. M. Ziegler and K. A. Doeg, Arch. Biochem. Biophys. 97, 41 (1962).

[139] T. P. Singer and E. P. Kearney, Biochim. Biophys. Acta 15, 151 (1954).

[140] R. E. Basford, H. D. Tisdale, and D. E. Green, Biochim. Biophys. Acta 24, 290 (1957).

[141] Y. Hatefi, Biochim. Biophys. Acta 31, 502 (1959).

[142] P. J. Russell and A. F. Brodie, Quinones Electron Transp., Ciba Found. Symp., 1960 p. 205 (1961).

[143] D. E. Griffiths and R. A. Chaplain, Biochem. Biophys. Res. Commun. 8, 501 (1962).

[144] K. Harrison, Nature (London) 181, 1131 (1958).

[145] V. M. Clark, D. W. Hutchinson, and A. R. Todd, J. Chem. Soc. London p. 715, 722 (1961).

K. Ubiquinone–Vitamin Interactions

The rise in liver ubiquinone content which occurs in the vitamin A-deficient rat has already been referred to (page 359). Thompson and Pitt[146, 147] reared three groups of rats on a basal diet free from vitamin A. One group was given vitamin A alcohol (210 μg/rat/week) and another received the sodium salt of vitamin A acid. When the third (unsupplemented diet) group began to lose weight, all the animals were killed and the livers were analyzed (Table V). The acid was as effective as the alcohol in maintaining normal low levels of Q and UC. (Table V).

TABLE V

EFFECT ON RAT LIVER UBIQUINONE (Q) AND UBICHROMENOL
(UC), VITAMIN A AND VITAMIN A ACID COMPARED WITH
UNSUPPLEMENTED VITAMIN A-FREE DIET

Group	Liver Q (μg/gm)	Liver UC (μg/gm)
Vitamin A-deficient rats	385	52.6
Vitamin A acid supplemented	129	23.3
Vitamin A alcohol supplemented	148	11.2

Vitamin A deficiency impairs adrenal function, but Phillips and Morton[148] found that the effects could not be simply related to raised liver levels of ubiquinone or ubichromenol.

Phillips[149] determined ubiquinone concentrations in rat liver on diets varying rather widely in respect to both vitamin A and vitamin E. It seems very unlikely that the effect of vitamin A status on ubiquinone rat liver levels is an indirect result of changes in tocopherol status. The work of J. Green's group (Edwin et al.,[150] Green et al.,[151–154] suggesting a fairly direct relationship between ubiquinone status and vitamin E intake, present an interesting but rather confused picture. Diplock et al.[155] found that the synthetic antioxidants santoquin and diphenyl-p-phenylenediamine (DPPD)

[146] J. N. Thompson and G. A. J. Pitt, Nature (London) 188, 672 (1960).
[147] J. N. Thompson and G. A. J. Pitt, Biochem. J. 79, 33P (1961).
[148] W. E. J. Phillips, and R. A. Morton, Biochem. J. 73, 430 (1959).
[149] W. E. J. Phillips, Can. J. Biochem. Physiol. 40, 1347 (1962).
[150] E. E. Edwin, A. T. Diplock, J. Bunyan, and J. Green, Biochem. J. 79, 91 (1961).
[151] J. Green, E. E. Edwin, A. T. Diplock, and J. Bunyan, Biochem. Biophys. Res. Commun. 2, 388 (1960).
[152] J. Green, E. E. Edwin, A. T. Diplock, and J. Bunyan, Biochim. Biophys. Acta 49, 417 (1961).
[153] J. Green, A. T. Diplock, J. Bunyan, and E. E. Edwin, Nature (London) 190, 318 (1961).
[154] J. Green, A. T. Diplock, J. Bunyan, and E. E. Edwin, Biochem. J. 79, 108 (1961).
[155] A. T. Diplock, E. E. Edwin, J. Bunyan, and J. Green, Brit. J. Nutr. 15, 425 (1961).

which are known to act in many respects as vitamin E substitutes, failed to influence the storage and apparently the biosynthesis of ubiquinone. Morton and Phillips[156] had already concluded that vitamin E status did not determine liver Q levels in rats, but scrutiny of the series of papers by Green's group indicates possibly a small fall in Q levels in various tissues as a result of vitamin E shortage. It must be remembered that ubiquinone is alkali labile and can be destroyed during alkali digestion. Pyrogallol[31] acts as a protective agent, and tocopherol might, as well, do so to some extent.

Dietary selenium (as sodium selenite) given to vitamin E-deficient rats raised liver Q levels from 101 to 233 μg/gm (Edwin et al.,[150] Diplock et al.[155]) but did not influence Q concentration in heart. In other experiments there were rises in various tissues when either selenium or tocopherol was administered. When selenium was added, tocopherol had no additional effect.

At present no full explanation of the possible E-Q relationship can be advanced.

The problematic vitamin E activity of ubichromenol is equally difficult. Some workers claim that the antioxidant property of α-tocopherol can account for most of its prophylactic or curative effects. Ubichromanol and ubichromenol are also effective as antioxidants, and it is not unexpected that vitamin E-replacing properties have been claimed. If ubiquinone can be converted to ubichromenol it would in this sense be a precursor substance. Sondergaard et al.[157] using chicks, found that oral Q-6 or Q-10 added to an E-deficient diet failed to prevent muscular dystrophy or encephalomalacia. If, however, phytylubichromenol (IX) (i.e., reduced UC-4) was used at 0.02% in the diet considerable prophylaxis occurred.

Dinning et al.[158] found that muscular dystrophy (and anemia) in the vitamin E-deprived rhesus monkey responded to intravenous injections of rather large doses of phytylubichromenol.

Johnson et al.[159] found that UC-10 injected into E-deficient female rats at 5–7 days after conception prevented the classic gestation resorption, but subsequent experience (Smith et al.[160]) failed to confirm this result. This variability may be due to some more subtle interconnection.

Ubiquinones have no vitamin K activity when given to chicks showing lengthened blood clotting time.

[156] R. A. Morton and W. E. J. Phillips, Biochem. J. 73, 427 (1959).

[157] E. Sondergaard, M. L. Scott, and H. Dam, J. Nutr. 78, 15 (1962).

[158] J. S. Dinning, C. D. Fitch, C. H. Shunk, and K. Folkers, J. Amer. Chem. Soc. 84, 2007 (1962).

[159] B. C. Johnson, Q. E. Crider, C. H. Shunk, B. O. Linn, E. L. Wong, and K. Folkers, Biochem. Biophys. Res. Commun. 5, 301 (1961).

[160] J. L. Smith, H. N. Bhagavan, R. B. Hill, S. Batani, P. B. Rama Rao, Q. E. Crider, B. C. Johnson, C. H. Shunk, A. F. Wagner, and K. Folkers, Arch. Biochem. Biophys. 101, 388 (1963).

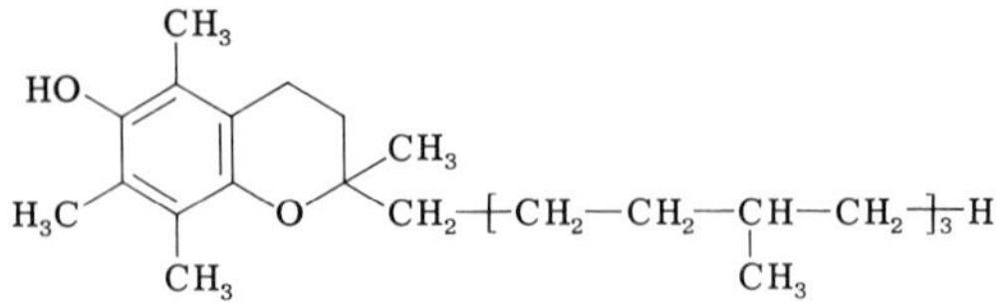

α-tocopherol
VIII

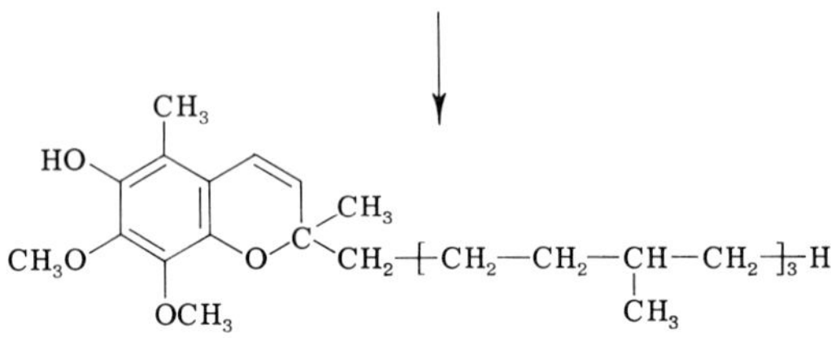

phytylubichromenol
(hexahydro UC-4)
IX

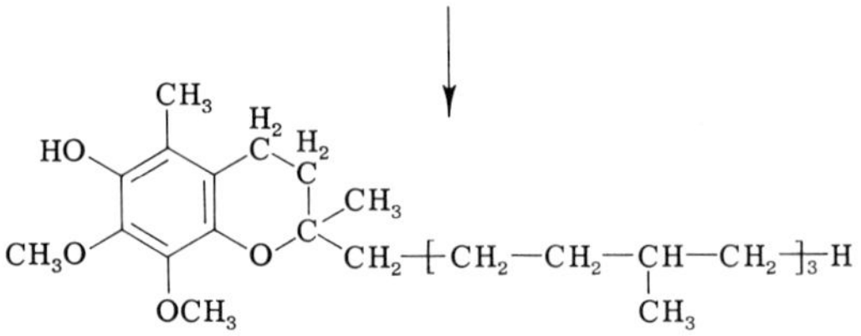

phytylubichromanol
X

FIG. 10. Structures of α-tocopherol, VIII phytylubichromenol IX, and phytylubichromanol.

Edwin *et al.*[161] found that thyroxine given orally raised Q and UC levels in livers of rats on normal and vitamin E-deficient diets with smaller rises in heart tissue. The effect has been confirmed (Beyer *et al.*,[162] Aiyar and Sreenivasan,[163] Pederson *et al.*[164]). The thyroxine-induced increase in metabolism may have caused the rise in Q levels, but against this thyroidectomy did not quickly influence tissue concentrations. Brain tissue levels of ubiquinone resisted change even when thyroxine was given.

In the guinea pig vitamin C deficiency did not appreciably influence liver

[161] E. E. Edwin, J. Green, A. T. Diplock, and J. Bunyan, *Nature* (*London*) **186**, 725 (1960).
[162] R. E. Beyer, W. M. Noble, and T. J. Hirschfeld, *Biochim. Biophys. Acta* **57**, 376 (1962).
[163] A. S. Aiyar and A. Sreenivasan, *Biochem. J.* **82**, 182 (1962).
[164] S. Pederson, J. R. Tata, and L. Ernster, *Biochim. Biophys. Acta* **69**, 407 (1963).

ubiquinone levels (Cunningham[165]) nor kidney levels (Thompson[166]) but Pofahl et al.[167] found that scorbutic guinea pigs had 70% of the Q levels found in heart, liver and kidney of control animals. Unless analytical procedures are accurate and specific, a decrease of 30% may be questionably significant.

Aiyar et al.[168] found that rats on a pantothenic acid-deficient diet showed a decrease in succinoxidase activity compared with control animals and a fall of 20% in ubiquinone. Aiyar and Sreenivassan[169, 170] observed reduced incorporation of ^{14}C from both acetate and mevalonate into Q in pantothenic acid deficiency. Addition of vanadium reduced Q synthesis by impairing coenzyme A-dependent processes. Wiss et al.[171] found that pantothenic acid-deficiency raised liver Q levels by 80% and a dietary supplement of calcium pantothenate restored nearly normal levels. There is here a contradiction which calls for further experimentation.

Droop and Pennock[172] have extended the work of Droop and Doyle[173] on Oxyrrhis marina Dujardin. This micro-organism is unusual in being phago-trophic and the only dinoflagellate with that mode of nutrition to have been cultivated under axenic conditions. It has now been shown to have an absolute requirement for a quinone and a need (possibly not absolute) for a steroid. The quinone must be a substituted benzoquinone possessing a polyprenyl side-chain of not less than 30 carbon atoms. The requirement is met equally well by a plastoquinone or an ubiquinone. Neither the chromanols nor the chromenols from either family are effective. Outside the Q-n and PQ-n families, modifications of substituents or of the side-chain cause disappearance of biological activity. A number of biosynthetic intermediates showed no activity and this indicated that the essentiality could arise from a severe block in biosynthesis at the stage of *para* substitution in the benzene ring, this being the first step leading to quinone formation. It is however more probable that Oxyrrhis cannot synthesise any part of the quinone molecule. For this organism plastoquinones and ubiquinones (with hexaprenyl or greater side chains) comply with the criteria for vitamins. It will be important to extend the investigation to other phagotrophic micro-organisms. In the meantime

[165] N. F. Cunningham, Ph.D. Thesis, Univ. of Liverpool, 1956.
[166] J. N. Thompson, Ph.D. Thesis, Univ. of Liverpool, 1962.
[167] T. R. Pofahl, W. E. Black, and E. A. Doisy, Jr., *Fed. Proc. Fed. Amer. Soc. Exp. Biol.* **22**, 489 (1963).
[168] A. S. Aiyar, G. A. Sulebele, D. V. Rege, and A. Sreenivasan, *Nature (London)* **184** 1867 (1959).
[169] A. S. Aiyar and A. Sreenivasan, *Nature (London)* **190**, 344 (1961).
[170] A. S. Aiyar and A. Sreenivasan, *Proc. Soc. Exp. Biol. Med.* **107**, 911, 914 (1961).
[171] O. Wiss, U. Gloor, and F. Weber, *Amer. J. Clin. Nutr.* **9**, 27 (1961).
[172] M. R. Droop and J. F. Pennock, *J. Mar. Biol. Assoc. U.K.* **51**, 455 (1971).
[173] M. R. Droop and J. Doyle, *Nature (London)* **212**, 1474 (1966).

the equal efficacy of plastoquinones and ubiquinones remains surprising.

Although ubiquinone can normally be synthesised in the animal organism and is indeed well-distributed in relatively large amounts, it may have therapeutic value under unusual circumstances. Majaj and Folkers[174] studied the macrocytic anaemia which often occurs in children suffering from nutritional deprivation as in kwashiorkor or marasmus, and obtained a definite beneficial effect with ubiquinone (Q-10). Even better results were obtained with hexahydro Q-4 (a ubiquinone with a hydrogenated tetraprenyl side-chain of the phytyl type) or the 6-chromanol obtained from it by cyclization. In protein-calorie malnutrition ubiquinone biosynthesis decreases, reflecting a shortage of aromatic amino acids.

Protein-starved monkeys also display anaemia and respond to Q-10 and hexahydro Q-4. Farley et al.[175] treated rabbits made dystrophic by nutritional lack and found Q-4 and hexahydro Q-4 to be very effective while Q-3, Q-6, Q-7 and Q-10 were not, presumably because of difficulties of absorption or assimilation. Scholler et al.[176] kept female rats on a vitamin E-deficient diet until they resorbed the foetal young; hexahydro Q-4 was then given in large doses and in due course normal litters were delivered. It seems very likely that the compound acted as a substitute for α-tocopherol. It also had a palliative but not curative effect on mice suffering from genetically-conditioned dystrophy.

An essential metabolite like ubiquinone made in the body from p-hydroxybenzoic acid by a biosynthetic pathway with 8 or more steps opens up a possibility of inborn errors of metabolism. The work of Folkers and his associates suggests that the main ubiquinone of animals (Q-10) may not itself be assimilable from food and this may also apply to the Q-7 and Q-8 produced by many micro-organisms. Either the genetic defect could be lethal or large doses of ubiquinone would be needed to compensate for poor absorption. On the other hand there could be pathological conditions such that the supply of Q-10 at, e.g. mitochondrial sites of action would be inadequate despite a normal intake of protein. Folkers' search for a therapeutic role might then succeed.

Skelton et al.[179] record the fact that ubiquinone (in the main Q-8) occurs in various types of malarial parasites (see Rietz et al.[177]; Skelton et al.[178]). The development of specific ubiquinone inhibitors of either the function or bio-

[174] A. S. Majaj and K. Folkers, Int. Z. Vitaminforsch. 38, 182 (1968).

[175] T. M. Farley, G. D. Daves, J. Scholler, and K. Folkers, Int. Z. Vitaminforsch. 38, 355 (1968).

[176] J. Scholler, T. M. Farley, and K. Folkers, Int. Z. Vitaminforsch. 38, 363, 369 (1968).

[177] P. J. Rietz, F. S. Skelton, and K. Folkers, Intern. J. Vit. Res. 37, 405 (1967).

[178] F. S. Skelton, K. D. Lunan, K. Folkers, J. V. Schnell, W. A. Siddiqui, and Q. M. Geiman, Biochemistry, 8, 1284 (1969).

[179] F. S. Skelton, C. M. Bowman, T. H. Porter, K. Folkers, and R. S. Paradini, Biochem. Biophys. Res. Commun. 43, 102 (1971).

synthesis of ubiquinone in *Plasmodium* affords a new approach to the chemotherapy of malaria. This thought would apply to any infection in which the causative organism utilises ubiquinone but clearly there will also be a possibility of damaging the host. The novelty of the work lies in the confluence of experience on antimalarial drugs and on electron transport studies. Certain naphthoquinones are active against *Plasmodium vivax* and two illustrative drugs 3-ω-cyclohexyloctyl-2-hydroxy-1,4-naphthoquinone and 3-ω-cyclo-hexyloctyl-6-hydroxy-5,8-quinolinequinone (Fig. 11).

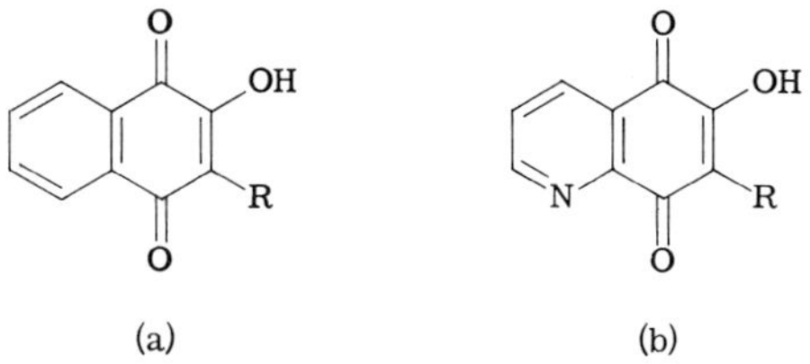

(a)   (b)

FIG. 11. Antiplasmodials that inhibit ultraquinone. R = ω-cyclohexyloctyl.

are effective ubiquinone inhibitors. Q-6 reverses the inhibition (0.76 parts of (a) being reversed by 3.0 of Q-6).

The impression gained from reviewing the literature on vitamin–ubiquinone interactions is that the original rat liver vitamin A effect is the best authenticated. Even this is not reproduced in the other species studied. It is to be expected that when biosynthetic pathways and catalytic mechanisms have elements in common verifiable interactions will be possible. Some such will be little more than examples of feedback processes lacking fundamental interest; others may be more significant, and only experiment can help us to distinguish the one type from the other.

L. Conclusion

The importance of Q as an almost ubiquitous catalyst for respiration makes certain its status as an essential metabolite. It may have other significant roles. For higher animals a simple precursor substance with an aromatic ring may have vitamin-like status, but dietary ubiquinone seems, on the whole, to be unimportant unless it provides the aromatic nucleus for endogenous synthesis.

V. Lyxoflavin

VERNON H. CHELDELIN

In 1947, Pellares et al.[1] isolated a pentose from human heart, which they identified as lyxose. Later,[2] these workers reported the isolation of lyxoflavin from the same source, although this was challenged by subsequent work.[3] This close relative of riboflavin (and of the corresponding moiety of vitamin B_{12}) was viewed by Emerson and Folkers[4,5] as a possible new member of the B complex, although they recognized that the experimental evidence for the reported existence of lyxoflavin was not as rigorous as might be desired. They therefore devised a ration based on soybean meal as the major constituent, to which had been added 0.5% desiccated thyroid, and observed the rate of growth of rats on this diet. The growth-depressing effect of large doses of thyroid was overcome by extracts of liver and by fish meal, or alternatively by synthetic lyxoflavin. The lyxoflavin effect was shown not to be due to conversion to riboflavin. The ability of lyxoflavin to completely replace the effect of liver or fish meal gave support for its classification as a vitamin for the rat, and its general importance was further suggested by the findings that it also stimulated swine and chick growth.[6,7] It seemed possible from this work that lyxoflavin might be related to or identical with the "stress factor" in liver observed by Ershoff,[8] which was capable of counteracting the growth-depressing effect of thyroid in rats fed a casein diet.

However, Ershoff has since shown[9] that lyxoflavin was ineffective as an antithyrotoxic factor when this diet was used. Since the diets employed in the two laboratories differed considerably in composition (soybean-dextrose versus casein-sucrose), the possibility has been raised (Cooperman et al.[10]) that lyxoflavin may act as a stimulant in liver factor synthesis by the intestinal flora when the soybean–dextrose diet is employed. Finally,

[1] E. S. Pellares, F. V. Orozco, and J. R. Carvallo, Arch. Inst. Cardiol. Mex. 17, 575 (1947).

[2] E. S. Pellares and H. M. Garza, Arch. Biochem. 22, 63, (1949).

[3] T. S. Gardner, E. Wenis, and J. Lee, Arch. Biochem. Biophys. 34, 98 (1951).

[4] G. A. Emerson and K. Folkers, J. Amer. Chem. Soc. 73, 2398 (1951).

[5] G. A. Emerson and K. Folkers, J. Amer. Chem. Soc. 73, 5383 (1951).

[6] R. C. Wahlstrom and B. C. Johnson, J. Anim. Sci. 10, 1065 (1951).

[7] H. W. Bruins, M. L. Sunde, W. W. Cravens, and E. E. Snell, Proc. Soc. Exp. Biol. Med. 78, 535 (1951).

[8] B. H. Ershoff, Proc. Soc. Exp. Biol. Med. 73, 459 (1950).

[9] B. H. Ershoff, Proc. Soc. Exp. Biol. Med. 79, 469 (1952).

[10] J. M. Cooperman, W. L. Marusich, J. Scheiner, L. Drekter, E. De Ritter, and S. H. Rubin, Proc. Soc. Exp. Biol. Med. 81, 57 (1952).

the latter authors were able to demonstrate a slight replacement of ribo-flavin in rat diets and *L. casei* growth media, and they concluded that the existing evidence did not warrant the classification of lyxoflavin as a new vitamin. Microbiological evidence is inconclusive, for lyxoflavin is stimulatory both in its own right[5] and as an adjuvant for riboflavin[10, 11] or is inhibitory.[11] Thus, the question whether lyxoflavin may be a member of the B complex remains unsettled. Of greater importance, however, is the question whether lyxoflavin can function in metabolism in *any* unique fashion. Further experiments are in order to definitely establish the natural occurrence of lyxoflavin, its possible presence in flavoproteins, and its effect upon growth and metabolism.

VI. Coenzyme III

VERNON H. CHELDELIN

Proteus vulgaris was shown by Singer and Kearney[12, 13] to require a previously undescribed cofactor for oxidation of cysteine-sulfinic acid to cysteic acid. Isolation of the factor from bakers' yeast produced a nucleotide which was thought by the authors to be identical with nicotinamideribose 5-pyrophosphate. Because of the similarity to the other nicotinamide coenzymes, the name coenzyme III was tentatively assigned. Coenzyme III was found in high concentration in yeast and in liver and kidney mitochondria.[14] In each of these systems, sulfinic dehydrogenase activity was demonstrated, and a fairly general requirement for this cofactor in cysteine metabolism appears possible.

[11] M. S. Shorb, *Proc. Soc. Exp. Biol. Med.* **79**, 611 (1952).
[12] E. B. Kearney and T. P. Singer, *Biochim. Biophys. Acta* **8**, 698 (1952).
[13] T. P. Singer and E. B. Kearney, *Biochim. Biophys. Acta* **8**, 700 (1952).
[14] T. P. Singer and E. B. Kearney, *Fed. Proc. Fed. Amer. Soc. Exp. Biol.* **12**, 269 (1953).

VII. Factors Required in Unheated Growth Media

VERNON H. CHELDELIN

In 1933 Orla-Jensen[15] observed that many lactic acid bacteria would not grow properly upon carbohydrates that had been sterilized in distilled water and added aseptically to a sterile yeast–casein medium. Heating of glucose with the medium resulted in normal growth, as did heating of small amounts of methylglyoxal, furfural, or pentoses with the yeast–casein mixture. These observations have been repeated and extended in later years,[16-19] so that it appears that at least two types of transformation occur during heating: one is the expulsion of oxygen and/or the formation of reducing substances,[17, 20-23] whereas the other involves interaction of carbohydrate with phosphate and/or the nitrogenous components of the medium. The compounds so produced were presumed to act as the stimulatory agents.

Studies in this laboratory[24] have revealed that products formed by heating glucose with inorganic phosphate and amino acids will greatly stimulate the growth of *Lactobacillus gayoni* 8289 (strain 45; cf. ref. 25 for description of organism) during a 12-hour incubation period. In a series of experiments, glycine was found to be consistently superior to other amino acids as a precursor of active material, whereas alanine produced substances that were strongly inhibitory. *N*-Glucosylglycine was then synthesized as the ethyl estel[26] and found to be as active as equal weights of yeast extract in a filter-sterilized medium, at levels up to 1 mg/10 ml of culture. Higher levels of yeast produced greater stimulation, whereas amounts of glucosylglycine above 5 mg became inhibitory. However, when glucosylglycine was heated separately and added aseptically to the basal medium, additional growth stimulation was provided which approached, although it did not equal, the

[15] A. D. Orla-Jensen, *J. Soc. Chem. Ind. London, Trans. Commun.* **52**, 374 (1933).
[16] K. L. Smiley, C. F. Niven, Jr., and J. M. Sherman, *J. Bacteriol.* **45**, 50 (1943).
[17] J. C. Rabinowitz and E. E. Snell, *J. Biol. Chem.* **169**, 631 (1947).
[18] E. E. Snell, E. Kitay, and E. Hoff-Jørgenson, *Arch. Biochem.* **18**, 495 (1948).
[19] C. E. Hoffman, E. L. R. Stokstad, B. L. Hutchings, A. C. Dornbush, and T. H. Jukes, *J. Biol. Chem.* **181**, 635 (1949).
[20] W. E. Shive, J. M. Ravel, and R. E. Eakin, *J. Amer. Chem. Soc.* **70**, 2614 (1948).
[21] V. Kocher, *Int. Z. Vitaminforsch.* **20**, 369 (1949).
[22] R. D. Greene, A. J. Brook, and R. B. McCormack, *J. Biol. Chem.* **178**, 999 (1949).
[23] L. K. Koditschek, D. Hendlin, and H. B. Woodruff, *J. Biol. Chem.* **179**, 1093 (1949).
[24] D. Rogers, T. E. King, and V. H. Cheldelin, *Proc. Soc. Exp. Biol. Med.* **82**, 140 (1953).
[25] V. H. Cheldelin and A. P. Nygaard, *J. Bacteriol.* **61**, 489 (1951).
[26] M. L. Wolfrom, R. D. Schuetz, and L. F. Cavalieri, *J. Amer. Chem. Soc.* **71**, 3518 (1949).

growth on yeast extract. Of approximately 20 species of lactic acid bacteria tested, 3 others were stimulated by unheated glucosylglycine: *Streptococcus zymogenes* 10100, *Lactobacillus acidophilus* (O.S.C. strain), and *Leuconostoc mesenteroides* P63. *L. gayoni* F20 responded only after the compound had been heated. Other organisms, such as *L. gayoni* 8289, strain 49.[25] *L. casei*, and *Saccharomyces cerevisiae* LM did not respond at all to glucosylglycine under these conditions, although they were stimulated by yeast extract.[27]

The relative superiority of glycine over other amino acids in producing a biologically active material with glucose, and the strong inhibition produced with alanine, appear to confer a measure of specificity upon the heat activation reaction and to raise the possibility that one or at most a few factors may be involved. Presumably these represent conversion products from glucosylglycine, since the latter compound possesses relatively low activity. The role of phosphate is not yet clear. Further research should disclose the nature of these factors, as well as their relation to the products of the Maillard " browning reaction."[28] The latter appears to be a more general reaction between carbohydrates and amino acids, resulting in a net *loss* of nutritional value of the amino acids toward higher animals.[29]

VIII. Guinea Pig Antistiffness Factor

VERNON H. CHELDELIN

A syndrome in guinea pigs has been described, whereby these animals developed characteristic joint stiffness on diets high in milk (Wulzen and Bahrs[30, 31]). When adequate greens were given, the animals maintained normal health. Intermediate degrees of stiffness at the wrist joints were detected in the animals on the milk diets, and an assay method was developed which attempted to place the stiffening (produced at least in part by the deposition of calcium phosphate in the joints) on a quantitative basis. Constituents of the diet were sought which might protect the animals against the onset of stiffness, and it was believed (van Wagtendonk and Wulzen[32]) that such a protective factor could be obtained in pure form, either from raw cream or from sugarcane juice. On the basis of this approach, the

[27] D. Rogers, T. E. King, and V. H. Cheldelin, unpublished observations.
[28] L. C. Maillard, *C. R. Acad. Sci.* **154**, 66 (1912).
[29] A. R. Patton, *Nutr. Rev.* **8**, 193 (1950).
[30] A. M. Bahrs and R. Wulzen, *Proc. Soc. Exp. Biol. Med.* **33**, 528 (1936).
[31] R. Wulzen and A. M. Bahrs, *Amer. J. Physiol.* **133**, 500P (1941).
[32] W. J. van Wagtendonk and R. Wulzen, *Arch. Biochem.* **1**, 373 (1943).

existence of a nutritional principle, the "antistiffness factor," was claimed, and methods were given for its isolation from cream[130] and from cane juice.[33]

The existence of the syndrome has been confirmed by other experimenters[34,35] and has been described in detail in a review of the subject by the principal authors.[36] The condition is accompanied by extensive calcification in the joints, body wall and cavity, and upper skeleton; profound changes have been observed in the skull and teeth. Hearing is impaired in the affected animals. Numerous changes have also been recorded for calcium, phosphorus, and protein levels in the blood.[36]

Beyond this, it is difficult, if not impossible, to make further positive statements regarding the "antistiffness factor," owing in the main to the fact that the assay method was developed and used without adequate controls. Later, a critical examination of the assay by Christensen et al.[37] and an examination[38] of the data of Oleson et al.[34] revealed that the assay method could not distinguish between concentrations of active materials that differed by 5 or even 10-fold. These discoveries necessarily vitiated the claims based on the wrist stiffness assay, whether for isolation of an active principle or for correlation of stiffness with peculiarities in metabolism. The fact that pure compounds have been isolated from cane juice[33,39,40] thus simply reflects the success of chemical separations of materials (chiefly steroid) in the ether-extractable fractions of sugarcane, with no connection between the chemical separations and any physiological index.

In spite of the unsatisfactory character of many of the studies, it appears possible that a variety of steroids may possess some antistiffness potency. Thus, positive results have been claimed for stigmasterol and various esters of ergostanol and ergostenol (although this is denied by the work of Smith et al.[41]). All these tests suffer from the inadequacies of the assay described above. It seems, however, that the assay is capable of detecting advanced stages of the condition; addition of these sterols to the "deficient" guinea pig diet over a period of several months might serve qualitatively to establish whether or not the compounds in question can serve as antistiffness agents.

[33] W. J. van Wagtendonk and R. Wulzen, J. Biol. Chem. 164, 597 (1946).
[34] J. J. Oleson, E. C. Van Donk, S. Bernstein, L. Dorfman, and Y. SubbaRow, J. Biol. Chem. 171, 1 (1947).
[35] H. G. Petering, L. Stubberfield, and R. A. Delor, Arch. Biochem. 18, 487 (1948).
[36] W. J. van Wagtendonk and R. Wulzen, Vitam. Horm. (New York) 8, 70 (1950).
[37] B. E. Christensen, M. B. Naff, V. H. Cheldelin, and R. Wulzen, J. Biol. Chem. 175, 275 (1948).
[38] In F. J. Stare, Nutr. Rev. 6, 107 (1948).
[39] D. H. Simonsen and W. J. van Wagtendonk, J. Biol. Chem. 170, 239 (1947).
[40] H. Rosenkrantz, A. T. Milhorat, M. Farber, and A. E. Milman, Proc. Soc. Exp. Biol. Med. 76, 408 (1951).
[41] S. E. Smith, M. A. Williams, A. C. Bauer, and L. A. Maynard, J. Nutr. 38, 87 (1949).

Finally, attention should be given to the question whether this is a nutritional or (perhaps more likely) a pharmacological principle, i.e., a condition brought about by high levels and imbalances of calcium and phosphorus in the diet. When cotton rats were maintained on diets high in calcium and phosphorus but low in several other minerals, especially magnesium, a similar "calcinosis" was observed, which led to extremely high (23–36%) ash contents in the heart tissue.[42] The condition, as in guinea pigs, was alleviated by feeding oatmeal but was aggravated by increasing the phosphate content of the diet. Vitamin E was ineffective. Microscopic appearance of the tissue lesions[43] was reported to be similar to those in guinea pigs.[44]

The gross similarities in guinea pig stiffness and human arthritis confer a continuing interest upon this unusual disease. It is hoped that studies will be resumed which will aim at the development of sound analytical procedures and the establishment of the nutritional and metabolic relationships that may exist.

[42] M. A. Constant and P. H. Phillips, *J. Nutr.* **47**, 317 (1952).
[43] M. A. Constant, P. H. Phillips, and D. M. Angevine, *J. Nutr.* **47**, 327 (1952).
[44] P. N. Harris and R. Wulzen, *Amer. J. Pathol.* **26**, 595 (1950).

IX. Unidentified Growth Factors

VERNON H. CHELDELIN AND ANNETTE BAICH

Sources of unidentified growth factors and organisms utilizing them are listed in Table VI.

TABLE VI
UNIDENTIFIED GROWTH FACTORS

	Source	References
Animals		
Chicks	Fish solubles, or fish meal of various kinds	1–18

[1] H. Menge, C. A. Denton, J. R. Sizemore, R. J. Lillie, and H. R. Bird, *Poultry Sci.* **32**, 863 (1953).

[2] J. Biely, B. E. March, and H. L. A. Tarr, *Fish. Res. Bd. Can., Progr. Rep. Pac. Coast Sta.* **92**, 10 (1952) [*Chem. Abstr.* **47**, 2849c].

[3] B. E. March, J. Biely, and H. L. A. Tarr, *Fish. Res. Bd. Can., Progr. Rep. Pac. Coast Sta.* **99**, 12 (1954) [*Chem. Abstr.* **48**, 14026d].

[4] G. F. Combs, G. H. Arscott, and H. L. Jones, *Poultry Sci.* **33**, 71 (1954).

[5] H. R. Bird and N. L. Karrick, *Commer. Fish. Rev.* **19**, No. 5A, 1 (1957) [*Chem. Abstr.* **51**, 18384g].

[6] B. L. Reid, R. L. Svacha, A. A. Kurnick, F. M. Salama, and J. R. Couch, *Proc. Distill. Feed Conf.* **11**, p. 68 (1956) [*Chem. Abstr.* **51**, 4520b].

[7] G. H. Arscott, *Poultry Sci.* **35**, 338 (1956).

[8] H. Morimoto, S. Ariyoshi, and H. Hoshii, *Poultry Sci.* **34**, 1392 (1955).

[9] H. M. Edwards, Jr., D. Chin, L. C. Norris, and G. F. Heuser, *J. Nutr.* **57**, 329 (1955).

[10] H. D. Tamimie, *Diss. Abstr.* **15**, 1959 (1955) [*Chem. Abstr.* **50**, 2778e].

[11] T. Tomiyama, Y. Yone, K. Hirowatori, S. T. Koyanagi, S. Uchida, and H. Tokuda, *Nippon Suisan Gakkaishi* **21**, 1806 (1955) [*Chem. Abstr.* **50**, 14064h].

[12] B. Laksesvela, *Meld. Sildolje-og Sildemelind. Forskningsinst.* **5**, 94 (1954) [*Chem. Abstr.* **49**, 5604c].

[13] A. A. Camp, H. T. Cartrite, J. H. Quisenberry, and J. R. Couch, *Poultry Sci.* **34**, 559 (1955).

[14] C. F. Peterson, A. C. Wiese, and A. R. Pappenhagen, *Poultry Sci.* **34**, 673 (1955).

[15] M. L. Scott and T. R. Zeigler, *Proc. Distill. Feed Conf.* **15**, 20 (1960) [*Chem. Abstr.* **54**, 20004e].

[16] W. W. Westerfield, and A. C. Hermans, *J. Nutr.* **76**, (4), 503 (1962).

[17] M. E. Mason, J. Sacks, and E. L. Stephenson, *J. Nutr.* **75**, 253 (1961).

[18] J. E. Savage, B. L. O'Dell, H. L. Kempster, and A. G. Hogan, *Poultry Sci.* **29**, 779 (1950).

TABLE VI—*continued*

Source	References
Dehydrated alfalfa	3, 19–24
Dried yeast and distillers dried solubles	15, 18, 19, 25–28
Dried whey	6, 13, 14, 27, 29–32
Mycelia of penicillin and streptomycin	33–35
Corn or vegetable oil	15, 36, 37
Animal fats	7
Petroleum wastes	38
Frog liver	39
Liver	9, 14, 22, 30–32, 40–43
Pigeon crop milk	44
Peanut meal	45
Casein	46

[19] M. G. Vavich, A. Wertz, and A. R. Kemmerer, *Poultry Sci.* 32, 433 (1953).
[20] H. M. Scott, H. Fisher, and J. M. Snyder, *Poultry Sci.* 32, 555 (1953).
[21] H. Fisher, H. M. Scott, and R. G. Hansen, *J. Nutr.* 52, 13 (1954).
[22] R. A. Rasmussen, P. W. Luthy, J. M. Van Lanen, and C. W. Boruff, *Poultry Sci.* 36, 46 (1957).
[23] B. E. March, J. Biely, and S. P. Touchburn, *Poultry Sci.* 34, 968 (1955).
[24] L. S. Jensen, *Diss. Abstr.* 15, 5 (1955).
[25] H. M. Scott, W. D. Morrison, and P. Griminger, *Poultry Sci.* 34, 1446 (1955).
[26] R. Dam, A. B. Morrison, and L. C. Norris, *J. Nutr.* 69, 277 (1959).
[27] J. A. Wakelam and W. P. Jaffe, *Nature (London)* 184, Suppl. No. 5, p. 272 (1959).
[28] W. W. Cravens, H. W. Bruins, M. L. Sunde, and E. E. Snell, *Fed. Proc. Fed. Amer. Soc. Exp. Biol.* 10, 379 (1951).
[29] H. L. Jones, G. F. Combs, and G. L. Romoser, *Poultry Sci.* 33, 930 (1954).
[30] J. R. Couch, O. Olcese, B. G. Sanders, and J. V. Halick, *J. Nutr.* 42, 473 (1950).
[31] H. Menge, G. F. Combs, P.-T. Hsu, and M. S. Shorb, *Poultry Sci.* 31, 237 (1952).
[32] H. Menge, G. F. Combs, and M. S. Shorb, *Poultry Sci.* 28, 775 (1949).
[33] H. M. Edwards, R. Dam, L. C. Norris, and G. F. Heuser, *Poultry Sci.* 32, 551 (1953) [Res. Notes].
[34] A. E. Schaefer, R. D. Greene, H. L. Sassaman, and S. Wind, *Poultry Sci.* 34, 851 (1955).
[35] J. C. Fritz, F. D. Wharton, Jr., R. M. Henley, and R. B. Schoene, *Poultry Sci.* 35, 552 (1956).
[36] D. C. Carver and E. L. Johnson, *Poultry Sci.* 32, 701 (1953).
[37] E. L. Johnson, *Feedstuffs* 24, No. 49, p. 48 (1952). [*Chem. Abstr.* 49, 7671a].
[38] M. A. Akhundov, *Dokl. Akad. Nauk Azerb. SSR* 12, 575 (1956) [*Chem. Abstr.* 51, 2965c].
[39] E. I. Shaw and J. R. Shaver, *Experientia* 9, 140 (1953).
[40] H. Menge and G. F. Combs, *Poultry Sci.* 31, 994 (1952).
[41] T. Tomiyama and Y. Yone, *Proc. Jap. Acad.* 29, 178 (1953) [*Chem. Abstr.* 48, 5961e].
[42] R. L. Atkinson and F. H. Kratzer, *Poultry Sci.* 39, 631 (1960).
[43] M. L. Scott, *Poultry Sci.* 31, 175 (1952).
[44] D. M. Pace, P. A. Landolt, and F. E. Mussehl, *Growth* 16, 279 (1953).
[45] R. J. Young, M. B. Gillis, and L. C. Norris, *J. Nutr.* 50, 291 (1953).
[46] F. A. Csonka, R. J. Lillie, and W. Martin, *J. Nutr.* 52, 285 (1954).

TABLE VI—*continued*

Source	References
Egg yolks	7, 47–49
Assorted	50–55
Chick embryo extract (for fibroblast	56, 57
cultures)	80
Swine intestinal tract	58
Venerupis philippinarum	59
Feather meal	60, 61
Corn fermentation solubles	62, 63
Corn steepwater	64, 65
Undialyzed serum	66
Soy proteins	16
Cow milk	67
Mouse glands	68
Bran	28
Grass juice	69, 70

[47] H. Menge, R. J. Lillie, and C. A. Denton, *J. Nutr.* **63**, 499 (1957).

[48] G. H. Arscott, P. H. Weswig, and J. R. Schubert, *Poultry Sci.* **36**, 513 (1957).

[49] J. H. Hopper, H. M. Scott, and B. C. Johnson, *Poultry Sci.* **35**, 195 (1956).

[50] L. S. Dietrich, W. J. Monson, and C. A. Elvehjem, *Arch. Biochem. Biophys.* **38**, 91 (1952).

[51] J. E. Savage, *Diss. Abstr.* **16**, 615 (1956).

[52] L. R. Berg, *Diss. Abstr.* **15**, 2370 (1955).

[53] J. M. Snyder, *Diss. Abstr.* **15**, 660 (1955).

[54] G. B. Sweet, *Diss. Abstr.* **16**, 200 (1956).

[55] R. Dam, *Diss. Abstr.* **20**, 1 (1959).

[56] R. J. Kutsky and M. Harris, *J. Cell. Comp. Physiol.* **43**, 193 (1954).

[57] J. O. Ely, *J. Franklin Inst.* **258**, 521 (1954).

[58] H. J. Anderson, J. J. Vacanti, and M. C. Lind, *Poultry Sci.* **36**, 675 (1957) [Res. Notes].

[59] T. Tomiyama, Y. Yone, Y. Harada, Y. Kato, M. Okamoto, M. Yamaoka, Y. Murakami, S. Tanaka, and S. Matsuo, *Nippon Suisan Gakkaishi* **21**, 937 (1955) [*Chem. Abstr.* **50**, 13322b].

[60] H. Menge, R. J. Lille, J. R. Sizemore, and C. A. Denton, *Poultry Sci.* **35**, 244 (1956).

[61] R. J. Lille, J. R. Sizemore, and C. A. Denton, *Poultry Sci.* **35**, 316 (1956).

[62] J. M. Russo and V. Heiman, *Poultry Sci.* **38**, 26 (1959).

[63] J. M. Russo and V. Heiman, *Poultry Sci.* **38**, 1324 (1959).

[64] A. A. Camp, H. T. Cartrite, B. L. Reid, J. H. Quisenberry, and J. R. Couch, *Poultry Sci.* **36**, 1354 (1957).

[65] C. R. Creger, M. A. Zavala, R. H. Mitchell, R. E. Davies, and J. R. Couch, *Poultry Sci.* **41**, 1928 (1962).

[66] M. Harris, *Proc. Soc. Exp. Biol. Med.* **102**, 468 (1959).

[67] P. N. Davis, L. C. Norris, and F. H. Kratzer, *J. Nutr.* **76**, 223 (1962).

[68] S. Cohen, *Natl. Cancer Inst. Monogr.* **13**, 13 (1964) [*Chem. Abstr.* **61**, 8595d].

[69] G. O. Kohler and W. R. Graham, *Poultry Sci.* **30**, 484 (1951).

[70] G. O. Kohler and W. R. Graham, *Poultry Sci.* **31**, 284 (1952).

TABLE VI—*continued*

	Source	References
Turkey poults	Fish meal, alfalfa	71–76
	Distillers dried solubles	71, 77
	Streptomycin fermentation products	78
	Yeast	43, 72, 79
	Liver	74–76
	Soybean oil	
Rats and mice	Liver	81–86
	Dried whey	81
	Fish solubles	81, 87
	Butter	88
	Distillers dried solubles	89
	Colostrum	90
	Meat meal	91, 92
	Laminaria japonica	93
	Pollen	94
	"Growth hormones"	95

[71] P. E. Waibel, *Poultry Sci.* **37**, 1144 (1958).
[72] R. L. Atkinson, T. M. Ferguson, and J. R. Couch, *Poultry Sci.* **34**, 855 (1955).
[73] R. L. Atkinson, B. L. Reid, J. H. Quisenberry, and J. R. Couch, *J. Nutr.* **51**, 53 (1953).
[74] R. L. Atkinson and J. R. Couch, *J. Nutr.* **44**, 249 (1951).
[75] J. McGinnis, L. R. Berg, J. R. Stern, M. E. Starr, R. A. Wilcox, and J. S. Carver, *Poultry Sci.* **31**, 100 (1952).
[76] G. M. Briggs, *Trans. Amer. Ass. Cereal Chem.* **10**, 31 (1952).
[77] H. Menge and G. F. Combs, *Poultry Sci.* **31**, 994 (1952).
[78] G. A. Donovan, W. K. Warden, and W. M. Reynolds, *Poultry Sci.* **37**, 422 (1958).
[79] O. F. Hixson and L. Rosner, *Poultry Sci.* **33**, 66 (1954).
[80] C. Gilvarg and E. Katchalski, *J. Biol. Chem.* **240**, 3093 (1965).
[81] W. C. Sherman, H. L. Schilt, and H. C. Schaefer, *J. Nutr.* **55**, 255 (1955).
[82] E. Tria and O. Barnabei, *Ric. Sci.* **24**, 1703 (1954) [*Chem. Abstr.* **49**, 7015e].
[83] L. P. Dryden, G. H. Riedel, and A. M. Hartman, *J. Nutr.* **70**, 547 (1960).
[84] D. K. Bosshardt and J. W. Huff, *J. Nutr.* **50**, 117 (1953).
[85] B. H. Ershoff, *Proc. Soc. Exp. Biol. Med.* **73**, 459 (1950).
[86] E. Tria, *Ric. Sci.* **30**, 268 (1960) [*Chem. Abstr.* **54**, 25115b].
[87] R. H. King and S. M. Hauge, *Arch. Biochem.* **24**, 350 (1949).
[88] C. Nieman, E. H. Groot, and B. C. P. Jansen, *Proc. Kon. Ned. Akad. Wetensch., Ser. C* **55**, 587 (1952) [*Chem. Abstr.* **47**, 7048d].
[89] K. Torigoe, *Bitamin* **9**, 463 (1955) [*Chem. Abstr.* **50**, 10896d].
[90] P. Gyorgy, M. I. Mello, F. E. Torres, and L. A. Barness, *Proc. Soc. Exp. Biol. Med.* **84**, 464 (1953).
[91] C. J. Ackerman, *J. Nutr.* **63**, 131 (1957).
[92] C. J. Ackerman, *J. Nutr.* **67**, 589 (1959).
[93] M. Tsuji, T. Yamanishi, and F. Yoshimatsu, *Natur. Sci. Rep. Ochanomizu Univ.* **4**, 100 (1953) [*Chem. Abstr.* **51**, 2142i].
[94] R. Chauvin, *C. R. Acad. Sci.* **244**, 120 (1957).
[95] A. Lacassagne and H. Tuchmann-Duplessis, *Acta Radiol. Interamer.* (*Buenos Aires*) **3**, 3 (1953) [*Chem. Abstr.* **49**, 13494c].

TABLE VI—*continued*

	Source	References
	Rat embryo extract	96
	Mouse salivary gland	68, 97
	Rice beans	98
	Grass juice	99
	Cornstarch	100
	Yeast	101
	Cottonseed	84
	Mycelia of *Aspergillus, oryzae*	102
	"Moslin" aspergillopeptidase A	103
Swine	Distillers dried solubles	104, 105
	Grass juice	106
	Yeast	104
	Whey	104
	Fish solubles	104, 107
	Nocardia rugosa mycelia	108
Beef calves	Grass juice	109
Infantile animals	*Streptococcus lactis*	110
Guinea pigs	"Growth hormones"	95
Ducks	Fish meal, whey, fish solubles, distillers solubles	111
Young animals	Lipid from animal tissue and egg yolk	112

[96] G. C. Velley and M. Rostin, *C. R. Soc. Biol.* **152**, 1660 (1958) [*Chem. Abstr.* **53**, 15260b].

[97] S. Cohen, *Proc. Nat. Acad. Sci. U.S.* **46**, 302 (1960).

[98] Y. Majima, *Seikagaku* **29**, 485 (1957) [*Chem. Abstr.* **54**, 17590f].

[99] G. O. Kohler, C. A. Elvehjem, and E. B. Hart, *J. Nutr.* **15**, 445 (1938).

[100] J. H. Baxter, *J. Nutr.* **34**, 333 (1947).

[101] K. Schwarz, *Proc. Soc. Exp. Biol. Med.* **78**, 852 (1951).

[102] T. Kamihara, M. Fukano, and E. Tozaki, *Bitamin* **25**, 317 (1962) [*Chem. Abstr.* **62**, 8182e].

[103] K. Hashimoto and F. Yoshida, *Chem. Pharm. Bull.* **13**, 612 (1965) [*Chem. Abstr.* **63**, 4734a].

[104] W. M. Beeson, D. L. Jeter, and J. H. Conrad, *Proc. Distill. Feed. Conf.* **14**, 62 (1959) [*Chem. Abstr.* **53**, 17259b].

[105] D. L. Jeter, J. H. Conrad, M. P. Plumlee, and W. M. Beeson, *J. Anim. Sci.* **19**, 226 (1960).

[106] D. I. Gard, D. E. Becker, S. W. Terrill, H. W. Norton, and A. V. Nalbandov, *J. Anim. Sci.* **14**, 532 (1955).

[107] D. I. Gard, *Diss. Abstr.* **15**, 4 (1955).

[108] Società Farmaceutici Italia (by R. Faustini, G. Gasparini, A. Tardani, and R. Barchielli), *Ger.* **1**, 168, 233 [*Chem. Abstr.* **61**, 4881a].

[109] E. E. Bartley, F. W. Atkeson, F. C. Fountaine, J. J. Radisson, and H. C. Freyer, *J. Dairy Sci.* **40**, 652 (1957).

[110] C. Lingen, O. Lindberg, and L. Ernster, *Exp. Cell Res. Suppl.* **3**, 244 (1955).

[111] M. L. Scott, E. H. Parsons, Jr., and E. Dougherty, III, *Poultry Sci.* **36**, 1181 (1957).

[112] J. Hradec and A. Stroufova, *Biochim. Biophys. Acta* **40**, 32 (1960).

TABLE VI—*continued*

	Source	References
Egg weight	Corn grain	113
Embryos	*Triturus cristatus* extract	114
Rhabiditus briggrae	Yeast, liver	115
Caenorhabiditus briggrae	Liver	116
Animals	Tryptose	117
Mink	Liver, whey	118, 119
Monkey	—	120
Foxes	—	121
Donovania granulomatis	Egg yolks	122
Tetramitus rostratus	*Bacillus cereus*	123
Endamoeba histolytica	*Streptobacillus*	124
Tetrahymena pyriformis	*Colpidium campylum*	125
Plants		
Avena coleoptile	*Phaseolus vulgaris*	126
	Coleus helianthus	127
Oat coleoptile	Oat coleoptile	128, 129
Lemna paucicostata	Liver	130
Apple trees	Linseed oil	131

[113] L. S. Jensen, J. B. Allred, R. E. Fry, and J. McGinnis, *J. Nutr.* **65**, 219 (1958).

[114] G. K. Roussen, *Experientia* **17**, 260 (1961).

[115] E. C. Dougherty, *J. Parasitol.* **39**, 371 (1953).

[116] F. W. Sayre, E. Hansen, T. J. Starr, and E. A. Yarwood, *Nature (London)* **190**, 1116 (1961).

[117] M. Lee, S. S. Kang, C. W. Kim, and K. C. Park, *Tachan Naekwa Hakhoe Chapchi* **6** (3), 169 (1963) [*Chem. Abstr.* **59**, 10591h].

[118] A. E. Schaefer, S. B. Tove, C. K. Whitehair, and C. A. Elvehjem, *J. Nutr.* **35**, 157 (1948).

[119] S. B. Tove, R. J. Lalor, and C. A. Elvehjem, *J. Nutr.* **42**, 433 (1950).

[120] J. M. Cooperman, H. A. Waisman, K. B. McCall, and C. A. Elvehjem, *J. Nutr.* **30**, 45 (1945).

[121] A. E. Schaefer, C. K. Whitehair, and C. A. Elvehjem, *J. Nutr.* **35**, 147 (1948).

[122] W. K. Hall, R. B. Dienst, and C. H. Chen, *Proc. Soc. Exp. Biol. Med.* **84**, 370 (1953).

[123] M. M. Brent, *Biol. Bull.* **106**, 269 (1954).

[124] J. L. Karlsson, M. B. James, and H. H. Anderson, *Exp. Parisitol.* **1**, 347 (1952).

[125] D. M. Lilly and R. H. Stillwell, *Science* **147**, 747 (1965).

[126] I. Feldmeier and H. v. Guttenberg, *Planta* **42**, 1 (1953).

[127] H. von Guttenberg, I. Eifler, and G. Nehring, *Planta* **42**, 209 (1953) [*Chem. Abstr.* **48**, 812e].

[128] H. Söding and E. Raadts, *Planta* **43**, 25 (1953) [*Chem. Abstr.* **48**, 3475h].

[129] L. J. Audus, *Congr. Int. Bot., Rapp. Commun., Paris* **8**, Sect. 11/12, p. 139 (1954) [*Chem. Abstr.* **48**, 10852i].

[130] Y. Yone and T. Tomiyama, *Nippon Suisan Gakkaishi* **17**, 329 (1952) [*Chem. Abstr.* **48**, 2207h].

[131] U. N. Rao, V. S. Rangacharlu, and B. S. Kuppuswamy, *Indian J. Hort.* **9**, No. 4, p. 59 (1952) [*Chem. Abstr.* **48**, 2305i].

TABLE VI—*continued*

	Source	References
Parthenocissus tricuspidata	Tomato juice	132
Quercus sessiliflora	*Agrilus biguttatus* extract	133
	Insects	
Trifolium confusum	Yeast	134–138
	Casein	139
Corcyra	Yeast	140, 141
Drosophila melanogaster	Yeast	142
Drosophila melanogaster	Pancreas	142
Phormia regina	Yeast	143
Cornborer	Corn leaf	144
Grasshoppers	Bran and wheat germ oil	145
	Lettuce	146
Acheta domesticus	Liver, kidney, yeast, and royal jelly	147
Larvae of amphibians	Placenta	148
Potato eelworm	Low molecular weight acid-lactone	149
	Microorganisms	
Lactic acid bacteria		
Lactobacilli	Peptides	150–152

[132] S. Demetriades and J. P. Nitsch. *C. R. Soc. Biol.* **147**, 1711 (1953).
[133] C. Jacquiot and J. Guillemain-Gouvernel, *C. R. Acad. Sci.* **238**, 924 (1954).
[134] G. Fröbrich, *Z. Vitam. Hormon Fermentforsch.* **6**, 1 (1954) [*Chem. Abstr.* **48**, 13106g].
[135] R. Charbonneau and A. Lemonde, *Can. J. Zool.* **38**, 443 (1960).
[136] R. Charbonneau and A. Lemonde, *Arch. Int. Physiol. Biochim.* **70**, 379 (1962).
[137] A. Lemonde and R. Charbonneau, *Laval Med.* **33**, 621 (1962). [*Chem. Abstr.* **59**, 7681g].
[138] R. Charbonneau and A. Lemonde, *Can. J. Zool.* **38**, 87 (1960).
[139] K. Offhaus, *Z. Vitamin. Hormon Fermentforsch.* **9**, 196 (1957–1958) [*Chem. Abstr.* **52**, 16624d].
[140] R. Sivaramakrishnan and P. S. Sarma, *J. Sci. Ind. Res., Sect. C* **17**, 4 (1958) [*Chem. Abstr.* **52**, 10437e].
[141] K. R. P. Singh, *Sci. Cult.* **20**, 339 (1955) [*Chem. Abstr.* **49**, 7760g].
[142] M. Begg, *J. Exp. Biol.* **33**, 142 (1956).
[143] M. Brust and G. Fraenkel, *Physiol. Zool.* **28**, 186 (1955).
[144] S. D. Beck, *J. Gen. Physiol.* **36**, 317 (1953).
[145] J. K. Nayar, *Can. J. Zool.* **42**, 11 (1964) [*Chem. Abstr.* **60**, 12425d].
[146] J. B. Kreasky, *J. Insect Physiol.* **8**, 493 (1962).
[147] P. F. Neville, P. C. Stone, and T. D. Luckey, *J. Nutr.* **74**, 265 (1961).
[148] A. Ninni, *Boll. Soc. Ital. Biol. Sper.* **31**, 97 (1955). [*Chem. Abstr.* **49**, 14208h].
[149] C. T. Calam, H. Raistrick, and A. R. Todd, *Biochem. J.* **45**, 513 (1949).
[150] E. Kitay and E. E. Snell, *J. Bacteriol.* **60**, 49 (1951).
[151] F. A. Robinson, B. W. Williams, and L. H. Brown, *J. Pharm. Pharmacol.* **4**, 27 (1952).
[152] G. Östling and W. Nyberg, *J. Pharm. Pharmacol.* **5**, 46 (1953).

TABLE VI—*continued*

	Source	References
L. leichmanii	Peptides	153
L. bifidus	Peptides	154–157
Fusobacteria	Peptides	158
Pythiogeton	Peptides	159
L. casei	Fish meal	160
L. arabinosus	Yeast	161
	Liver	152, 161
L. bifidus	Milk	162–165
L. parabifidus	Milk	157, 166
L. bulgaricus	Milk	167
	Spleen and urine protein	168
L. casei	Edam cheese	169
L. bifidus	Plant material	170
Streptococcus agalactiae	Milk	171
Lactic streptococci	Milk	172
Acetic acid bacteria	Yeast	173
Hemolytic streptococci	Yeast	174

[153] H. T. Peeler and L. C. Norris, *J. Biol. Chem.* **188**, 75 (1951).

[154] H. Gyllenberg, M. Rossander, and P. Roine, *Acta Chem. Scand.* **7**, 694 (1953).

[155] M. S. Shorb and F. A. Veltre, *Poultry Sci.* **32**, 924 (1953).

[156] G. F. Springer and P. György, *Fed. Proc. Fed. Amer. Soc. Exp. Biol.* **12**, 272 (1953).

[157] C. S. Rose, R. Kuhn, and P. György, *Fed. Proc. Fed. Amer. Soc. Exp. Biol.* **12**, 428 (1953).

[158] R. R. Omata, *J. Bacteriol.* **65**, 326 (1953).

[159] D. Perlman, *Amer. J. Bot.* **38**, 652 (1951).

[160] W. N. Sumerwell, *Commer. Fish. Rev.* **17** (8), 11 (1955) [*Chem. Abstr.* **50**, 12401f].

[161] W. G. Jaffe, *Rev. Sanid. Asistencia Soc.* **16**, 533 (1951) [*Chem. Abstr.* **47**, 7595e].

[162] F. Petuely and G. Kristen, *Öesterr. Z. Kinderheilk. Kinderfuersorge* **6**, 173 (1951) [*Chem. Abstr.* **47**, 178g].

[163] P. György, *Pediatrics* **11**, 98 (1953).

[164] F. Petuely, *Naturwissenschaften* **40**, 349 (1953).

[165] P. György, C. S. Rose, and G. F. Springer, *J. Lab. Clin. Med.* **43**, 543 (1954).

[166] E. Frisell, *Acta Paediat. (Stockholm)* **39**, 460 (1950) [*Chem. Abstr.* **48**, 2840d].

[167] R. Irie, N. Yano, T. Morichi, and H. Kembo, *Nippon Saikingaku Zasshi* **17**, 413 (1962) [*Chem. Abstr.* **63**, 3348e].

[168] G. Agren, *Acta Pathol. Microbiol. Scand.* **35**, 91 (1954).

[169] F. Tokita and T. Nakanishi, *Nippon Chikusan Gakkai-Ho* **33**, 156 (1962) [*Chem. Abstr.* **59**, 6901f].

[170] M. S. Shorb and F. A. Veltre, *Proc. Soc. Exp. Biol. Med.* **86**, 140 (1954).

[171] J. E. Auclair, *Int. Dairy Congr., Proc. 13th, The Hague* **3**, 1402 (1953) [*Chem. Abstr.* **47**, 11586e].

[172] A. W. Anderson and P. R. Elliker, *J. Dairy Sci.* **36**, 608 (1953).

[173] M. R. R. Rao and J. L. Stokes, *J. Bacteriol.* **65**, 405 (1953).

[174] T. A. Nevin, *J. Bacteriol.* **67**, 217 (1954).

TABLE VI—*continued*

	Source	References
Corynebacterum diptheriae	Yeast	175
Streptococcus faecalis	Yeast	161
Fusobacterium nucleatum	Yeast	176
Mycobacterium flavum	Yeast	177, 178
Sporovibrio desulfuricans	Yeast	179
Lactic streptococci	Liver	172
Saccharomyces cerevisiae	Liver	82, 180–182
Streptomyces faecalis	Liver	161
Mycobacterium flavum	Liver	177
Leuconostoc mesenteroides	Oatmeal, peanut butter	183
Bacteria	Petroleum wastes	184
Mycobacterium flavum	Asparagus juice	177
Paramecium aurelia	Lemon juice	185
Pleuropneumonia-like organisms	Chick embryo extract	186
M. johnei	*Mycobacterium phlei*	187
Tubercule bacteria	*Mycobacterium phlei*	188
Arthobacter terregens	*Arthobacter pascens*	189
Salmonella typhosa	Bile	190
Treponemata	Enzymatic protein digests	191, 192
Trypanosoma cruzi	Blood	193

[175] F. W. Chattaway, D. E. Dolby, D. A. Hall, and F. C. Happold, *Int. Congr. Biochem., 1st Congr., Cambridge, Eng. Abstr. Commun.* p. 294 (1949).

[176] R. R. Omata, *J. Bacteriol.* **65**, 326 (1953).

[177] R. W. Bishop, M. S. Shorb, and M. J. Pelczar, *Proc. Soc. Exp. Biol. Med.* **81**, 407 (1952).

[178] E. Brand and D. K. Bosshardt, *Abstr. Amer. Chem. Soc., 114th Meet.* p. 38C (1948).

[179] A. Baumann and V. Denk, *Arch. Mikrobol.* **15**, 283 (1950) [*Chem. Abstr.* **48**, 12891d].

[180] E. Tria, and O. Barnabei, *Boll. Soc. Ital. Biol. Sper.* **28**, 1569 (1952) [*Chem. Abstr.* **47**, 4442e].

[181] E. Tria and O. Barnabei, *Minerva Med.* p. 1763 (1958) [*Chem. Abstr.* **52**, 14726e].

[182] E. Tria, *Ric. Sci.* **25**, 933 (1955) [*Chem. Abstr.* **49**, 14943c].

[183] M. J. Horn and H. W. Warren, *J. Nutr.* **83**, 267 (1964).

[184] D. M. Guseïnov, N. N. Edigarova, and G. S. Kasimova, *Fiziol. Rast.* **3**, 149 (1956) [*Chem. Abstr.* **50**, 10323d].

[185] R. L. Conner, W. J. van Wagtendonk, and C. A. Miller, *J. Gen. Microbol.* **9**, 434 (1953).

[186] J. G. Leece, W. R. Stinebring, and H. E. Morton, *J. Bacteriol.* **66**, 622 (1953).

[187] J. Francis, H. M. Macturk, J. Madinaveitia, and G. A. Snow, *Biochem. J.* **55**, 596 (1953).

[188] J. Marks, *J. Pathol. Bacteriol.* **67**, 254 (1954). [*Chem. Abstr.* **48**, 7695f].

[189] M. O. Burton, F. J. Sowden, and A. G. Lochhead, *Can. J. Biochem. Physiol.* **32**, 400 (1954).

[190] T. Takatori, *Nippon Saikingaku Zasshi* **7**, 311 (1952) [*Chem. Abstr.* **48**, 12885a].

[191] H. Eagle and H. G. Steinman, *J. Bacteriol.* **56**, 163 (1948).

[192] H. G. Steinman and H. Eagle, *J. Bacteriol.* **60**, 57 (1950).

[193] W. L. McRay, E. R. Noble, and E. L. Tondenold, *Science* **115**, 288 (1952).

TABLE VI—*continued*

	Source	References
Trichomonas vaginalis	Pancreas	194
Clostridium	Peptide	195, 196
Pleuropneumonia-like organisms	Protein	197, 198
Staphylococcus albus	Glycopeptide	199, 200
Pilobolus	Fermentation liquors	201, 202
Pilobolus kleinii	"Coprogen"	203
	Cow dung	204
E. coli	*E. coli* peptide	205
Streptococcus lactis	Casein	206
Streptococcus faecalis	*Bacillus subtilis*	207
Yeast	Radish leaf	208
L-cells	Chick extract	209
	Hepatoma extract	210
Leptospira canicola	Egg yolk	211
Mycobacterium tuberculosis	Serum lipid	212
Escherichia histolytica	*Escherichia coli*	213
Bacillus subtilis	*Bacillus stearothermophilus*	214
Milk cultures	Pancreas extract	215

[194] H. Sprince, E. L. Gilmore, and R. S. Lowry, *Arch. Biochem.* **22**, 483 (1949).

[195] B. C. J. G. Knight and P. Fildes, *Brit. J. Exp. Pathol.* **14**, 112 (1933).

[196] L. W. Jones and C. E. Clifton, *H. Bacteriol.* **65**, 540 (1953).

[197] F. F. Tang, H. Wei, D. L. McWhirter, and J. Edgar, *J. Pathol. Bacteriol.* **40**, 391 (1935).

[198] P. F. Smith and H. E. Morton, *Arch. Biochem. Biophys.* **38**, 23 (1952).

[199] T. P. Hughes, *J. Bacteriol.* **23**, 437 (1932).

[200] N. H. Sloane and R. W. McKee, *J. Amer. Chem. Soc.* **74**, 987 (1952).

[201] C. W. Hesseltine, C. Pidacks, A. R. Whitehill, N. Bohonos, B. L. Hutchings, and J. H. Williams, *J. Amer. Chem. Soc.* **74**, 1362 (1952).

[202] J. B. Neilands, *J. Amer. Chem. Soc.* **74**, 4846 (1952).

[203] C. Pidacks, A. R. Whitehall, L. M. Pruess, C. W. Hesseltine, B. L. Hutchings, N. Bohonos, and J. H. Williams, *J. Amer. Chem. Soc.* **75**, 6064 (1953).

[204] R. M. Page, *Amer. J. Bot.* **39**, 731 (1952).

[205] S. Simmonds, M. T. Dowling, and D. Stone, *J. Biol. Chem.* **208**, 701 (1954).

[206] L. A. Liberman, *Mikrobiol. Zh.* (Kiev) **23**, (6), 54 (1961) [*Chem. Abstr.* **57**, 5110a].

[207] W. A. Zygmunt, E. E. Haley, H. P. Sarett, H. E. Conrad, P. A. Tavorrmina, and H. E. Staveley, *Can. J. Microbiol.* **8**, 429 (1962).

[208] M. Akaki, *Hakko Kogaku Zasshi* **39**, 419 (1961) [*Chem. Abstr.* **59**, 4288a].

[209] M. Kuru, G. Kosaki, and H. Watanabe, *Gann* **54**, 119 (1963) [*Chem. Abstr.* **59**, 1866b].

[210] E. Ito, *Osaka Daigaku Igaku Zasshi* **35**, 315 (1961) [*Chem. Abstr.* **59**, 2041e].

[211] I. Mifuchi, M. Hosoi, and Y. Yanagihara, *Jap. J. Microbol.* **5**, 215 (1961) [*Chem. Abstr.* **59**, 9361h].

[212] I. Mifuchi, *Kekkaku* **28**, 193 (1953) [*Chem. Abstr.* **48**, 803a].

[213] A. K. Mukherjea, *Proc. Nat. Acad. Sci. India, Sect.* **20**, 660 (1954) [*Chem. Abstr.* **49**, 12488b].

[214] E. H. C. Sie, H. Sobotka, and H. Baker, *Biochem. Biophys. Res. Commun.* **6**, 205 (1961).

[215] M. L. Speck, and R. A. Ledford, *Milk Dealer* **48** (8), 53, 84 (1959) [*Chem. Abstr.* **53**, 20604e].

TABLE VI—*continued*

Source		References
Slime molds	Gram-negative bacteria	216
Streptococcus faecalis	Mycelia of *Aspergillus oryzae*	217
	Fish	
Trout fingerlings	Fish meal, milk	218
Carp	"H" factor	219
	Tissue Cell Cultures	
	Addition	
Plant cells		
Carrot cells	Coconut milk	220–225
Plant cells	Coconut milk	226
Tobacco cells	Coconut milk	221
	Crown gall, *Vinca rosea*	227
Artichoke tissue	Corn	228
Wheat roots	Peptone	229
Animal cells		
Fibroblast cultures	Chick embryo extract	230–234

[216] M. Sussman and S. G. Bradley, *Arch. Biochem. Biophys.* **51**, 428 (1954).

[217] T. Kamihara, *Bitamin* **24**, 101 (1961) [*Chem. Abstr.* **62**, 4370d].

[218] L. E. Wolf, *Progr. Fish Cult.* **14**, 148 (1952).

[219] Y. Hashimoto, *Nippon Suisan Gakkaishi* **19**, 899 (1953).

[220] F. C. Steward and S. M. Caplin. *Ann. Bot. (London)* **16**, 477 (1952).

[221] J. R. Mauney, W. S. Hillman, C. O. Miller, F. Skoog, R. A. Clayton, and F. M. Strong, *Physiol. Plant.* **5**, 485 (1952).

[222] R. S. DeRopp, J. C. Vitucci, B. L. Hutchings, and J. H. Williams, *Proc. Soc. Exp. Biol. Med.* **81**, 704 (1952).

[223] J. van Overbeek, M. E. Conklin, and A. F. Blakeslee, *Science* **94**, 350 (1941).

[224] L. Duhamet and R. J. Gautheret, *C. R. Soc. Biol.* **144**, 177 (1950).

[225] F. C. Steward and S. M. Caplin, *Science* **113**, 518 (1951).

[226] E. M. Shantz and F. C. Steward, *J. Amer. Chem. Soc.* **74**, 6133 (1952).

[227] A. C. Braun and U. Naf, *Proc. Soc. Exp. Biol. Med.* **86**, 212 (1954).

[228] G. Netien and G. Beauchesne, *C. R. Acad. Sci.* **237**, 1026 (1953).

[229] A. Fujiwara and K. Ojima, *Nippon Dojo-Hiryogaku Zasshi* **32**, 371 (1961) [*Chem. Abstr.* **59**, 8362b].

[230] C. Rizzoli and M. Gliozzi, *Bull. Soc. Ital. Biol. Sper.* **33**, 215 (1957) [*Chem. Abstr.* **52**, 2133e].

[231] Y. Ito and A. Ohyama, *Acta. Sch. Med. Univ. Kioto* **33**, 86 (1955) [*Chem. Abstr.* **51**, 9797e].

[232] R. Kutsky and R. Underwood, *Science* **125**, 741 (1957).

[233] H. Maganini, G. M. Hass, A. W. Schweitzer, and B. Wallace, *Lqb. Invest.* **9**, 239 (1960) [*Chem. Abstr.* **55**, 9490h].

[234] M. Harris, *Growth* **16**, 215 (1952) [*Chem. Abstr.* **47**, 82222d].

TABLE VI—*continued*

	Source	References
Tumor cells	Nucleopeptide exudates	235–237
Human cells	Serum protein	238, 239
	Bovine serum albumin	240, 241
	Serum	242–245
	Mouse glands	246, 247
	Pancreatic extract	241
	Mouse fibroblasts	248–250
	HeLa cells	251
Rat cells	Human cancerous serum	252
Nerve cells	Protein from various sources	253, 254
	Liver	255
	Yeast	255

Table VII recapitulates most of the activities now known to be associated with the various vitamins. As close inspection will reveal, the alphabet is nearly filled with "accessory food factors," and the proposed closing of this chapter of research thus seems poetically more appropriate. One may wish a corresponding degree of success for other fields, as the assembled artisans scatter, and bring to their chosen new tasks the experience that has been accumulated in solving this one.

[235] V. Menkin, *Amer. J. Pathol.* **35**, 707 (1959) [*Chem. Abstr.* **56**, 13425g].
[236] V. Menkin, *Acta Unio Int. Contra Cancrum* **16**, 1231 (1960) [*Chem. Abstr.* **54**, 25218g].
[237] V. Menkin, *Proc. Soc. Ex. Biol. Med.* **104**, 312 (1960).
[238] I. Lieberman and P. Ove, *Biochim. Biophys. Acta* **25**, 449 (1957).
[239] H. Eagle, *Science* **122**, 501 (1955).
[240] I. Lieberman and P. Ove, *J. Biol. Chem.* **233**, 634 (1958).
[241] H. Eagle, *Proc. Nat. Acad. Sci. U.S.* **46**, 427 (1960).
[242] S. J. Pirt, *Proc. Roy. Soc. Med.* **56**, 1061 (1963) [*Chem. Abstr.* **60**, 11139h].
[243] D. P. Metzgar, Jr. and M. Moskowitz, *Proc. Soc. Exp. Biol. Med.* **104**, 363 (1960).
[244] I. Lieberman and P. Ove, *J. Biol. Chem.* **234**, 2574 (1959).
[245] R. B. L. Gwatkin, *Nature (London)* **186**, 984 (1960).
[246] A. I. Cohen, E. C. Nicol, and W. Richter, *Proc. Soc. Exp. Biol. Med.* **116**, 784 (1964).
[247] R. Levi-Montalcini and B. Booker, *Proc. Nat. Acad. Sci. U.S.* **46**, 373 (1960).
[248] L. J. Alfred and R. W. Pumper, *Biochem. Biophys. Res. Commun.* **7**, 284 (1962).
[249] L. J. Alfred, *Diss. Abstr.* **23**, 4516 (1963) [*Chem. Abstr.* **59**, 10547d].
[250] L. J. Alfred and R. W. Pumper, *Proc. Soc. Exp. Biol. Med.* **103**, 688 (1960).
[251] J. F. Foley, B. J. Kennedy, and J. D. Ross, *Cancer Res.* **23**, 368 (1963) [*Chem. Abstr.* **60**, 9720d].
[252] T. Inoue, K. Masuda, S. Tanabe, Y. Matsuoka, N. Itou, and Y. Fukai, *Nara Igaku Zasshi* **14**, 149 (1963) [*Chem. Abstr.* **60**, 14952a].
[253] R. Levi-Montalcini and P. V. Angeletti, *Reg. Neurochem., Reg. Chem., Physiol. Pharmacol. Nerv. Syst., Proc. Int. Neurochem. Symp.*, 4th Varenna 1960 p. 362 (1961).
[254] R. Levi-Montalcini, *Pubbl. Staz. Zool. Napoli* **29**, 1 (1957) [*Chem. Abstr.* **54**, 19929c].
[255] J. F. Morgan, M. E. Campbell, and H. J. Morton, *J. Nat. Cancer Inst.* **16**, 557 (1955) [*Chem. Abstr.* **50**, 1998i].

TABLE VII

NAMES FOR VITAMINS AND GROWTH FACTORS (4, 363)

Factor	Remarks	References
A, including A_1, A_2, A_3, etc.	Chemically, physiologically similar forms of the antixerophathalmic vitamin	256, 257
B_1 (thiamine)	Original water-soluble B, the anti-beriberi vitamin	256, 257
B_2 (riboflavin)	Also known as G (Goldberger)	256, 257
B_3	Probably pantothenic acid	258, 259
B_4	Replaceable by arginine + glycine or riboflavin + B_6	256, 257, 260
B_5	A growth stimulator for pigeons probably identical with nicotinic acid	256, 257
B_6	Name for activity produced by the closely related forms pyridoxal, pyridoxamine, pyridoxol	256, 257
B_7	Prevents digestive disturbances in the pigeon; also known as vitamin I	256, 257
B_8	Adenylic acid	261
B_9	Unused designation	257
B_{10} and B_{11}	Chick feathering and growth factors	256, 257
B_{12}	Also known as the "animal protein factor." Several compounds exist which have activity	256, 257
$B_{12a, b, d}$	Aquocobalamin	256, 257
B_{12c}	Nitritobalamin	256, 257
B_{13}	Unconfirmed	256, 257
B_{14}	Unconfirmed	256, 257
B_{15}	Unconfirmed	256
B_c	A form of folic acid, active for the chick	256, 257
B_p	Antiperosis factor for chicks, replaceable by Mg, choline	256, 257, 262
B_t	Probably identical with carnitine, active for insect growth	256, 257

[256] A. F. Wagner and K. Folkers, "Vitamins and Coenzymes," Wiley (Interscience), New York, 1964. pp. 244–63.

[257] V. H. Cheldelin, *Nutr. Rev.* **9**, 289 (1951).

[258] J. G. Lee and A. G. Hogan, *M. Agr. Exp. Sta. Bull.* **342** (1942).

[259] R. R. Williams and R. E. Waterman, *J. Biol. Chem.* **78**, 311 (1928).

[260] V. Reader, *Biochem. J.* **23**, 689 (1929).

[261] H. von Euler, F. Schlenk, L. Melzer, and B. Högberg, *Hoppe-Seyler's Z. Physiol. Chem.* **258**, 212 (1939).

[262] A. G. Hogan, N. B. Guerrant, and H. L. Kempster, *J. Biol. Chem.* **64**, 113 (1925).

TABLE VII—*continued*

Factor	Remarks	References
B_w, B_x	Activities associated with biotin; pantothenic acid and *p*-aminobenzoic acid	257
Biotin	Prevents egg-white injury (rat); vitamin H (obsolete)	256, 257
C	Synonymous with ascorbic acid	256, 257
C_2	Antipneuomonia principle	256
Choline	Antiperosis agent for poultry; of doubtful status as a vitamin	256, 257
Citrovorum factor	N^5-Formyl-5, 6, 7, 8-tetrahydro-pteroylmonoglutamic acid. A naturally occurring form of folic acid	256
D, including $D_2, D_3, D_4,$ etc.	The antirachitic vitamin, composed of chemically related sterols	256, 257
E	Include: α-, β-, γ-tocopherol; also over 50 products of laboratory synthesis. Most prevent sterility, muscular dystrophy in animals	256, 257
F	Obsolete designation for essential fatty acids. Also an abandoned term for thiamine	256, 257
Folic acid	A common vitameric name for pteroylglutamic acid and related compounds.	256
Vitamin G	*See* riboflavin	256, 257
Vitamin H	An obsolete term for biotin	256, 257
Vitamin I	(Obsolete) *see* B_7	256, 257
Vitamin J	(Obsolete); an antipneumonia principle	256, 257
Vitamin K	Antihermorrhagic; about 100 vitamers are known to exist	256, 257
Vitamin L_1, L_2	Liver (or yeast) filtrate, reported active for lactation	256, 257
Lipoic acid	Participates in oxidative carboxylation, cooperating in enzymatic activity with: DPN, diphospho-thiamine, coenzyme A. Vitamin status not yet proved	256
M	Active in monkeys; promotes healthy blood picture. An active form of folic acid	256, 257
N	(Obsolete) a term used to describe anticancer activity from brain or stomach	256, 257
Nicotinic acid, amide	The pellagra-preventive factor	256, 257

TABLE VII—*continued*

Factor	Remarks	References
Pantothenic acid	See vitamin B_3; a compound that prevents rat achromotrichia, chick dermatitis	256, 257
Pteroylmonoglutamic acid	The preferred vitameric name: folic acid	256, 257
Coenzyme Q	Synonymous with "ubiquinone." It is a series of combined forms of vitamin K-like quinones in which the quinone is combined with 5–50 carbon atoms arranged in isoprenoid structures about the naphthalene ring. May be important for cellular oxidations	256
Vitamin R	A bacterial growth promoter; apparently related to folic acid	256, 257
Vitamin S	A chick growth activity, possibly related to strepogenin	256, 257
Vitamin T	Isolated factor(s) from termites	256, 257, 263
Factor U	Probably a mixture, containing B_6 and folic acid activity	256, 257
Factor V	A bacteriol growth factor. Contains DPN	256, 257
Factor X	(Obsolete); equivalent to biotin	264
Factor Y	(Obsolete); equivalent to pyridoxine	264
Growth factors for guinea pigs GRF-1 GRF-2 GRF-3		264, 265
Factors for *L. helveticus*, *S. lactis*, HL 1, 2, 3, 4	Chloroform-soluble fractions from liver; may be related to folic acid group, also lipoic acid	264, 266
L. gayoni factor	Partly replaced by nucleotides, plus high levels of glutamine or asparagine; glucosylglycine active	264
Xanthine oxidase factor	Obsolete; replaceable by inorganic molybdate	264

[263] W. Goetsch, *Experientia* **3**, 326 (1947).

[264] V. H. Cheldelin, *in* "The Vitamins" (W. H. Sebrell, Jr. and R. S. Harris, eds.), Vol. 3, pp. 575–600. Academic Press, New York, 1954.

[265] D. W. Woolley and H. Sprince, *J. Biol. Chem.* **153**, 687 (1944).

[266] E. C. Barton-Wright, W. B. Emery, and F. A. Robinson, *Biochem. J.* **39**, 334 (1945).
R. A. Wilcox, C. W. Carlson, W. Kohlmeyer, and G. F. Gastler, *Poultry Sci.* **40**, 1353 (1961).
S. D. Beck, J. H. Lilly, and J. F. Stauffer, *Ann. Entomol. Soc. Amer.* **42**, 483 (1949).
G. R. Jago, *J. Dairy Res.* **21**, 111 (1954).
L. G. Colis and V. Babb, *J. Biol. Chem.* **174**, 405 (1948).

AUTHOR INDEX

Numbers in parentheses are reference numbers and indicate that an author's work is referred to, although his name is not cited in the text. Numbers in italics show the pages on which the complete reference is listed.

SUBJECT INDEX

449